# WEBSTER'S NEW WORLD™

# Medical Dictionary

*From the Doctors and Experts at MedicineNet.com*

*Edited by Mitzi Waltz*

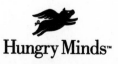

## Hungry Minds™

Best-Selling Books • Digital Downloads • e-Books • Answer Networks • e-Newsletters • Branded Web Sites • e-Learning

New York, NY ◆ Cleveland, OH ◆ Indianapolis, IN

Webster's New World™ Medical Dictionary

Copyright © 2000 by Hungry Minds, Inc.

Hungry Minds, Inc.
909 Third Avenue
New York, NY 10022

For general information on Hungry Minds' products and services please contact our Customer Care Department within the U.S. at 800-762-2974, outside the U.S. at 317-572-3993 or fax 317-572-4002.

A Webster's New World™ Book

Library of Congress Control Number: 99-75537

ISBN: 0-02-863734-8

Manufactured in the United States of America

10 9 8 7 6 5 4 3

# Acknowledgments

A very special thanks to my dear friend and MedicineNet.com co-editor for this dictionary, Frederick Hecht, M.D. His relentless drive and talents have been catalysts for the development of the *Webster's New World*™ *Medical Dictionary*. It has been an honor to work with such a professional. On Ted's behalf, I also wish to thank his lovely wife, Barbara, for supporting the expression of such talents.

I am grateful to Kenneth Kaye, M.D., a longtime friend, colleague, and MedicineNet.com assistant editor, whose tender poise and meticulous skill contributed greatly to fine-tuning this project.

At MedicineNet.com, we made an assumption that readers are truly interested in understanding medical topics. Accordingly, we have addressed medical terms with a sensitivity to those who are potentially acutely and chronically involved with disease and health issues. Without you, the public, there would be no MedicineNet.com.

On behalf of MedicineNet.com, I wish to thank the staff at IDG Books for bringing this dictionary to those who need it. I also thank the officers of MedicineNet.com, especially Peter Whyte and Gene Lu, who allowed the dictionary project to happen.

I applaud the incomparable professionalism and talents of the editors at IDG Books, especially Cynthia Kitchel, Renee Wilmeth, and Mitzi Waltz, each of whom made this project a pleasure.

The excellence of the technical and editorial staffs at MedicineNet.com facilitated the entire project, especially that of Dan Griffith, whose publishing software development made it all possible. Vic Sangveraphunsri, Spencer Lee, and Tony Jezek were intimately involved in data transmission. Julie Shapiro and Cynde Lee maintained communication between editors and writers. David Sorenson and Tanya Buchanan from marketing have been so helpful. Donna Whyte's sensitive MedicineNet.com radar vigilantly kept us apprised of what information people were seeking.

A special thanks to the children of my San Juan Capistrano, California neighborhood (Mollie, Chris, Jeffery, Brad, Kevin, and my own) who helped inspire the original common terms for MedicineNet's dictionary years ago on a summer Saturday afternoon. I cannot thank enough my own children, Cara, Daniel, and Tim, who endured the apparent inattentiveness of a distracted father. With endless love I thank my wife, Catherine, whose existence makes me whole.

Thank you all.

—*William C. Shiel Jr., M.D., F.A.C.P.*

# EDITORIAL STAFF

*Co-Editors in Chief:*
Frederick Hecht, M.D., F.A.A.P.
www.MedicineNet.com

William C. Shiel Jr., M.D., F.A.C.P.
www.MedicineNet.com

*Special Development Editor:*
Mitzi Waltz

*Acquisitions Editor:*
Joyce Pepple

*Production Editors:*
Suzanne G. Snyder, Ph.D.
Heather Gregory

*Associate Editor:*
Kenneth Kaye, M.D.
www.MedicineNet.com

*Assistant Editors:*
Dennis Lee, M.D.
www.MedicineNet.com

Barbara Hecht, Ph.D.
www.MedicineNet.com

Jay Marks, M.D.
www.MedicineNet.com

Catherine Shiel, J.D.
www.MedicineNet.com

*Research & Office Assistants:*
Julie Shapiro
www.MedicineNet.com

Donna Whyte
www.MedicineNet.com

*Special Contributing Editor:*
Renee Wilmeth

# About the Authors

## FREDERICK HECHT, M.D., F.A.A.P., CO-EDITOR IN CHIEF

Frederick Hecht, M.D. lives in Jacksonville, Florida and Berkeley, California. He is a Pediatrician and Medical Geneticist and is board-certified by the American Boards of Pediatrics and of Medical Genetics. Dr. Hecht was born in Baltimore and raised nearby in Pikesville, Maryland. After graduating from Baltimore Friends School, he attended Dartmouth College in Hanover, N.H. and the Sorbonne at the University of Paris, receiving his B.A. degree *cum laude* with distinction from Dartmouth. He then studied at Middlebury College in Vermont (in French); the Defense Language School (in Russian) in Monterey, California; the University of Maryland (in German); and Boston University (in biomedical sciences) before entering the University of Rochester School of Medicine and Dentistry. He received his M.D. degree from Rochester with honors. He trained first in Pediatrics at Strong Memorial Hospital in Rochester and University Hospital in Seattle, and then in Medical Genetics at the University of Washington. He has been on the medical school faculty at the Universities of Rochester, Washington, Oregon, Arizona and Nevada. He has been a Traveling Fellow of the Royal Society of Medicine in Great Britain. He founded and served as President and Director of the Southwest Biomedical Research Institute in Arizona and Director of the Genetics Center and Cancer Center, now part of Genzyme, Inc. He has held administrative and research positions including that of Principal Investigator for grants and contracts from the National Institutes of Health. Dr. Hecht has taught at a number of medical schools including the University of Washington, the Oregon Health Sciences University, and Harvard Medical School. Recently, he served as Professor of Medicine at the University of Nice, France for three years. There he worked in the Laboratory for the Molecular Genetics of Human Cancers, a unit of the CNRS (the French National Center for Scientific Research). He is President of Hecht Associates, consultants in Medical Genetics. He has served on the editorial boards of medical journal and reviewed articles for distinguished journals including the Proceedings of the National Academy of Sciences, Nature, Science; the *New England Journal of Medicine; Pediatrics;* the *Journal of Pediatrics;* the *American Journal of Human Genetics;* and *The Lancet*. He has published extensively and authored and co-authored more than 700 articles and books.

## WILLIAM SHIEL JR., M.D., F.A.C.P., CO-EDITOR IN CHIEF

Dr. Shiel received a Bachelor of Science degree with honors from the University of Notre Dame. There he was involved in research in radiation biology and received the Huisking Scholarship. After graduating from St. Louis University School of Medicine, he completed his Internal Medicine residency and Rheumatology fellowship at University of California, Irvine. He is board-certified in Internal Medicine and Rheumatology, and is a Fellow of the American Colleges of Physicians and Rheumatology. Dr. Shiel is in active practice in the field of rheumatology at the Arthritis Center of Southern Orange County, California. He is currently an active Associate Clinical Professor of Medicine at University of California, Irvine. He has served as chairman of the Department of Internal Medicine at Mission Hospital Regional Medical Center. Dr. Shiel has authored numerous articles on subjects related to arthritis for prestigious peer-reviewed medical journals, as well as many expert medical-legal reviews. He has lectured in person and on television both for physicians and the community. He is a contributor for questions for the American Board of Internal Medicine, and has reviewed board questions on behalf of the American Board of Rheumatology Subspecialty. He served on the Medical and Scientific Committee of the Arthritis Foundation, and is currently on the Medical Advisory Board of the Lupus Foundation of America. Dr. Shiel is proud to have served as Chief Editor for MedicineNet.com since its founding in 1996.

## KENNETH KAYE, M.D., ASSOCIATE EDITOR

Dr. Kaye received a Bachelor of Arts degree with honors from the University of California, San Diego, in Applied Mechanics and Engineering Sciences. After graduating from New York Medical College, he completed his internship and residency training in pathology at Harbor—UCLA Medical Center. Following residency, he joined Mission Pathology Medical Associates, and currently practices general pathology and is Blood Bank Director at Mission Hospital Regional Medical Center, Mission Viejo, California. He is board-certified in Anatomical and Clinical Pathology and a fellow of the College of American Pathologists and American Society of Clinical Pathologists.

## BARBARA K. HECHT, Ph.D., ASSISTANT EDITOR

Dr. Barbara Kaiser-McCaw Hecht is Director of Hecht Associates, Inc., consultants in Medical Genetics based in Jacksonville, Florida. Dr. Hecht lives in Jacksonville and in Berkeley, California. She is board-certified in her fields of expertise, and is a Diplomate of the American Board of Medical Genetics, both in Clinical Cytogenetics (Chromosome Genetics) and in Medical Genetics (Genetic Counseling). Dr. Hecht earned both her B.A. degree and an M.A. degree in Biology from Stanford University. Her master's thesis on cell physiology and radiation was done at Stanford under Prof. Arthur Giese. Following receipt of her M.A., she was Research Assistant in the Department of Biology at Stanford. She then worked as an Exobiologist for NASA, doing research on the chemistry of extraterrestial life, with a special interest in Mars. She earned her Ph.D. in Biology (Genetics) at the University of Oregon, Eugene, under Prof. Edward Novitski. Her doctoral thesis was on the clonal origin of human tumors, using the diseases ataxia-telangiectasia, Burkitt's lymphoma, and ovarian teratomas as models. She did an NIH Postdoctoral Research Fellowship in Medical Genetics under Dr. Robert D. Koler at the Oregon Health Sciences University. Dr. Hecht was Research Associate both there and at Portland State University. Her subsequent teaching positions included Clinical Assistant Professor of Obstetrics and Gynecology at the University of Nevada School of Medicine, Associate Professor of Biology at Arizona State University, and Professor of Medicine at the University of Missouri-Kansas City. She has served on numerous scientific committees and published extensively in a number of fields, including Cell Biology, Biochemistry, Human and Medical Genetics, and Oncology. Dr. Hecht was cofounder of the Southwest Biomedical Research Institute (now part of Genzyme, Inc.) in Arizona and served as its Senior Associate Director and Director of Laboratories. She has held positions in both diagnostic and research genetic laboratories in the United States, Australia, and France. She was recipient of an ARC (French Cancer Society) Fellowship for Cancer Research at the University of Nice, and was a staff member of the Laboratory for the Molecular Genetics of Human Cancers, a unit of the CNRS (the French National Center for Scientific Research) in France. Dr. Hecht has reviewed articles for distinguished biomedical journals, served on their editorial boards, and published hundreds of scientific and medical articles.

## DENNIS LEE, M. D., ASSISTANT EDITOR

Dennis Lee, M.D. was born in Shanghai, China, and received his college and medical training in the United States. He is fluent in English and three Chinese dialects. He graduated with chemistry departmental honors from Harvey Mudd College. He was appointed president of AOA society at UCLA School of Medicine. He underwent internal medicine residency and gastroenterology fellowship training at Cedars Sinai Medical Center. Board certified in Internal Medicine and Gastroenterology, he is currently a member of Mission Internal Medical Group, a multispecialty medical group serving south Orange County. Dennis has maintained an interest in technology and medical education. He is a regular guest lecturer at Saddleback College in Orange County, California.

# JAY W. MARKS, M.D., ASSISTANT EDITOR

Jay W. Marks, M.D. is a board-certified internist and gastroenterologist. He graduated from Yale University School of Medicine and trained in internal medicine and gastroenterology at UCLA/Cedars-Sinai Medical Center in Los Angeles. For 20 years he was Associate Director of the Division of Gastroenterology at Cedars-Sinai Medical Center and an Associate Professor of Medicine, In Residence, at UCLA. At Cedars Sinai he co-directed the Gastrointestinal Endoscopy Unit, taught physicians during their graduate and postgraduate training, and performed specialized, nonendoscopic, gastrointestinal testing. He carried out Public Health Service–sponsored (National Institutes of Health) clinical and basic research into mechanisms of the formation of gallstones and methods for the nonsurgical treatment of gallstones. He is the author of 36 original research manuscripts and 24 book chapters. Dr. Marks presently directs an independent Gastrointestinal Diagnostic Unit where he continues to perform specialized tests for the diagnosis of gastrointestinal diseases.

## CONTRIBUTING AUTHORS

Kent Adamson, M.D., Orthopedic Surgery • Leon Baginski, M.D., Obstetrics & Gynecology • Edward Block, M.D., Gastroenterology • James Bredencamp, M.D., Otolaryngology • Steve Ehrlich, M.D., Cardiology • Manuel Fernandez, M.D., Endocrinology • Ronald Gehling, M.D., Allergy & Immunology • Gus Gialamas, M.D., Orthopedic Surgery • Mitchell J. Gitkind, M.D., Gastroenterology • Mark Graber, M.D., Family Practice • David Kaminstein, M.D., Gastroenterology • Eric Lee, M.D., Gastroenterology • Margaret Lee, DDS, Dentistry • Ralph Maeda, M.D., Surgery • Murray Margolis, M.D., Internal Medicine • Randy Martin, M.D., Pulmonary/Infectious Diseases • James Meaglia, M.D., Urology • John Mersch, M.D., Pediatrics • Michael Miyamoto, M.D., Cardiology • John R. Morris, M.D., Orthopedic Surgery • Mim Mulford, M.D., Endocrinology • Omudhome Ogbru, Pharm.D., Pharmacy • Dennis Philips, M.D., Pediatrics • Donald Pratt, M.D., Internal Medicine • Donald Rediker, M.D., Cardiology • Emmanuel Saltiel, Pharm.D, Pharmacy • Michael Santoro, M.D., Gastroenterology • George Schiffman, M.D., Pulmonary • Leslie J. Schoenfield, M.D. Ph.D., Gastroenterology • Melvin Shiffman, M.D., Cosmetic Surgery • David Simon, M.D., Internal Medicine • Robert Simon, M.D., Neurology • Mark Sullivan, M.D., Urology • Bruce Tammelin, M.D., Pulmonary • Michael Truong, M.D., Endocrinology • Theodore Van Dam, M.D., Internal Medicine • Edward J. White, M.D., General Surgery • Leslie Williams, Ed. D, Psychology • David Zachary, M.D., Family Medicine

# Introduction

*Webster's New World™ Medical Dictionary* has been conceived and developed by the staff of the health information website MedicineNet.com. One of the earliest health information sites on the Internet, MedicineNet.com has devoted a number of years to creating an online medical dictionary. This dictionary now contains a wealth of contemporary medical terms.

Like all of the medical content from MedicineNet.com, this dictionary was written by physicians to be used by anyone concerned about their own health or the health of those who matter to them.

All the medical information found on MedicineNet.com has been developed by a network of physicians. The doctors select the topics, and review and edit all written content. These physicians also make use of medical specialists and health writers throughout the United States. The editorial staff page earlier in this book lists the primary editors for both MedicineNet.com and IDG books, as well as the administrative staff who organized *Webster's New World™ Medical Dictionary*. The authorship pages provide abbreviated biographies of the editors and specialists who contributed content to the MedicineNet.com online dictionary.

Medicine is a field that is advancing rapidly on many fronts, and its language is continually evolving. In today's health industry, there is constant communication between and among consumers and providers of healthcare. There is consequently a need for a high-quality, contemporary medical dictionary.

In today's complex health-care environment, patients and their physicians, nurses, and allied health professionals must be able to discuss the ever-changing aspects of health, disease, and biotechnology. An accurate understanding of medical terminology can assist communication and improve care for patients, as well as help to alleviate the concerns of families and friends.

The fact that the content of this dictionary is 100 percent doctor-produced by MedicineNet.com ensures an unusual degree of professional expertise, reliability, and perspective.

*Webster's New World™ Medical Dictionary* is designed in an easy-to-read format with cross-referencing of terms that readers will find helpful. Moreover, from a technical standpoint, the CD-ROM introduces a dynamic updating capability as well as rapid ease of use for computers in the office or home. The CD serves to enhance many of the terms found in this dictionary, and it provides an Internet link to MedicineNet.com for readers who want even more detailed information on the latest medical issues.

We hope that you will find this *Webster's New World™ Medical Dictionary* a valuable addition to your family or office library, and a source of both information and illumination in any medical situation.

Frederick Hecht, M.D., F.A.A.P.
William C Shiel, Jr., M.D., F.A.C.P.
Co-Editors in Chief

# Aa

**A** In genetics, **A** stands for adenine, one member of the adenine-thymine (A-T) base pair in DNA.

**a-** Prefix indicating the absence or depletion of something: for example, aphagia (not eating) or aphonia (voiceless). The related prefix an- is usually used before a vowel, as in anemia (without blood) or anoxia (without oxygen).

**a.c.** Abbreviation of the Latin phrase *ante cibum,* meaning before meals. See also *Appendix A, "Prescription Abbreviations."*

**AA** 1 Alcoholics Anonymous. 2 Amino acid.

**AAA** 1 American Association of Anatomists. 2 *Abdominal aortic aneurysm.*

**AAAS** Pronounced "triple-A-S," AAAS is an acronym for the American Association for the Advancement of Science, a professional organization.

**AAD** American Association of Dermatology, a professional organization.

**AAFP** American Association of Family Physicians, a professional society for American doctors who treat both adults and children.

**AAMC** The Association of American Medical Colleges.

**AAO** 1 American Association of Ophthalmology. 2 American Association of Orthodontists. 3 American Academy of Otolaryngology.

**AAOS** American Academy of Orthopaedic Surgeons, a professional organization. See also *orthopaedics.*

**AAP** 1 American Academy of Pediatrics, a professional organization for pediatricians that also supervises the Board certification Fellow of the American Academy of Pediatrics (FAAP). 2 American Academy of Pedodontics, a professional organization. 3 American Academy of Periodontology, a professional organization. 4 American Association of Pathologists, a professional organization.

***ab ovo*** From the beginning, from a Latin expression meaning "from the egg."

**ab-** Prefix used to to indicate from, away from, or off, as in abduction (movement of a limb away from the midline of the body) or abnormal (away from normal).

**ABC** Aneurysmal bone cyst.

**abdomen** The part of the body that contains all of the structures between the chest and the pelvis: the belly. The abdomen is anatomically separated from the chest by the diaphragm, the powerful muscle spanning the body cavity below the lungs. See also *abdominal cavity.*

**abdomen, acute** See *acute abdomen.*

**abdominal aorta** The final section of the largest artery in the body. The abdominal aorta begins at the diaphragm as a continuation of the thoracic aorta. At its end, the abdominal aorta splits in two, forming the common iliac arteries. It supplies oxygenated blood to all the abdominal and pelvic organs, as well as to the legs. Also known as the aorta abdominalis, pars abdominalis aortae. See also *aorta.*

**abdominal aortic aneurysm** See *aneurysm, abdominal aortic.*

**abdominal cavity** The cavity within the abdomen. This space between the abdominal wall and the spine contains a number of crucial organs, including the lower part of the esophagus, the stomach, small intestine, colon, rectum, liver, gallbladder, pancreas, spleen, kidneys, and bladder. See also *abdomen.*

**abdominal guarding** Tensing of the abdominal wall muscles to guard inflamed organs within the abdomen from the pain of pressure upon them. Abdominal guarding is detected when the abdomen is pressed. Guarding is a characteristic finding in the physical examination for an abruptly painful (acute) abdomen with inflammation of the inner abdominal (peritoneal) surface due, for example, to appendicitis or diverticulitis. The tensed muscles of the abdominal wall automatically go into spasm to keep the tender underlying tissues from being touched.

**abdominal hysterectomy** See *hysterectomy, abdominal.*

**abdominal muscles** A large group of muscles in the front of the abdomen that assists in maintaining regular breathing movements, supports the muscles of the spine while lifting, and keeps abdominal organs in place. Abdominal muscles are the target of many exercises, such as sit-ups. Informally known as the abs.

**abdominal pain** Pain in the belly. Abdominal pain can be acute or chronic. It may reflect a major problem with one of the organs in the abdomen, such as appendicitis or a perforated intestine, or it may result from a fairly minor problem, such as excess buildup of intestinal gas.

**abducens nerve**   See *abducent nerve*.

**abducent nerve**   The sixth cranial nerve, which emerges from the skull to operate the lateral rectus muscle. This muscle draws the eye toward the side of the head. Paralysis of the abducent nerve causes inward turning of the eye.

**abduction**   The movement of a limb sideways, away from the midline of the body. The opposite of abduction is adduction, the movement of a limb toward the midline of the body.

**abductor muscle**   See *muscle, abductor*.

**ABG**   Arterial blood gas.

**abiotrophy**   Loss of function, or degeneration for reasons unknown.

**ablate**   To remove. See *ablation*.

**ablatio placentae**   See *abruptio placentae*.

**ablation**   Removal or excision. Ablation is usually carried out surgically. For example, surgical removal of the thyroid gland (a total thyroidectomy) is ablation of the thyroid.

**abnormal**   Outside the expected norm, or uncharacteristic of a particular patient.

**ABO blood group**   The major human blood group system. The ABO type of a person depends on the presence or absence of two genes, A and B. These genes determine the configuration of the red blood cell surface. A person who has two A genes has red blood cells of type A. A person who has two B genes has red cells of type B. If the person has one A and one B gene, the red cells are type AB. If the person has neither the A nor B gene, the red cells are type O. It is essential to match the ABO status of both donor and recipient in organ transplants and blood transfusions.

**abortifacient**   A medication or substance that causes, or is suspected of causing, pregnancy to end prematurely.

**abortion**   Premature exit of the products of the fetus, fetal membranes, and placenta from the uterus. Abortion can be a natural process, as in a miscarriage; an induced procedure, using medication or other substances that cause the body to expel the fetus; or a surgical procedure that removes the contents of the uterus. See also *dilatation, curettage*.

**abortion, habitual**   The miscarriage of three or more consecutive pregnancies with no intervening pregnancies. Habitual abortion is a form of infertility. In about 5 percent of couples who have had two or more spontaneous abortions, one member of the couple is carrying a chromosome translocation responsible for the miscarriages. In other cases there is an Rh conflict between mother and fetus, a physical problem that prevents carrying the fetus to term, or causes unknown. There are many medical treatments and procedures available to help couples prevent reoccurence of spontaneous abortion. Treatment should begin with consulting a fertility specialist. Also known as multiple abortion, recurrent abortion.

**abortion, multiple**   See *abortion, habitual*.

**abortion, recurrent**   See *abortion, habitual*.

**abortion, spontaneous**   Miscarriage.

**abortive**   **1** Tending to cut short, as in abortive polio. **2** Causing abortion, as in a medication that induces abortion. See also *abortifacient*.

**abortive polio**   See *polio*.

**abrasion**   **1** A wearing away of the upper layer of skin as a result of applied friction force. See also *scrape*. **2** In dentistry, the wearing away of tooth surfaces.

**abruptio placentae**   Premature separation (abruption) of the placenta from the wall of the uterus, often in association with high blood pressure or preeclampsia. Abruption is a potentially serious problem both for mother and fetus, as the area where it occurs bleeds and the uterus begins to contract. Shock may occur. Also called ablacio placentae. See also *placenta, preeclampsia*.

**abs**   Slang term for the abdominal muscles.

**abscess**   A local accumulation of pus anywhere in the body. See also *boil, pus*.

**abscess, perianal**   An abscess that forms next to the anus, causing tenderness, swelling, and pain on defecation.

**abscess, peritonsillar**   An abscess behind the tonsils that pushes one of the tonsils toward the uvula (the prominent soft tissue dangling from the back of the palate in the back of the mouth). A peritonsillar abscess is generally very painful, and is usually associated with a decreased ability to open the mouth. If left untreated, the infection can spread deep into the neck, causing airway obstruction and other life-threatening complications.

**abscess, skin**   Medical term for a common boil.

**abscission**   To remove tissue by cutting it away, as in surgery.

**absence of the breast**   See *amastia*.

**absence of the nipple**   See *athelia*.

**absinthe**   Once a major medical hazard, absinthe is an emerald-green liqueur flavored with extracts of the wormwood plant, licorice, and aromatic flavorings in an alcohol base. Absinthe was manufactured, commercialized, and popularized in France in the late 1700s by Henri-Louis Pernod. It was an extremely addictive drink. Prolonged drinking of absinthe causes convulsions, blindness, hallucinations, and mental deterioration. Absinthe has been banned, but something of its taste is still available in such drinks as Greek ouzo and French pastis. Homemade absinthe may still be illicitly consumed in some areas.

**absolute CD4 count**   The number of "helper" T-lymphocytes in a cubic millimeter of blood. With HIV, this number declines as the infection progresses. The absolute CD4 count is frequently used to monitor the extent of immune suppression in persons with HIV. Also called a T4 count.

**absorption**   Uptake. Intestinal absorption is the uptake of food (or other substances) from the digestive tract.

**abuse, child**   See *child abuse*.

**abuse, elder**   See *elder abuse*.

**abuse, emotional child**   See *child abuse*.

**abuse, physical child**   See *child abuse*.

**abuse, psychological child**   See *child abuse*.

**abuse, sexual child**   See *child abuse*.

**abuse, verbal child**   See *child abuse*.

**AC joint**   See *acromioclavicular joint*.

**acapnia**   Lower than normal level of carbon dioxide in the blood. The opposite of acapnia is hypercapnia.

**accelerated phase of leukemia**   Chronic myelogenous leukemia that is progressing. In this phase, the number of immature, abnormal white blood cells in the bone marrow and blood is higher than in the chronic phase, but not as high as in the blast phase.

**accessory nerve**   The eleventh cranial nerve, which emerges from the skull and receives an additional (accessory) root from the upper part of the spinal cord. It supplies the sternocleidomastoid and trapezius muscles.

**accessory neuropathy**   Disease of the accessory nerve. Paralysis of the accessory nerve prevents rotation of the head away from one or both sides, and causes the

shoulder to droop. Damage can be confined to the accessory nerve, or may also involve the ninth and tenth cranial nerves, which exit the skull through the same opening.

**accessory placenta**   See *placenta, accessory*.

**acclimatization to altitude**   The process of adapting to the decrease in oxygen concentration at a specific altitude. A number of changes must take place for the body to operate with decreased oxygen. These changes include increasing the depth of respiration; increasing the pressure in the pulmonary arteries, forcing blood into portions of the lung that normally are not used at sea level; manufacture of additional oxygen-carrying red blood cells; manufacture of extra 2,4-DPG, a substance that facilitates the release of oxygen from hemoglobin to the body tissues. Acclimatization generally takes one to three days at each new altitude.

**accoucheur**   French for a male obstetrician.

**accoucheuse**   French for a female obstetrician, sometimes also used to refer to a midwife.

**ACE**   Angiotensin converting enzyme. This enzyme converts an angiotensin to its activated form, angiotensin II, enabling it to function.

**ACE inhibitors**   Drugs that inhibit ACE. ACE inhibitors lower the blood pressure by inhibiting the formation of angiotensin II. This relaxes the arteries, consequently not only lowering blood pressure, but also improving the pumping efficiency of a failing heart and improving cardiac output in patients with heart failure. ACE inhibitors are therefore used for blood pressure control and congestive heart failure. Popular ACE inhibitors include benazepril (brand name: Lotensin), captopril (Capoten), lisinopril (Zestril, Prinivil), quinapril (Accupril), and ramipril (Altace). Interestingly, the ACE inhibitors were developed from the venom of a Brazilian snake.

**acentric chromosome**   A fragment of a chromosome that is lacking a centromere, and so is lost when the cell divides.

**acetabulum**   The cup-shaped socket of the hip joint. The acetabulum is a feature of the pelvis. The head (upper end) of the femur (thighbone) fits into the acetabulum and articulates with it, forming a ball-and-socket joint.

**acetaminophen**   A nonaspirin analgesic, acetaminophen may be given alone to relieve pain and inflammation. It may also be combined with other drugs. For example, the migraine medication Fioricet contains acetaminophen, a barbituate, and caffeine.

**acetone**   A volatile liquid used as an industrial solvent. Acetone is also one of the so-called ketone bodies formed when the body uses fat instead of glucose (sugar) for energy. The formation of acetone is usually a sign that cells lack insulin or cannot effectively use the insulin that is available, as occurs in diabetes. Acetone is excreted via the urine.

**acetone breath**   The breath of a person with a lot of acetone in his or her body smells fruity. Acetone breath is a telltale sign of diabetes. See also *diabetes mellitus*.

**acetylcholine**   A neurotransmitter released by the parasympatheic nervous system, acetylcholine is essential for communication between the nerves and muscles.

**acetylsalicylic acid**   See *aspirin*.

**achalasia**   A rare disease of the esophagus, usually diagnosed in young adults. Abnormal function of nerves and muscles of the esophagus causes difficulty swallowing, and sometimes chest pain. Regurgitation of undigested food can occur, as can coughing, or breathing problems related to entry of food material into the lungs. The underlying problem is weakness of the lower portion of the esophagus, and failure of the lower esophageal sphincter to open and allow passage of food. Diagnosis may be made by an X-ray, endoscopy, or esophageal manometry. Treatment includes medication, dilation (stretching) to widen the lower part of the esophagus, and surgery to open the lower esophagus. A new approach involves injecting medicines into the lower esophagus to relax the sphincter.

**Achilles heel**   See *Achilles tendon*.

**Achilles tendon**   One of the longest tendons in the body, the Achilles tendon is a tough sinew that attaches the calf muscle to the back of the calcaneus (heel bone). The name comes from Greek mythology: The hero Achilles was invulnerable to injury except for his heel, which proved his downfall when it was pierced by Paris' arrow. Also known as the tendo Achilles, tendo calcaneus.

**achlorhydria**   A lack of hydrochloric acid in the digestive juices in the stomach.

**achondroplasia**   A genetic disorder of bone growth, achondroplasia is the most common cause of short stature (dwarfism) with disproportionately short arms and legs. Typically, the individual with achondroplasia has a large head with a prominent forehead (frontal bossing); underdevelopment (hypoplasia) of the midface, with cheekbones that lack prominence; and a low nasal bridge, with narrow nasal passages. The fingers are short, and the ring and middle fingers diverge to give the hand a trident (three-pronged) appearance. The brain is entirely normal in people with achondroplasia, but complications can hurt the brain and spinal cord. Although the parents

of children with achondroplasia are usually normal, it is inherited as an autosomal dominant trait, affecting boys and girls equally. Most cases are due to new mutations that appear for the first time in the affected child. Achondroplasia is caused by a mutation of the fibroblast growth factor receptor 3 (FGFR3) gene, and prenatal diagnosis is possible. See also *dwarfism; dwarfism, hydrochondroplastic*.

**acid phosphatase**   An enzyme that works under acid conditions, acid phosphatase is made in the liver, spleen, bone marrow, and prostate gland. Abnormally high serum levels of the enzyme may indicate infection, injury, or cancer of the prostate.

**acid, pantothenic**   Vitamin B5. See also *Appendix C, "Vitamins."*

**acidophilus**   Bacteria found in yogurt with "live cultures" that can help restore a supportive bacterial environment to an intestinal tract whose normal bacterial population (flora) has been disturbed by disease or antibiotics. Eating yogurt with acidophilus may also be useful in preventing overgrowth of Candida yeast in the intestinal tract, mouth (candidiasis, thrush), and vagina (yeast infection). See also *probiotics*.

**acidosis**   Too much acid in the blood and body. This distinctly abnormal condition results from either the accumulation of acid or the depletion of alkaline reserves. The pH of the acidotic body is below normal. For a person with diabetes, this can lead to diabetic ketoacidosis. The opposite of acidosis is alkalosis.

**ACL**   Anterior cruciate ligament.

**acne**   Localized skin inflammation resulting from overactivity of the oil glands at the base of hair follicles, or as a response to contact with irritating substances. See also *acne vulgaris*.

**acne rosacea**   See *rosacea*.

**acne vulgaris**   The common form of acne seen most often in teenagers or young adults, acne vulgaris is the result of overactive oil glands that become plugged and inflamed. Most outbreaks of acne can be treated by keeping the skin clean and avoiding irritating soaps, foods, drinks, and cosmetics. Severe acne and acne in those who are prone to scarring can be treated with topical creams and anti-inflammatory medications. Skin damaged by acne can be improved via treatment by a dermatologist or facial technologist. Techniques include dermabrasion (sanding), removal of scar tissue via laser, and chemical peels. Also known as pimples. See also *keloid*.

**ACOG** The American College of Obstetricians and Gynecologists, a professional organization.

**acquired** In medicine, new, or not inherited; or added, in the sense that a condition was not present at birth (congenital). For example, AIDS is an acquired, not an inherited, form of immune deficiency.

**acquired immunodeficiency disease** Disease caused by infection with the human immunodeficiency virus (HIV): AIDS. This term could also be used to describe other forms of acquired immune-system deficiency. See *AIDS*.

**acquired immunodeficiency syndrome** AIDS.

**acquired mutation** A change in a gene or chromosome that occurs in a single cell after the conception of an individual. That change is then passed along to all cells descended from that cell. Acquired mutations are involved in the development of cancer.

**acrocentric chromosome** A chromosome in which the centromere is located quite near one end of the chromosome. Humans normally have five pairs of acrocentric chromosomes. Down syndrome is caused by an extra acrocentric chromosome, namely chromosome 21.

**acrocephalosyndactyly** An inherited disorder causing abnormalities of the skull, face, hands, and feet. It begins with premature closure of some sutures of the skull (craniosynostosis). This results in an abnormally shaped head, which is unusually tall and peaked; and an abnormally shaped face with shallow eye sockets and an underdeveloped midface. There is fusion of fingers and toes (syndactyly), and the thumbs and big toes have broad ends. Acrocephalosyndactyly is an autosomal dominant trait, with boys and girls affected equally. An affected parent can transmit the gene for the disorder, or it can occur due to a new mutation. Surgery is often useful to correct the abnormalities of the skull, face, hands, and feet. See also *Apert syndrome, Crouzon syndrome, Pfeiffer syndrome*.

**acrochordon** See *skin tag*.

**acrocyanosis** Blueness of the hands and feet, usually due to sluggish circulation.

**acrodermatitis enteropathica** A progressive, hereditary disease of children, acrodermatitis enteropathica is characterized by the simultaneous occurrence of skin inflammation (dermatitis) and diarrhea. The skin on the cheeks, elbows, and knees is inflamed, as is tissue about the mouth and anus. There is also balding of the scalp, eyebrows, and lashes; delayed wound healing; and recurrent bacterial and fungal infections due to immune defi-

ciency. The key laboratory finding in acrodermatitis enteropathica is an abnormally low blood zinc level, reflecting impaired zinc uptake. Treatment with zinc by mouth is curative. It is an autosomal recessive disorder. See also *zinc, zinc deficiency*.

**acromegaly** Enlargement of the tongue, forehead, hands, and feet due to the production of too much growth hormone (somatotropin) by the pituitary gland, or by a tumor of the pituitary gland. Removal or radiation therapy can be used to treat the tumor. See also *gigantism*.

**acromioclavicular joint** Located between the acromion (a projection of the scapula that forms the point of the shoulder) and the clavicle (the collar bone), this is a gliding joint. It is served and supported by the capsular, superior, and inferior acromioclavicular ligaments; the articular disk; and the coracoclavicular (trapezoid and conoid) ligaments.

**acrosyndactaly** Fused or webbed fingers or toes. Acrosyndactyly can be partial or complete, and can usually be corrected via surgery. It is associated with several birth-defect syndromes. See also *Apert syndrome, Pfeiffer syndrome*.

**ACS** The American College of Surgeons.

**actinic keratosis** Thick and scaly patches of skin, considered a precancerous condition. Also called solar or senile keratosis.

**active euthanasia** The active acceleration of a terminally ill patient's death by use of drugs or other means, with the aid of a doctor. Currently, active euthanasia is openly practiced in the Netherlands and in the US state of Oregon. The patient's request to the doctor must be voluntary, explicit, and carefully considered, and it must have been made repeatedly. Moreover, the patient's suffering must be unbearable and without any prospect of improvement. Suicide for other reasons, whether irrational or rational, is not active euthanasia. The forced killing of an ill or disabled person, as has occurred in eugenics programs, is also not active euthanasia. And although medications administered for pain relief may hasten death, aggressive pain relief is a normal medical decision in terminal care, not active euthanasia. See also *assisted suicide, eugenics, euthanasia*.

**active immunity** Immunity produced by the body in response to stimulation by a disease-causing organism or other agent.

**activities of daily living** Things people normally do, including self-care (eating, bathing, dressing, grooming), work, homemaking, and leisure. The ability or inability to perform these activities can be used as a very practical measure of ability or disability, and may be used by insurers and HMOs as a rationale for approving or denying physical therapy or other treatments. Abbreviated as ADLs.

**acuity, auditory**  The clarity or clearness of hearing, a measure of how well a person hears.

**acuity test, visual**  The familiar eye chart test, which measures how well a person can see at various distances.

**acuity, visual**  The clarity or clearness of a person's vision, a measure of how well one sees.

**acupressure**  Similar in concept to acupuncture but done without needles, this alternative therapy involves putting pressure on specific points on the body to achieve a therapeutic aim.

**acupuncture**  The practice of inserting needles into specific points on the body with a therapeutic aim, such as to reduce pain or to induce anesthesia without the use of drugs. Traditional Chinese acupuncturists say the practice unblocks the flow of a life force called *ch'i;* Western researchers believe acupuncture may affect production of endorphins, the body's natural painkillers.

**acupuncturist**  A person skilled in the practice of acupuncture, who may or may not be credentialed by a national accrediting body.

**acute**  Of short duration, rapid, and abbreviated in onset. A condition is termed acute in comparison to a subacute condition, which lasts longer or changes less rapidly; or to a chronic condition, with may have indefinite duration or virtually no change. Of course, each disease has a unique time scale: An acute myocardial infarction (heart attack) may last a week, whereas an acute sore throat may last only a day or two.

**acute abdomen**  Medical shorthand for the acute onset of abdominal pain. A potential medical emergency, an acute abdomen may reflect a major problem with one of the organs in the abdomen, such as appendicitis (inflamed appendix), cholecystitis (inflamed gallbladder), a performated ulcer in the intestine, or a ruptured spleen.

**acute esophageal stricture**  See *esophageal stricture, acute.*

**acute fatty liver of pregnancy**  Liver failure in late pregnancy, usually from unknown cause. Abbreviated as AFLP, this typically occurs in first-time pregnancies during the last trimester. Symptoms include nausea and vomiting; abdominal pain, especially in the upper abdomen (epigastrium); yellowing of the skin and eyes (jaundice); frequent thirst (polydipsia) and increased urination

(polyuria); fatigue, headache, and altered mental state. Laboratory features of AFLP include profoundly low blood sugar (hypoglycemia), elevated liver enzymes, and low levels of blood platelets. These findings indicate that the liver is infiltrated with fat. Untreated AFLP can cause complete liver failure, bleeding due to impaired blood clotting, and death of the mother and fetus. AFLP is treated by delivering the baby as soon as possible, often by inducing early labor. Women with AFLP generally improve soon after delivery, unless the liver damage is severe. AFLP does not usually recur during subsequent pregnancies. In some cases AFLP is associated with an abnormality of fatty-acid metabolism. This abnormality is a deficiency of the enzyme long-chain-3-hydroxyacyl-CoA dehydrogenease (LCHAD). In such cases the mother and father have half the normal LCHAD activity, and the fetus has no LCHAD activity. This metabolic disease in the baby's liver apparently causes the fatty liver disease in the mother. In cases of AFLP due to LCHAD deficiency, there is a 25 percent or greater risk of AFLP in each pregnancy.

**acute HIV infection**  See *HIV infection, acute.* See also *AIDS, AIDS-related complex.*

**acute idiopathic polyneuritis**  See *Guillain-Barre syndrome.*

**acute illness**  A disease with an abrupt onset and, usually, a short course.

**acute leukemia**  Cancer of the blood cells that characteristically comes on abruptly and, if not treated, progresses rapidly.

**acute membranous gingivitis**  A progressive and painful infection of the mouth and throat due to the spread of infection from the gums. Symptoms include ulceration, swelling, and sloughing off of dead tissue from the mouth and throat. Certain germs (including fusiform bacteria and spirochetes) have been thought to be involved, but the actual cause is not yet known. As with most poorly understood diseases, acute membranous gingivitis goes by many other names, including acute necrotizing ulcerative gingivitis (ANUG), fusospirillary gingivitis, fusospirillosis, fusospirochetal gingivitis, necrotizing gingivitis, phagedenic gingivitis, trench mouth, ulcerative gingivitis, Vincent angina, Vincent gingivitis, Vincent infection, and Vincent stomatitis.

**acute mountain sickness**  The physical effect of being in a high altitude environment. Abbreviated as AMS, it is common at altitudes above 8,000 feet. Three-quarters of people will have mild symptoms of AMS at altitudes over 10,000 feet. Occurrence depends on the altitude, the rate of ascent, and individual susceptibility. Symptoms of mild AMS begin 12 to 24 hours after arrival at a new altitude, and include headache, dizziness, fatigue, shortness of breath, loss of appetite, nausea, disturbed sleep, and a general feeling of malaise. These symptoms tend to be worse at night, when the respiratory drive is decreased. Symptoms should subside within two to four days, and can be treated by using pain medications such as aspirin. Diamox, a drug that allows one to breathe faster and so metabolize more oxygen, can also be used to minimize symptoms caused by poor oxygenation. Diamox may be taken in advance. Moderate AMS has the same symptoms, but the headaches cannot be relieved with medication, and both breathing and coordinated movements become difficult. The only remedies are advanced medications and descent to a lower altitude. Severe AMS is indicated by greater shortness of breath at rest, inability to walk, decreasing mental status, and fluid buildup in the lungs. Severe AMS requires immediate descent to lower altitudes: 2,000 to 4,000 feet. See also *acclimatization to altitude*.

**acute myocardial infarction** A heart attack that occurs when the heart muscle is suddenly deprived of circulating blood. Abbreviated as AMI. See also *myocardial infarction, acute*.

**acute necrotizing ulcerative gingivitis** See *acute membranous gingivitis*.

**acute otitis media** Painful inflammation of the middle ear. Acute otitis media typically causes fluid in the middle ear, accompanied by signs or symptoms of ear infection: a bulging eardrum usually accompanied by pain; or a perforated eardrum, often with drainage of pus. The customary treatment for acute otitis media is antibiotics for 7 to 10 days. About 90 percent of children will respond within the first 48 hours of treatment. After antibiotic treatment, 40 percent are left with some fluid in the middle ear, which can cause temporary hearing loss for up to 6 weeks. In most children, the fluid eventually disappears on its own. If a child has a bulging eardrum and is experiencing severe pain, a myringotomy (surgical incision of the eardrum) to release the pus may be done. The eardrum usually heals within a week. Tubes may be placed in the ear to drain fluid. See also *ear infection*.

**acute respiratory distress syndrome** Respiratory failure of sudden onset due to fluid in the lungs (pulmonary edema), following an abrupt increase in the permeability of the normal barrier between the capillaries in the lungs and the air sacs. The muscles of the lungs are forced to work harder, causing labored and inefficient breathing. An abnormally low level of oxygen in the blood (hypoxemia) occurs. Acute respiratory distress syndrome (ARDS) is the most serious response to acute lung injury. The types of acute lung injury that may lead to ARDS are diverse. They include, but are by no means limited to, aspiration of food or other items into the lungs, inhalation

of a toxic substance, widespread infection of the lungs, blood infection (sepsis), and near-drowning. Treatment frequently involves temporary use of a mechanical ventilator to help the patient breathe.

**acute thrombocytopenic purpura** Sudden onset of low blood platelet levels, with bleeding into the skin and elsewhere. Acute thrombocytopenic purpura (ATP) can have many causes. For example, it can be a potentially serious complication during the acute phase of measles infection.

**acute-phase proteins** Proteins whose plasma concentrations increase or decrease by 25 percent or more during certain inflammatory disorders. Perhaps the best known of these is C-reactive protein (CRP).

**acyclovir** A potent antiviral (brand name: Zovirax) that works against several human herpes viruses, Epstein-Barr virus, herpes zoster, varicella (chicken pox), cytomegalovirus, and other viruses. It is part of the AIDS drug AZT. See also *AZT*.

**ad-** Latin prefix meaning "toward" and "in the direction of." For example, adduction is the movement of a limb toward the midline of the body, and adrenal means toward the kidney.

**ad lib** Abbreviation from the Latin term *ad libitum*, meaning "as much as one desires" or "at your discretion." See also *Appendix A, "Prescription Abbreviations."*

**ADA** 1 American Dental Association. 2 The American Diabetes Association. 3 Adenosine deaminase.

**Adam's apple** This familiar feature on the front of the neck is the forward protrusion of the largest cartilage of the larynx, the thyroid cartilage. It tends to enlarge at adolescence, particularly in males. It is usually said to take its name from the story that a piece of the forbidden fruit stuck in Adam's throat. Also known as prominentia laryngea or pomum Adami.

**ADD** 1 Attention deficit disorder. 2 Adenosine deaminase deficiency.

**Addison anemia** See *anemia, pernicious*.

**Addison disease** Long-term underfunction of the outer portion of the adrenal gland. Causes can include physical trauma to the adrenal gland, hemorrhage, tuberculosis, and destruction of the pituitary gland cells that secrete adrenocorticotropic hormone (ACTH), which normally controls the adrenal gland. Addison disease is characterized by bronzing of the skin, anemia, weakness, and low blood pressure.

**addisonian anemia** See *anemia, pernicious*. See also *Addison disease*.

**adducted thumbs** Clasped thumbs, caused by absence of the extensor pollicis longus and/or brevis muscles to the thumb. When associated with mental retardation, it is part of an X-linked syndrome that affects mainly boys. See *MASA syndrome*.

**adduction** Movement of a limb sideways toward the midline of the body. The opposite of adduction is abduction.

**adductor muscle** See *muscle, adductor*.

**adenine** One member of the base pair adenine-thymine (A-T) in DNA.

**adenocarcinoma** A cancer that develops in the lining or inner surface of an organ. More than 95 percent of prostate cancers are adenocarcinomas. An adenocarcinoma resembles or arises in glandular tissue.

**adenoidectomy** The surgical removal of the adenoids.

**adenoiditis** Infection of the adenoids.

**adenoids** Masses of lymphoid tissue in the upper part of the throat, behind the nose. When the adenoids are enlarged due to frequent infections, breathing through the nose may become difficult. Surgical removal is the usual remedy, often accompanied by removal of the tonsils. Also called the pharyngeal tonsils.

**adenoma** A benign tumor that arises in or resembles gladular tissue. If it becomes cancerous, it is called an adenocarcinoma.

**adenomyoma** A nodule that forms around endometrial tissue in cases of adenomyosis. See *adenomyosis*.

**adenomyomata** Plural form of adenomyoma.

**adenomyosis** A common, benign condition of the uterus in which the mucous membrane lining the inside of the uterus (endometrium) grows into the adjacent uterine musculature located just outside the endometrium (myometrium). The myometrium may respond to this intrusion with muscular overgrowth. If an island of endometrial tissue is contained and circumscribed within the myometrium, it forms an adenomyoma. Also known as endometriosis interna, endometriosis uterina, adenomyosis uteri, and adenomyometritis.

**adenomyosis uteri** Adenomyosis.

**adenosine deaminase** An enzyme that plays a key role in salvaging purine molecules. Abbreviated as ADA.

**adenosine deaminase deficiency** A genetic (autosomal recessive) condition that results in severe combined immunodeficiency disease. The first successful gene therapy for this condition in humans was done in 1990 by infusing patients with genetically engineered blood cells.

**adenosine triphosphate** A nucleotide compound, ATP is of critical importance for the storage of energy within cells, and in the synthesis of RNA.

**adenovirus** One of a group of viruses that can cause infections of the lung, stomach, intestine, and eyes. Symptoms resemble those of the common cold. There are no effective medications for treating adenovirus infection. Adenovirus infection typically does not cause death or permanent problems. Over 40 types of adenoviruses have been recognized, all of them extremely tiny. Adenoviruses are being used in research as a vehicle for gene therapy and as a vector for vaccines.

**ADH** Antidiuretic hormone.

**ADH secretion, inappropriate** Inappropriate secretion of antidiuretic hormone (ADH) results in the inability to produce dilute urine, and disturbs normal balance of fluids and electrolytes in the body. Symptoms include nausea, vomiting, muscle cramps, confusion, and convulsions. This syndrome may occur with oat-cell lung cancer, pancreatic cancer, prostate cancer, and Hodgkin disease, among other disorders.

**ADHD** See *attention deficit hyperactivity disorder*.

**adhesion** The union of two opposing tissue surfaces. This term is often used to refer to the sides of a wound, as well as to scar tissue strands that can form in the area of a previous operation, such as within the abdomen after a laparotomy.

**adiposis dolorosa** See *Dercum disease*.

**adjuvant** A substance that helps and enhances the pharmacological effect of a drug, or increases the ability of an antigen to stimulate the immune system.

**adjuvant chemotherapy** Chemotherapy given after removal of a cancerous tumor. Many chemotherapy drugs are more effective after the main tumor has been removed and any remaining cancer is in small amounts (microscopic metastases).

**adjuvant therapy** Any treatment that is given in addition to the primary (initial) treatment.

**ADLs** See *activities of daily living*.

**adnexa** Latin word used to refer to appendages. For example, in gynecology the adnexa are the appendages of the uterus, namely the ovaries, the Fallopian tubes, and the ligaments that hold the uterus in place.

**adrenal glands** A pair of small glands located on top of each kidney. The adrenal glands produce hormones that help control heart rate, blood pressure, the way the body uses food, and other vital functions.

**adrenaline** A substance produced within the adrenal gland, adrenaline is synonymous with epinephrine. It is a sympathomimetic catcholamine that quickens the heart beat, strengthens the force of the heart's contraction, and opens up the bronchioles in the lungs, among other effects. The secretion of adrenaline is part of the human "fight or flight" response to fear, panic, or perceived threat.

**adult respiratory distress syndrome** See *acute respiratory distress syndrome*.

**adult-onset Still disease** Although Still disease was first described in children, it is known to begin in adults. See *Still disease*.

**advance directives** Documents drawn up by a patient or, in some cases, the patient's representative to set treatment preferences and to designate a surrogate decision-maker should the patient become unable to make medical decisions. Advance directives include the living will, power of attorney, and health care proxy.

**adverse event** In pharmacology, any unexpected or dangerous reaction to a drug or vaccine.

**aer-, aero-** Prefix indicating a problem due to air or gas, such as aerogastria (excess stomach gas).

**aerobic exercise** Brisk exercise that promotes the circulation of oxygen through the blood. Examples include running, swimming, and bicycling.

**aerophagia** Literally meaning "to eat air," aerophagia is a common cause of stomach gas. Everyone swallows small amounts of air when eating or drinking. However, rapid eating or drinking, chewing gum, smoking, or ill-fitting dentures may cause a significant increase in swallowed air.

**aerosinusitis** Sinus troubles, particularly with pain, due to changing atmospheric pressures. This is the cause of sinus pain when going up or down in a plane. Also known as barosinusitis, sinus barotrauma.

**aerosol** A fine spray or mist. Medications in aerosol form can be administered via a nebulizer and inhaled.

**aerotitis** Middle ear problems due to changing atmospheric pressures, as when a plane descends to land. It is caused by changing pressure in the sinuses. Symptoms include ear pain, ringing ears, diminished hearing and, sometimes, dizziness. Also known as aerotitis media, barotitis, barotitis media, otic barotrauma.

**aerotitis media** See *aerotitis*.

**Aesculapius** The ancient Roman god of medicine, whose staff with a snake curled around it is commonly used as a symbol of medicine. Followers of Aesculapius established temples of healing called asclepions, where the sick rested while proper remedies were revealed to temple priests in their dreams. According to mythology, Aesculapius' children included Hygieia, the goddess of health, and Panaceia, the goddess of healing.

**affective disorder** Psychiatric disorders that affect the control of mood. See *bipolar disorders, cyclothymia, depression, seasonal affective disorder*.

**afferent** Carrying away. A vein is an afferent vessel, since it carries blood from the body toward the heart. The opposite of afferent is efferent.

**afferent nerve** A nerve that carries impulses away from the body and toward the central nervous system.

**afferent vessel** A vessel carrying blood toward the heart. A vein or venule.

**AFO** Ankle-foot orthosis.

**AFP** Alpha-fetoprotein.

**African tapeworm** See *Taenia saginata*.

**African tick typhus** See *typhus, African tick*. See also *rickettsia, rickettsial diseases*.

**afterbirth** The placenta and the fetal membranes that are normally expelled from the uterus after the birth of the baby. See also *placenta*.

**agammaglobulinemia** Total or near-total absence of infection-fighting proteins belonging to the class called gamma globulins. Agammaglobulinemia can be due to certain genetic diseases, or caused by acquired diseases, including AIDS.

**agenesis** Lack of development. For example, agenesis of a toe means the toe failed to form.

**agenesis of the gallbladder** A condition in which the gallbladder fails to develop. It occurs in approximately one out of every 1,000 people, usually without additional birth defects.

**agenesis, sacral** See *caudal regression syndrome*. See also *sacral agenesis*.

**agent, antihypertensive**   See *antihypertensive*.

**agent, anti-infective**   A medication or other substance that can act against infection, either by inhibiting the spread of an infectious agent, or by killing the infectious agent outright.

**agent, antiviral**   See *antiviral agent*.

**aggressive fibromatosis**   See *desmoid tumor*.

**Aging, National Institute on**   See *National Institutes of Health*.

**agonist**   A substance that acts like another substance, and therefore stimulates an action. An agonist is the opposite of an antagonist, which acts against and blocks an action.

**agranulocytosis**   A marked decrease in the number of granulocytes. Agranulocytosis results in frequent chronic bacterial infections of the skin, lungs, throat, and other areas. It can be an inherited genetic condition or acquired as, for example, an aspect of leukemia. See also *agranulocytosis, infantile genetic; granulocytopenia; severe congenital neutropenia*.

**agranulocytosis, infantile genetic**   Children born with this condition lack neutrophils, a type of white blood cell that is important in fighting infection, and suffer frequent bacterial infections. In the past, three-quarters died before three years of age. Also known as Kostmann disease or syndrome, genetic infantile agranulocytosis. See also *agranulocytosis, granulocytopenia, severe congenital neutropenia*.

**agreement, arbitration**   See *arbitration agreement*.

**Aicardis syndrome**   A rare genetic disorder that occurs only in females. It is caused by congenital absence of the corpus callosum, a large bundle of nerves that normally connects the left and right sides of the brain. Features include epilepsy that emerges in infancy and is difficult to control, vision problems due to maldeveloped retinas, developmental delay, and sometimes physical deformities of the spine, face, and/or heart. Diagnosis is by observation, eye exam, CAT scan, and EEG. Treatment is by medication for epilepsy, and sometimes surgery for physical problems. See also *epilepsy, seizure disorders*.

**AID**   Artificial insemination by donor.

**AIDS**   Acquired immunodeficiency syndrome. This syndrome is characterized by infection with the human immunodeficiency virus (HIV) and ensuing compromise of the body's immune system. Symptoms include deficiency of certain types of leukocytes, especially T cells; infection with any of a number of opportunistic infections

that take advantage of the impaired immune response, such as tuberculosis, bacterial pneumonia, human herpes virus, or toxoplasmosis; certain types of cancer, particularly Kaposi sarcoma; inability to maintain body weight (wasting); and in advanced cases, AIDS dementia complex. Diagnosis of AIDS in most countries requires a positive HIV test, accompanied by other symptoms. Treatment for AIDS has advanced rapidly, to the extent that in developed nations some people with AIDS appear to be recovering immune function. Antiviral, antibacterial, and immune-boosting medications, among other treatments, are part of current treatment protocols.

**AIDS dementia complex**   A brain disorder that occurs in people with AIDS, causing loss of cognitive capacity, and affecting the ability to function in a social or occupational setting. The exact mechanism by which HIV triggers AIDS dementia complex has not been determined, but it may result from HIV infection of cells in the brain or from an inflammatory reaction to such an infection. Another possibility is opportunistic infection of the brain by any of many viruses known to cause neuropsychiatric symptoms. The AIDS dementia complex is considered an AIDS-defining illness: one of the serious illnesses that occurs in HIV-positive individuals and warrants an AIDS diagnosis, according to the Centers for Disease Control's definition of AIDS.

**AIDS-related complex**   In the early years of the AIDS epidemic, this term (abbreviated as ARC) was used to describe people with HIV infection who had only mild symptoms of illness, such as swollen lymph glands. It is rarely used today.

**airway obstruction**   Partial or complete blockage of the breathing tubes to the lungs due to the presence of foreign bodies, allergic reactions, infections, anatomical abnormalities, trauma, or other causes. The onset of respiratory distress may be sudden, with only a cough for warning. There is often agitation in the early stages. Other signs include labored, ineffective breathing, until the person is not longer breathing (apneic). Loss of consciousness occurs if the obstruction is not relieved. Treatment of airway obstruction due to a foreign body includes the Heimlich maneuver for adults, a series of five abdominal thrusts for children over one year of age, and a combination of five back blows with the flat of the hand and five abdominal thrusts with two fingers on the upper abdomen for infants.

**AKA**   Above the knee amputation.

**akasthisia**   An intense internal sensation of physical restlessness and jumpiness. A person with akasthisia will look and feel uncomfortable if he or she tries to be still. Can be a side effect of some psychiatric medications.

**akinesia**  The state of being without movement.

**akinetic**  Related to the loss of the normal ability to move the muscles.

**akinetic epilepsy**  See *epilepsy, akinetic*.

**akinetic mutism**  See *mutism, akinetic*.

**Alagille syndrome**  A genetic disorder initially characterized by jaundice in the newborn period. A stagnant flow of bile from the liver (cholestasis) then develops, with puritis (itching), stools without the usual yellowing brown color, and enlargement of the liver and spleen. The face of a person with Alagille sysndrome has deep-set eyes, broad forehead, long nose with flat tip, prominent chin, and low-set or malformed ears. The outlook depends on the degree of congenital heart disease. Alagille syndrome is an autosomal dominant trait, meaning that the gene for it is carried on an autosome, and a single edition of the Alagille gene is sufficient to produce the disease. The gene has been discovered on chromosome 20 in band 20p12. Also known as arteriohepatic dysplasia. See *congenital heart disease*.

**alanine aminotransferase**  An enzyme that is normally present in liver and heart cells, abbreviated as ALT. ALT is released into blood when the liver or heart is damaged, and some medications can raise ALT levels. Also known as serum glutamic pyruvic transaminase (SGPT).

**alb-**  Prefix from the Latin root for the color white, *albus*.

**albinism**  A pigmentation disorder characterized by partial or total lack of the pigment melanin in the skin, hair, and iris. Albinism is caused by an autosomal recessive gene, and can occur in people of any race. People with albinism have delicate skin that sunburns and develops skin cancer easily, and may suffer from eye disorders as well. Albinism may be partial or complete (tyrosinase-negative albinism).

**albinism with hemorrhagic diathesis and pigmented reticuloendithelial cells**  See *Hermansky-Pudlak syndrome*.

**albino**  A person with albinism. The term was first applied by the Portuguese to people in West Africa, who may have had partial or complete albinism.

**albuginea**  Tough white fibrous tissue. The tunica albuginea of the testis, for example, is the layer of dense whitish inelastic tissue that surrounds the testis.

**albumen**  The white of an egg.

**albumin**  The main protein in human blood, albumin is key to regulating the osmotic pressure of blood. Chemically, albumin is soluble in water, precipitated by acid, and coagulated by heat.

**albuminuria**  A condition characterized by more than the normal amount of albumin in the urine. Albuminuria can be a sign that protein is leaking through the kidney, most often through the glomeruli; or a sign of significant kidney disease. It may also be the harmless result of vigorous exercise. Synonymous with proteinuria.

**alcohol**  An organic substance formed when a hydroxyl group is substituted for a hydrogen atom in a hydrocarbon. The type of alcohol used in alcoholic beverages, ethanol, derives from fermenting sugar with yeast. Once ingested, it is converted to sugar-based fuel by the body. Alcohol acts as a central nervous system depressant, and has many medicinal uses. It may be part of solutions used as preservatives, antiseptics, or medications.

**alcohol abuse**  Use of alcoholic beverages to excess, either on individual occasions (binge drinking) or as a regular practice. For some individuals—children or pregnant women, for example—almost any amount of alcohol use may be legally considered "alcohol abuse," depending on local laws. Heavy alcohol abuse can cause physical damage and death.

**alcohol poisoning**  A condition in which a toxic amount of alcohol has been consumed, usually in a short period of time. The individual may become extremely disoriented, unresponsive, or unconscious, with shallow breathing. Because alcohol poisoning can be deadly, emergency treatment is necessary.

**alcohol use in pregnancy**  The consumption of alcohol during pregnancy, which can damage the fetus. See also *fetal alcohol effect, fetal alcohol syndrome*.

**Alcoholics Anonymous**  A free, self-help organization founded to assist people addicted to alcohol in breaking old behavior patterns and gaining support for living a sober lifestyle.

**alcoholism**  Physical dependance on alcohol to the extent that stopping alcohol use will bring on withdrawal symptoms. In popular and therapeutic parlance, the term may also be used to refer to ingrained drinking habits that cause health or social problems. Treatment requires first ending the physical dependance, then making lifestyle changes that help the individual avoid relapse. In some cases, medication or hospitalization are necessary. Alcohol dependance can have many serious effects on the brain, liver, and other organs of the body, some of which can lead to death.

**aldosterone**  Hormone produced by the outer portion (cortex) of the adrenal gland. Aldosterone regulates the balance of water and electrolytes in the body, encouraging the kidney to excrete potassium into the urine and retain sodium, thereby retaining water. It is classified as a mineralocorticoid hormone.

**aldosteronism**   Overproduction of the hormone aldosterone by the adrenal gland or by a tumor containing that type of tissue. Excess aldosterone results in low potassium levels (hypokalemia), underacidity of the body (alkalosis), muscle weakness, excess thirst (polydipsia), excess urination (polyuria), and high blood pressure (hypertension). Also known as hyperaldosteronism, Conn syndrome.

**alexia**   Loss of the ability to read or understand the written word, due either to brain damage that disconnects these functions, or to temporary dysfunction caused by unusual electrical or chemical activity in the brain.

**alienist**   French term for a psychologist, psychiatrist, or other practitioner who cares for the mentally ill.

**alkaline phosphatase**   An enzyme made in the liver, as well as in bone and other tissues. Alkaline phosphatase can be measured in a routine blood test. Abnormally high serum levels of alkaline phosphatase may indicate bone disease, liver disease, or bile duct obstruction.

**alkalosis**   Relatively too much base in the blood and body. This distinctly abnormal condition results from either the accumulation of base or the depletion of acid. The pH of the alkalotic body measures above normal. The opposite of alkalosis is acidosis.

**allele**   An alternative form of a gene.

**allergen**   A substance that can cause an allergic reaction. Common allergens include ragweed pollen, animal dander, and mold.

**allergic conjunctivitis**   Inflammation of the whites of the eyes (conjunctivae) with itching, redness, and tearing, due to allergy.

**allergic granulomatosis**   See *Churg-Strauss syndrome*.

**allergic granulomatous angiitis**   See *Churg-Strauss syndrome*.

**allergic reaction**   A hypersensitive immune response to a substance. This reaction can occur when the immune system attacks a normally harmless substance. The immune system calls upon a protective antibody called immunoglobulin E (IgE) to fight these invading substances. Although everyone has some IgE, an allergic person has an unusually large army of IgE defenders. These

IgE antibodies engage and attack the invading allergens. In the melee, special cells, called mast cells, are injured or irritated. The mast cells then release a variety of strong chemicals, including histamine, into the tissues and blood. These chemicals are very irritating, and cause itching, swelling, and fluid leakage from nearby cells. They may also cause muscle spasms, and can lead to lung, airway, and throat tightening, as is found in asthma; and to loss of voice. They are also the cause of allergic rhinitis and some cases of pink eye (conjunctivitis). See also *allergic conjunctivitis, allergic rhinitis, anaphylactic shock, asthma*.

**allergic rhinitis**   Medical term for hay fever, an allergic reaction that mimics a chronic cold. Symptoms include nasal congestion, a clear runny nose, sneezing, nose and eye itching, and tearing eyes. Post-nasal dripping of clear mucus frequently causes a cough. Loss of smell is common, and loss of taste occurs occasionally. Nosebleeds may occur if the condition is severe.

**allergic rhinitis, perennial**   Allergic rhinitis that occurs throughout the year.

**allergic rhinitis, seasonal**   Allergic rhinitis that occurs during a specific season.

**allergic salute**   The characteristic gesture of a person with allergic rhinitis: rubbing his or her nose with the index finger.

**allergic vasculitis**   See *Churg-Strauss syndrome*.

**allergy**   A hypersensitivity of the body's immune system in response to exposure to specific substances (antigens), such as pollen, bee stings, poison ivy, drugs, or foods. See also *allergic reaction, anaphylactic shock*.

**Allergy and Infectious Diseases, National Institute of**   See *National Institutes of Health*.

**allergy desensitization**   Stimulation of the immune system with gradually increasing doses of the substances to which a person is allergic, the aim being to modify or stop the allergic response by reducing the strength of the IgE and its effect on the mast cells. This form of treatment is very effective for allergies to pollen, mites, animal dander, and stinging insects, including bees, hornets, yellow jackets, wasps, velvet ants, and fire ants. Allergy immunotherapy may take six months to a year to become effective, and injections are usually required for three to five years. New methods of allergy desensitization that do not involve injections are currently under development.

**allergy scratch test**   See *allergy skin test*.

**allergy skin test**  In this test, a small drop of the suspected allergy-provoking substance (allergen) is placed on the skin. The skin is then gently scratched through the drop with a special sterile needle. If the skin reddens and, more important, if it swells, the test is read as positive and allergy to that substance is considered probable.

**allergy to cockroaches**  A condition that manifests as an allergic reaction when one is exposed to tiny protein particles shed or excreted by cockroaches. Asthma can be due to exposure to cockroach allergens. Removing cockroach allergens from the home is not an easy job, but can go far in reducing the frequency and severity of asthma and other allergic reactions.

**alopecia**  Baldness. Temporary hair loss may occur as a result of chemotherapy. Permanent hair loss may result from any of several conditions, including common male-pattern baldness. Radiation therapy administered to the head can also cause permanent baldness due to irreversible damage to the hair follicles. See also *alopecia areata; alopecia capitis totalis; alopecia universalis; alopecia, traumatic.*

**alopecia areata**  Patchy baldness that typically begins with hair loss on discrete areas of the scalp. It sometimes progresses to complete baldness, and even loss of body hair. The hair loss tends to be rather rapid and asymmetrical, in contrast to male-pattern baldness. The characteristic diagnostic finding in alopecia areata is "exclamation point" hairs. These short, broken hairs are narrower closer to the scalp, and therefore look like an exclamation point. In some cases a biopsy is necessary for diagnosis. Alopecia areata affects both males and females. It tends to occur most often in children and young adults, but older individuals can also be affected. It appears to be caused by an autoimmune mechanism, wherein the body's own immune system attacks the hair follicles and disrupts normal hair formation. Biopsies of affected skin show lymphocytes (one of the body's immune system cells) inside hair follicles, where lymphocytes normally are not present. Alopecia areata is sometimes associated with allergic disorders, thyroid disease, vitiligo, lupus, rheumatoid arthritis, ulcerative colitis, and other conditions, and some forms may be genetically transmitted. In about half of cases, the hair regrows within a year without any treatment. The longer the period of time of hair loss, the less chance that it will regrow. A variety of treatments can be tried, including steroid injections and creams, drugs like minoxidil, irritants, topical immunotherapy, and even aromatherapy using essential oils.

**alopecia capitis totalis**  Loss of all scalp hair, with normal hair elsewhere on the body remaining.

**alopecia universalis**  Loss of all hair on the entire body.

**alopecia, traumatic**  Hair loss caused by injury to the scalp. Common causes include the use of caustic hair straighteners, especially those that include lye as an ingredient; stress traction injury from tight rollers and braiding; overheating of the hair shafts; or compulsive pulling out of hair (trichotillomania). Vigorous combing, chemical bleaches, and some styling products can further irritate the scalp, increasing the rate of hair loss. Traumatic alopecia commonly occurs on both sides of the scalp, and the broken-off hairs are frequently visible. In the US, traumatic alopecia is a common form of hair loss in African-American women. To treat traumatic alopecia, discontinue all styling practices that may be causing the hair and scalp injury. Partial or complete regrowth of hair may follow, although permanent loss of hair can occur if the roots of the hair have been severely damaged. To minimize the risk of scalp injury, either opt for "natural" hair styles, or choose styling products carefully, use looser and larger wrappings and braids to reduce scalp and hair tension, apply any chemicals to the hair only, and unbraid the hair at least every two weeks. See also *alopecia.*

**Alpers disease**  A progressive disease of the nervous system characterized by muscle tightness (spasticity), muscle spasms (myoclonus), dementia, and liver problems with jaundice and cirrhosis. This disorder usually begins with convulsions early in life. A continuous seizure (status epilepticus) is often the final event. Alpers disease has more than one cause. Some cases are inherited as autosomal recessive traits, with both parents appearing normal but carrying one Alpers gene. Each child of such unions has a one-in-four risk of this disease. Other causes are disorders of oxidative phosphorylation, including mitochondrial DNA depletion syndromes. Also known as Alpers progressive infantile poliodystrophy, Alpers diffuse degeneration of cerebral gray matter with hepatic cirrhosis, diffuse degeneration of cerebral gray matter with hepatic cirrhosis, progressive infantile poliodystrophy.

**alpha-1 antitrypsin deficiency**  An inherited disease that results in low or no production of an important protein, alpha-1 antitrypsin. Lack of this protein leads to damage of various organs, especially the lung and liver. Symptoms may become apparent at a very early age or in adulthood, manifesting either as shortness of breath, or liver-related symptoms such as jaundice, fatigue, fluid in the abdomen, mental changes, or gastrointestinal bleeding. There are several options for treatment of the lung disease, including replacement of the missing protein. Treatment of the liver disease is a well-timed liver transplant.

**alpha cell, pancreatic**  A type of cell found in areas, called the islets of Langerhans, within the pancreas. Alpha cells make and release glucagon, which raises the level of glucose (sugar) in the blood.

**alpha error** The statistical error made in testing an hypothesis when it is concluded that a result is positive when it really is not. Alpha error is often referred to as a false positive.

**alpha interferon** One of the three main classes of interferons: specialized proteins (lymphokines) produced by the body in response to an infection. These substances interfere with cell infection. The other two main classes are beta and gamma.

**Alpha Omega Alpha** An honor society, the medical school equivalent of Phi Beta Kappa.

**alpha thalassemia** See *thalassemia, alpha*. See also *thalassemia*.

**alpha-fetoprotein** A plasma protein normally produced by a fetus. Abbreviated as AFP, it is manufactured principally in the fetus's liver, the fetal gastrointestinal (GI) tract, and the yolk sac, a structure temporarily present during embryonic development. The level of AFP is typically high in the fetus's blood. It goes down in the baby's blood after birth. By one year of age, it is virtually undetectable. During pregnancy, AFP crosses the placenta from the fetal circulation and appears in the mother's blood. The level of AFP in the mother's blood (the maternal serum AFP, or MSAFP) provides an opportunity to screen for a number of disorders, including open neural tube defects (anencephaly and spina bifida), Down syndrome, and other chromosome abnormalities. MSAFP tends to be high in the presence of open neural tube defects, and low in Down syndrome. After infancy, renewed AFP production can be stimulated by some diseases in the liver, such as viral hepatitis and cirrhosis. AFP is also made by primary liver tumors (hepatomas) and by germ cell tumors (teratocarcinoma and embryonal cell carcinomas). A person's serum AFP level can therefore be used to help detect these conditions and monitor their treatment.

**ALS** Amyotropic lateral sclerosis (Lou Gehrig's disease).

**ALT** Alanine aminotransferase.

**alternative medicine** Healing arts not generally taught in Western medical schools or typically practiced in Western hospitals. This term is used to cover a wide variety of practices, ranging from the use of traditional Chinese medicine to healing prayer. Some alternatives that appear to be effective have been embraced by mainstream physicians, who may mix them with Western practices: This practice is known as "complementary medicine." Some other alternative therapies are useless or even potentially harmful. See *acupressure, acupuncture, aromatherapy, biofeedback, bodywork, chiropractic,* *craniosacral therapy, dietary supplement, guided imagery, herbal remedy, homeopathy, iridology, massage, naturopathy, orthomolecular medicine, osteopathy, vision therapy.*

**altitude illness** See *altitude sickness*.

**altitude sickness** Sickness caused by being at a high altitude, usually above 8,000 feet. The cause of altitude sickness is a matter of oxygen physiology. At sea level the concentration of oxygen is about 21 percent, and the barometric pressure averages 760 mmHg. As altitude increases, the concentration remains the same but the number of oxygen molecules per breath is reduced. At 12,000 feet above sea level, the barometric pressure is only 483 mmHg, so there are roughly 40 percent fewer oxygen molecules per breath. In order to oxygenate the body effectively, the breathing rate must increase. This extra ventilation increases the oxygen content in the blood, but not to sea level concentrations. Since the amount of oxygen required for activity is the same, the body must adjust to having less oxygen. In addition, high altitude and lower air pressure cause fluid to leak from the capillaries, which can cause fluid buildup in both the lungs and the brain. Prevention measures for altitude sickness include avoiding or retreating from high altitude areas, gradual acclimatization, and medication. The acclimatization process is inhibited by dehydration, overexertion, and the use of alcohol and other depressant drugs. Preventive medications include acetazolamide (brand name: Diamox) and dexamethasone (a steroid). See also *acclimatization to altitude, acute mountain sickness*.

**altitude, acclimatization to** See *acclimatization to altitude*.

**altitude, high** High altitude is defined as 8,000 to 12,000 feet above sea level; very high altitude as 12,000 to 18,000 feet above sea level; and extremely high altitude as over 18,000 feet above sea level.

**alveoli** Tiny air sacs at the end of the bronchioles.

**Alzheimer disease** A progressive degenerative disease of the brain that leads to dementia. On a cellular level, Alzheimer is characterized by the finding of unusual helical protein filaments in nerve cells (neurons) of the brain. These odd, twisted filaments are called neurofibrillary tangles. On a functional level, there is degeneration of the cortical regions, especially the frontal and temporal lobes, of the brain. There is currently no cure for Alzheimer disease, but new medications and therapies appear to slow its progress and improve the patient's ability to function.

**AMA**   American Medical Association.

**amastia**   A rare condition wherein the normal growth of the breast or nipple does not occur. Unilateral amastia occurs on one side only, and is often associated with absence of the pectoral muscles. Bilateral amastia (absence of both breasts) is associated in 40 percent of cases with multiple birth defects involving other parts of the body. See also *amazia*.

**amaurotic familial idiocy**   An outdated term for Tay-Sachs disease (TSD). See *Tay-Sachs disease*.

**amazia**   A condition wherein the breast tissue is absent, but the nipple is present. Amazia typically is a result of radiation or surgery.

**amblyopia, nocturnal**   Night blindness, also called day sight. See *nyctalopia*.

**ambulance**   Today, a special vehicle equipped with medications and devices intended to stabilize patients while speeding them to a hospital. In its original sense, this term denoted a mobile field hospital.

**ambulant**   Ambulatory, or a patient who is ambulatory.

**ambulatory**   Able to walk about, not bedridden or immobile.

**ambulatory care**   Medical care provided on an outpatient basis, including diagnosis, observation, treatment, and rehabilitation services.

**ameba**   A single-celled, protozoan organism that constantly changes shape. Amebae can infect the bowels, causing diarrhea. They can also infect the liver, causing abscesses to form.

**amebiasis**   The state of being infected with amebae, especially with the ameba *Entamoeba histolytica*.

**amebic colitis**   Amebic dysentery with ulcers in the colon due to infection with the ameba *Entamoeba histolytica*. This single-celled parasite is transmitted to humans via contaminated water and food.

**amebic dysentery**   Inflammation of the intestine due to infection with the ameba *Entamoeba histolytica*. Amebic dysentery can be accompanied by amebic infection of the liver and other organs.

**amelioration**   Improvement in a patient's condition, or the activity of making an effort to correct, or at least make more acceptable, conditions that are difficult to endure.

**amenia**   See *amenorrhea*.

**amenorrhea**   Absence or cessation of menstruation. See also *amenorrhea, physiologic; amenorrhea, primary; amenorrhea, secondary*.

**amenorrhea, physiologic**   The cessation of menstruation for completely normal reasons. The lack of menstruation during pregnancy and lactation are forms of physiologic amenorrhea.

**amenorrhea, primary**   The failure of menstruation to occur at puberty.

**amenorrhea, secondary**   The cessation of menstruation for abnormal reasons. Causes include anorexia nervosa; inflammation, disease, or cancer of the female reproductive tract; and overexercise. Secondary amenorrhea can also be caused by certain medications, notably the birth control medication Depo-Provera. In this case, amenorrhea is an expected effect.

**American College of Obstetricians and Gynecologists**   A professional organization for women's health care providers that also does advocacy work to improve the care of female patients. Pronounced "a cog," and abbreviated as ACOG.

**American College of Surgeons**   A professional organization that administers standards of practice for surgeons. Those who meet the group's standards can call themselves Fellows of the ACS.

**American Dental Association**   A professional organization for dentists. Its Council on Dental Education and Commission on Dental Accreditation are responsible for accrediting schools of dentistry and allied professions.

**American Diabetes Association**   A nonprofit health organization that sponsors diabetes research, provides information about diabetes and diabetes prevention to patients and others, and advocates for improved treatment of people with diabetes.

**American Medical Association**   A professional organization for physicians that sets widely accepted standards of practice and ethics.

**American Type Culture Collection**   Although little known to the general public, ATTC is the world's premier biological culture repository, and a key resource for medical research. The ATCC assures medical and other biological scientists a reliable source of over 60,000 authenticated, viable cultures of everything from cultured cell lines to recombinant DNA for use in the lab.

**AMI**   Acute myocardial infarction.

**amine**   A chemical compound containing nitrogen. Amines are derived from ammonia.

**amino acid** One of the 20 building blocks from which proteins are assembled. Isoleucine, leucine, lysine, phenylalanine, threonine, tryptophan, and valine are deemed "essential" amino acids because the human body cannot make them. These must be obtained in the diet. Amino acids are sometimes taken orally in supplement form.

**amino acid assay** A lab test that returns information about the levels of various amino acids in the body. It may be useful in diagnosing certain metabolic conditions.

**aminotransferase** An enzyme that catalyzes the transfer of an amino group from a donor molecule to a recipient molecule (acceptor). The donor molecule is usually an amino acid, whereas the recipient molecule is usually an alpha-2 keto acid. Two of the better known enzymes in this class are serum glutamic oxaloacetic transaminase (SGOT) and serum glutamic pyruvic transaminase (SGPT). Both are normally found primarily in cells in the liver and heart, are released into the bloodstream as the result of liver or heart damage, and so are used as liver and heart tests. Also called a transaminase.

**amitryptyline** A tricyclic antidepressant drug (brand name: Elavil) prescribed to treat depression, chronic pain, migraine, eating disorders, and a wide variety of other conditions. See also *tricyclic antidepressant*.

**amnesia** An impairment to or lack of memory.

**amnesia, antegrade** Amnesia after a traumatic event in which the lack of memory relates to events occurring after the event.

**amnesia, retrograde** Amnesia after a traumatic event in which the lack of memory relates to events occurring before the event.

**amniocentesis** A prenatal diagnostic procedure in which a long needle is used to obtain amniotic fluid from within the womb. This fluid can be used for genetic and other diagnostic tests. Informally called an amnio.

**amnion** A thin membrane surrounding the fetus during pregnancy. The amnion is the inner of the two fetal membranes (the chorion is the outer one). It contains the amniotic fluid.

**amniotic fluid** The fluid bathing the fetus within the womb, which serves as a shock absorber.

**amoeba** Alternative spelling for ameba, used mainly in the UK. See *ameba*.

**amphetamine** A drug with a stimulant effect on the central nervous system.

**amplification** Event producing multiple copies of a gene or of any sequence of DNA. Gene amplification plays a role in cancer. Amplification can occur in vivo (in the living individual) or in vitro (in the laboratory).

**ampulla of Vater** A small projection into the duodenum through which bile and pancreatic secretions flow to mix with food for digestion.

**amputation** Surgery to remove all or part of an arm, leg, finger, or toe.

**AMS** 1 Atypical measles syndrome. 2 Acute mountain sickness.

**amygdala** An almond-shaped structure within the basal ganglia of the brain, the amygdala is believed to impact the sense of smell, mood, emotion, instinctive behavior, and short-term memory.

**amyloidosis** Disorder due to deposits of abnormal protein (amyloid) in body tissues.

**amyotrophic lateral sclerosis** A progressive chronic disease of the motor neurons, the nerves that come from the spinal cord. These nerves are responsible for supplying electrical stimulation to the muscles, a necessary process for the movement of body parts. Abbreviated as ALS, amyotrophic lateral sclerosis is progressive and fatal in two to seven years, usually as a result of additional illnesses that occur as the body becomes weaker. ALS occurs most often in adults over 50. The cause of ALS is unknown. It is sometimes called Lou Gehrig's disease after a great baseball player who was its best-known victim.

**an-** See *a-*.

**ANA** 1 Antinuclear antibodies. 2 Anti-Nuclear Antibody screen, a blood test that looks for antinuclear antibodies. The ANA test presents different patterns depending on how the cell nucleus was stained in the laboratory: homogeneous, or diffuse; speckled; nucleolar; and peripheral or rim. While these patterns are not specific for any one illness, certain illnesses can more frequently be associated with one pattern or another. For example, the nucleolar pattern is more commonly seen in the disease scleroderma. The speckled pattern is seen in many conditions and in persons who do not have any autoimmune disease. ANAs can be found in approximately 5 percent of the normal population, usually in low titers (low levels). These persons have no disease. Titers of lower than 1:80 are less likely to be significant. Even higher titers are often insignificant in those over 60. ANA results must be interpreted in the specific context of an individual patient's symptoms and other test results. 3 Anti-Neuronal Antibody screen, a test that searches for antibodies to brain tissue in the bloodstream. Their presence is a general indicator for lupus and some other autoimmune inflammatory diseases.

**anal fissure** A tear in the anal canal, one of the most common causes of red blood in the stool.

**anal itching** Irritation of the skin at the exit of the rectum, accompanied by the desire to scratch. The intensity of anal itching is increased by moisture, pressure, and abrasion caused by clothing and sitting. At its most intense, anal itching causes intolerable discomfort. It may be caused by irritating chemicals in food (as in spices, hot sauces, and peppers); irritation due to frequent liquid stools, as in diarrhea; diseases, such as diabetes mellitus or HIV infection, that increase the possibility of yeast infections; and psoriasis. Abnormal passageways (fistulas) from the intestine to the skin around the anus can form as a result of Crohn disease and other conditions. These fistulas bring irritating fluids to the anal area. Other causes of anal itching include hemorrhoids, anal fissures, abnormal local growth of anal skin (anal papillae), and skin tags. Treatment is directed first toward relieving the burning and soreness. Clean and dry the anus thoroughly, and avoid leaving soap in the anal area. Shower gently without direct rubbing or irritation of the skin. Use moist pads rather than toilet paper to clean the anus after bowel movements. Local application of cortisone cream may help. If anal itching persists, an examination by a doctor can rapidly identify most causes of anal itching. Also known as pruritus ani.

**analgesia** The inability to feel pain.

**analgesic** A drug that relieves pain.

**analysis** A psychology term for conversation-based therapeutic processes used to gain understanding of complex emotional or behavioral issues.

**anaphylactic shock** A widespread and very serious allergic reaction. Symptoms include dizziness, loss of consciousness, labored breathing, swelling of the tongue and breathing tubes, blueness of the skin, low blood pressure, and heart failure, and can result in death. Immediate emergency treatment is required, including administration of antivenom in the case of bee or wasp stings. See also *allergic reaction.*

**anaphylactoid purpura** A form of blood vessel inflammation that affects small capillaries in the skin and the kidneys. It results in skin rash associated with joint inflammation (arthritis) and cramping pain in the abdomen. Anaphylactoid purpura frequently follows a bacterial or viral infection of the throat or breathing passages, and is an unusual reaction of the body's immune system to this infection. It occurs most commonly in chil-

dren. Generally a mild illness that resolves spontaneously, anaphylactoid purpura can sometimes cause serious problems in the kidneys and bowels. Treatment is directed toward the most significant area of involvement. Joint pain can be relieved by antiinflammatory medications, such as aspirin or ibuprofen. Some patients may require steroid medications, such as prednisone. Also known as Henoch-Schonlein purpura (HSP).

**anaphylaxis** Allergic reaction. In severe cases, this can include potentially deadly anaphylactic shock. See also *allergic reaction, anaphylactic shock.*

**anastomosis** A procedure to reconnect healthy sections of the colon or rectum after a cancerous portion has been surgically removed.

**anat.** Abbreviation for anatomy.

**anatomy** The study of human or animal form, by observation or examination of the living being, examination or dissection of dead specimens, or microscopic examination.

**anatomy, gross** The study of structures that can be seen with the naked eye. Better known among medical students simply as "gross."

**anatomy, microscopic** Known among medical students simply as "micro," this is the study of normal structures as seen under the microscope. Also known as histology.

**anatripsis** The use of friction as a treatment modality for a medical condition. Anatripsis may or may not also involve the application of a medicament.

**Anderson-Fabry disease** A genetic disease that causes a deficiency of the enzyme alpha-galactosidase A. This enzyme is essential to the metabolism of molecules known as glycosphingolipids. Without it, glycosphingolipids accumulate in the kidneys, heart, nerves, and throughout the body, impairing function. Males with Fabry disease are more severely affected than females, since the gene for Fabry disease is on the X chromosome. Males have only one X, whereas females have a second X and therefore some enzyme activity. Females with partial enzyme activity may not show any symptoms, or symptoms may not emerge until late in life. Diagnosis is made by determining the level of alpha-galactosidase A in blood plasma, or by genetic testing to detect the abnormal gene. Treatment is available only for the signs and symptoms of the disorder. Gene therapy may someday make this a curable disease. Also known as Fabry disease, Fabry-Anderson disease, angiokeratoma corporis diffusum universale.

**androgen**  A group of hormones, including androsterone, that promote the development and maintenance of male sex characteristics. Androgen production is stimulated by the hormone testosterone. See also *testosterone*.

**androsterone**  See *androgen*.

**android pelvis**  See *male pelvis*.

**anemia**  The condition of having less than the normal number of oxygen-transporting red blood cells. Patients with anemia may feel tired, fatigue easily, appear pale, develop palpitations, and become short of breath. There are many causes of anemia, including bleeding, abnormal hemoglobin formation, as in sickle cell anemia; a deficiency of vitamin B12 or folate (iron); rupture of red blood cells (hemolytic anemia); and bone marrow diseases.

**anemia, Addison**  See *anemia, pernicious*.

**anemia, addisonian**  See *anemia, pernicious*.

**anemia, aplastic**  Anemia due to failure of the bone marrow to produce blood cells, including red and white blood cells as well as platelets. Aplastic anemia frequently occurs without a known cause. Causes can include exposure to chemicals (benzene, toluene in glues, insecticides, solvents), drugs (chemotherapy, gold, seizure medications, antibiotics, and others), viruses (for instance, HIV and Epstein-Barr) radiation, immune conditions (systemic lupus erythematosus, rheumatoid arthritis), pregnancy, paroxysmal nocturnal hemoglobinuria, and inherited disorders (Fanconi anemia). Symptoms can include fatigue, bruising, bleeding, shortness of breath, fever, chills and, less frequently, bone pain. Diagnosis is based on the presence of low red blood cell, white blood cell, and platelet counts, as well as a decrease in the normal cells of the bone marrow. Treatment of aplastic anemia is based on the severity of the condition and the age of the patient affected. All medications that could suppress the bone marrow are discontinued. Male hormones (androgens) are sometimes given to stimulate the suppressed bone marrow. Bone marrow stimulating factors are now manufactured in laboratories, and are often given intravenously. Blood transfusions can be required. Patients must avoid infections and even antibiotics while the white blood cell count is severely lowered. Bone marrow transplantation is considered when genetically matched marrows are available. For older patients, suppression of the immune system may be necessary. Immunosuppression therapy can include antithymocyte globulin, cortisone medications, and cyclosporine.

**anemia, Biermer**  See *anemia, pernicious*.

**anemia, Cooley**  See *thalassemia*.

**anemia, Fanconi**  A genetic disease characterized by a progressive decline in blood cells and a tendency to develop leukemia. See also *anemia, aplastic*.

**anemia, iron deficiency**  Iron is necessary to make hemoglobin, the key molecule in red blood cells responsible for the transport of oxygen. In iron deficiency anemia, the red cells are unusally small (microcytic) and pale (hypochromic). Characteristic features of iron deficiency anemia in children include failure to thrive (grow) and increased infections. The treatment of iron deficiency anemia, whether it be in children or adults, is with iron and iron-containing foods. Food sources of iron include meat, poultry, eggs, vegetables, and cereals, especially those fortified with iron. Iron supplements may also be taken, although they should never be given to children without a doctor's recommendation.

**anemia, Mediterranean**  See *thalassemia*.

**anemia, pernicious**  A blood disorder caused by a lack of vitamin B12. Patients who have this disorder do not produce intrinsic factor (IF), a substance that allows the body to absorb vitamin B12. Pernicious anemia (PA) is characterized by the presence in the blood of large, immature, nucleated cells (megaloblasts) that are forerunners of red blood cells. It is thus a type of megaloblastic anemia. It can be treated by injection of vitamin B12: oral administration will not work, since people with PA absorb vitamin B12 taken by mouth. There is some evidence that PA may be genetic, although its mode of inheritance is poorly documented. One form is clearly inherited as an autosomal recessive trait inherited from both parents. The IF gene itself has been localized to human chromosome 11. The word "pernicious" means highly injurious, destructive, or deadly, and pernicious anemia was once quite deadly. Today, fortunately, it is not. Also known as addisonian anemia, Addison anemia, and Biermer anemia.

**anemia, refractory**  Anemia that is unresponsive to treatment.

**anemia, sickle cell**  A genetic blood disorder caused by the presence of an abnormal, sickle-shaped form of hemoglobin. These hemoglobin molecules tend to aggregate after unloading oxygen, forming long, rod-like structures that force the red cells to assume a sickle shape. Unlike normal red cells, which are usually smooth and deformable, the sickle red cells cannot squeeze through small blood vessels. When the sickle cells block small blood vessels, the organs are deprived of blood and oxygen. This leads to periodic episodes of pain, and damages the vital organs. In addition, sickle red cells die after only about 10 to 20 days, instead of the usual 120 days or so. Because they cannot be replaced fast enough, the blood is chronically short of red blood cells, causing anemia. The gene for sickle cell anemia must be inherited from both parents for the illness to occur in children; otherwise the child may carry the sickle-cell trait but have no symptoms of illness. Sickle cell disease affects millions of people. It is particularly common among people whose ancestors came from sub-Saharan Africa; Spanish-speaking regions (South America, Cuba, Central America); Saudi Arabia; India; and Mediterranean countries, such as Turkey, Greece, and Italy. In the US, sickle cell disease occurs in about 1 in every 500 African-American births and 1 in every 1,000 to 1,400 Hispanic-American births. It is believed that the sickle-cell error in the hemoglobin gene results from a genetic mutation that occurred many thousands of years ago, when malaria epidemics caused the death of great numbers of people. In areas where malaria was a problem, children with one sickle hemoglobin gene—and who therefore carried the sickle cell trait—had a survival advantage. See also *sickle cell trait*.

**anencephaly**　Absence of the cranial vault and of most or all of the cerebral hemispheres of the brain. Anencephaly is due to abnormal development of the neural tube, the structure that gives rise to the central nervous system, during very early pregnancy. Specifically, the upper end of the neural tube fails to close. Anencephaly is a uniformlly lethal malformation. The risk of all neural tube defects, including anencephaly, can be decreased if the mother's diet during pregnancy contains ample folic acid. See also *neural tube defect*.

**anesthesia**　Loss of feeling or awareness, as when an anesthetic is administered before surgery.

**anesthesiologist**　A physician or, less often, a dentist who is specialized in the practice of anesthesiology.

**anesthesiology**　The branch of medicine specializing in the use of drugs or other agents that cause insensibility to pain.

**anesthetic**　A substance that causes lack of feeling or awareness, dulling pain to permit surgery and other painful procedures.

**anesthetic, epidural**　An anesthetic injected into the epidural space surrounding the fluid-filled sac (the dura) around the spine. It partially numbs the abdomen and legs. Most commonly used during childbirth.

**anesthetic, general**　An anesthetic that puts the person to sleep.

**anesthetic, local**　An anesthetic that causes loss of feeling in a part of the body.

**anesthetist**　A nurse or technician trained to administer anesthetics.

**aneuploidy**　One or a few chromosomes above or below the normal chromosome number. For example, having three copies of a chromosome 21, which is characteristic of Down syndrome, is a form of aneuploidy.

**aneurysm**　A localized widening (dilatation) of an artery, a vein, or the heart. At the area of an aneurysm, there is typically a bulge. The wall of the blood vessel or organ is weakened, and may rupture.

**aneurysm, abdominal**　An aneurysm situated within the abdomen (belly). See *aneurysm, abdominal aortic*.

**aneurysm, abdominal aortic**　A balloon-like swelling in the wall of the largest artery in the abdomen. This swelling weakens the aorta's wall. Because of the great volume of blood flowing under high pressure in the aorta, this condition can result in a dangerous rupture. Surgery is often recommended if the aneurysm is five centimeters in diameter or larger.

**aneurysm, aortic**　An aneurysm of the largest artery in the body, the aorta, involving that vessel in its course above the diaphragm (thoracic aortic aneurysm) or, more commonly, below the diaphragm (abdominal aortic aneurysm). Because of the volume of blood flowing under relatively high pressure within the aorta, a ruptured aneurysm of the aorta is a catastrophy. See also *aneurysm, abdominal aortic; aneurysm, thoracic*.

**aneurysm, arterial**　An aneurysm involving an artery.

**aneurysm, arteriosclerotic**　An aneurysm that occurs because the vessel wall is weakened by arteriosclerosis. Also called an atherosclerotic aneurysm.

**aneurysm, atherosclerotic**　See *aneurysm, arteriosclerotic*.

**aneurysm, berry**　See *aneurysm, brain*.

**aneurysm, brain**　A small aneurysm that looks like a berry, and classically occurs at the point at which a cerebral artery departs from the circular artery (the circle of Willis) at the base of the brain. Brain aneurysms frequently rupture and bleed. Also known as a berry aneurysm.

**aneurysm, cardiac**　Outpouching of an abnormally thin portion of the heart wall. Heart aneurysms tend to involve the left ventricle, as the blood there is under greatest pressure.

**aneurysm, dissecting**　An aneurysm in which the wall of an artery rips (dissects) longitudinally. This occurs because bleeding into the weakened wall splits the wall. Dissecting aneurysms tend to affect the thoracic aorta. They are a particular danger in Marfan syndrome.

**aneurysm, fusiform**   An aneurism that is shaped like a spindle, widening an artery or vein.

**aneurysm, miliary**   A tiny, millet-seed–sized aneurysm that tends to affect minute arteries in the brain and, in the eye, the retina.

**aneurysm, racemose**   An aneurysm that looks like a bunch of grapes.

**aneurysm, renal**   An aneurysm involving the kidney.

**aneurysm, saccular**   An aneurysm that resembles a small sack. A berry aneurysm is typically saccular.

**aneurysm, thoracic**   An aneurysm situated within the thorax (chest). See also *aneurysm, aortic*.

**aneurysm, venous**   An aneurysm involving a vein.

**aneurysmal bone cyst**   A tumor-like lesion that develops on one of the long bones, usually in children. It contains blood and connective tissue, surrounded by a thin, bony shell. Abbreviated as ABC.

**Angelman syndrome**   A rare genetic disorder characterized by distinctive facial features, including a wide, upturned mouth with a thin upper lip, and deep-set eyes. People with Angelman syndrome often have very pale eyes, hair, and skin. Other symptoms include autistic-like behaviors, including hand-flapping and severe speech disorders; attention deficits; hyperactivity; a stiff gait; mental retardation; and in some cases self-injurious behavior. See also *autism*.

**angiitis**   Inflammation of the walls of small blood vessels. Also known as vasculitis.

**angiitis, allergic granulomatous**   See *Churg-Strauss syndrome*.

**angina**   Chest pain due to an inadequate supply of oxygen to the heart muscle. The pain is typically severe and crushing, and is characterized by a feeling of pressure and suffocation just behind the breastbone.

**angina pectoris**   See *angina*.

**angina trachealis**   See *croup*.

**angina, exudative**   See *croup*.

**angina, Printzmetal**   Chest pain due to coronary artery spasm, a sudden constriction of one of the vessels that supply the heart muscle with oxygen-rich oxygen.

This spasm deprives the heart muscle of blood and oxygen. Coronary artery spasm can be triggered by emotional stress, medicines, street drugs (particularly stimulants and cocaine), or exposure to cold. Treatments include beta-blocker medications and, classically, nitroglycerin to open up the coronary arteries. Also known as variant angina.

**angina, variant**   See *angina, Printzmetal*.

**angina, Vincent**   See *acute membranous gingivitis*.

**angioedema**   A swollen skin eruption that resembles hives but affects a deeper skin layer. See also *angioedema, hereditary*.

**angioedema, hereditary**   A genetic form of angioedema. Persons with it are born lacking C1 esterase inhibitor, a protein that normally inhibits activation of a cascade of proteins. Without this inhibitor protein, angioedema occurs. Patients can develop recurrent attacks of swollen tissues, pain in the abdomen, and swelling of the voice box (larynx), which can compromise breathing. The diagnosis is suspected with a history of recurrent angioedema. It is confirmed by finding abnormally low levels of C1 esterase inhibitor in the blood. Treatment and prevention options include antihistamines and male steroids (androgens). Also known as hereditary angioneurotic edema, Quinke disease. See also *angioedema*.

**angiogenesis**   The process of developing new blood vessels. Angiogenesis is important during normal development of the embryo and fetus in a mother's womb. It also appears to be important during tumor formation. Certain proteins secreted by tumors, including angiostatin and endostatin, appear to interfere with the blood supply that tumors need.

**angiogram**   An X-ray of blood vessels. The vessels can be seen because of an injection of a dye that shows up in the X-ray pictures.

**angioid streaks**   Tiny breaks in the elastin-filled tissue in the back of the eye (retinae). These abnormalities are visible during an examination using a viewing instrument called an ophthalmoscope. Angioid streaks are seen in patients with pseudoxanthoma elasticum, a rare disorder of degeneration of the elastic fibers with tiny areas of calcification in the skin, retinae, and blood vessels. Angioid streaks can be associated with blindness.

**angiokeratoma corporis diffusum universale**   See *Anderson-Fabry disease*.

**angioneurotic edema, hereditary**   See *angioedema, hereditary*.

**angiopathy**　Disease of the arteries, veins, and capillaries. There are two types of angiopathy: microangiopathy and macroangiopathy. In microangiopathy, the walls of small blood vessels become so thick and weak that they bleed, leak protein, and slow the flow of blood. For example, diabetics may develop microangiopathy with thickening of capillaries in many areas, including the eye. In macroangiopathy, fat and blood clots build up in the large blood vessels, stick to the vessel walls, and block the flow of blood. Macroangiopathy in the heart is coronary artery disease; in the brain, it is cerebrovascular disease. Peripheral vascular disease is macroangiopathy that affects, for example, vessels in the legs.

**angioplasty**　Procedure that uses a balloon-tipped catheter to enlarge a narrowing in a coronary artery. Also known as percutaneous transluminal coronary angioplasty (PTCA).

**angiosarcoma**　A sarcoma that arises in blood-vessel (vascular) tissue, often as a bone lesion. See also *sarcoma*.

**angiostatin**　A fragment of a protein, plasminogen, used in blood clotting. This fragment is normally secreted by tumors. It appears to halt the process of developing new blood vessels, which is necessary to tumor development. Angiostatin may represent the prototype for a new class of cancer-treatment agents.

**angiotensin**　A family of peptides that constrict blood vessels. Narrowing the diameter of the blood vessels sends up the blood pressure.

**angiotensin converting enzyme**　See *ACE*.

**angle-closure glaucoma**　Increased pressure in the front (anterior) chamber of the eye due to blockage of the normal fluid circulation within the eye. The blockage takes place at the angle of the anterior chamber, which is formed by the junction of the cornea and the iris. If the iris is retracted and thickened when the pupil of the eye is wide open (dilated), it blocks the canal of Schlemm, a key component of the drainage pathway for fluid within the eye. This sends the pressure within the eye (intraocular pressure, or IOP) soaring, due to the buildup of fluid. High pressure can damage the optic nerve and lead to blindness. The elevated pressure is best detected before the appearance of symptoms, so IOP is routinely checked in eye exams. When symptoms of acute angle-closure glaucoma do develop, they include severe eye and facial pain, nausea and vomiting, decreased vision, blurred vision, and seeing a halo effect around lights. In advanced cases, the eye appears red with a clouded cornea and a fixed (nonreactive), dilated pupil. Acute angle-closure glaucoma is an emergency, because optic nerve damage

and vision loss can occur within hours of its onset. Angle-closure glaucoma tends to affect people born with a narrow angle, particularly people of Asian or Eskimo/Aleut ancestry. Age, family history, and female gender are also risk factors. Chronic angle-closure glaucoma, like the more common open-angle glaucoma, may cause vision damage without symptoms. See also *glaucoma*.

**anhidrosis**　Not sweating. Anhidrosis creates a dangerous inability to tolerate heat.

**anisocoria**　A condition in which the left and right pupils of the eyes are not of equal size. The pupil may appear to open (dilate) and close (constrict), but it is really the iris that is the prime mover: the pupil is merely the absence of iris. The size of the pupil determines how much light is let into the eye. With anisocoria, the larger pupil lets more light enter the eye.

**ankle**　A complex structure made up of two joints: the true ankle joint and the subtalar joint. The ends of the bones in the joints of the ankle are covered by cartilage. The ankle's movement is constrained and controlled by ligaments, including the anterior tibiofibular ligament that connects the tibia to the fibula, the lateral collateral ligaments that attach the fibula to the calcaneus to give the outside of the ankle stability, and the deltoid ligaments on the inside of the ankle that connect the tibia to the talus and calcaneus, providing medial stability to the ankle. In popular usage, the ankle is often taken to be the ankle joint proper plus the surrounding region, including the lower end of the leg and the tarsus, the start of the flat of the foot. See also *ankle joint*.

**ankle joint**　The true ankle joint is composed of three bones: the tibia, the fibula, and the talus. The true ankle joint is responsible for the up-and-down motion of the foot. The subtalar joint is under the true ankle joint, and consists of the talus on top and calcaneus on the bottom. The subtalar joint is responsible for the side-to-side motion of the foot.

**ankle pain**　The ankle is a "hinged" joint, so there are many potential causes for ankle pain. Ankle sprains resulting from accident or misuse can range from mild, resolving within 24 hours; to severe, possibly requiring surgical repair. Tendinitis of the ankle is an inflammation of one or more tendons in the ankle, and may be caused by trauma or certain forms of arthritis.

**ankle-foot orthosis**　A brace, usually made of plastic, that is worn on the lower leg and foot to support the ankle, hold the foot and ankle in the correct position, and correct foot drop. Abbreviated AFO.

**ankylosing spondylitis**　A type of arthritis that causes chronic inflammation of the spine.

**ankyrin deficiency** See *spherocytosis, hereditary*.

**Annexin V** A substance that normally forms a shield around certain phospholipid molecules in the blood, blocking their entry into coagulation (clotting) reactions. Annexin V is the cause of antiphospholipid antibody syndrome, a condition characterized by abnormal blood clotting. In the antiphospholipid antibody syndrome, the formation of this shield is disrupted by abnormal antibodies. Without the shield, there is an increased quantity of phospholipid molecules on cell membranes, speeding up coagulation reactions and causing abnormal blood clotting.

**annexins** A family of proteins that bind calcium and phospholipids.

**anomaly** Something abnormal or unusual.

**anomoly, congenital** A birth defect.

**anorexia** A decreased appetite or aversion to food, resulting in disturbed eating habits and weight loss. Anorexia may be caused by some medications and medical conditions, particularly in elderly or hospitalized patients.

**anorexia nervosa** An eating disorder characterized by extreme attempts to control the diet, and/or an aversion to food. It affects young women most often, but may also be seen in men, children, and older adults. Symptoms can include extreme weight loss, weakness, and dulling of hair and skin. Recent research indicates that in some cases anorexia nervosa may be a form of obsessive-compulsive disorder. Treatment may include medication, therapy, dietary counseling and, in extreme cases, hospitalization. Untreated anorexia can cause organ failure and death. See also *body dysmorphic disorder, bulimia nervosa, obsessive-compulsive disorder*.

**anosmia** The failure of development or loss of the sense of smell.

**anotia** The absence from birth of the external, visible part of the ear (the auricle).

**anoxia** Lack of oxygen.

**ant stings** See *fire ants*.

**antagonist** In medical biochemistry, an antagonist acts against and blocks an action. An antagonist is the opposite of an agonist, which acts like and stimulates an action. Antagonists and agonists are key players in the chemistry of the human body and in pharmacology.

**antegrade amnesia** See *amnesia, antegrade*.

**anterior** The front, as opposed to the posterior. The breastbone is part of the anterior surface of the chest. See also *Appendix B, "Anatomic Orientation Terms."*

**anterior cruciate ligament** A ligament in the knee that crosses from the underside of the femur to the top of the tibia. Injuries to the anterior cruciate ligament can occur in a number of situations, including sports, and can be quite serious. Surgery may be needed. Abbreviated as ACL. See also *knee*.

**anteroposterior** From front to back, as opposed to posteroanterior. When a chest X-ray is taken with the patient's back against the film plate and the X-ray machine in front of the patient, it is referred to as an anteroposterior (AP) view. The opposite of anteroposterior is posteroanterior: from back to front. See also *Appendix B, "Anatomic Orientation Terms."*

**anthrax** A serious infection to which cattle, sheep, horses, mules, and some wild animals are highly susceptible. Humans (and swine) are generally resistant to anthrax. Anthrax can take different forms. With the lung form of the disease, anthrax spores are inhaled. Untreated patients are likely to die. An intestinal form is caused by eating meat contaminated with anthrax. Cutaneous (skin) anthrax is the most common form in humans, and was once well-known among people who handled infected animals, like farmers, wool-sorters, and tanners. The hallmark of skin anthrax is a cluster of boils that ulcerates in an ugly way. Typically this lesion has a hard black center surrounded by bright red inflammation. Anthrax has been in the news recently as a possible biological warfare agent.

**anthrax immunization** A series of six shots over a six-month period, followed by annual booster shots. This vaccination is given routinely to veterinarians and others working with livestock. In 1997 it was announced that all US military personnel would receive the vaccine, as do soldiers in the UK and Russia, out of concern that anthrax might be used as a biological warfare agent.

**anti-angiogenesis drugs** Drugs, including angiostatin and endostatin, that halt the process of developing new blood vessels (angiogenesis).

**antibiotic** A substance produced by one microorganism that selectively inhibits the growth of another microorganism. Wholly synthetic antibiotics, usually chemically related to natural antibiotics, are made that accomplish comparable tasks. Antibiotics are used to treat bacterial infections. See also *cephalosporin antibiotics, penicillin*.

**antibiotic resistance** The ability of bacteria and other microorganisms to withstand an antibiotic to which they were once sensitive. Also known as drug resistance.

**antibodies** Specialized proteins produced by white blood cells. Antibodies circulate in the blood, seeking and attaching to foreign proteins, microorganisms, or toxins in order to neutralize them. See also *immune system*.

**antibodies, antinuclear** See *antinuclear antibodies*.

**anticholinergic** Adjective used to describe drugs and other substances that inhibit the neurotransmitter acetylcholine, which inhibits the transmission of parasympathetic nerve impulses, thereby reducing spasms of smooth muscle (for example, muscles in the bladder).

**anticholinergic side effects** A set of side effects that include dry mouth and related dental problems, blurred vision, tendency toward overheating (hyperpyrexia), and in some cases, dementia-like symptoms.

**anticipation** The progressively earlier appearance and increased severity of a disease from generation to generation. The phenomenon of anticipation was once thought to be an artifact, but a biological basis for it has been discovered in a number of genetic disorders, such as myotonic dystrophy and Huntington disease.

**anticoagulant agents** Medications used to thin the blood, thus preventing blood clots and maintaining open blood vesssels.

**antidepressant** A medication that prevents or reduces the symptoms of clinical depression. Some antidepressants may also be prescribed for their other medical effects, including increasing blood flow within the brain and treating chronic pain. See also *MAO inhibitor, SSRI, tricyclic antidepressant*.

**antidiuretic hormone** A relatively small molecule (peptide), ADH is made in the hypothalamus and then released at the base of the brain by the nearby pituitary gland. ADH prevents the production of dilute urine, and so is antidiuretic. It can also stimulate contraction of arteries and capillaries, and may have effects on mental function. Also known as vasopressin. See also *ADH secretion, inappropriate*.

**antiDNAse B** A blood test for antibodies to the streptococcus B bacteria.

**antidote** A drug that counteracts a poison.

**antifungal** Medication used to reduce or prevent the growth of yeasts and other fungal organisms in or on the body.

**antigen** A substance that the immune system perceives as foreign or dangerous, combating it with the production of antibodies.

**antigen, prostate specific** See *prostate specific antigen test*.

**antihistamines** Drugs that combat the histamine released during an allergic reaction by blocking the action of the histamine on the tissue. Antihistamines do not stop the formation of histamine, but protect tissues from some of its effects. Antihistamines frequently cause dry mouth and sleepiness. Newer, nonsedating antihistamines are generally thought to be somewhat less effective. Antihistamine side effects that may occur include urine retention in males, and increased heart rate.

**antihypertensive** A medication or other substance that reduces high blood pressure (hypertension).

**anti-infective** Something capable of acting against infection, either by inhibiting the spread of an infectious agent or by killing the infectious agent outright.

**antinuclear antibodies** Unusual antibodies that are directed against the structures within the nucleus of cells. Abbreviated as ANAs, these antibodies are found in patients whose immune systems may attack their own body tissues. ANAs are found in patients with a number of autoimmune diseases, such as systemic lupus erythematosus, rheumatoid arthritis, juvenile diabetes mellitus, and pulmonary fibrosis. ANAs can also be found in patients with chronic infections and cancer. Many medications can stimulate their production, including procainamide (brand name: Procan SR), hydralazine, and dilantin. See also *ANA, autoimmune disorders*.

**antiphospholipid antibody syndrome** An immune disorder characterized by the presence of abnormal antibodies in the blood. Abbreviated as APLS, it is associated with abnormal blood clotting, migraine headaches, recurrent pregnancy losses, and low blood platelet counts (thrombocytopenia). The abnormal antibodies are directed against phospholipids, fats that contain phosphorous. APLS can occur by itself (primary APLS) or be caused by an underlying condition (secondary APLS), such as systemic lupus erythematosus. About a third of persons with primary APLS have heart-valve abnormalities. Antiphospholipid antibodies reduce the levels of Annexin V, a protein that binds phospholipids and has potent anticoagulant activity. The reduction of Annexin V levels is thought to be a possible mechanism underlying the increased tendency of blood to clot and the propensity to pregnancy loss in antiphospholipid antibody syndrome. See also *Annexin V*.

**antiplatelet agents** Medications that reduce the tendency of platelets in the blood to clump and clot.

**antiseptic** Something that discourages the growth of microorganisms. Commonly used to refer to antiseptic preparations used during medical procedures or to maintain sanitary conditions in nursing homes, barbershops, tattoo parlors, and other facilities where unchecked microorganism growth could transmit disease. By contrast, aseptic refers to the absence of microorganisms.

**antispasmodic** 1 A medication that lowers the incidence of or prevents seizures. 2 A medication that lowers the incidence of or prevents muscle spasms. See also *epilepsy, seizure disorders*.

**antitoxin** 1 An antibody naturally produced to counteract a toxin, such as a bacterial infection. 2 An antibody from the serum of an animal stimulated with specific antibodies that is administered to humans or other animals to provide passive immunity to a disease. Such antitoxins are of short-term value only, and are used for treatment rather than prevention.

**antiviral agent** A medicine or other agent that kills viruses, or that inhibits their capability to reproduce.

**antro-duodenal motility study** A study designed to detect and record the contractions of the muscles of the stomach and the first part of the small intestine (duodenum). An antro-duodenal motility study requires passage of a tube through the nose, throat, esophagus, and stomach until the tip of the tube lies in the small intestine. The tube senses when the muscles of the stomach and small intestine contract and squeeze the tube tightly. The contractions are recorded for analysis by a computer. The study is performed to diagnose motility disorders of the stomach and small intestine.

**antrum** A general term for cavity or chamber. The antrum of the stomach (gastric antrum) is a portion before the outlet, which is lined by mucosa that does not produce acid. The paranasal sinuses can be referred to as the frontal antrum, ethmoid antrum, and maxillary antrum.

**ants, fire** See *fire ants*.

**ants, velvet** See *velvet ant stings*.

**ANUG** See *acute membraneous gingivitis*.

**anus** The opening of the rectum to the outside of the body.

**anus, imperforate** Birth defect in which the rectum is a blind alley, and there is no anus. Imperforate anus occurs in about 1 in 5,000 births, and can be corrected by surgery.

**aorta** The largest artery in the body, the aorta arises from the left ventricle of the heart, ascends a little, arches over, and then descends through the chest and then the abdomen. It ends by dividing into two arteries called the common iliac arteries, which go to the legs. Anatomically, the aorta is traditionally divided into the ascending aorta, the aortic arch, and the descending aorta. The descending aorta is, in turn, subdivided into the thoracic aorta, which descends within the chest, and the abdominal aorta, which descends within the belly. The aorta gives off branches that go to the head and neck, the arms, the major organs in the chest and abdomen, and the legs. It serves to supply them all with oxygenated blood. The aorta is the central conduit from the heart to the body.

**aorta, abdominal** See *abdominal aorta*.

**aorta, ascending** See *ascending aorta*.

**aorta, coarctation of the** Pinching or constriction of the aorta. The sides of the aorta at the point of a coarctation appear pressed together. Flow of blood is impeded below the level of the constriction, and blood pressure is increased above the constriction. Symptoms may not be evident at birth, but develop as soon as the first week after birth with congestive heart failure or high blood pressure that call for early surgery. Surgery can otherwise be delayed. The outlook after surgery is favorable. Some cases have been treated by balloon angioplasty.

**aorta, descending** See *descending aorta*.

**aorta, thoracic** See *thoracic aorta*.

**aortic aneurysm** See *aneurysm, aortic*.

**aortic arch** The second section of the aorta. It gives off, in order, the brachiocephalic trunk, and the left common carotid and subclavian arteries. The brachiocephalic trunk, the first branch off the aortic arch, subsequently splits to form the right subclavian and the right common carotid arteries, which supply blood to the right arm and right side of the neck and head. The left common carotid artery and left subclavian artery, the second and third branches off the aortic arch, perform parallel functions on the left side.

**aortic insufficiency** Sloshing of blood back down from the aorta into the left ventricle due to incompetency of the aortic valve. Also known as aortic regurgitation.

**aortic regurgitation** See *aortic insufficiency*.

**aortic stenosis** Narrowing (stenosis) of the heart valve between the left ventricle of the heart and the aorta. This narrowing impedes the delivery of blood to the body through the aorta, and makes it tough for the heart to carry out this herculean task. A normal aortic valve has three flaps (cusps), but a stenotic valve may have only one cusp (unicuspid) or two cusps (bicuspid), which are thick, stiff, and stenotic. Some children with aortic stenosis have chest pain, unusual fatigue, dizziness, or fainting. Many have few or no symptoms. The need for surgery depends on the degree of stenosis. Although surgery may enlarge the stenotic valve, the valve remains deformed and eventually may need to be replaced with an artificial one. A procedure called balloon valvuloplasty has been used in some children with aortic stenosis. Persons with aortic stenosis need medical follow-up all their lives, as even mild stenosis may worsen over time.

**aortic valve** One of the four valves in the heart, the aortic valve is positioned at the beginning of the aorta. It permits blood from the left ventricle to flow into the aorta, but prevents blood in the aorta from returning to the heart. See also *heart valves*.

**aortic valve, bicuspid** An abnormal aortic valve with only two cusps. See *aortic stenosis*.

**AP** **1** Angina pectoris. **2** Arterial pressure. **3** In endocrinology, anterior pituitary gland. **4** In anatomy, anteroposterior.

**Apert syndrome** The best-known type of acrocephalosyndactyly, Apert syndrome is due to a mutation in the fibroblast growth factor receptor 2 (FGFR2) gene on chromosome 10. Different mutations in FGFR2 are responsible for two other genetic diseases, Pfeiffer syndrome and Crouzon syndrome. All three are autosomal dominant traits. See also *acrocephalosyndactyly, fibroblast growth factor receptor 2*.

**Apert syndrome acrocephalosyndactyly** See *acrocephalosyndactyly, Apert syndrome*.

**apex** From the Latin word for summit, the apex is the tip of a pyramidal or rounded structure, such as the lung or the heart. The apex of the lung is indeed its tip, its rounded most superior portion. The apex of the heart is likewise its tip, but that is formed by the left ventricle, so it is essentially the most inferior portion of the heart.

**Apgar** See *Apgar score*.

**Apgar score** A number arrived at by scoring the heart rate, respiratory effort, muscle tone, skin color, and response to a catheter in the nostril. Each of these objective signs can receive 0, 1, or 2 points. An Apgar score of 10 means an infant is in the best possible condition. The Apgar score is done routinely 60 seconds after the complete birth of the infant. An infant with a score of 0 to 3 needs immediate resuscitation. The Apgar score is commonly repeated 5 minutes after birth, and in the event of a difficult resusitation, the Apgar may be done again at 10,

15, and 20 minutes. An Apgar score of 0 to 3 at 20 minutes of age is predictive of high morbidity (disease) and mortality. The test is named for its inventor, American anesthesiologist Virginia Apgar.

**aphagia** Inability to eat.

**aphasia** Literally, aphasia means no speech, but the term may also be used to describe defects in spoken expression or comprehension of speech.

**aphonia** Inability to speak.

**apical** The adjective for apex, the tip of a pyramidal or rounded structure, like the lung or the heart. For example, an apical lung tumor is a tumor located at the top of the lung.

**aplasia** Failure to develop. Conversely, if something develops and then wastes away, that is atrophy.

**aplasia of the breast** See *amastia*.

**aplastic anemia** See *anemia, aplastic*.

**APLS** See *antiphospholipid antibody syndrome*.

**apnea** The absence of breathing (respiration).

**apnea, central sleep** See *sleep apnea*.

**apophysitis calcaneus** Inflammation of the growth plate of the calcaneus, the bone at the back of the heel, where the Achilles tendon attaches. It occurs mainly in older children and adolescents, especially active boys. It can be very painful, although it may be dismissed as "growing pains." Treatment includes activity limitation, medication, shoe inserts, heel lifts, and sometimes casting if it becomes especially severe. Fortunately, it usually disappears as the child gets older. Also known as Sever condition. See also *Achilles tendon*.

**appendectomy** Surgical removal of the appendix. An appendectomy is performed because of probable appendicitis, inflammation of the wall of the appendix generally associated with infection. Appendicitis usually is suspected because of the medical history and physical examination. The pain of developing appendicitis is not confined to one spot at first, but as the inflammation extends through the appendix to its outer covering and then to the lining of the abdomen, the pain changes and becomes localized to one small area between the front of the right hip bone and the belly button. If the appendix ruptures and infection spreads throughout the abdomen, the pain becomes diffuse again as the entire lining of the abdomen becomes inflamed. Ultrasonography and computerized tomography also may be helpful in diagnosis.

Due to the varying size and location of the appendix, and the proximity of other organs to the appendix, it may be difficult to differentiate appendicitis from other intra-abdominal diseases.

**appendicitis** Inflammation of the appendix. Appendicitis usually also involves infection of the appendix. Appendicitis often causes fever, loss of appetite, and pain.

**appendix** A small outpouching from the beginning of the large intestine.

**appendix epididymis** A small cystic projection from the surface of the epididymis (a structure within the scrotum that is attached to the backside of the testis), which represents a remnant of the embryologic mesonephros.

**appendix epiploica** A finger-like projection of fat attached to the colon.

**appendix testis** A small solid projection of tissue on the outer surface of the testis, which is a remnant of the embryologic mullerian duct.

**apposition** The act of adding or accretion, and the act of putting things in juxtaposition or side by side. Growth by apposition is characteristic of many tissues in the body by which nutritive matter from the blood is transformed on the surface of an organ into a solid unorganized substance. To lose a pair of apposed teeth is to lose teeth that are next to each other.

**apraxia of speech** A severe speech disorder characterized by inability to speak, or a severe struggle to speak clearly. Apraxia of speech occurs when the oral-motor muscles do not or cannot obey commands from the brain, or when the brain cannot reliably send those commands. It is believed to be caused by a difference in or damage to Broca area in the brain, possibly with inheritable, genetic underpinnings. Children with apraxia can be helped significantly with intensive speech therapy. See also *dyspraxia of speech*.

**apthous ulcers** See *canker sores*.

**aqueduct** A channel for the passage of fluid.

**aqueduct of Sylvius** A canal between the third and fourth ventricles in the brain within the system of four communicating cavities that are continuous with the central canal of the spinal cord. The ventricles are filled with cerebrospinal fluid, which is carried by the aqueduct of Sylvius.

**aqueduct of the midbrain** See *aqueduct of Sylvius*.

**arachnodactyly** Long, spider-like fingers and toes, a frequent finding in Marfan syndrome.

**arbitration agreement** An arrangement in which the patient waives the right to sue the doctor and, instead, agrees to submit any dispute to arbitration. Arbitration agreements are legal and binding. The arguments in their favor are that, for patients, the case can be settled faster and more money can go to them (not to a lawyer). Doctors can often get a discount on their malpractice insurance if the majority of their patients sign such an agreement.

**arborvirus** A type of virus transmitted to humans by mosquitoes and ticks. The arborvirus category includes the Bunyaviridae, Flaviviridae, Filoviridae, and Togaviridae virus families. See also *hemorrhagic fever with renal syndrome*.

**arch, aortic** See *aortic arch*.

**archaea** A unique group of microorganisms. They are called bacteria (Archaeobacteria), but are genetically and metabolically different from all other known bacteria. They appear to be living fossils, the survivors of an ancient group of organisms that bridged the gap in evolution between bacteria and multicellular organisms (eukaryotes).

**arcus senilis** A cloudy opaque arc or circle around the edge of the eye, often seen in the eye of the elderly.

**ARDS** Acute respiratory distress syndrome.

**areola** 1 The small, darkened area around the nipple of the breast. 2 The colored part of the iris around the pupil of the eye. 3 Any small space in a tissue.

**arginine** An essential amino acid and a key component of protein, arginine causes the release of human growth hormone. Lack of arginine in the diet impairs growth, and in adult males it decreases the sperm count. Arginine is available in turkey, chicken, and other meats; and as L-arginine in supplements. Babies born without an enzyme called phosphate synthetase have arginine deficiency syndrome; adding arginine to their diet permits normal growth and development.

**argyria** Silver poisoning, resulting in ashen, gray, discolored skin, and damage to other tissues of the body. Caused by long-term use of silver salts or other preparations containing silver.

**arm** In popular usage, the arm extends from the shoulder to the hand. However, the medical definition refers to the upper extremity extending from the shoulder only to the elbow, excluding the forearm, which extends from the elbow to the wrist. The arm contains one bone: the humerus.

**arm, wrist, and hand bones**    See *bones, appendicular*.

**armed tapeworm**    See *Taenia solium*.

**aromatherapy**    A form of alternative medicine in which essential oils or other scents are inhaled to achieve therapeutic benefit. The mechanism of action is unknown, but recent studies have shown that aromatherapy may be beneficial for some health problems.

**arrector pili**    A microscopic band of muscle tissue that connects a hair follicle to the dermis. When stimulated, the arrector pili will contract and cause the hair to become more perpendicular to the skin surface (stand on end).

**arrectores pilorum**    Tiny muscles that act as the hair erector muscles. The arrectores pilorum play a key role in goose bumps, a temporary local change in the skin. See also *goose bumps*.

**arrhythmias**    Abnormal heart rhythms. The heartbeats may be too slow, too rapid, irregular, or too early. When a single heartbeat occurs earlier than normal, it is called a premature contraction. See also *bradycardia, tachycardia*.

**arrhythmias, atrial**    Abnormal heart rhythm due to electrical disturbances in the the upper chambers of the heart (atria) or the AV node "relay station," leading to fast heart beats. Examples of atrial arrhythmias include atrial fibrillation, atrial flutter, and paroxysmal atrial tachycardia.

**arrhythmias, rapid**    Abnormally rapid heart rhythms. See *tachycardia*.

**arrhythmias, slow**    Abnormally slow heart rhythms. See *bradycardia*.

**arrhythmias, ventricular**    Abnormal rapid heart rhythms that originate in the lower chambers of the heart (ventricles). Ventricular arrhythmias include ventricular tachycardia and ventricular fibrillation. Both are life-threatening arrhythmias most commonly associated with heart attacks or scarring of the heart muscle from previous heart attack.

**arterial anastomosis**    A joining of two arteries.

**arterial aneurysm**    See *aneurysm, arterial*.

**arterial blood gas**    Sampling of the blood levels of oxygen and carbon dioxide within the arteries, as opposed to the levels of oxygen and carbon dioxide in

veins. Typically, the acidity, or pH, is also simultaneously measured. Abbreviated as ABG.

**arterial tension**    The pressure of the blood within an artery, the arterial pressure. Also called intra-arterial pressure.

**arteries**    The blood vessels that carry oxygen-rich blood from the heart to the rest of the body.

**arteries, coronary**    See *coronary arteries*.

**arteriogram**    An X-ray of blood vessels, which can be seen after an injection of a dye that shows up in the X-ray pictures.

**arteriohepatic dysplasia**    See *Alagille syndrome*.

**arteriole**    A small branch of an artery leading to a capillary. The oxygenated hemoglobin (oxyhemoglobin) makes the blood in arteries and arterioles look bright red.

**arteriosclerosis**    Hardening and thickening of the walls of the arteries.

**arteriosclerotic aneurysm**    See *aneurysm, arteriosclerotic*.

**arteritis, cranial**    A serious disease characterized by inflammation of the walls of the blood vessels (vasculitis). It can lead to blindness and/or stroke. Patients are usually over 50 years of age. The disease is detected by a biopsy of an artery. It is treated with high dose cortisone-related medications. Also known as temporal arteritis and as giant cell arteritis.

**arteritis, giant cell**    See *arteritis, cranial*.

**arteritis, temporal**    See *arteritis, cranial*.

**artery**    A blood vessel that carries blood high in oxygen away from the heart to the body. The oxygenated hemoglobin (oxyhemoglobin) in arterial blood makes it look bright red. Arteries are part of the efferent wing of the circulatory system.

**artery spasm, coronary**    See *coronary artery spasm*.

**artery, brachial**    See *brachial artery*.

**artery, carotid**    See *carotid arteries*.

**artery, ophthalmic**    See *ophthalmic artery*.

**artery, radial**    See *radial artery*.

**artery, splenic**    See *splenic artery*.

**artery, vertebral**    See *vertebral artery*.

**arthralgia**  Pain in the joints.

**arthritis**  Inflammation of a joint. When joints are inflamed they can develop stiffness, warmth, swelling, redness, and pain. There are over 100 types of arthritis. See also *ankylosing spondylitis; arthritis, degenerative; arthritis, gout; arthritis, Lyme; arthritis, psoriatic; arthritis, Reiter; arthritis, rheumatoid; arthritis, spondylitis; gout; lupus; pseudogout.*

**Arthritis and Musculoskeletal and Skin Diseases, National Institute of**  See *National Institutes of Health.*

**arthritis in children**  Arthritis can affect children, usually in the form of juvenile/pediatric arthritis or rheumatoid arthritis.

**arthritis, degenerative**  A type of arthritis caused by inflammation, breakdown, and eventual loss of the cartilage of the joints. It is the most common form of arthritis, usually affecting the hands, feet, spine, and large weight-bearing joints, such as the hips and knees. Also known as osteoarthritis.

**arthritis, gout**  Joint inflammation caused by uric acid crystal deposits in the joint space. An attack is usually extremely painful. The uric acid crystals are deposited in the joint fluid (synovial fluid) and joint lining (synovial lining). Intense joint inflammation occurs as white blood cells engulf the uric acid crystals, causing pain, heat, and redness of the joint tissues. The term "gout" commonly is used to refer to these painful arthritis attacks, but gouty arthritis is only one manifestation of gout.

**arthritis, Lyme**  Inflammation of the joints associated with Lyme disease, a bacterial disease spread by ticks. See also *Lyme disease.*

**arthritis, psoriatic**  Joint inflammation associated with psoriasis.

**arthritis, Reiter**  The combination of inflammation of the joints (arthritis), eyes (conjunctivitis), and genitourinary and/or gastrointestinal systems. See also *Reiter syndrome.*

**arthritis, rheumatoid**  An autoimmune disease characterized by chronic inflammation of the joints, it also can cause inflammation of tissues in other areas of the body, such as the lungs, heart, and eyes. Because it can affect multiple organs of the body, rheumatoid arthritis is referred to as a systemic illness, and is sometimes called rheumatoid disease. Although rheumatoid arthritis is a chronic illness, patients may experience long periods without symptoms.

**arthritis, septic**  Inflammation of the joints caused by infection: either from sepsis (blood poisoning), from infection within the affected joint itself, or as a side-effect of infection in other body tissues. Treatment is by anti-inflammatory medication and physical therapy.

**arthritis, spondylitis**  A form of arthritis causing chronic inflammation of the spine.

**arthritis, systemic-onset chronic rheumatoid**  See *arthritis, systemic-onset juvenile rheumatoid.*

**arthritis, systemic-onset juvenile rheumatoid**  A form of joint disease that presents with systemic signs and symptoms, including high intermittent fever, a salmon-colored skin rash, swollen lymph glands, enlargement of the liver and spleen, inflammation of the lungs (pleuritis), and inflammation around the heart (pericarditis). The arthritis itself may not be immediately apparent, but in time it surfaces and may persist after the systemic symptoms are long gone. Also known as systemic-onset juvenile chronic arthritis, Still disease. See also *Still disease.*

**arthrocentesis**  Joint aspiration, a procedure whereby a sterile needle and syringe are used to drain fluid from the joint. This is usually done as an office procedure or at the bedside in the hospital. The skin over the joint is sterilized with a liquid. Local anesthetic is applied to the area of the joint either by injection or topical liquid freezing, or both. A needle with a syringe attached is inserted in the joint and fluid is sucked back (aspirated). For certain conditions, medication is put into the joint after fluid removal. The needle is then removed, and a bandage or dressing is applied over the entry point. Joint fluid is typically sent for examination to the lab to determine the cause of the joint swelling, such as infection, gout, and rheumatoid disease. Arthrocentesis can be helpful in relieving joint swelling and pain. Occasionally, cortisone medications are injected into the joint during the arthrocentesis in order to rapidly relieve joint inflammation and further reduce symptoms.

**arthrogryposis**  Joint contractures that develop before birth and are evident at birth. A newborn with arthrogryposis lacks the normal range of motion in one or more joints. Neurologic deficits are thought to be the leading causes of arthrogryposis, including brain defects, such as anencephaly; defects of the spine such as spina bifida (meningomyelocele); and nerve deficiencies. Prenatal limitation of joint mobility can also result from muscle problems, such as failure of muscle development (agenesis of muscle), diseases of fetal muscle (fetal myopathies), and a condition called myotonic dystrophy; connective tissue and skeletal defects, such as fusion of two or more bones (synostosis), failure of a joint to develop, prenatal fixation of a joint, excess laxity of joints with dislocation of joints, and fixation of soft tissue around the joint; or fetal-crowding or constraint, as may occur in multiple births.

**arthrogryposis multiplex congenita**  A disorder that develops before birth, is present at birth, and is characterized by reduced mobility of multiple joints. The range of motion of the joints in the arms and legs is usually limited or fixed. Joints affected may include the shoulders, elbows, wrists, and fingers, and the hips, knees, ankles, feet, or any other joints. The impairment of joint mobility is often accompanied by overgrowth of fibrous tissue in the joints (fibrous ankylosis). Once thought to be a single disease, it is clearly many. The mechanisms responsible are presumed to be the same as for all arthrogryposis, irrespective of the number of joints involved.

**arthroscopic**  Refers to the surgical technique of arthroscopy.

**arthroscopy**  A surgical technique whereby a doctor inserts a tube-like instrument into a joint to inspect, diagnose, and repair tissues. It is most commonly performed in patients with diseases of the knees or shoulders.

**arthrosis**  See *joint*.

**articulation**  **1** In medicine, the joint where bones come together. See *joint*. **2** In dentistry, the occlusal surfaces of the teeth, where the teeth come together. **3** In speech, the production of intelligible words and sentences by joining together the lips, tongue, palate, and other structures.

**articulation disorder**  Any speech disorder involving difficulties in articulating specific types of sounds. Articulation disorders often involve substitution of one sound for another, slurring of speech, or indistinct speech. Treatment is with speech therapy.

**articulations of the body, principal**  See *joints of the body, principal*.

**artificial heart**  A man-made heart.

**artificial insemination**  A procedure in which a fine catheter (tube) is inserted through the natural opening of the uterus (cervix) to directly deposit a sperm sample. The purpose of this relatively simple procedure is to achieve fertilization and pregnancy. Also known as intrauterine insemination (IUI).

**artificial insemination by donor**  A procedure in which a fine catheter (tube) is inserted through the natural opening of the uterus (cervix) into the uterus to directly deposit a sperm sample from a donor other than the woman's mate. The purpose of this procedure is to achieve fertilization and pregnancy. Abbreviated as AID. Also known as heterologous insemination.

**artificial insemination by husband**  A procedure in which a fine catheter (tube) is inserted through the natural opening of the uterus (cervix) into the uterus to deposit a sperm sample from the woman's mate directly into the uterus. The purpose of this procedure is to achieve fertilization and pregnancy. Abbreviated as AIH. Also known as homologous insemination.

**artificial pacemaker**  A device that uses electrical impulses to regulate the heart rhythm or reproduce it. An internal pacemaker is one in which the electrodes into the heart, the electronic circuitry, and the power supply are implanted internally, within the body. Although there are different types of pacemakers, all are designed to treat a heart rate that is too slow (bradycardia). Pacemakers may function continuously and stimulate the heart at a fixed rate, or they may function at an increased rate during exercise. A pacemaker can also be programmed to detect an overly long pause between heartbeats and then stimulate the heart.

**artificial pancreas**  A machine that constantly measures glucose (sugar) in the blood and, in response to an elevated level of glucose, releases an appropriate amount of insulin. In this respect, the machine functions like a pancreas.

**asbestos**  A natural material made up of tiny fibers.

**asbestosis**  A scarring of the lungs caused by inhaling asbestos fibers. When these fibers lodge in the lungs, it can also lead to cancer, such as mesothelioma.

**ascaris**  Intestinal roundworms.

**ascending aorta**  The first section of the aorta. The ascending aorta starts from the left ventricle of the heart and extends to the arch (the bend) of the aorta. The right and left coronary arteries that supply blood to the heart muscle arise from the ascending aorta.

**ascites**  Abnormal buildup of fluid in the abdomen. Ascites can occur as a result of severe liver disease.

**ASD**  Atrial septal defect.

**aseptic**  In the absence of microorganisms. In contrast, something that discourages the growth of microorganisms is antiseptic.

**aseptic bursitis**  See *bursitis, aseptic*.

**aseptic necrosis**  Condition in which poor blood supply to an area of bone leads to bone death. Also called avascular necrosis and osteonecrosis.

**Asian cholera**   See *cholera*.

**ASO**   A blood test that looks for antibodies to the streptococcus A bacteria. Also abbreviated as ASLO.

**aspartate aminotransferase**   An enzyme that is normally present in liver and heart cells, aspartate aminotransferase (AST) is released into the blood when the liver or heart is damaged. The blood AST levels are thus elevated with liver damage (for example, from viral hepatitis) or with an insult to the heart (for example, from a heart attack). Some medications can also raise AST levels. Also known as serum glutamic oxaloacetic transaminase (SGOT).

**Asperger syndrome**   A disorder related to autism, characterized by obsessive interests and behavior, but without speech delay or mental retardation. Other symptoms include physical clumsiness, and/or moderate to severe social deficits. Also called Asperger disorder, and sometimes misdiagnosed as borderline peronality disorder, obsessive-compulsive personality disorder, or schizotypal personality disorder. See also *autism*.

**Aspergillus**   A family of fungal organisms and molds, some of which can cause disease.

**aspergillosis**   Infection with Aspergillus fumigatus, rarely seen except in people with compromised immune systems.

**asphyxia**   Impaired or impeded breathing.

**aspirate**   To suck in. For example, a patient may aspirate by accidentally drawing material from the stomach into the lungs, whereas a doctor can aspirate fluid from a joint. See also *arthrocentesis, aspiration*.

**aspiration**   Removal of a sample of fluid and cells through a needle. Aspiration also refers to the accidental sucking of food particles or fluids into the lungs.

**aspiration pneumonia**   Inflammation of the lungs due to aspiration.

**aspiration, joint**   See *arthrocentesis*.

**aspirin**   Once the Bayer trademark for acetylsalicylic acid, aspirin has since become a common synonym for this anti-inflammatory pain reliever.

**assay**   **1** An analysis done to determine the presence of a substance and the amount of that substance. For example, an assay may be done to determine the level of thyroid hormones in the blood of a person suspected of being hypothyroid. **2** An analysis done to determine the biological or pharmacological potency of a drug. For example, an assay may be done of a vaccine to determine its potency. **3** As a verb, the act of trying or attempting. For example, "She assayed this operation for the first time, and so was understandably nervous." **4** The act of analyzing a mixture for one or more of its components. **5** The act of judging the value or worth of something.

**assay, CEA**   A blood test for carcinoembryonic antigen (CEA), a protein found in many types of cells but primarily associated with tumors and the developing fetus. The normal range is <2.5 ng/ml in an adult nonsmoker, and <5.0 ng/ml in a smoker. Conditions that can increase CEA include smoking, infection, inflammatory bowel disease, pancreatitis, cirrhosis of the liver, and some benign tumors (in the same organs that have cancers with increased CEA). Benign disease does not usually cause a CEA increase over 10 ng/ml. However, the main use of CEA is as a tumor marker, especially with intestinal cancer. The most common cancers that elevate CEA are in the colon and rectum. Others include cancer of the pancreas, stomach, breast, lung, and certain types of thyroid and ovarian cancer. Levels over 20 ng/ml before therapy are associated with cancer that has already spread (metastasized). CEA is useful in monitoring the treatment of CEA-rich tumors. If the CEA is high before treatment, it should fall to normal after successful therapy. A rising CEA level usually indicates progression or recurrence of the cancer, although chemotherapy and radiation therapy can themselves cause a rise in CEA due to death of tumor cells and release of CEA into the blood stream. That rise is typically temporary.

**assay, NSE**   A blood test for neuron-specific enolase (NSE), a substance that has been detected in patients with certain tumors, namely neuroblastoma, small cell lung cancer, medullary thyroid cancer, carcinoid tumors, endocrine tumors of the pancreas, and melanoma. Studies of NSE as a tumor marker have concentrated primarily on patients with neuroblastoma and small cell lung cancer. Measurement of NSE levels in patients with these two diseases can provide information about the extent of the disease and the patient's prognosis, as well as about the patient's response to treatment.

**assistant, physician**   See *physician assistant*.

**assisted living**   Used to describe a type of long-term care facility for elderly or disabled people who are able to get around on their own but who may need help with some activities of daily living, or simply prefer the convenience of having their meals in a central cafeteria and having nursing staff on call.

**assisted suicide**   Deliberate hastening of death performed by a terminally ill patient with assistance from a doctor, family member, or other individual. See also *active euthanasia*.

**assistive device**   Any device that is designed, made, or adapted to help a person perform a particular task. For example, canes, crutches, walkers, wheelchairs, and shower chairs are all assistive devices. See also *assistive technology*.

**assistive technology**   This term may be used to mean an assistive device, but more commonly denotes some kind of electronic or computerized device that helps a disabled person to function more easily in the world. Examples of assistive technology include devices that allow people to control a computer with the mouth, keyboards that can "speak" for mute individuals, and closed captioning systems that help the hearing impaired enjoy television shows and videos. See also *augmentative communication device*.

**association**   **1** In the study of birth defects (dysmorphology), association means the nonrandom occurrence in two or more individuals of a pattern of multiple anomalies not known to be a malformation syndrome (such as Down syndrome), a malformation sequence of events, or what is called a polytopic field defect, in which all of the defects are concentrated in one particular area of the body. An example of an association in dysmorphology is the VATER association. **2** In genetics, the occurrence together of two or more characteristics more often than would be expected by chance alone. Association is to be distinguished from linkage (the tendency for certain genes to be inherited together because they are on the same chromosome). An example of association involves a feature on the surface of white blood cells, the HLA (human leukocyte antigen) type. A particular HLA type, HLA type B-27, is associated with an increased risk for a number of diseases, including ankylosing spondylitis. The extent of the association is enormous. The disease is 87 times more likely in bearers of HLA B-27 than in the rest of the population.

**Association of American Medical Colleges**   A nonprofit association of accredited medical schools in the US and Canada, more than 400 major teaching hospitals and health systems, and over 90 academic and professional societies representing medical students, residents, and faculty members at these and other institutions. The AAMC is responsible for the Medical College Admission Test (MCAT), an entrance exam required to enter medical school in the US and Canada.

**association, VATER**   See *VATER association*.

**AST**   Aspartate aminotransferase.

**asthma**   Reversible narrowing of the airways (bronchospasm), causing breathing difficulties that can range from mild to life-threatening. Asthma is usually due to an allergic reaction. Treatment may include lifestyle changes, activity reduction, allergy shots, and medication, including inhalers for rapid relief.

**asthma, exercise-induced**   Asthma triggered by vigorous physical activity. It primarily affects children and young adults because of their high level of physical activity, but it can occur at any age. Exercise-induced asthma is initiated by respiratory heat exchange, the fall in airway temperature during rapid breathing followed by rapid reheating with lowered ventilation. The more heat transferred, the cooler the airways become, and the more rapidly they rewarm, the more the bronchi are narrowed. Acute attacks can be minimized by warming up before strenuous activity. If need be, an inhalator may also be used before exertion. The condition is common and usually treatable. Exercise-induced asthma is also known as exercise-induced bronchospasm or thermally induced asthma.

**asthma, thermally induced**   See *asthma, exercise-induced*.

**astigmatic**   A person with astigmatism.

**astigmatism**   A common form of visual impairment in which part of an image is blurred due to an irregularity in the curvature of the front surface of the eye, the cornea. The curve of the cornea is shaped somewhat like an American football. Light rays entering the eye there are not uniformly focused on the retina. Rays entering through the more-curved surface are focused before the rays coming through the less-curved surface. The light is focused clearly along one plane but is blurred along the other. The result is blurred vision at all distances. Only part of what the person is looking at is in clear focus at any one time. Almost everyone has some degree of astigmatism, usually so slight that it causes no problems. Significant astigmatism can cause headaches and eye strain, and seriously blur vision. Astigmatism may contribute to poor school performance but is often not detected during routine eye screening in schools. It may coexist with other refractive errors like nearsightedness or farsightedness. Astigmatism is corrected with slightly cylindrical lenses that have greater light-bending power in one direction than the other. Use of these lenses elongates objects in one direction and shortens them in the other, much like looking into a distorting wavy mirror at a circus.

**asymptomatic**   To have a disease or condition without showing outward symptoms.

**AT**   **1** The adenine-thymine base pair in DNA. **2** Ataxia-telangiectasia.

**ataxia**   Poor coordination and unsteadiness due to the brain's failure to regulate the body's posture and regulate the strength and direction of limb movements. Ataxia is usually a consequence of disease in the brain, specifically in the cerebellum, which lies beneath the back part of the cerebrum.

**ataxia, cerebellar**   See *ataxia*.

**ataxia-telangiectasia**   A genetic disease characterized by a wobbly gait and eyes that look red because of widening of small blood vessels in the conjunctiva of the eye. AT carries with it an increased risk of leukemia and lymphoma.

**ATCC**   American Type Culture Collection.

**atelectasis**   Failure of full expansion of the lung at birth, or lung collapse thereafter.

**atelectasis, primary**   Failure of full expansion of the lung at birth.

**atelectasis, secondary**   Partial or complete collapse of a previously expanded lung. Secondary atelectasis may occur in a variety of situations, including after chest surgery.

**athelia**   Absence of the nipple. Athelia tends to occur on one side (unilaterally) in children with the Poland syndrome, and on both sides (bilaterally) in certain types of ectodermal dysplasia. Athelia also occurs in association with progeria (premature aging) and Yunis-Varon syndrome. See also *amastia, amazia, Poland syndrome, progeria*.

**atherectomy**   A procedure to remove plaque (atheroma) from the inside of a blood vessel. Most commonly, atherectomy is done in major arteries, such as the coronary arteries, the carotid ateries, or the vertebral arteries, that have experienced the occlusive effects of atherosclerosis. Atherectomy may be accomplished by various means, including a balloon-tipped catheter (angioplasty), laser surgery, conventional surgical incision, or with a small drill-tipped catheter. In the US, atherectomy is nicknamed the "Rotorooter" procedure, after a company that reams out drainage pipes.

**atherosclerotic aneurysm**   See *aneurysm, arteriosclerotic*.

**athetosis**   Involuntary writhing movements, particularly of the arms and hands. Athetosis is associated with several neurological disorders, particularly cerebral palsy and Rett syndrome.

**athlete's foot**   A skin infection caused by a fungus called Trichophyton, athlete's foot thrives within the upper layer of the skin when it remains moist, warm, and irritated. The fungus can be found on floors, and in socks

and clothing, and can be spread from person to person by contact with these objects. However, without proper growing conditions, the fungus will not infect the skin. It can be treated with topical antifungal preparations. Also called tinea pedis, athlete's foot is a form of ringworm.

**atlas**   The first vertebra in the neck. It supports the head.

**atlas and axis joint**   The joint between the first and second neck vertabrae. The axis has what is called the odontoid process about which the atlas rotates. The joint between the atlas and axis is a pivot type of joint. It allows the head to turn from side to side. This joint is supported and strengthened by the capsular, anterior and posterior atlantoaxial, and transverse ligaments. Also known as the atloaxoid joint.

**ATP**   **1** Acute thrombocytopenic purpura. **2** Adenosine triphosphate.

**atresia**   Failure of a structure to be tubular. Esophageal atresia is a birth defect in which part of esophagus is not hollow. With anal atresia, there is no hole at the bottom end of the intestine.

**atria**   The plural of atrium.

**atrial arrhythmias**   See *arrhythmias, atrial*.

**atrial fibrillation**   See *fibrillation, atrial*.

**atrial septal defect**   A hole in the wall (septum) between the upper chambers of the heart (atria), commonly called an ASD. ASDs constitute a major class of heart-formation abnormalities that are present at birth (congenital). Normally, when clots in veins break off (embolize), they travel first to the right side of the heart and then to the lungs, where they lodge. The lungs act as a filter to prevent the clots from entering the arterial circulation. When there is an ASD, however, a clot can cross from the right to the left side of the heart, then pass into the arteries as a paradoxical embolism. Once in the arterial circulation, a clot can travel to the brain, block a vessel there, and cause a stroke. Because of the risk of stroke from paradoxical embolism, it is usually recommended that even small ASDs be closed.

**atrial septum**   The wall between the right and left atria of the heart.

**atrioventricular**   Pertaining to the the upper chambers of the heart (atria) and the lower chambers of the heart (ventricles).

**atrioventricular node**   The electrical relay station between the upper and lower chambers of the heart. Electrical signals from the atria must pass through the atrioventricular node (usually called the AV node) to reach the ventricles. The AV node is one of the major elements in the cardiac conduction system, which controls the heart rate. The AV node serves as an electrical relay station, slowing the electrical current sent by the sinoatrial (SA) node before the signal is permitted to pass down through to the ventricles. This delay ensures that the atria have a chance to fully contract before the ventricles are stimulated. After passing the AV node, the electrical current travels to the ventricles along special fibers embedded in the walls of the lower part of the heart.

**atrium**  An entry chamber. On both sides of the heart, the atrium is the chamber leading to the ventricle.

**atrophic vaginitis**  Thinning of the lining (endothelium) of the vagina due to decreased production of estrogen. This may occur with menopause.

**atrophy**  Wasting away or diminuition. Muscle atrophy is decrease in muscle mass, often as a result of extended immobility.

**atropine**  A drug, made from belladonna, that is administered via injection, eye drops, or in oral form to relax muscles by inhibiting nerve responses.

**atropine psychosis**  A syndrome characterized by dry mouth, blurred vision, forgetfulness, and difficulty with urination that can be set off by the anticholinergic effects of some drugs, particularly antipsychotic medications. Treatment requires reducing or stopping the medication.

**Atrovent**  See *ipratropium*.

**attack, vasovagal**  See *vasovagal reaction*.

**attention**  The act of attending to discrete stimuli in the environment. Learning is most efficient when a person is paying attention. Poor attention can be a key sign of behavior disorders in children.

**attention deficit disorder**  An inability to control behavior due to difficulty in processing neural stimuli. A child with ADD may appear to be distracted or daydreaming much of the time. ADD is diagnosed by using a combination of parent and/or patient interview, observation of the patient, and sometimes use of standardized screening instruments. Treatments include making adjustments to the environment to accomodate the disorder, behavior modification, and the use of medications. Stimulants are the most common drugs used, although certain medications developed for high blood pressure and some antidepressants are also effective in some patients.

**attention deficit hyperactivity disorder**  An inability to control behavior due to difficulty in processing neural stimuli, accompanied by an extremely high level of motor activity. A child with ADHD may be extremely distractable, unable to remain still, and very talkative. ADHD is diagnosed by using a combination of parent and/or patient interview, observation of the patient, and sometimes use of standardized screening instruments. Treatments include making adjustments to the environment to accomodate the disorder, behavior modification, and the use of medications. Stimulants are the most common drugs used, although certain medications developed for high blood pressure and some antidepressants are also effective in some patients.

**attenuate**  To attenuate is to weaken, or to make (or become) thin.

**attenuated virus**  An attenuated virus is a weakened, less vigorous virus, and may be used to make a vaccine capable of stimulating an immune response and creating immunity, but not of causing illness.

**atypical**  Unusual, or not fitting a single diagnostic category.

**atypical measles syndrome**  An altered expression of measles, atypical measles syndrome begins suddenly with high fever, headache, cough, and abdominal pain. The rash may appear one to two days later, often beginning on the limbs. Swelling (edema) of the hands and feet may occur. Pneumonia is common, and may persist for three months or more. Abbreviated as AMS, this syndrome occurs in persons who were incompletely immunized against measles, such as those given the old killed-virus measles vaccine (which is no longer available) or attenuated live measles vaccine that inactivated during improper storage. In such cases, immunization does not prevent measles virus infection, but may instead sensitize the person so that the expression of the disease is altered. AMS may also occur when a person with a compromised immune system is vaccinated. AMS can be confused with Rocky Mountain spotted fever, meningococcal infection, pneumonia, appendicitis, juvenile rheumatoid arthritis, and other entities. See also *measles*.

**audiogram**  A test of hearing at a range of sound frequencies.

**audiology**  The study of hearing.

**audiometry**  The measurement of hearing.

**auditory acuity**  The clarity or clearness of hearing, a measure of how well a person hears. Auditory acuity is what is measured when determining the need for a hearing aid.

**auditory integration training**  An experimental procedure for reducing painful hypersensitivity to sound. It has proved beneficial for some people with autism and other neuropsychiatric disorders.

**auditory tube**   See *Eustachian tube.*

**augmentative communication device**   A physical, mechanical, or electronic device that helps a person with a speech impairment to communicate. Augmentative communication devices range from books of pictures or words that the patient can show to express thoughts, to computers capable of synthesizing complex speech.

**aura**   A premonition-like sensation that is a symptom of brain malfunction. An aura often occurs before a migraine or seizure. It may consist of flashing lights, a gleam of light, blurred vision, an odor, the feeling of a breeze, numbness, weakness, or difficulty in speaking. Aura-like phenomena may also be seizures themselves: seizures that affect areas of the brain other than the motor cortex.

**aural vertigo, recurrent**   See *Ménière disease.*

**auricle**   **1** The principal projecting part of the ear, also called the pinna. **2** Something that is ear-shaped, like the atrium of the heart.

**auricular**   Of or pertaining to the outer ear, or to something else that is ear-shaped, such as the atrium of the heart.

**auricular fibrillation**   See *fibrillation, auricular.*

**auscultate**   To listen, for diagnostic purposes, to the sounds made by the internal organs of the body. For example, nurses and doctors auscultate the lungs and heart of a patient by using a stethoscope placed on the patient's chest.

**autism**   A spectrum of neuropsychiatric disorders characterized by deficits in social interaction and communication, and unusual and repetitive behavior. Some, but not all, people with autism are nonverbal. Autism is normally diagnosed before age six, and may be diagnosed in infancy in some cases. The cause of autism is currently unknown, although it is believed to involve an inherited or acquired genetic defect involving multiple chromosomes, possibly including chromosomes 6, 15, 17, and/or the X chromosome. Researchers believe that immune-system, metabolic, and environmental factors may play an important part as well. Autism is not caused by emotional trauma, as was once theorized. Autistic or autistic-like behavior may be caused by other neurological conditions, particularly the seizure disorder Landau-Kleffner syndrome, certain forms of encephalitis, and several genetic disorders, including Angelman syndrome and Rett syndrome. Also known as Kanner syndrome or infantile

autism. See also *Angelman syndrome, Asperger syndrome, elective mutism, Fragile X syndrome, Landau-Kleffner syndrome, Prader-Willi syndrome, Rett syndrome.*

**autistic disorder**   Autism, particularly the most serious form of the disorder.

**autoantibodies**   Antibodies that attack the patient's own body tissues.

**autoclave**   A chamber for sterilizing with steam under pressure. The original autoclave was essentially a pressure cooker. The steam tightened the lid.

**autogenous**   Self-produced.

**autoimmune disorders**   Illnesses that occur when body tissues are mistakenly attacked by the patient's own immune system. The immune system is a complex organization within the body that is designed to seek and destroy invaders of the body, particularly infectious viruses and bacteria. Autoimmune diseases are characterized by the abnormal production of antibodies (autoantibodies) directed against the tissues of the body instead of against these foreign invaders. Autoimmune diseases typically feature inflammation of various tissues of the body.

**autoimmune thyroiditis**   See *Hashimoto disease.*

**automotism**   Unconscious movements associated with temporal lobe (complex partial) epilepsy. Automotisms may resemble simple repetitive tics, or may be complex sequences of natural-looking movements. See also *epilepsy, seizure disorders.*

**autonomic nervous system**   This part of the nervous system regulates key functions of the body, including the activity of the heart muscle; the smooth muscles, including the muscles of the intestinal tract; and the glands. The autonomic nervous system has two divisions: the sympathetic nervous system, which accelerates the heart rate, constricts blood vessels, and raises blood pressure; and the parasympathetic nervous system, which slows the heart rate, increases intestinal and gland activity, and relaxes sphincter muscles.

**autopsy**   Postmortem examination. Also known as a necropsy.

**autosome**   Any chromosome other than the X and Y sex chromosomes. People normally have 22 pairs of autosomes (44 autosomes) in each cell.

**aux-**   Prefix indicating growth or increase.

**AV**   Standard medical abbreviation for atrioventricular.

**AV node**   Atrioventricular node.

**avascular necrosis**   A condition in which poor blood supply to an area of bone leads to bone death. Also known as osteonecrosis.

**Avenytl**   See *nortrypyline*.

**avulsion**   Tearing away. A nerve can be avulsed by an injury, as can part of a bone.

**axilla**   Armpit.

**axillary dissection**   Removal of a portion of the lymph nodes under the arm.

**axis**   The second cervical vertebra. The first cervical vertebra rotates about the odontoid process of the axis.

**axon**   A long fiber of a nerve cell (neuron) that acts somewhat like a fiber-optic cable to carry outgoing messages. The neuron sends electrical impulses from its cell body through the axon to target cells. Each nerve cell has one axon. An axon can be over a foot in length. See also *dendrite, neuron.*

**azotemia**   A higher than normal blood level of urea or other nitrogen-containing compounds. The hallmark test is the serum blood urea nitrogen (BUN) level. Azotemia is usually caused by the inability of the kidney to excrete these compounds.

**AZT**   Azidothymidine, now renamed zidovudine, but still best-known by the acronym AZT. This antiviral drug is prescribed, usually in combination with protease inhibitors and other drugs, to treat AIDS.

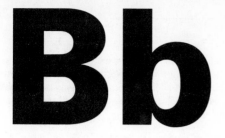

**B cell**  A lymphocyte (a type of white blood cell) that may mature into a plasma cell, which produces antibodies to infection; or a memory B cell. In humans, B cells mature largely in the bone marrow. See also *memory B cells, plasma cells*.

**B cells, memory**  See *memory B cells*.

**B variant GM2-gangliosidosis**  See *Tay-Sachs disease*.

**B. quintana**  See *Bartonella quintana*.

**b.i.d.**  On a prescription, twice a day. See also *Appendix A, "Prescription Abbreviations."*

**Babinski reflex**  An important neurologic test characterized by extension of the great toe and also by fanning of the other toes. The Babinski reflex is obtained by stimulating the external portion (the outside) of the foot's sole. The examiner begins the stimulation at the heel and goes forward to the base of the toes. Most newborn babies and young infants are not neurologically mature, and therefore show a Babinski reflex. A Babinski reflex in an older child or adult is abnormal. It is a sign of a problem in the central nervous system (CNS), most likely in a part of the CNS called the pyramidal tract. When the Babinski reflex is present on one side but not the other, that is also abnormal. It can tell the doctor which side of the CNS is involved. Also known as the plantar response; toe or big toe sign or phenomenon; Babinski phenomenon, response, or sign.

**Babinski response**  See *Babinski reflex*.

**Babinski sign**  See *Babinski reflex*.

**bacillemia**  See *bacteremia*.

**bacillus**  A large family of bacteria that have a rod-like shape. They include the bacteria that cause food to spoil, and also those responsible for some types of diseases. Helpful members of the bacillus family are used to make antibiotics, or colonize the human intestinal tract and aid with digestion.

**back pain, low**  Pain in the lower back area can relate to problems with the lumbar spine, the discs between the vertebrae, the ligaments around the spine and discs, the spinal cord and nerves, muscles of the low back, internal organs of the pelvis and abdomen, or the skin covering the lumbar area. See also *sciatica*.

**backbone**  The spine. A flexible row of bones stretching from the base of the skull to the tailbone. See also *vertebral column*.

**bacteremia**  Infection of the blood, as demonstrated by the presence of bacteria in the bloodstream. Also known as bacillemia. See also *septicemia*.

**bacteria**  Single-celled microorganisms that can live as independent organisms or as parasites. For example, the streptococcus pyogenes bacteria (strep B) is responsible for the common throat infection known as strep throat.

**bactericide**  Substances or solutions that can kill bacteria, as used in medical facilities, barber shops, and other facilities where bacterial infestation could transmit disease. Antibiotics, antiseptics, and disinfectants are all bactericidal.

**bacteriophage**  A virus that lives within a bacteria, replicating itself and eventually destroying the bacterial cell. Bacteriophages have been very helpful in the study of bacterial and molecular genetics. They are sometimes simply called phages.

**bag of waters**  The amniotic sac and amniotic fluid.

**Baker cyst**  A swelling in the space behind the knee (the popliteal space) composed of a membrane-lined sac filled with synovial fluid that has escaped from the joint. Also called a synovial cyst of the popliteal space.

**balanitis**  Inflammation of the rounded head (the glans) of the penis. Inflammation of the foreskin is called posthitis. In the uncircumcised male, balanitis and posthitis generally occur together as balanoposthitis: inflammation of both the glans and foreskin.

**balanitis, circinate**  A form of skin inflammation around the penis in males with Reiter syndrome. The skin around the shaft and tip of the penis can become inflamed and scaly. This inflammation can be helped by cortisone creams. See also *balanitis, keratodermia blennorrhagicum, Reiter syndrome*.

**balanoposthitis**  In the uncircumcised male, balanitis and posthitis (inflammation of the foreskin) usually occur together as balanoposthitis: inflammation of both the glans and foreskin. An uncircumcised boy should be taught to clean his penis with care to prevent infection and inflammation of the foreskin and the glans. Cleaning of the penis is done by gently, not forcibly, retracting the foreskin. The foreskin should be retracted only to the point where resistance is met. Full retraction of the foreskin may not be possible until after the age of three. Circumcision prevents balanoposthitis. Without a foreskin, there can be no posthitis, and hence no balanoposthitis. See also *balanitis, posthitis*.

**baldness**   Lack or loss of hair on the scalp. See *alopecia*.

**ball-and-socket joint**   A joint in which the round end of a bone fits into the cavity of another bone. The hip joint is a ball-and-socket joint.

**balloon angioplasty**   Coronary angioplasty is accomplished by using a balloon-tipped catheter inserted through an artery in the groin or arm to enlarge a narrowing in a coronary artery. Angioplasty is successful in opening coronary arteries in 90 percent of patients. Forty percent of patients with successful coronary angioplasty will develop recurrent narrowing at the site of balloon inflation. See also *coronary artery disease*.

**balloon tamponade**   A procedure in which a balloon is inflated within the esophagus or stomach to apply pressure on bleeding blood vessels, compress the vessels, and stop the bleeding. It is used in the treatment of bleeding veins in the esophagus (esophageal varices) and stomach. The balloon used in the esophagus is shaped like a sausage, whereas that in the stomach is rounded. Balloon tamponade is also called esophagogastric tamponade.

**banding of chromosomes**   Treatment of chromosomes to reveal characteristic patterns of horizontal bands. Thanks to these banding patterns, which resemble bar codes, each human chromosome is distinctive and can be identified without ambiguity.

**barbiturate**   A class of drugs that depress activity in the central nervous system, including many sleeping pills, sedatives, antispasmodics, and anesthetics. Barbiturates are addictive, carry a high risk of overdose, and should never be used with alcohol or with other CNS depressants.

**barium enema**   An enema given with a white, chalky solution containing barium in preparation for series of X-rays of the lower intestine. The barium outlines the intestines on the X-rays.

**barium solution**   A liquid containing barium sulfate, which shows up on X-rays. It outlines organs of the body so they can be seen on X-ray film.

**barium sulfate**   An odorless, tasteless barium salt. Barium is a metallic chemical element. See *barium enema, barium solution, barium swallow*.

**barium swallow**   A test that involves filling the esophagus, stomach, and small intestines with a barium solution in preparation for an X-ray test to define the anatomy of the upper digestive tract. Women who are or may be pregnant should notify the doctor requesting the procedure and the radiology staff. Also called an upper gastrointestinal series.

**Barlow syndrome**   See *mitral valve prolapse*.

**barosinusitis**   See *aerosinusitis*.

**barotitis**   Middle ear problems due to changing atmospheric pressures, as when a plane descends to land. The problems include ear pain, ringing, diminished hearing, and sometimes dizziness. Also known as aerotitis, aerotitis media, barotitis media, and otic barotrauma.

**barotitis media**   See *barotitis*.

**barotrauma, otic**   See *barotitis*.

**barotrauma, sinus**   See *aerosinusitis*.

**Barr body**   A microscopic feature of female cells caused by the presence of two X chromosomes in the female. One of these X chromosomes is inactive, and crumples up to form the Barr body.

**Barrett esophagus**   A change in the cells of the tissue that lines the bottom of the esophagus. The esophagus may become irritated when the contents of the stomach back up, a condition known as reflux. Reflux that happens often over a period of time can lead to Barrett esophagus, which is a risk factor in esophageal cancer.

**barrier method**   A birth control method that employs a barrier which prevents sperm from entering the cervix, thereby preventing conception. See also *cervical cap; condom; condom, female; diaphragm*.

**Bartholin glands**   A pair of glands between the vulva and the vagina that produce lubrication in response to stimulation. With a second pair of nearby glands called the lesser vestibular glands, they act to aid in sexual intercourse. Also known as the greater vestibular glands.

**Bartonella henselae**   Bacterium responsible for causing cat scratch fever. See *cat scratch fever*.

**Bartonella quintana**   A parasitic microorganism in the rickettsiae family, Bartonella quintana can multiply within the gut of the body louse and then can be transmitted to humans. Transmission to people can occur by rubbing infected louse feces into abraded skin or into the whites of the eyes. Abbreviated as B. quintana, it is the cause of trench fever. Trench fever was first recognized in the trenches of World War I, and also occurs among homeless people, injection drug users, street alcoholics, and others who may live in cramped, unhygienic quarters.

B. quintana also has been found responsible for a disease called bacillary angiomatosis in people infected with HIV, and for infection of the heart and great vessels (endocarditis) with bloodstream infection (bacteremia). The full spectrum of disease caused by B. quintana is still unfolding. Also known as Rochalimaea quintana. See also *trench fever*.

**basal cell carcinoma** A type of skin cancer in which the cancer cells resemble the basal cells of the epidermis.

**basal cells** Small, round cells found in the lower part, or base, of the epidermis, the outer layer of the skin.

**basal ganglia** A set of structures within the cerebellum that are involved in the control of involutary movement and other functions. The basal ganglia include the amygdala, and the caudate nucleus and lentricular nucleus (known together as the corpus striatum). They are located to each side of the thalamus glands. Differences in or damage to the basal ganglia are implicated in Tourette syndrome, obsessive-compulsive disorder, and other neurological disorders.

**basal metabolic rate** The rate of metabolism, as measured by the amount of heat given off when a person is at rest; it is expressed as calories of energy per hour per square meter of skin. The basal metabolic rate can offer clues as to underlying health problems: For example, someone with an overly active thyroid will have an elevated basal metabolic rate.

**basal temperature** 1 Usually, a person's temperature on awakening in the morning. As changes in basal temperature accompany ovulation, it is often tracked by women who wish to ensure or avoid pregnancy. 2 A measure of thyroid function achieved by taking and comparing basal temperatures. Also known as the Broda test.

**basal thermometer** Colloquially used as a synonym for basal temperature. Any thermometer can be used to take the basal temperature, although special digital thermometers capable of storing and tracking basal temperatures over a period of time are available.

**base** A unit of DNA. There are four bases in DNA: adenine (A), guanine (G), thymine (T), and cytosine (C). The sequence of bases (for example, CAG) is the genetic code.

**base pair** Two DNA bases complementary to one another (A and T, or G and C) that join in strands to form the double-helix shape that is characteristic of DNA.

**base sequence** The order of nucleotide bases in a DNA molecule.

**base sequence analysis** A method for determining the order of nucleotide bases in DNA.

**battered child syndrome** Skeletal fractures, especially multiple injuries of various ages, as a result of child abuse. The term "battered child syndrome" entered medicine in 1962. By 1976 all states in the US had adopted laws mandating the reporting of suspected instances of child abuse. See also *child abuse*.

**battle fatigue** The World War II name for what is known today as post-traumatic stress disorder (PTSD). See also *post-traumatic stress disorder*.

**BCG** See *tuberculosis vaccination*.

**bedbug** A blood-sucking bug in the Cimex family that lives hidden in bedding or furniture, coming out at night to bite its victims.

**bedsore** A painful, often reddened area of degenerating, ulcerated skin caused by pressure and lack of movement, and worsened by exposure to urine or other irritating substances on the skin. Untreated bedsores can become seriously infected or gangrenous. Bedsores are a major problem for patients who are confined to a bed or wheelchair, and can be prevented by moving the patient frequently, changing bedding, and keeping the skin clean and dry. Also known as a pressure sore, decubitus sore, or decubitus ulcer.

**bedwetting** Involuntary urination in bed after the usual age of toilet training, also called nighttime enuresis or noctural enuresis. It may be caused by incomplete development of bladder control, a sleep or arousal disorder, bladder or kidney disease, neurological problems, or occasionaly psychological causes (such as fear of the dark that prevents the child from leaving the bed). About 20 percent of five-year-olds wet the bed at least once a month; surprisingly, 1 to 2 percent of teenagers have nighttime enuresis. Treatment depends on the cause, and may include education, behavior modification techniques, the use of alarms, bladder-retention training, or medication. See also *enuresis*.

**bee stings** Stings from bees and other large stinging insects such as yellow jackets, hornets, and wasps can trigger allergic reactions, up to and including life-threatening anaphylactic shock. Avoidance and prompt treatment are essential. Inspect and eliminate sites of possible colonization (holes, junk piles, and so on). Self-injectible adrenaline can be carried by persons known to be allergic when in risk areas. Hikers should wear long pants and shirts in risk areas. If attacked, run for shelter, covering face to prevent airway stings. Treatment depends on the severity of symptoms. Stingers should be removed promptly, and the area cleansed with soap and water. Ice packs, pain medications, and anti-itching medications can be helpful for local reactions. Victims with more serious symptoms or multiple stings are often hospitalized for observation and treatment. They can require intravenous fluids, oxygen, cortisone medicine, or epinephrine, as well as medications to open the breathing passages. In very severe reactions, the venom is removed from the blood by plasmapheresis or hemodialysis. In selected cases, allergy injection therapy is highly effective for prevention. For those who are not allergic, stings are a minor nuisance unless they come in multiples. The lethal dose of honeybee venom, for example, is about 19 stings per kilogram of body weight (that is, 1,300 stings for a 150-pound person).

**bee stings, Africanized** Stings from Africanized ("killer") bees, a species of large honey bees found in South and Central America, and now in some parts of the US. This species of bees has an unusual and dangerous natural defense mechanism when disturbed. A loud noise or vibration near a hive, such as a barking dog or lawn mower, may cause the bees to display aggressive behavior. They attack in large numbers and for a longer period of time than is typical of the common European honey bee. As a result, Africanized honeybees inflict more stings, injecting a higher dosage of bee venom into their victims. See also *bee stings*.

**beef tapeworm** See *Taenia saginata*.

**behavior modification** The use of rewards and/or punishments to encourage desirable behavior.

**behavior therapy** See *behavior modification; cognitive behavior therapy*.

**behavioral disorder** Technically, a condition characterized by undesirable behavior that is within the patient's control: for example, substance abuse and antisocial behavior. The term is also used as a euphemism for psychiatric disorder.

**behaviorism** The science of studying and modifying animal or human behavior, often through behavior modification techniques.

**Behcet syndrome** A chronic inflammatory disorder involving the small blood vessels. It is classically characterized by a triad of features, namely, ulcers in the mouth, ulcers of the genitalia, and inflammation of the eye (uveitis). The ulcers of the mouth are typically recurring crops of aphthous ulcers. Arthritis is also commonplace in this disorder. The cause of Behcet syndrome is not known. The disease is more frequent and severe in patients from the Eastern Mediterranean and Asia than in those of European descent.

**belching** A normal process of releasing through the mouth air that accumulates in the stomach, thereby relieving distention. Upper abdominal discomfort associated with excessive swallowed air may extend into the lower chest, producing symptoms that suggest heart or lung disease.

**Bell palsy** Paralysis of the nerve that supplies the facial muscles on one side of the face. Bell palsy typically starts suddenly, and causes paralysis of the muscles of the same side as the affected facial nerve. The cause of Bell palsy is not known, but it is thought to be related to viral infection. Treatment is directed toward protecting the eye on the affected side from dryness during sleep. Massage of affected muscles can reduce soreness. Sometimes cortisone medication, such as prednisone, is given to reduce inflammation during the first weeks of illness. The outlook for patients with Bell palsy is generally good: about 80 percent of patients recover within weeks to months.

**belly** That part of the body that contains all the structures between the chest and the pelvis. See also *abdomen*.

**belly button** The navel or umbilicus; the onetime site of attachment of the umbilical cord.

**benign** Not cancerous; a condition that does not invade surrounding tissue or spread to other parts of the body.

**benign cortical defect** The presence of noncancerous bone lesions in children. These lesions are found most frequently in the femur and tibia, and disappear over time as the bone grows. Also known as a nonossifying fibroma.

**benign lymphoreticulosis** See *cat scratch fever*. See also *Bartonella henselae*.

**benign partial epilepsy with centro-temporal spikes** See *epilepsy, benign rolandic*. See also *seizure, partial*.

**benign prostatic hyperplasia** A noncancerous prostate problem in which the normal elements of the prostate gland grow in size and number. Their sheer bulk may compress the urethra, which courses through the center of the prostate, impeding the flow of urine from the bladder through the urethra to the outside. This leads to urine retention and the need for frequent urination. If severe enough, complete blockage can occur. Abbreviated as BPH, this disorder generally begins in a man's 30s, evolves slowly, and only causes symptoms after age 50. BPH is very common. Half of men over age 50 develop symptoms of PBH, but only 10 percent need medical or surgical intervention. Watchful waiting with medical monitoring once a year is appropriate for most men with BPH. Medical therapy includes drugs, such as finasteride and terazosin. Prostate surgery has traditionally been seen as offering the most benefits for BPH, and also the most risks. BPH is not a sign of prostate cancer. Also known as benign prostatic hypertrophy, nodular hyperplasia of the prostate.

**benign prostatic hypertrophy**   See *benign prostatic hyperplasia*.

**benign rolandic epilepsy of childhood**   See *epilepsy, benign rolandic*. See also *seizure, partial*.

**benzodiazepine tranquilizer**   A family of medications (brand names include Ativan, Clonazepam, Valium) that are useful against severe anxiety and insomnia (unlike the others, Clonazepam is an antispasmodic). The benzodiazepines tend to be sedating, and can interact with or potentiate other central nervous system depressants. With long-term use, addiction is possible.

**Bernard syndrome**   See *Horner syndrome*.

**Bernard-Horner syndrome**   See *Horner syndrome*.

**Bernard-Soulier syndrome**   A disorder in which the platelets lack the ability to stick adequately to injured blood vessel walls. As this is a crucial aspect of the process of forming a blood clot, abnormal bleeding occurs. Bernard-Soulier syndrome usually presents in the newborn period, infancy, or early childhood with bruises, nosebleeds (epistaxis), and/or gum (gingival) bleeding. Problems can occur later with anything that induces bleeding, such as menstruation, trauma, surgery, or stomach ulcers. Bernard-Soulier syndrome is an inherited disease, and is transmitted in an autosomal recessive pattern. Both parents must carry a gene for the Bernard-Soulier syndrome and transmit that gene to the child for the child to have the disease. The molecular basis is known, and is due to a deficiency in platelet glycoproteins Ib, V, and IX. The Bernard-Soulier gene has been mapped to the short (p) arm of chromosome 17. There is no specific treatment for Bernard-Soulier syndrome. Bleeding episodes may require platelet transfusions. The abnormal platelets in the Bernard-Soulier syndrome are usually considerably larger than normal platelets when viewed on blood films or sized by automated instruments. However, this is not the only syndrome with large platelets. Specific platelet function tests, as well as tests for the glycoproteins, can confirm the diagnosis. Also known as giant platelet syndrome.

**berry aneurysm**   See *aneurysm, brain*.

**beta adrenergic blocking drugs**   See *beta blockers*.

**beta blockers**   A class of drugs that block beta-adrenergic substances such as adrenaline (epinephrine), a key agent in the sympathetic portion of the autonomic (involuntary) nervous system. By blocking the action of the sympathetic nervous system on the heart, these agents relieve stress on the heart. They slow the heartbeat, lessen the force with which the heart muscle contracts, and reduce blood vessel contraction in the heart, brain, and body. Beta blockers are used to treat abnormal heart rhythms (cardiac arrhythmias), specifically to prevent abnormally fast heart rates (tachycardias) or irregular heart rhythms, such as premature ventricular beats. Since beta blockers reduce the demand of the heart muscle for oxygen, they can be useful in treating angina. They have also become an important drug in improving survival after a person has had a heart attack. Thanks to their effect on blood vessels, beta blockers can lower the blood pressure and be of value in the treatment of hypertension. Other uses include the prevention of migraine headaches and the treatment of familial or hereditary essential tremors. Beta blockers reduce the pressure within the eye (intraocular pressure), probably by reducing the production of the liquid (aqueous humor) within the eye, and so are used to lessen the risk of damage to the optic nerve and loss of vision in glaucoma. The beta blockers include acebutolol (brand name: Sectral), atenolol (Tenormin), bisoprolol (Zebeta), metoprol (Lopressor, Lopressor LA, Toprol XL), nadolol (Corgard), and timolol (Bloacadren). Beta blockers are also available in combination with a diuretic; for example, with bisoprolol and hydrochlorothiazide (Ziac). Eye-specific beta blockers include timolol ophthalmic solution (Timoptic) and betaxolol hydrochloride (Betoptic).

**beta carotene**   A protective antioxidant vitamin. See also *Appendix C, "Vitamins."*

**beta cell, pancreatic**   A cell found in the areas of the pancreas called the islets of Langerhans. The beta cells are important because they make insulin. Degeneration of the beta cells is the main cause of type I (insulin-dependent) diabetes mellitus. See also *diabetes mellitus*.

**beta error**   The statistical error (said to be "of the second kind," or type II) made in testing when it is concluded that something is negative when it really is positive. Beta error is often referred to as a false negative.

**beta-2 microglobulin**   A test that measures the amount of cell destruction present. It is considered to be one of the best ways to measure the progression of HIV-related disease, although it may also indicate cell destruction due to cytomegalovirus or other causes. Results over 5 are considered very significant.

**bezoar**   A clump or wad of swallowed food and/or hair. Bezoars can sometimes be found to cause blockage of the digestive system, especially at the exit of the stomach. When a bezoar is composed of hair, it is referred to as a hairball or trichobezoar. When a bezoar is composed of vegetable materials, it is referred to as a phytobezoar or foodball. When a bezoar is composed of hair and food, it is referred to as a trichophytobezoar or hairy foodball.

**BF** Doctor's shorthand for black female.

**bi-** Prefix meaning two, as in biceps or bicuspid.

**bias** In a clinical trial, bias refers to effects that may cause an incorrect conclusion. Common examples of bias include advanced knowledge of the treatment being given, strong desire in the researcher for a specific outcome, or improper study design. To avoid bias, a blinded study may be done. See also *blinded study, double-blinded study*.

**Biaxin** See *clarithromycin*.

**biceps** A muscle that has two heads, or origins. There is more than one biceps muscle. The biceps brachii is the well-known flexor muscle in the upper arm, and bulges when the arm is bent in a C-shape with the fist toward the forehead. The biceps femoris is in the back of the thigh.

**bicarbonate** In medicine, bicarbonate usually refers to bicarbonate of soda (sodium bicarbonate, baking soda), a white powder that is a common ingredient in antacids.

**bicornuate** Having two horns or horn-shaped branches. The uterus is normally unicornuate, but can sometimes be bicornuate.

**bicuspid** Having two flaps or cusps.

**bicuspid aortic valve** Whereas the normal aortic valve in the heart has three flaps (cusps) that open and close, a bicuspid valve has only two. There may be no symptoms of this difference in childhood, but in time the valve may become narrowed (stenotic), making it harder for blood to pass through it, or blood may start to leak backward through the valve (regurgitate). Treatment depends on how the valve is working.

**bicuspid valve** See *mitral valve*.

**Biermer anemia** See *anemia, pernicious*.

**bifid** Split in two. For example, a bifid (cleft) uvula is split into two sections.

**bifid uvula** See *cleft uvula*.

**big toe sign** See *Babinski reflex*.

**bilateral** Affecting both sides. For example, bilateral lung reduction would reduce both the left and right lobes of the lung in size.

**bile** A yellow-green fluid that is made by the liver, bile is stored in the gallbladder and passes through the common bile duct into the duodenum, where it helps digest fat. The principal components of bile are cholesterol, bile salts, and the pigment bilirubin. Cholesterol is normally kept in liquid form by the dissolving action of the bile salts; an increased amount of cholesterol in the bile overwhelms the dissolving capacity of the bile salts and leads to the formation of cholesterol gallstones. Similarly, a deficiency of bile salts promotes cholesterol gallstone formation. Pigment gallstones are frequently associated with chronic infection in the bile, especially in certain Asian countries where parasitic infection of the bile ducts is common. Patients with blood diseases that cause excessive breakdown of red blood cells can have increased amounts of bilirubin in the bile, thus causing bilirubin gallstone formation. See also *gallstones*.

**bile acid resin** Bile acid resins are substances that bind in the intestines with bile acids that contain cholesterol, and are then eliminated in the stool. The major effect of bile acid resins is to lower LDL-cholesterol by about 10 to 20 percent. Small doses of resins can produce useful reductions in LDL-cholesterol. Bile acid resins are sometimes prescribed with a statin for patients with heart disease, to increase cholesterol reduction. When these two drugs are combined, their effects are added together, lowering LDL-cholesterol by over 40 percent. Cholestyramine (brand name: Questran) and colestipol (Colestid) are the two main bile acid resins currently available. These two drugs are available as powders or tablets. Bile acid resin powders must be mixed with water or fruit juice and taken once or twice (rarely three times) daily with meals. Tablets must be taken with large amounts of fluids to avoid gastrointestinal symptoms. Resin therapy may produce a variety of symptoms, including constipation, bloating, nausea, and gas. The bile acid resins are not prescribed as the sole medicine to lower cholesterol in patients with high triglycerides or a history of severe constipation. Although resins are not absorbed, they may interfere with the absorption of other medicines if taken at the same time. Therefore, other medications should be taken at least one hour before or four to six hours after the resin.

**bile sludge** See *biliary sludge*.

**bilharzia** Disease caused by trematode worms (flukes) that parasitize people. Three main species of these worms—Schistosoma haematobium, S. japonicum, and S. mansoni—cause disease in humans. Larval forms of the parasite live in freshwater snails. When the parasite is liberated from the snail, it burrows into the skin, transforms to the schistosomulum stage, and migrates to the urinary tract (S. haematobium), or liver or intestine (S. japonicum or S. mansoni), where the adult worms develop. Eggs are shed into the urinary tract or the intestine, hatch to form another form of the parasite called miracidia that can then infect snails again, completing the parasite's life cycle. Adult schistosome worms can seriously damage tissue. Also known as schistosomiasis. See also *bilharziasis, schistosoma haematobium, schistosoma japonicum, schistosoma mansoni*.

**bilharziasis** A parasite infection by a trematode worm acquired from infested water. Species that live in man can produce liver, bladder, and gastrointestinal problems. Species of the schistosomiasis parasite that cannot live in man cause swimmer's itch. Also known as schistosomiasis. See also *bilharzia*.

**biliary** Having to do with bile, a fluid made by the liver and stored by the gallbladder. See also *bile*.

**biliary cirrhosis, primary** See *cirrhosis, primary biliary*.

**biliary sand** A term used by surgeons to describe uncountable, small particles in bile that are visible to the naked eye in a gallbladder that has been removed. Biliary sand may be looked upon as a stage of growth between sludge, which is made up of microscopic particles, and gallstones, which are large enough to be counted easily. The composition of biliary sand varies, but is similar to that of gallstones. The most common components are cholesterol crystals and calcium salts. Biliary sand may cause no symptoms or cause intermittent symptoms, including pain in the abdomen, nausea, and vomiting, particularly after a fatty meal. Biliary sand can cause complications, including inflammation of the pancreas (pancreatitis) and inflammation of the gallbladder (cholecystitis). Biliary sand often can be detected by an ultrasound of the abdomen. If patients with biliary sand develop symptoms or complications, gallbladder removal (cholecystectomy) is performed.

**biliary sludge** A mixture of microscopic particulate matter in bile that occurs when particles of material precipitate from bile. The composition of biliary sludge varies. The most common particulate components of biliary sludge are cholesterol crystals and calcium salts. Biliary sludge has been associated with certain conditions, including rapid weight loss, fasting, pregnancy; the use of certain medications (for example, ceftriaxone or octreotide); and bone marrow or solid organ transplantation. However, it most commonly occurs in individuals with no identifiable condition. Biliary sludge can be looked upon as a condition of microscopic gallstones, although it is not clear at what size the particles in biliary sludge should be considered gallstones. Biliary sludge usually causes no symptoms and may appear and disappear over time. It may, however, cause intermittent symptoms, most commonly pain in the abdomen, often associated with nausea and vomiting. This occurs when the particles obstruct the ducts leading from the gallbladder to the intestine. On occasion, the particles may grow in size to become larger gallstones. Biliary sludge also may cause more serious complications, including inflammation of the pancreas (pancreatitis) and inflammation of the gallbladder (cholecystitis). Biliary sludge can be detected with ultrasound of the abdomen, or by directly examining bile content under a microscope (bile microscopy). If patients with biliary sludge develop symptoms or complications, gallbladder removal (cholecystectomy) is performed. Because sludge usually does not cause symptoms, every effort should be made before the gallbladder is removed to ascertain that a patient's symptoms are due to sludge

**bilirubin** A yellow-orange compound produced by the breakdown of hemoglobin from red blood cells.

**binge drinking** The dangerous practice of consuming large quantities of alcoholic beverages in a single session. Binge drinking carries a serious risk of harm, including alcohol poisoning. See also *alcohol poisoning*.

**binge eating disorder** An eating disorder characterized by periods of extreme overeating, but not followed by purging behaviors as in bulimia. Binge eating can occur alone, or in conjunction with a lesion of the hypothalamus gland, Prader-Willi disorder, or other medical conditions. It can contribute to high blood pressure, weight gain, diabetes, and heart disease. Treatment depends on the patient and the underlying disorder, but may include therapy, dietary education and advice, and medication.

**binocular vision** The ability to maintain visual focus on an object with both eyes, creating a single visual image. Lack of binocular vision is normal in infants. Adults without binocular vision experience distortions in depth perception and visual measurement of distance.

**bio-** Prefix indicating living plants or creatures, as in biology, the study of living organisms.

**biofeedback** A technique for increasing personal control over physical or emotional processes, such as pain or heart rate, by using a device that returns immediate data for self-training purposes.

**bioflavinoids** Antioxidant compounds found in various plants, which may also be available in supplement form. Once known as vitamin P.

**biologic evolution** Biologic evolution occurs with all forms of life. This process is mediated by genes, shows a slow rate of change, employs random variation (mutations) and selection as agents of change. New variants are often harmful, and when these new variants are transmitted from parents to offspring, the mode of transmission is simple. Complexity is achieved by the rare formation of new genes by chromosome duplication. The biology of humans requires cultural as well as biological evolution. See also *cultural evolution*.

**biological response modifiers**  Substances that stimulate the body's response to infection and disease. The body naturally produces small amounts of these substances, which are abbreviated as BRMs. Scientists can produce some of them in the laboratory in large amounts for use in treating cancer, rheumatoid arthritis, hepatitis, and other diseases. BRMs used in biological therapy include monoclonal antibodies, interferon, interleukin-2 (IL-2), and several types of colony-stimulating factors (for example, CSF, GM-CSF, and G-CSF). Side effects of BRM therapy often include flu-like symptoms, such as chills, fever, muscle aches, weakness, loss of appetite, nausea, vomiting, and diarrhea. Some patients develop a rash, and some bleed or bruise easily. Interleukin therapy can cause swelling. Depending on the severity of these problems, patients may need to stay in the hospital during treatment. These side effects usually go away gradually after treatment stops.

**biological therapy**  Treatment to stimulate or restore the ability of the immune system to fight infection and disease. Biological therapy is thus any form of treatment that uses the body's natural abilities that cause the immune system to fight infection, or to protect the body from side effects of treatment. Biological therapy often employs substances called biological response modifiers (BRMs). For example, biological therapy to block the action of instruments of inflammation called tumor necrosis factor (TNF) is being explored to treat conditions such as Crohn disease and rheumatoid arthritis. Also called biotherapy or immunotherapy.

**biomarker**  A biochemical feature or facet that can be used to measure the presence or progress of disease, or the effects of treatment.

**biopsy**  The removal of a sample of tissue for examination under a microscope to check for cancer cells or other abnormalities. A physical exam, imaging, endoscopy, and lab tests can show that something abnormal is present, but a biopsy is the only sure way to know whether the problem is cancer. In a biopsy, the doctor may remove a sample of tissue from the abnormal area, or may remove the whole tumor for examination by a pathologist. If cancer is present, the pathologist can usually tell what kind of cancer it is, and may be able to judge whether the cells are likely to grow slowly or quickly.

**biopsy, endometrial**  A common and very valuable procedure for sampling the lining of the uterus (the endometrium). Endometrial biopsy is usually done to learn the cause of abnormal uterine bleeding, but may be used to determine the cause of infertility, test for uterine infections, and even to monitor response to certain medications. The procedure can be done in the doctor's office. There are few risks, the leading risks being cramping and pain. In some cases vaginal bleeding or infection occurs, as can, very rarely, perforation of the uterus. Oral pain medications taken beforehand may help reduce cramping and pain. See also *biopsy*.

**biopsy, needle**  The taking of small amounts of tissue for examination by using a hollow needle. See also *biopsy; biopsy, stereotactic needle*.

**biopsy, punch**  See *punch biopsy*.

**biopsy, sentinel-lymph–node**  Examination of the first lymph node that receives lymphatic drainage from a tumor to learn whether that node does or does not have tumor cells within it. The sentinel node's identity is determined by injecting around the tumor a tracer substance that will travel through the lymphatic system to the first draining node, thereby identifying it. The tracer substance may be blue dye that can be visually tracked, or a radioactive colloid that can be radiologically followed. If the sentinel node contains tumor cells, removal of more nodes in the area may be warranted. If the sentinel node is normal, this obviates the need for extensive dissection of the regional lymph-node basin. Sentinel-lymph–node biopsy has become a standard technique for determining the nodal stage of disease in some patients with malignant melanoma. See also *biopsy*.

**biopsy, stereotactic needle**  In a stereotactic needle biopsy, the spot to be biopsied is located three-dimensionally, the information is entered into a computer, and then the computer calculates the information and positions a needle to remove the biopsy sample. It can be done in a properly equipped doctor's office, and carries a minimal amount of pain and risk, compared to other types of biopsy. See also *biopsy*.

**biotechnology**  The fusion of biology and technology, biotechnology is the application of biological techniques to product research and development. In particular, biotechnology involves the use by industry of recombinant DNA, cell fusion, and new bioprocessing techniques.

**biotherapy**  See *biological therapy*.

**bipolar disorders**  A neurological disorder, formerly called manic-depressive illness, in which the patient cycles through uncontrollable mood states. Less prevalent than simple clinical depression, bipolar disorders involve cycles of depression, hypomania (elevated mood), mania (extremely elevated mood), and in some cases psychosis. Sometimes the mood switches are dramatic and rapid, but most often they are gradual. Both depression and mania affect thinking, judgment, and social behavior in ways that cause serious problems. For example, unwise business, financial, and personal decisions may be made when an individual is in a manic phase. Bipolar disorder is usually a chronic recurring condition, with serious impairment and suicide common in untreated cases. The cause is as yet unknown, although bipolar disorders appear to have a strong genetic basis, and may be influenced by seasonal patterns, hormones, or viral infection. Diagnosis of bipolar disorder is based on observation, patient and family history, and sometimes the use of standardized symptom scales. Primary treatment is with medication, particularly lithium or anticonvulsants. See *bipolar I, bipolar II, bipolar III, cyclothymia, seasonal affective disorder.* See also *depression, mania, mixed mania.*

**bipolar I**   Bipolar disorder characterized by episodes of both depression and mania.

**bipolar II**   Bipolar disorder characterized by cyclical episodes of clinical depression and perhaps by hypomania, but not by mania.

**bipolar III**   A colloquial term used by some doctors to describe patients with genetic "loading" for bipolar disorders but no sympyoms, or subclinical symptoms. These patients need to exercise care when taking medications that can cause depression or mania.

**birth**   The process of delivering a fetus from the uterus. Normally, the fetus is expelled through the cervix and birth canal with the assistance of rhythmic muscle contractions. Birth may instead be a surgical procedure: a Caesarian section. See also *Caesarian section.*

**birth control**   The practice of exercising some level of control over contraception. Birth control methods are many, and they vary in effectiveness. The most effective method is abstinence from sex, followed by oral, injectible, or implanted contraceptives; barrier methods used consistently and with spermicidal gel; and the basal temperature method, if used carefully and consistently. See also *barrier method; cervical cap; condom; condom, female; contraceptive; contraceptive, emergency; contraceptive, implanted; Depo-Provera; diaphragm; intrauterine device; natural family planning; oral contraceptive.*

**birth defect**   A physical abnormality that is present at birth (congenital). Birth defects may be caused by inherited genetic disorders, by spontaneous genetic mutations, or by exposure to toxic substances in the womb. Many of the most common birth defects, such as cleft palate, can be easily corrected with surgery. Some, such as anencephaly (absence of a brain) are always deadly. Others are not deadly but do cause deformity or disability, and may or may not respond to currently available treatments.

**birth defects, study of**   See *dysmorphology.*

**birth rate**   The number of live births divided by the average population, or by the population at midyear. In 1995, for example, the crude birth rate per 1,000 population was 14 in the United States and 16.9 in Australia. Also known as crude birth rate.

**birthmark**   A discoloration of the skin that may or may not be raised, and is present at birth. Most birthmarks are harmless. Occasionally a specific type of birthmark can be a visible marker for a more serious health problem. See also *café au lait spots, port-wine stain.*

**bite**   In dental terms, how well the teeth fit together (occlude) in the mouth.

**bite-wing X-ray**   A dental X-ray that shows how the teeth fit together on one side of the mouth.

**BKA**   Below-the-knee amputation.

**black death**   See *bubonic plague.*

**black eye**   Bruising of the eyelid and/or under-eye area as a result of trauma to the eye. Colloquially known as a shiner.

**black lung disease**   A disease of the lungs caused by inhaling coal dust, which in some patients can lead to progressive massive fibrosis of the lungs and severely impaired lung function. Also known as anthracosis, coal miner's pneumoconiosis.

**Black Plague**   See *bubonic plague.*

**bladder**   The organ that stores urine. The bladder is a hollow organ in the lower abdomen. The kidneys filter waste from the blood and produce urine, which enters the bladder through two tubes called ureters. Urine leaves the bladder through another tube, the urethra. In women, the urethra is a short tube that opens just in front of the vagina. In men, it is longer, passing through the prostate gland and then the penis.

**bladder cancer**   The most common warning sign of bladder cancer is blood in the urine. The diagnosis of bladder cancer is supported by findings in the medical history and examination, blood, urine, and X-ray tests, and confirmed with a biopsy (usually during a cystoscope exam). Smoking is a major risk factor. Cigarette smokers develop bladder cancer two to three times more often than do nonsmokers. Quitting smoking reduces the risk of bladder cancer, lung cancer, several other types of cancer, and a number of other diseases as well. Workers in some occupations are at higher risk of developing bladder cancer because of exposure to carcinogens (cancer-causing substances) in the workplace. These workers include people in the rubber, chemical, and leather industries, as well as hairstylists, machinists, metal workers, printers, painters, textile workers, and truck drivers. Treatment of bladder cancer depends on the growth, size, and location of the tumor.

**bladder infection** Some people are at greater risk for bladder and other urinary tract infections (UTIs) than others. One woman in five develops a UTI during her lifetime. Not everyone with a UTI has symptoms. Common symptoms include a frequent urge to urinate, and a painful burning when urinating. Underlying conditions that impair the normal urinary flow can lead to more complicated UTIs.

**bladder inflammation** See *cystitis*.

**bladder pain** Among the symptoms of bladder infection are feelings of pain, pressure, and tenderness around the bladder, pelvis, and perineum (the area between the anus and vagina or anus and scrotum), which may increase as the bladder fills and decrease as it empties; decreased bladder capacity; an urgent need to urinate; painful sexual intercourse; and, in men, discomfort or pain in the penis and scrotum.

**Blalock-Taussig operation** Operation named for the American surgeon Alfred Blalock and the pediatric cardiologist Helen B. Taussig, and designed to treat children born with a heart malformation (tetralogy of Fallot).

**blast crisis** See *blast phase*.

**blast phase** A phase of advanced chronic myelogenous leukemia in which the number of immature, abnormal white blood cells in the bone marrow and blood is extremely high. Also known as blast crisis. See also *leukemia*.

**blastoma** A tumor that arises in embryonic tissue.

**blasts** Immature blood cells.

**bleb** A bladderlike structure more than 5 mm in diameter with thin walls that may be full of fluid. Also known as a bulla.

**bleeding** The process of blood loss, usually caused by minor injury to the small blood vessels known as capillaries. In typical cases of bleeding, simply cleaning the site of injury and applying mild pressure or a bandage is sufficient treatment. If bleeding is caused by injury to a major blood vessel, emergency care is necessary. Bleeding through the skin without visible injury is a very serious condition and also requires emergency care. Menstrual bleeding does not involve injury; it is the normal expulsion of uterine contents and does not involve the blood vessels at all. See also *hemorrhage, menstruation*.

**bleeding, uncontrolled** See *hemorrhage*.

**blepharospasm** The involuntary, forcible closure of the eyelids. The first symptoms may be uncontrollable blinking. Only one eye may be affected initially, but eventually both eyes are usually involved. The spasms may leave the eyelids completely closed, causing functional blindness even though the eyes and vision are normal. Blepharospasm is a form of focal dystonia.

**blind** Unable to see. See also *blindness*.

**blinded study** Clinical trials of drugs in which the test subjects do not know whether they are receiving the product being tested or a control/placebo. This blinding is intended to ensure that the results of a study are not affected by the power of suggestion (the placebo effect). See also *double-blinded study*.

**blindness** Loss of useful sight. Blindness can be temporary or permanent. There are many causes of blindness. Damage to any portion of the eye, the optic nerve, or the area of the brain responsible for vision can lead to blindness.

**blindness, night** See *nyctanopia*.

**blister** A collection of fluid underneath the top layer of skin (epidermis). There are many causes of blisters, including burns, friction forces, and diseases of the skin.

**Bloch-Sulzberger syndrome** See *incontinentia pigmenti*.

**blocker, beta adrenergic** See *beta blockers*.

**blockers, beta** See *beta blockers*.

**blood** The fluid in the body that contains red and white cells as well as platelets, proteins, plasma and other elements. It is transported throughout the body by the circulatory system.

**blood cell** One of several different types of cells that make up the blood. The erythrocytes (red blood cells) contain hemoglobin, which carries oxygen in the blood. The leukocytes (white blood cells) are a blood-borne part of the immune system. The platelets help blood to clot. Together, these three types of cells make up about half of blood volume. The remainder is made up of plasma, a yellowish liquid. Also known as a blood corpuscle. See also *erythrocyte, leukocytes, plasma, platelets*.

**blood clot** A mass of coagulated blood. A blood clot can block a major blood vessel, causing stroke or other major trouble.

**blood clots, estrogen-associated** Blood clots are occasional but serious side effects of estrogen therapy.

They are dose-related; that is, they occur more frequently with higher doses of estrogen. Cigarette smokers on estrogen therapy are at a higher risk for blood clots than non-smokers are. Therefore, patients requiring estrogen therapy are strongly encouraged to quit smoking. See also *estrogen, estrogen replacement therapy*.

**blood coagulation**   The aggregation of blood platelets and other components to form a semisolid clot. Coagulation takes place due to the influence of clotting factors fibrinogen, prothrombin, and thrombin, which are normally activated in response to injury. Working together, these substances not only thicken the blood, but also produce fibrin, a substance that closes off the wound. When blood coagulates abnormally, dangerous blood clots can enter the bloodstream.

**blood conservation**   Actions taken during medical treatment and surgery to limit the amount of donor blood needed.

**blood count**   A test that measures how many of a certain type of cell are found in the blood. See also *blood count, complete; hematocrit*.

**blood count, complete**   A standard blood test that measures the number of both red and white blood cells in a cubic millimeter of blood. Abbreviated as CBC.

**blood culture**   A procedure in which a blood sample obtained using sterile technique is then placed into a culture medium that will support the growth of bacteria. If bacteria grow, they can be identified as to type and tested against different antibiotics for proper treatment of infection.

**blood group**   An inherited feature on the surface of the red blood cells. A series of related blood types constitute a blood group system, such as the Rh or ABO system.

**blood group, ABO**   See *ABO blood group*.

**blood in the urine**   Blood in the urine is termed hematuria. Gross hematuria refers to blood that is so plentiful in the urine that the blood is visible grossly, with just the naked eye. Gross hematuria is in contrast to microhematuria, in which the blood is visible only under a microscope: there is so little blood that it cannot be seen without magnification. Hematuria, whether gross or microscopic, is abnormal and should be further investigated. It may or may not be accompanied by pain. Painful hematuria can be caused by a number of disorders, including infections and stones in the urinary tract. Painless hematuria can also be due to a large number of causes, including cancer.

**Blood Institute, National Heart, Lung, and**   See *National Institutes of Health*.

**blood poisoning**   See *sepsis*.

**blood pressure**   The pressure of the blood within the arteries. It is produced primarily by the contraction of the heart muscle. Its measurement is recorded by two numbers. The first (systolic pressure) is measured after the heart contracts, and is the higher. The second (diastolic pressure) is measured before the heart contracts, and is the lower. A blood pressure cuff is used to measure the pressure. See also *hypertension, hypotension*.

**blood pressure, high**   See *hypertension*.

**blood pressure, low**   See *hypotension*.

**blood sugar, high**   See *hyperglycemia*. See also *diabetes mellitus*.

**blood sugar, low**   See *hypoglycemia*.

**blood test**   A test that requires withdrawing a sample of blood for examination. Some tests require only a finger-stick, others require venipuncture.

**blood titre**   A blood test that looks for the level or amount (titre) of something in the blood. For example, a strep titre looks for the level of streptococcus antibodies in the blood.

**blood transfusion**   The transfer of blood or blood products from one person (the donor) into the bloodstream of another person (the recipient). In most situations, this is done as a lifesaving maneuver to replace blood cells or blood products lost through severe bleeding. Transfusion of your own blood (autologous) is the safest method but requires planning ahead, and not all patients are eligible. Directed donor blood allows the patient to receive blood from known donors. Volunteer donor blood is usually most readily available and, when properly tested, has a low incidence of adverse events.

**blood urea nitrogen**   Abbreviated as BUN, this is a measure primarily of the urea level in blood. Urea is cleared by the kidney. Diseases that compromise the function of the kidney frequently lead to increased blood urea nitrogen levels.

**blood, urinary**   See *hematuria*.

**blood-brain barrier**   A protective network of blood vessels and cells that filters blood flowing to the brain. The blood-brain barrier normally prevents infectious agents and foreign substances from getting into the brain. Drugs designed to work within the central nervous system have to cross the blood-brain barrier, or influence the behavior of a natural substance that can, such as a neurotransmitter.

**blood-thinner** An anticoagulant agent: a medication that works against coagulating factors in the blood.

**bloody nose** See *nosebleed; nosebleed, treatment of.*

**bloody show** Literally, the appearance of blood, a classic sign of impending labor. The bloody show consists of blood-tinged mucus created by extrusion and passage of the mucous plug that filled the cervical canal during pregnancy.

**blot, Northern** A technique in molecular biology, used mainly to separate and identify pieces of RNA. Called a Northern blot only because it is similar to a Southern blot.

**blot, Southern** A common test for checking for a match between DNA molecules. DNA fragments are separated by agarose gel electrophoresis, transferred (blotted) onto membrane filters, and hybridized with complementary radio-labeled probes. The aim is to detect specific base sequences with the probes. The Southern blot is named after its inventor, British biologist M.E. Southern.

**blot, Western** A technique in molecular biology, used to separate and identify proteins. Called a Western blot merely because it has some similarity to a Southern blot.

**Blount disease** See *tibia vara.*

**blue baby** See *cyanosis.*

**blush** Redness of the skin, typically over the cheeks or neck. A blush is temporary, and is brought on by excitement, exercise, fever, or embarrassment. Blushing is an involuntary response of the nervous system that leads to widening of the capillaries in the involved skin. Also referred to as a flush.

**BM** Doctor's shorthand for black male.

**BMI** Body mass index.

**BMJ** The British Medical Journal.

**BMRs** Biological response modifiers.

**BMT** Bone marrow transplantation.

**Board certified** In medicine, "Board certified" means a physician has taken and passed a medical specialty examination by one of several recognized boards of specialists. Before obtaining Board certification, the physician must become Board eligible.

**Board eligible** In medicine, "Board eligible" means that a physician has completed the requirements for admission to a medical specialty board examination, but has not taken and passed that examination. For example,

a physician must have three years of training in an approved pediatric residency to be eligible for certification by the American Board of Pediatrics.

**body dysmorphic disorder** A psychiatric disorder characterized by excessive preoccupation with imagined defects in physical appearance. It is classified as an anxiety disorder, and is believed to be a variant of obsessive-compulsive disorder. Also called somatoform disorder, dysmorphophobia.

**body mass index** A key index for relating weight to height. The body mass index is a person's weight in kilograms (kg) divided by his or her height in meters (m) squared. The National Institutes of Health now defines normal weight, overweight, and obesity according to BMI rather than the traditional height/weight charts. Since the BMI describes the body weight relative to height, it correlates strongly with total body fat content in adults. Overweight is defined by NIH as a BMI of 27.3 percent or more for women and 27.8 percent or more for men. Obesity is defined as a BMI of 30 or above (about 30 pounds overweight). Some very muscular people may have a high BMI without health risks.

**body type** A somewhat old-fashioned term used to classify the human shape into three primary types: ectomorphic, mesomorphic, or endomorphic.

**bodywork** Any of a number of therapeutic or simply relaxing practices that involve the manipulation, massage, or regimented movement of body parts. Examples include massage, craniosacral therapy, and Pilates. Bodywork may be used as an adjunct to medical treatment, or it may be prescribed as a form of physical therapy for certain conditions.

**boil** A skin abcess: a collection of pus that forms inside the body. The main treatments include hot packs and draining (lancing) the boil, once it is soft. Antibiotics are usually not very helpful. If you have a fever or long-term illness, such as cancer or diabetes, or are taking medications that suppress the immune system, contact your health care practitioner if you develop a boil.

**bone** The hard connective tissue that forms the skeleton of the body. It is composed chiefly of collagen fibers containing calcium phosphate and calcium carbonate. Bones also serve as a storage area for calcium, playing a large role in calcium balance in the blood. The 206 bones in the human body serve a wide variety of purposes. They support and protect internal organs: for example, the ribs protect the lungs. Muscles pull against bones to make the body move. Bone marrow, the spongy tissue in the center of many bones, makes and stores blood cells.

**bone cancer** Cancers that begin in bone. Bone cancer is rare, but it is not unusual for cancers to spread to bone from other parts of the body. These cancers are named for the organ or tissue in which they began. Pain is the most frequent symptom of cancer of the bone. Diagnosis is supported by a medical history and examination, blood tests, and X-rays. It is confirmed with a biopsy. Treatment of bone cancer depends on the type, location, size, and extent of the tumor, as well as the age and health of the patient.

**bone cyst, aneurysmal**   See *aneurysmal bone cyst.*

**bone cyst, simple**   A lesion on a bone, most commonly on the humerus. This type of bone cyst can cause pain in or near the area where it occurs. Also known as a unicameral bone cyst or solitary bone cyst.

**bone density**   The amount of bone tissue in a certain volume of bone. It can be measured by using a special X-ray called a quantitative computed tomogram.

**bone marrow**   The soft substance that fills bone cavities and makes blood cells. It is composed of mature blood cells, immature blood cells, and fat. The blood cells include white blood cells, red blood cells, and platelets. Diseases or drugs that affect the bone marrow can affect the total counts of these cells.

**bone marrow aspiration**   The removal through a needle of a small sample of bone marrow (usually from the hip) for microscopic examination, to see whether cancer cells are present.

**bone marrow biopsy**   The examination of an aspirated sample of bone marrow under a microscope to see whether cancer cells are present.

**bone marrow transplantation**   A procedure in which doctors replace diseased or damaged bone marrow with healthy bone marrow. The bone marrow to be replaced may be deliberately destroyed by high doses of chemotherapy and/or radiation therapy. Replacement marrow may come from another person, or the patient's own marrow may be removed and stored before treatment for later use. When marrow from an unrelated donor is used, the procedure is called an allogeneic bone marrow transplantation. If the marrow is from an identical twin, it is termed syngeneic. Autologous bone marrow transplantation uses the patient's own marrow. Abbreviated as BMT.

**bone scan**   A technique for creating images of bones on a computer screen or on film. A small amount of radioactive material is injected, and travels through the bloodstream. It collects in the bones, especially in abnormal areas of the bones, and is detected by a special instrument called a scanner. Bone scans are used by doctors for the detection and monitoring of disorders affecting the bones, including Paget disease, cancer, infections, and fractures.

**bone, cuboid**   The outer bone in the instep of the foot. It is called the cuboid bone because it is shaped like a cube. The cuboid bone is jointed in back with the heel bone (calcaneus) and in front with bones just behind the fourth and fifth toes (metatarsals).

**bone, heel**   A more or less rectangular bone at the back of the foot. Also called the calcaneus.

**bone, sesamoid**   A little bone that is embedded in a joint capsule or tendon: for example, the kneecap (patella).

**bone, shin**   The larger of the two bones in the lower leg, the shinbone is anatomically known as the tibia. Its smaller companion is the fibula.

**bones of the arm, wrist, and hand**   There are 64 bones in the upper extremities. They consist of 10 shoulder and arm, 16 wrist, and 38 hand bones. The 10 shoulder and arm bones are the clavicle, scapula, humerus, radius, and ulna on each side. The 16 wrist bones are the scaphoid, lunate, triquetrum, pisiform, trapezium, trapezoid, capitate, and hamate on each side. The 38 hand bones are the 10 metacarpal bones and 28 finger bones (phalanges). Also known as the appendicular bones.

**bones of the head**   There are 29 bones in the human head. They include 8 cranial bones, 14 facial bones, the hyoid bone, and 6 ear (auditory) bones. The 8 cranial bones are the frontal, 2 parietal, occipital, 2 temporal, sphenoid, and ethmoid bones. The 14 facial bones are the 2 maxilla, the mandible, 2 zygoma, 2 lacrimal, 2 nasal, 2 turbinate, vomer, and 2 palate bones. The hyoid bone is the horseshoe-shaped bone at the base of the tongue. The 6 small auditory bones (ossicles) are the malleus, incus, and stapes in each ear. Along with the bones of the trunk, also known as the axial bones.

**bones of the leg, ankle, and foot**   There are 62 lower extremity bones. They consist of 10 hip and leg, 14 ankle, and 38 foot bones. The 10 hip and leg bones are the innominate or hip bone (fusion of the ilium, ischium, and pubis), femur, tibia, fibula, and patella (kneecap) on each side. The 14 ankle bones are the talus, calcaneus (heel bone), navicular, cuboid, internal cuneiform, middle cuneiform, and external cuneiform on each side. The 38 foot bones are the 10 metatarsals and 28 toe bones (phalanges).

**bones of the skeleton**   The human body has 206 bones. These consist of 80 axial (head and trunk) bones and 126 appendicular (upper and lower extremity) bones. See *bones of the arm, wrist, and hand; bones of* *the head; bones of the leg, ankle, and foot; bones of the trunk.*

**bones of the trunk**  The 51 trunk bones consist of 26 vertebrae, 24 ribs, and the sternum. The 26 vertebrae comprise 7 cervical, 12 thoracic, and 5 lumbar vertebrae, plus the sacrum and the coccyx. The 24 ribs comprise 14 true ribs, 6 false ribs, and 4 floating ribs. The sternum is the breastbone. Along with the bones of the head, also known as the axial bones.

**bones, appendicular**  See *bones of the arm, wrist, and hand.*

**bones, axial**  See *bones of the head, bones of the trunk.*

**bones, lower extremity**  See *bones of the leg, ankle, and foot.*

**bony syndactyly**  A condition in which the bones of the fingers or toes are joined together. Bony syndactyly is not the same as cutaneous syndactyly, which only involves webbing of the skin between the digits.

**bony tarsus**  A structure made up of seven bones situated between the bones of the lower leg and the metatarsus bones. The seven bones of the bony tarsus are the calcaneus, talus (astragalus), cuboid, and navicular (scaphoid), plus the first, second, and third cuneiform bones. The bony tarsus contributes to the broad, flat framework of the foot.

**borborygmus**  A gurgling, rumbling, or squeaking noise from the abdomen that is caused by the movement of gas through the bowels. When your stomach is rumbling, that's a borborygmus. The plural is borborygmi.

**borderline personality disorder**  A personality type characterized by difficulty forming and keeping stable relationships; highly emotional or aggressive behavior; impulsivity; and rapid shifts in values, self-image, mood, and behavior.

**Bornholm disease**  A temporary illness resulting from viral infection. Symptoms include fever, intense abdominal and chest pain, and headache. The chest pain is caused by inflammation of the tissue lining the lungs, and is typically worsened by breathing or coughing. The illness usually lasts from 3 to 14 days. The virus most commonly implicated in Bornholm disease is an enterovirus called Coxsackie B. Also known as epidemic myalgia, pleurodynia.

**botulism**  Food poisoning caused by the bacteria Clostridium botulinium, which produces a potentially fatal toxin when it infests foodstuffs. Mild symptoms include nausea, but symptoms can progress to heart and lung failure. Botulism occurs in unrefrigerated foods and foods without preservatives, especially uncooked or undercooked meats. It can be prevented by careful use of refrigeration and preservative techniques, and the toxin can be destroyed with heat. See also *food poisoning.*

**boutonneuse**  See *typhus, African tick.* See also *rickettsial diseases.*

**bowel**  The small and large intestine.

**bowel disease, inflammatory**  A group of chronic illnesses that cause inflammation of the bowel. The portion of the intestine affected becomes irritated and swollen. Ulcers may form. Inflammatory bowel disease can be limited to the intestine, or it can be associated with disease involving the skin, joints, spine, liver, eyes, and other organs. The cause is not always known, although it can be caused or made worse by infection. Symptoms include abdominal pain and persistent diarrhea. These are far from being specific signposts, so a physician usually has to exclude other illnesses, including bowel infections, before making a firm diagnosis of inflammatory bowel disease. Although people of any age can be affected, the diagnosis is most commonly made in young adults. The course of inflammatory bowel disease is unpredictable. Symptoms tend to wax and wane, and long remissions and even spontaneous resolution of symptoms are well known. Treatment involves dietary changes, the use of medicines, and sometimes surgery, depending on the type and course of the disease under care. Effective therapy exists for the majority of cases. Research in this area is bringing new and promising treatments to patients. The most common types of inflammatory bowel disease are ulcerative colitis and Crohn disease. See also *celiac sprue; colitis; colitis, amebic; colitis, pseudomembranous; colitis, ulcerative; Crohn disease; diverticulosis; irritable bowel syndrome.*

**bowel disorders and fiber**  High-fiber diets help delay the progression of and number of bouts with diverticulosis. In many cases, this type of diet helps reduce the symptoms of irritable bowel syndrome (IBS). It is generally accepted that a diet high in fiber is protective, or at least reduces the incidence of colon polyps and colon cancer.

**Bowen disease**  See *cancer, skin; carcinoma in situ, squamous cell.*

**bowlegs**  A condition in which the legs curve out to leave a gap between the knees after the period of infancy has passed. It can be corrected with surgery or casting. Also known as genu varum, tibia vara.

**bp**  **1** In genetics, base pair. **2** In general medicine, blood pressure.

**BP**   **1** Blood pressure. On a medical chart, you might see "BP90/60 T98.6 Ht60/reg R15," which signifies that the blood pressure (BP) is 90/60 mm Hg, the temperature (T) is 98.6 degrees Fahrenheit, the heart rate (Ht) is 60 beats per minute and regular, and respirations are occuring at 15 per minute.   **2** Bipolar.

**BPH**   Benign prostatic hyperplasia, benign prostatic hypertrophy. See also *benign prostatic hyperplasia*.

**brace, foot drop**   See *ankle-foot orthosis*.

**brachial artery**   The artery that runs from the shoulder down to the elbow. See also *artery*.

**brachial plexus**   A bundle of nerves beginning in the back of the base of the neck, and extending through the axilla. It is formed by the union of portions of the fifth through eighth cervical spinal nerves and first thoracic spinal nerve. Damage to the brachial plexus can affect nerves supplying the arm and chest.

**brachial vein**   A vein that accompanies the brachial artery between the shoulder and the elbow. The route of the brachial artery is from the shoulder down to the elbow, whereas that of the brachial vein is in the reverse direction.

**brachy-**   Prefix indicating shortness.

**brady-**   Prefix indicating slowness, as in bradycardia.

**bradycardia**   A slow heart rate, usually defined as less than 60 beats per minute.

**bradykinesia**   Slowed ability to start and continue movements, and impaired ability to adjust the body's position. Can be a symptom of neurological disorders, particularly Parkinson disease, or a side effect of medications.

**bradyphrenia**   Slowed thought processes. Can be a side effect of certain psychiatric medications.

**brain**   The portion of the central nervous system that is located within the skull. It functions as a primary receiver, organizer, and distributor of information for the body. It has a right and left half, each of which is called a hemisphere.

**brain aneurysm**   See *aneurysm, brain*.

**brain death**   The permanent, irreversable cessation of all brain functions. Brain death is not the same thing as a coma or vegetative state. The presence of brain death is legally synonymous with death in most states.

**brain malleability**   See *brain plasticity*.

**brain plasticity**   The phenomenon of change and learning in the adult brain. Also known as brain malleability.

**brain stem**   The stemlike part of the brain that is connected to the spinal cord.

**brain stem glioma**   A type of brain tumor involving the glial cells.

**brain tumors**   Primary brain tumors initially form in brain tissue. Secondary brain tumors are cancers that have spread (metastasized) to the brain tissue from tissue elsewhere in the body. Brain tumors can be malignant or benign, and can occur at any age.

**brain ventricle**   One of a system of four communicating cavities within the brain that are continuous with the central canal of the spinal cord. There are four ventricles: two lateral ventricles, the third ventricle, and the fourth ventricle. The lateral ventricles are in the cerebral hemispheres. Each lateral ventricle consists of a triangular central body and four horns. The lateral ventricles communicate with the third ventricle through what is called the interventricular foramen (opening). The third ventricle is a median (midline) cavity in the brain, bounded by the thalamus and hypothalamus on either side. In front, the third ventricle communicates with the lateral ventricles, and in back it communicates with the aqueduct of the midbrain (the aqueduct of Sylvius). The fourth ventricle is the lowest of the four venticles of the brain. It extends from the aqueduct of the midbrain to the central canal of the upper end of the spinal cord, with which it communicates by the two foramina (openings) of Luschka and the foramen of Magendie. The ventricles are filled with cerebrospinal fluid, which is formed by structures, called choroid plexuses, located in the walls and roofs of the ventricles.

**brain, fornix of the**   One of a pair of arching fibrous bands in the brain that connects the two lobes of the cerebrum.

**brain, water on the**   See *hydrocephalus*.

**branchial cleft cyst**   A cavity that is a remnant from embryologic development present at birth in one side of the neck, just in front of the large angulated muscle on either side (the sternocleidomastoid muscle). The cyst may not be recognized until adolescence, as it enlarges its oval shape. Sometimes it develops a sinus or drainage pathway to the surface of the skin, from which mucus can be expressed. Total surgical excision is the treatment of choice. Recurrence is not expected. Also known as a branchial cyst.

**branchial cyst**   See *branchial cleft cyst*.

**BRCA1** A gene that normally acts to restrain the growth of cells. (The symbol BRCA comes from BReast CAncer).

**BRCA1 breast cancer susceptibility gene** This mutated (changed) version of the BRCA1 gene makes a person susceptible to developing breast cancer.

**BRCA2** Breast cancer 2, a gene that conveys susceptibility to an inherited form of breast cancer. It is located on chromosome 13. See also *breast cancer susceptibility genes.*

**BRCA2 breast cancer susceptibility gene** A mutated form of the BRCA2 gene. More than one such mutation has been identified. One BRCA2 mutation, known as the 6174delT base-pair deletion mutation, has so far been found only in women of Ashkenazi Jewish descent.

**breakbone fever** See *dengue fever.*

**breast** The front of the chest or, more specifically, the mammary gland. The mammary gland is a milk-producing gland that is composed largely of fat. Within the mammary gland are sac-like structures called lobules, which produce the milk, as well as a complex network of branching ducts. These ducts exit from the lobules at the nipple. The lobules and ducts are supported in the breast by surrounding fatty tissue and ligaments. The breast contains blood vessels and lymphatics, but no muscles. The lymphatics are thin channels similar to blood vessels; they do not carry blood, but collect and carry tissue fluid, which ultimately reenters the bloodstream. Breast tissue fluid drains through the lymphatics into the lymph nodes located in the underarm (axilla) and behind the breastbone (sternum). The appearance of the normal female breast differs greatly between individuals and at different times during a woman's life: before, during, and after adolescence; during pregnancy; during the menstrual cycle; and after menopause. The nipple of the breast becomes erect because of cold, breastfeeding, and sexual activity. The pigmented area around the nipple is called the areola. See also *gland, mammary.*

**breast absence** See *amastia.*

**breast aplasia** See *amastia.*

**breast augmentation** Enlargement of the breasts. Augmentation of the breast typically consists of insertion of a silicone bag (prosthesis) under the breast (submammary), or under the breast and chest muscle (subpectoral), after which the bag is filled with saline solution. This prosthesis expands the breast area to give the appearance of a fuller breast (increased cup size).

**breast cancer** There are many types of breast cancer, and the various types differ in their capability for spreading to other body tissues (metastasis). Breast cancer can occur in both men and women, although it is more common in women. Some forms of breast cancer appear to be linked to genetic differences, some are linked to exposure to cancer-causing substances, and others occur for unknown reasons. Risk factors for breast cancer may include genetic predisposition, as indicated by a history of breast cancer in close relatives; overexposure of the chest to radiation; smoking; childlessness; induced abortion; obesity and diet; and exposure to carcinogenic substances. Breast cancer is diagnosed with self- and physician-examination of the breasts, mammography, ultrasound testing, and biopsy. Treatment depends on the type and location of the breast cancer, as well as the age and health of the patient. Options may include lumpectomy (removal of the small, cancerous area only), chemotherapy, radiation, and partial or total mastectomy. The American Cancer Society recommends that all women should perform regular breast self-exams, and that women should have a baseline mammogram done between the ages of 35 and 40 years. Between 40 and 50 years of age, mammograms are recommended every other year. After age 50, yearly mammograms are recommended. Breast cancer prevention includes diet changes, avoiding carcinogens when possible, and screening. When caught early, most breast cancers are treatable and survival rates are high. See also *breast cancer susceptibility genes; breast cancer, familial; breast, infiltrating ductal carconoma of; breast, infiltrating lobular carcinoma of; mastectomy.*

**breast cancer susceptibility genes** Inherited factors that predispose an individual to breast cancer. Two of these genes, BRCA1 and BRCA2, have been identified. Several other genes (those for the Li-Fraumeni syndrome, Cowden disease, Muir-Torre syndrome, and ataxia-telangiectasia) are also known to predispose women to breast cancer. However, since all of these known breast cancer susceptibility genes together do not account for more than a minor fraction of breast cancer that clusters in families, it is clear that more breast cancer genes remain to be discovered. See *BRCA1 breast cancer susceptibility gene, BRCA2 breast cancer susceptibility gene.*

**breast cancer, familial** A number of factors have been identified that increase the risk of breast cancer. One of the strongest is a history of breast cancer in a relative. About 15 to 20 percent of women with breast cancer have such a family history of the disease, clearly reflecting the participation of inherited (genetic) components in the development of some breast cancers. Dominant breast cancer suceptibility genes, including BRCA1 and BRCA2, appear to be responsible for about 5 percent of all breast cancer. See *breast cancer susceptibility genes, BRCA1, BRCA1 breast cancer susceptibility gene, BRCA2, BRCA2 breast cancer susceptibility gene.*

**breast cancer, male** Breast cancer is much less common in men than in women. Fewer than 1 percent of persons with breast cancer are male. (In the US, about 175,000 women are diagnosed with breast cancer each year, as compared to 1,300 men.) However, breast cancer is no less dangerous in males than females. Once the diagnosis of breast cancer is made, the mortality rates are virtually the same for men and women.

**breast, infiltrating ductal carcinoma of** One of several recognized specific patterns of cancer of the breast, so named because it begins in the cells forming the ducts of the breast. It is the most common form of breast cancer, comprising 65 to 85 percent of all cases. On a mammogram, invasive ductal carcinoma is usually visualized as a mass with fine spikes radiating from the edges (spiculation). It may also appear as a smooth-edged lump in the breast. On physical examination, this lump usually feels much harder or firmer than benign lumps in the breast, which are usually cysts. On microscopic examination, the cancerous cells that are invading and replacing normal breast tissue can be seen.

**breast, infiltrating lobular carcinoma of the** Infiltrating lobular carcinoma is the second most common type of invasive breast cancer, accounting for 5 to 10 percent of breast cancer. Infiltrating lobular carcinoma starts in the lobules, the glands that secrete milk, and then infiltrates surrounding tissue. On a mammogram, a lobular carcinoma can look similar to a ductal carcinoma. However, on physical examination of the breast, a lobular carcinoma is usually not a hard mass like a ductal carcinoma, but rather a vague thickening of the breast tissue. Lobular carcinoma can occur in more than one site in the breast (a multicentric tumor) or in both breasts at the same time (a bilateral lobular carcinoma).

**breastbone** See *sternum*.

**breastfeeding** The highly recommended practice of feeding infants with the mother's natural milk. Breast milk contains vitamins, minerals, and enzymes that aid the baby's digestion, and immunity factors in breast milk can help infants fight off infections. Breast milk can be expressed, manually or with the assistance of a breast pump, for use while the mother is away, or breastfeeding and formula-feeding can be used together. The activity of breastfeeding has strong benefits for mothers as well as infants: It encourages the release of hormones that improve uterine muscle tone, and may help to prevent breast cancer. The ability of the breast to produce milk diminishes soon after childbirth without the stimulation of breastfeeding. Also known as nursing. See also *lactation*.

**breathing** The process of respiration, during which air is inhaled into the lungs through the mouth or nose due to muscle contraction, and then exhaled due to muscle relaxation.

**BREC** Benign rolandic epilepsy of childhood. See *epilepsy, benign rolandic*.

**breech** The buttocks.

**breech birth** Literally, birth of a baby with the buttocks, rather than the head, emerging first. Breech birth is more likely to cause injury to the mother or the infant. In many cases a baby in the breech position can be "turned" before delivery by using repeated, gentle massage.

**breech delivery** See *breech birth*.

**breech presentation** See *breech birth*.

**bridge** A set of one or more false teeth supported by a metal framework, used to replace one or more missing teeth.

**Brill-Zinsser disease** Infection with epidemic typhus that occurs years after an earlier attack of the disease. Rickettsia prowazekii, the agent that causes epidemic typhus, remains viable for many years. When the host's defenses are down, it can be reactivated. See also *rickettsial diseases; typhus, epidemic*.

**Brissaud infantilism** See *hypothyroidism, infantile*.

**brittle bone disease** A group of genetic diseases that affect collagen, a key component of connective tissue in tissues such as bone, tendon and skin. See *osteogenesis imperfecta, osteogenesis imperfecta type I, osteogenesis imperfecta type II*.

**Broca area** An area of the cerebral motor cortex in the frontal lobe of the brain that is responsible for speech development. Damage to Broca area can cause speech disorders, including aphasia, apraxia, and dyspraxia. See also *aphasia, apraxia of speech, dyspraxia of speech*.

**Broda test** See *basal temperature*.

**bronchi** The large air tubes that begin at the end of the trachea and then branch into the lungs. They have supporting walls made up in part of cartilage.

**bronchioles** The tiny branches of air tubes within the lungs that are the continuation of the bronchi. The bronchioles connect to the alveoli (air sacs).

**bronchiolitis** A childhood disease characterized by inflammation of the bronchioles, usually due to viral infections.

**bronchitis** Inflammation and swelling of the bronchi. Bronchitis can be acute or chronic.

**bronchitis, chronic** A daily cough with production of mucus (sputum) for three months, lasting for two years in a row. In chronic bronchitis, there is inflammation and swelling of the lining of the airways, leading to narrowing and obstruction of the airways. The inflammation stimulates production of mucus, which can cause further obstruction of the airways. Obstruction of the airways, especially with mucus, increases the likelihood of bacterial lung infections.

**bronchopulmonary dysplasia** Chronic lung disease in infants who received mechanical respiratory support with high oxygenation in the neonatal period.

**bronchopulmonary segments** A subdivision of one lobe of a lung, based on the connection to the segmental bronchus. For example, the right upper lobe has apical, anterior, and posterior segments.

**bronchoscope** A thin, flexible instrument used to view the air passages of the lung.

**bronchoscopy** A test that permits the doctor to see the breathing passages through a lighted tube.

**bronchospasm** A temporary narrowing of the airways in the lung. Bronchospasm causes the breathing difficulties seen in asthma. See also *asthma*.

**bronchospasm, exercise-induced** See *asthma, exercise-induced*.

**Brown syndrome** An eye abnormality that is present at birth, characterized by an inability to elevate the eyeball when trying to move the eyeball to the outside. Brown syndrome can also be caused by other conditions that affect the normal function of the eye muscles.

**Brucellosis** An infectious disease characterized by rising and lowering (undulant) fever, sweating, muscle and joint pains, and weakness. Brucellosis is caused by a bacterium called Brucella, which can be transmitted in unpasteurized milk from cattle, sheep, and goats; cheese made from this unpasteurized milk; or contact with diseased animals. Antibiotics are used to treat Brucellosis. Also known as undulant fever.

**bruise** A traumatic injury of the soft tissues, resulting in breakage of the local capillaries and leakage of red blood cells. In the skin it can be seen as a reddish-purple discoloration that does not blanch when pressed. When a bruise fades, it becomes green and brown as the body metabolizes the blood cells in the skin. It is best treated with local application of a cold pack immediately after injury. Also known as a contusion.

**Brushfield spots** Little white spots that are slightly elevated on the surface of the iris, and arranged in a ring concentric with the pupil. These spots occur in normal children, but are far more frequent in Down syndrome (trisomy 21). They are due to aggregation of a normal iris element (connective tissue). Also called speckled iris.

**bubo** An enlarged lymph node that is tender and painful, particularly in the groin and armpit (the axillae). These swollen glands are seen in a number of infectious diseases, including gonorrhea, syphilis, tuberculosis, and the eponymous bubonic plague. The plural is buboes.

**bubonic plague** An infectuous disease caused by the bacterium Yersinia pestis, which is transmitted to humans from infected rats by the oriental rat flea. It is named for the characteristic feature of buboes (painfully enlarged lymph nodes) in the groin, armpits (axillae), neck, and elsewhere. Other symptoms of the bubonic plague include headache, fever, chills, and weakness. Bubonic plague can lead to gangrene (tissue death) of the fingers, toes, and nose, the so-called "black death."

**buccal mucosa** The inner lining of the cheeks and lips.

**bulimia nervosa** An eating disorder characterized by periods of extreme overeating, often interrupted by periods of anorexia. Bulimia is usually accompanied by self-induced vomiting or other forms of purging, including the use of laxatives, exercise, or fasting. It can be life-threatening due to dehydration, and can cause permanant damage to the bowels, liver, kidney, teeth, and heart. It also raises a person's risk of seizures. Believed to be closely related to obsessive-compulsive disorder. Treatment may include cognitive behavior therapy, dietary and health education, and antidepressant medication. See also *anorexia nervosa, body dysmorphic disorder, obsessive-compulsive disorder*.

**bulla** See *bleb*.

**bullous** Characterized by blistering, such as a second-degree burn.

**bullous pemphiguoid** A disease characterized by tense, blistering eruptions of the skin. It is caused by antibodies abnormally accumulating in a layer of the skin called the basement membrane. Can be chronic and mild without affecting the general health. It is diagnosed by skin biopsy showing the abnormal antibodies deposited in the skin layer. Treatment is with topical cortisone creams, but sometimes requires high doses of cortisone (steroids) taken internally.

**bumps** A raised area resulting from blood leaking from injured blood vessels into the tissues, as well as from the body's response to the injury. A purplish, flat bruise that occurs when blood leaks out into the top layers of skin is referred to as an ecchymosis.

**BUN** Blood urea nitrogen.

**bunion** A localized, painful swelling at the base of the big toe. The joint becomes enlarged due to new bone formation, and the toe is often misaligned. It is frequently associated with inflammation. It can be related to inflammation of the nearby bursa (bursitis), or degenerative joint disease (osteoarthritis). Bunions most commonly affect women, particularly those who wear tight-fitting shoes and high heels. Treatment includes rest, a change in shoes, foot supports, medications, or surgery.

**Burkitt lymphoma** A type of non-Hodgkin lymphoma that most often occurs in young people between the ages of 12 and 30. The disease usually causes a rapidly growing tumor in the abdomen.

**burning mouth syndrome** An intense burning sensation on the tongue, often at the tip of the tongue. Burning mouth syndrome tends to develop in "supertasters"— people with an unusually large density of taste buds, each surrounded by pain fibers—and in postmenopausal women, who may lose their ability to sense bitter tastes as a result. Clonazepam (brand name: Klonopin), an anti-seizure drug, is reportedly effective in treating burning mouth syndrome in more than 70 percent of patients.

**burns** Damage to the skin or other body parts caused by extreme heat, flame, contact with heated objects, or chemicals. Burn depth is generally categorized as first, second, or third degree. The treatment of burns depends on the depth, area, and location of the burn, as well as additional factors, such as material that may be burned onto or into the skin. Options range from simply applying a cold pack to emergency treatment to skin grafts.

**burns, first degree** A first-degree burn is superficial, and has similar characteristics to a typical sunburn. The skin is red in color, and sensation is intact. In fact, the burn is usually somewhat painful.

**burns, second degree** Second-degree burns are also red and sensation is intact; however, the damage is severe enough to cause blistering of the skin, and the pain is usually somewhat more intense.

**burns, third degree** In third-degree burns the damage has progressed to the point of skin death. The skin is white and without sensation. In extreme cases damage may extend beyond the skin and into underlying tissue. In these cases the skin may be blackened or burned away. Unless skin grafts are feasible, loss of the affected limb, permanent disfigurement, and even death are likely in such severe cases.

**bursa** A closed, fluid-filled sac that functions as a gliding surface to reduce friction between tissues of the body. When the bursa becomes inflamed, the condition is known as bursitis.

**bursitis** Inflammation of a bursa, causing joint pain and restriction of movement. See also *bursa; bursitis, aseptic; bursitis, calcific; bursitis, elbow; bursitis, hip; bursitis, knee; bursitis, septic; bursitis, shoulder*.

**bursitis, aseptic** Bursitis that is not due to an infectious condition. Treatment of noninfectious bursitis includes rest, ice, and medications for inflammation and pain.

**bursitis, calcific** Chronic bursitis with calcification of the bursa. The calcium deposition can occur as long as the inflammation is present.

**bursitis, elbow** Inflammation of the bursa at the tip of the elbow, called the olecranon bursa. The olecranon bursa is a common site of bursitis.

**bursitis, hip** Inflammation of a bursa of the hip. There are two major bursae of the hip, a common location for bursitis.

**bursitis, knee** Inflammation of a bursa of the knee. There are three major bursae of the knee, a common site for bursitis.

**bursitis, septic** Inflammation of a bursa due to infection with bacteria. Infectious bursitis is treated with antibiotics, aspiration, and surgery.

**bursitis, shoulder** Inflammation of a bursa of the shoulder. There are two major bursae of the shoulder, making it a common area for the development of bursitis.

**butterfly rash** A red, flat, butterfly-shaped facial rash over the bridge of the nose. Over half of patients with systemic lupus erythematosus (SLE) develop this characteristic rash. The butterfly rash of lupus is typically painless and does not itch. Along with inflammation in other organs, the rash can be precipitated or worsened by exposure to sunlight. This photosensitivity can be accompanied by a worsening of inflammation throughout the body, causing a flare-up of the disease. A similar rash can also occur in other conditions, such as rosacea. Also known as a malar rash. See also *lupus; lupus, discoid; lupus erythematosis, systemic*.

**bypass** An operation in which the surgeon creates a new pathway for the movement of substances in the body.

**bypass, cardiopulmonary** Bypass of the heart and lungs as, for example, in open heart surgery. Blood returning to the heart is diverted through a heart-lung machine (a pump-oxygenator) before returning to the arterial circulation.

**bypass, coronary** A form of bypass surgery that can create new routes around narrowed and blocked arteries, permitting increased blood flow to deliver oxygen and nutrients to the heart muscles. Coronary artery bypass graft (CABG) surgery is advised for selected groups of patients with significant narrowings and blockages of the heart arteries. The bypass graft for a CABG can be a vein from the leg, or an inner chest-wall artery. CABG surgery is one of the most commonly performed major operations. Coronary artery disease develops because of hardening of the arteries (atherosclerosis) that supply blood to the heart muscle. Diagnostic tests include an electrocardiogram (EKG), stress test, echocardiography, and coronary angiography.

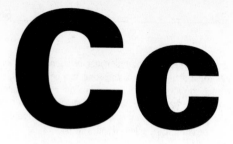

# Cc

**C** In genetics, cytosine.

**C-reactive protein** An acute-phase plasma protein whose blood concentration can rise as high as 1000-fold with inflammation. Abbreviated as CRP. Conditions that commonly lead to marked increases in CRP include infection, trauma, surgery, burns, inflammatory conditions, and advanced cancer. Moderate changes occur after strenuous exercise, heatstroke, and childbirth. Small changes occur after psychological stress and in several psychiatric illnesses. C-reactive protein is therefore a blood test that reflects the presence and intensity of inflammation, although an elevation in C-reactive protein is not a telltale sign of any particular condition.

**C-section** See *Caesarian section.*

**C1** Abbreviation for the first cervical (neck) vertebra, which supports the head.

**C2** The second cervical (neck) vertebra, also called the axis

**C3** The third cervical vertebra.

**C4** The fourth cervical vertebra.

**C5** The fifth cervical vertebra.

**C6** The sixth cervical vertebra.

**C7** The seventh cervical (neck) vertebra, sometimes called the prominent vertebra because of the long projection that emerges from the back of the vertebral body.

**CA 125** Cancer antigen 125, a protein normally made by certain cells in the body, including those of the Fallopian tubes, uterus, cervix, and the lining of the chest and abdominal cavities (the pleura and peritoneum). When it is found in larger than normal amounts, it is considered a marker for cancer.

**CA 125 test** A test for CA 125 that uses a blood sample or fluid from the chest or abdominal cavity. All tests in current use are based upon the use of an antibody directed against CA 125 (this is called the monoclonal

antibody technique). The normal value for CA 125 is usually less than 35 kU/ml. Without additional information, it is impossible to interpret a high CA 125, since it is increased in so many conditions. In someone being evaluated for a pelvic mass, a CA 125 level greater than 65 is associated with malignancy in approximately 90 percent of cases. Without a demonstrable pelvic mass, the association is much weaker. Increases in CA 125 can also occur with malignancies of the Fallopian tubes, the lining of the uterus, or the lung, breast, or gastrointestinal tract. With a known malignancy, the CA 125 level may be monitored periodically. A decreasing level indicates effective therapy, whereas an increasing level indicates tumor recurrence. Because of test variation, small changes are usually not considered significant. A doubling or halving of the previous value would be important. Benign conditions that can raise CA 125 include infections of the lining of the abdomen and chest (peritonitis and pleuritis), menstruation, pregnancy, endometriosis, and liver disease. Benign tumors of the ovaries can also cause an abnormal test result. See also *CA 125.*

**CABG** Coronary artery bypass graft. See *bypass, coronary.*

**cachexia** Weight loss and weakness caused by disease, or as a side effect of illness.

**caduceus** A staff with two snakes entwined about it, topped by a pair of wings. The caduceus was carried by the Greek messenger god Hermes, whose Roman counterpart was Mercury, and is therefore the sign of a herald. By a curious misconception, the caduceus also became the insignia of the US Army Medical Corps and a well-known symbol of doctors and medicine. The Corps should have chosen the symbol of medicine: the rod of Aesculapius, which has only one snake and no wings. No wings were necessary, since the essence of medicine was not speed. The single serpent that could shed its skin and emerge in full vigor represented the renewal of youth and health. That said, the ancient caduceus with its pair of snakes coiled about each other is reminiscent of the double helix structure of DNA, which was not discovered until modern times.

**caecal** Pertaining to the caecum. See *caecum.*

**caecum** The first portion of the large bowel, which is situated in the lower right quadrant of the abdomen. The caecum receives fecal material from the small bowel (ileum), which opens into it. The appendix is attached to the caecum.

**Caesarian section** Procedure in which an infant is surgically removed from the uterus rather than being born vaginally. As the name "Caesarian" suggests, this is not exactly a new procedure. It was done in ancient civilizations to salvage the baby upon the death of a near-full–term pregnant woman. Julius Caesar is said to have been born by this procedure, hence the name. The term "section" in surgery refers to the division of tissue. What is being divided here is the abdominal wall of the mother, as well as the wall of the uterus, in order to extract the baby. Also known as a C-section.

**Caesarian section, lower segment** A Caesarian section in which the surgical incision is made in the lower segment of the uterus. Abbreviated as LSCS.

**Caesarian section, vaginal birth after** It was once the rule that after a C-section, the next delivery also had to be by C-section. Now vaginal delivery after Caesarian section (VBAC) is frequently feasible.

**café au lait spots** Flat spots on the skin that have a color similar to that of coffee with cream in persons with light skin, or a darker appearance than the surrounding skin in persons with dark skin. About 10 percent of the general population have café au lait spots, and they can be removed with a Yag laser technique. Café au lait spots are normally harmless, but in some cases they are a sign of neurofibromatosis. See also *neurofibromatosis, Yag laser surgery*.

**caffeine** An alkaloid stimulant found naturally in coffee, and also present in cola drinks. Caffeine can help to relieve headaches, so a number of over-the-counter and prescription pain relievers include it as an ingredient, usually with aspirin or another analgesic.

**Caffey disease** An inflammatory bone disorder seen only in newborn and very young babies, characterized by swelling of soft tissues, irritability, fever, and paleness. Also known as infantile cortical hyperostosis.

**calamine** An astringent made from zinc carbonate or zinc oxide, customarily used in lotion form to treat skin problems or insect bites that cause itching or discomfort.

**calcaneal spur** A bony spur projecting from the back or underside of the heel bone (the calcaneus) that may make walking painful. Calcaneal spurs are associated with inflammation of the Achilles tendon (Achilles tendinitis), and cause tenderness and pain at the back of the heel, which is made worse by pushing off the ball of the foot. Spurs under the sole (the plantar area) are associated with inflammation of the plantar fascia, which is the bowstring-like tissue stretching from the heel underneath the sole. These spurs cause localized tenderness and a type of pain that is made worse by stepping down on the heel. Not all heel spurs cause symptoms. Some are discovered on X-rays taken for other purposes. Heel spurs and plantar fasciitis can occur alone, or may be related to underlying diseases that cause arthritis, such as Reiter disease, ankylosing spondylitis, and diffuse idiopathic skeletal hyperostosis. Treatment is designed to decrease the inflammation and avoid reinjury. Icing reduces pain

and inflammation. Anti-inflammatory agents, such as ibuprofen or injections of cortisone, can help. Heel lifts reduce stress on the Achilles tendon and relieve painful spurs at the back of the heel. Donut-shaped shoe inserts take pressure off plantar spurs. Infrequently, surgery is done on chronically inflamed spurs. Also known as a heel spur.

**calcaneocuboid joint** The joint located in the foot between the calcaneus bone and the cuboid bone. It is a gliding type of joint. The ligaments that serve to support and strengthen this joint are called the capsular, dorsal calcaneocuboid, bifurcated, long plantar, and plantar calcaneocuboid ligaments.

**calcaneus** The heel bone, a more or less rectangular bone at the back of the foot. Also known as the os calcis.

**calcific bursitis** Chronic inflammation of a bursa (bursitis) that leads to calcium deposition (calcification) of the bursa. The calcification can occur as long as the inflammation is present. See also *bursa, bursitis*.

**calcification** The process of building bone by suffusing tissues with calcium salts. Also known as ossification.

**calcification, nonarteriosclerotic cerebral** See *cerebral calcification, nonarteriosclerotic*.

**calcified granuloma** A node-like type of tissue inflammation (granuloma) containing calcium deposits. Since it usually takes some time for calcium to be deposited in a granuloma, it is generally assumed that a calcified granuloma is an old granuloma. For example, a calcified granuloma in the lung may be due to tuberculosis contracted years earlier that is now dormant.

**calcinosis** The presence of an abnormal deposit of calcium salts in body tissues, as is seen in some forms of disease.

**calcitonin** A thyroid hormone involved in calcium metabolization and bone strength. Findings of excess calcitonin can indicate medullary thyroid cancer.

**calcium** A mineral found mainly in the hard part of bones, where it is stored. Calcium is added to bone by cells called osteoblasts, and removed from bone by cells called osteoclasts. Calcium is essential for healthy bones, and is also important for muscle contraction, heart action, and normal blood clotting. Food sources of calcium include dairy foods; some leafy green vegetables, such as broccoli and collards; canned salmon; clams; oysters; calcium-fortified foods; and soy foods, like tofu. According to the National Academy of Sciences, adequate intake of calcium is 1 gram daily for both men and women. The upper limit for calcium intake is 2.5 grams daily.

**calcium deficiency**  A low blood level of calcium (hypocalcemia), which can make the nervous system highly irritable, causing spasms of the hands and feet (tetany), muscle cramps, abdominal cramps, overly active reflexes, and so on. Chronic calcium deficiency contributes to poor mineralization of bones, soft bones (osteomalacia) and osteoporosis, and, in children, to rickets and impaired growth.

**calcium excess**  Overly high intake of calcium (hypercalcemia) may cause muscle weakness and constipation, affect the conduction of electrical impulses in the heart (heart block), lead to calcium stones in the urinary tract, impair kidney function through nephrocalcinosis, and interfere with the absorption of iron, predisposing the person to iron deficiency.

**calculi, renal**  See *kidney stone.*

**calculus, renal**  See *kidney stone.*

**caliper**  **1** A metal or plastic instrument used to measure the diameter of an object. The skin-fold thickness in several parts of the body can be measured with calipers, as can fat deposits. This measurement is done in medicine, especially in the diagnosis and treatment of obesity, and in physical anthropology. Calipers are also used to measure the diameter of the pelvis in pregnant women to ensure that it is large enough to permit birth. **2** A type of leg splint.

**callus**  **1** A localized, firm thickening of the upper layer of skin as a result of repetitive friction. A callus on the skin of the foot has often become thick and hard from rubbing against an ill-fitting shoe. Calluses of the feet may lead to other problems, such as serious infections. Shoes that fit well can keep calluses from forming on the feet. **2** Hard new bone substance that forms in an area of bone fracture. It is part of the natural bone-repair process.

**calorie**  A unit of food energy. The word calorie is ordinarily used instead of the more precise, scientific term kilocalorie. A kilocalorie represents the amount of energy required to raise the temperature of a liter of water one degree centigrade at sea level. Technically, a kilocalorie represents 1000 true calories of energy.

**Canavan disease**  A severe, progressive, inherited disorder of the central nervous system. Canavan disease is caused by a deficiency of the enzyme aspartoacylase, which leads to increased excretion of its substrate, a substance called N-acetylaspartic acid (NAA), in the urine. Diagnosis of Canavan disease is made by finding an increased level of urinary NAA via organic acid analysis. The abnormally high level of NAA leads to loss of insulation along nerve fibers (demyelination) and spongy degeneration of the brain. The signs of Canavan disease

usually appear when children are between three and six months of age. They include developmental delay, significant motor slowness, enlargement of the head (macrocephaly), loss of muscle tone (hypotonia), poor head control, and severe feeding problems. As the disease progresses, seizures, shrinkage of the nerve to the eye (optic atrophy) and often blindness develop, as do heartburn (gastrointestinal reflux), and deterioration of the ability to swallow. Canavan disease is inherited as an autosomal recessive condition, with both parents silently carrying a single Canavan gene and each of their children running a one-in-four risk of receiving both genes and, therefore, having the disease. Canavan disease is more prevalent among individuals of Eastern European Jewish (Ashkenazi) background than those of other communities. There is currently no cure or effective treatment. Most children with Canavan disease die in the first decade of life. Also known as spongy degeneration of the central nervous system, Canavan-Van Bogaert-Bertrand disease, and by several names of a biochemical nature, including aspartoacylase deficiency, ASPA deficiency, ASP deficiency, aminoacylase 2 deficiency, and ACY2 deficiency.

**cancer**  An abnormal, uncontrolled growth that can begin in or involve any tissue of the body, and that can have many different forms in each body area. Cancer is a group of more than 100 different diseases. Most cancers are named for the type of cell or organ in which they begin. Benign tumors are not cancer; malignant tumors are cancer. When cancer spreads (metastasizes), the new tumor has the same name as the original (primary) tumor. Skin cancer is the most common type of cancer in both men and women. The second most common are prostate cancer in men, and breast cancer in women. Lung cancer is the leading cause of death from cancer for both men and women in the US. Cancer is not contagious. Also known as malignancy. See also *cancer, causes.*

**Cancer Antigen 125**  See *CA 125.*

**Cancer Institute, National**  See *National Institutes of Health.*

**cancer of the penis**  A malignant tumor in which cancer cells are found on the skin of the penis or in the tissues of the penis. It is rare in the US. A doctor should be seen if any of the following problems occur: growths or sores on the penis, any unusual liquid coming from the penis (abnormal discharge), or bleeding. The doctor will examine the penis and feel for any lumps. If warranted, a small sample of tissue (a biopsy) will be removed from the penis and looked at under a microscope to see whether there are any cancer cells. If cancer is found, more tests will be done to find out whether the cancer has spread to other parts of the body (staging). Treatment options include surgery, radiation therapy, chemotherapy, and biological therapy. The chance of recovery and choice of treatment depend on the stage of the cancer and the patient's general state of health. Men who are not circumcised at birth may have a higher risk of getting cancer of the penis.

**cancer symptoms**   The following symptoms may be associated with cancer: changes in bowel or bladder habits, a sore that does not heal, unusual bleeding or discharge, thickening or a lump in the breast or any other part of the body, indigestion or difficulty swallowing, obvious change in a wart or mole, and a nagging cough or hoarseness. These symptoms are not always a sign of cancer; they can be caused by less serious conditions. Some forms of cancer cause little or no discomfort until the disease is far advanced, so it is important to see your doctor for regular checkups rather than wait for problems to occur. Only a doctor can make a diagnosis.

**cancer, bladder**   A malignant tumor of the hollow organ responsible for temporarily holding urine after it leaves the kidneys. The most common warning sign of bladder cancer is blood in the urine. Diagnosis of bladder cancer is supported by findings of the medical history, examination, and blood, urine, and X-ray tests; and can be confirmed with a biopsy, usually during a cystoscope exam.

**cancer, bone**   A malignant tumor of one or more areas of the skeleton. Pain is the most frequent symptom of cancer of the bone. Diagnosis is supported by findings of the medical history, examination, and blood and X-ray tests; and can be confirmed with a biopsy. Cancers that begin in bone are rare, but it is not unusual for cancers to spread (metastasize) into bone from other parts of the body. In such cases the disease is not called bone cancer, but is named for the organ or tissue in which the cancer began.

**cancer, brain**   A malignant tumor of the body's information-processing center. Tumors in the brain can be malignant or benign, and can occur at any age. Only malignant tumors are cancerous. Primary brain tumors initially form in the brain tissue; secondary brain tumors are cancers that have spread to the brain tissue (metastasized) from elsewhere in the body.

**cancer, breast**   See *breast cancer*. See also *breast cancer susceptibility genes; breast cancer, familial; breast, infiltrating ductal carconoma of; breast, infiltrating lobular carcinoma of; mastectomy.*

**cancer, breast, familial**   See *breast cancer, familial.* See also *BRCA1; BRCA2; breast cancer susceptibility genes.*

**cancer, breast, susceptibility genes**   See *breast cancer susceptibility genes.* See also *BRCA1; BRCA2.*

**cancer, causes**   In most individual cases, the exact cause of cancer is unknown. It's likely that each case represents an interplay of several factors. These may include increased genetic susceptibility; environmental insults, such as chemical exposure or smoking cigarettes; lifestyle factors, including diet; damage caused by infectious disease; and many more. Although they are not causes per se, many characteristics can influence the development of cancer. These include gender, race, age, and the health of the patient's immune system. When common causes for a type of cancer are discovered, this information can be very helpful in prevention, and sometimes in treatment. For example, the link between overexposure to the sun and skin cancer is well-known, and individuals can easily reduce their risk by avoiding suntanning and sunburns.

**cancer, cervical**   A malignant tumor of the cervix, the lower, narrow part of the uterus that forms a canal which opens into the vagina. Regular pelvic exams and Pap testing can detect precancerous changes in the cervix. The most common symptom of cervical cancer is abnormal bleeding. Cancer of the cervix can be diagnosed by using a Pap test or other procedures that sample the cervix tissue. Precancerous changes in the cervix may be treated with cryosurgery, cauterization, or laser surgery. Cancer of the cervix requires different treatment than cancer that begins in other parts of the uterus.

**cancer, colon**   A malignant tumor arising from the inner wall of the large intestine. In the US, colon cancer is the third leading cause of cancer in males, and the fourth in females. Risk factors for cancer of the colon and rectum (colorectal cancer) include heredity, colon polyps, and long-standing ulcerative colitis. Most colorectal cancers develop from polyps. Removal of colon polyps can prevent colorectal cancer. Colon polyps and early cancer can have no symptoms. Therefore, regular screening is important. Diagnosis can be made by barium enema or by colonoscopy, with biopsy confirmation of cancer tissue. Surgery is the most common treatment for colorectal cancer.

**cancer, esophagus**   A malignant tumor of the swallowing tube that passes from the throat to the stomach. The risk of cancer of the esophagus is increased by long-term irritation of the esophagus, such as by smoking, heavy alcohol intake, or Barrett esophagitis. Cancer of the esophagus can cause pain and difficulty with swallowing solid food. Diagnosis of esophageal cancer can be made by barium X-ray of the esophagus, and confirmed by endoscopy with biopsy of the cancer tissue.

**cancer, gastric** A malignant tumor of the stomach, the major organ that holds food for digestion. Stomach cancer (gastric cancer) can develop in any part of the stomach and spread to other organs. Stomach ulcers do not appear to increase a person's risk of developing stomach cancer. Symptoms of stomach cancer are often vague, such as loss of appetite and weight. The cancer is diagnosed with a biopsy of stomach tissue during an endoscopy.

**cancer, Hodgkin lymphoma** One of four subtypes of cancer of the lymphatic system; also known as Hodgkin disease. The most common symptom of Hodgkin disease is a painless swelling in the lymph nodes in the neck, underarm, or groin. Most patients are in their teens or 20s. Hodgkin disease is diagnosed when abnormal tissue is detected by a pathologist after a biopsy of an enlarged lymph node. Treatment usually includes radiation therapy or chemotherapy. Regular follow-up examinations are important after treatment for Hodgkin disease. Patients treated for Hodgkin disease have an increased risk of developing other types of cancer later in life, especially leukemia.

**cancer, kidney** A malignant tumor of the major organ responsible for removing toxins produced during metabolization from the blood. Childhood kidney cancer is different from adult kidney cancer. The most common symptom of kidney cancer is blood in the urine. The diagnosis of kidney cancer is supported by findings of the medical history and examination, blood, urine, and X-ray tests, and confirmed with a biopsy. Kidney cancer is treated with surgery, embolization, radiation therapy, hormone therapy, biological therapy, or chemotherapy.

**cancer, laryngeal** A malignant tumor of the voice box, which is located at the top of the windpipe (trachea). Cancer of the larynx occurs most often in people over the age of 55, especially those who have been heavy smokers. People who stop smoking can greatly reduce their risk. Painless hoarseness can be a symptom of cancer of the larynx. The larynx can be examined with a viewing tube called a laryngoscope. Cancer of the larynx is usually treated with radiation therapy or surgery. Chemotherapy can also be used for laryngeal cancers that have spread.

**cancer, larynx** See *cancer, laryngeal.*

**cancer, leukemia** See *leukemia.* See also *leukemia, accelerated phase of; leukemia, blastic phase of; leukemia, chronic phase of; leukemia, hairy cell; leukemia, lymphocytic; leukemia, myelogenous; leukemia, myeloid; leukemia, refractory; leukemia, smoldering.*

**cancer, lung** A malignant tumor of the major organ of respiration. Lung cancer kills more men and women than any other form of cancer. Since the majority of lung cancer is diagnosed at a relatively late stage, only 10 percent of all lung cancer patients are ultimately cured. Eight out of 10 lung cancers are due to damage caused by tobacco smoke. Lung cancers are classified as either small cell or nonsmall cell cancers. Persistent cough and bloody sputum can be symptoms of lung cancer. Diagnosis of lung cancer can be based on examination of sputum, or on tissue examination with biopsy, using bronchoscopy, needle through the chest wall, or surgical excision.

**cancer, lymphoma, Hodgkin** See *Hodgkin disease.*

**cancer, lymphoma, non-Hodgkin** See *lymphoma, non-Hodgkin.*

**cancer, male breast** See *breast cancer, male.*

**cancer, malignant melanoma** A skin cancer that begins in cells called melanocytes, which normally grow together to form benign (noncancerous) moles. A change in size, shape, or color of a mole can be a sign of melanoma. Melanoma can be cured if detected early. If you wait, it may spread to other areas of the body, and that can cause death. Diagnosis is confirmed with a biopsy of the abnormal skin. Sun exposure can cause skin damage, which can in turn lead to melanoma.

**cancer, melanoma** See *cancer, malignant melanoma.*

**cancer, multiple myeloma** A bone-marrow cancer involving a type of white blood cell called a plasma (or myeloma) cell; in this type of cancer the cells form many tumors. See also *cancer, myeloma.*

**cancer, myeloma** A bone-marrow cancer involving a type of white blood cell called a plasma (or myeloma) cell. The tumor cells can form a single collection (plasmacytoma) or many tumors (multiple myeloma). Plasma cells are part of the immune system, and make antibodies. Because myeloma patients have an excess of identical plasma cells, they have too much of one type of antibody. As myeloma cells increase in number, they damage and weaken the bones, causing pain and often fractures. When bones are damaged, too much calcium is released into the blood, leading to loss of appetite, nausea, thirst, fatigue, muscle weakness, restlessness, and confusion. Myeloma cells prevent the bone marrow from forming normal plasma cells and other white blood cells important to the immune system, so patients may not be able to fight infections. The cancer cells can also prevent the growth of new red blood cells, causing anemia. Excess antibody proteins and calcium may prevent the kidneys from filtering and cleaning the blood properly.

**cancer, non-Hodgkin lymphoma** See *lymphoma, non-Hodgkin.*

**cancer, oral**   A malignant tumor of the mouth area. A sore in the mouth that does not heal can be a warning sign of oral cancer. A biopsy is the only way to know whether an abnormal area in the oral cavity is cancerous. Oral cancer is almost always caused by tobacco (smoking and chewing) or alcohol use. Surgery to remove the tumor in the mouth is the usual treatment.

**cancer, ovarian**   A malignant tumor of the egg sac of females. There are several types of ovarian cancer. Symptoms of ovarian cancer can be vague. Detection involves physical examination (including pelvic exam), ultrasound, X-ray tests, CA-125 blood test, and biopsy of the ovary. Most ovarian growths (tumors) in women under age 30 are benign (noncancerous), fluid-filled cysts.

**cancer, ovary**   See *cancer, ovarian.*

**cancer, pancreatic**   A malignant tumor of the pancreas has been called a "silent" disease because early pancreatic cancer usually does not cause symptoms. If the tumor blocks the common bile duct and bile cannot pass into the digestive system, the skin and whites of the eyes may become yellow (jaundiced), and the urine may become darker as a result of accumulated bile pigment (bilirubin).

**cancer, prostate**   A malignant tumor of the gland that produces some of the components of semen fluid. Prostate cancer is the second leading cause of death of males in the US. It is often first detected as a hard nodule found during a routine rectal examination. The PSA blood test is a screening test for prostate cancer. Diagnosis of prostate cancer is established when cancer cells are identified in prostate tissue obtained by a biopsy. In some patients, prostate cancer is life-threatening. In many others, prostate cancer can exist for years without causing any health problems. Treatment options for prostate cancer include observation, radiation therapy, surgery, hormonal therapy, and chemotherapy.

**cancer, prostatic**   See *cancer, prostate.*

**cancer, rectal**   A malignant tumor arising from the inner wall of the end of the large intestine (rectum). In the US, it is the third leading cause of cancer in males, and the fourth in females. Risk factors include heredity, colon polyps, and long-standing ulcerative colitis. Most colorectal cancers develop from polyps in the colon. Removal of these polyps can prevent cancer. Colon polyps and early rectal cancer can have no symptoms, so regular screening is important. Diagnosis can be made by barium enema, or by colonoscopy with biopsy confirmation of cancer tissue. Surgery is the most common treatment.

**cancer, renal cell**   A malignant tumor that develops in the lining of the renal tubules, which filter the blood and produce urine. Also known as renal cell carcinoma.

**cancer, skin**   A malignant tumor of the outer surface of the body. Skin cancer is the most common cancer in the US. There are many types of skin cancer; Its main cause is ultraviolet light from sunlight. Unexplained changes in the appearance of the skin that last longer than two weeks should always be evaluated by a doctor. The cure rate for skin cancer could be 100 percent if all skin cancers were brought to a doctor's attention before they had a chance to spread. See also *cancer, malignant melanoma.*

**cancer, stomach**   See *cancer, gastric.*

**cancer, testicular**   A malignant tumor of the male sex organ (testicle) that normally produces the hormone testosterone. It is one of the most common cancers in young men. Most testicular cancers are found by men themselves, as a lump in the testicle. The risk of testicular cancer is increased in males whose testicles did not move down normally into the scrotum during childhood, a condition known as undescended testicles. When a growth in a testicle is detected, cancer is confirmed after surgical removal of the affected testicle (orchiectomy) and examination of the tissue under a microscope. Testicular cancer is almost always curable if it is found early.

**cancer, thyroid**   A malignant tumor of the gland in front of the neck that normally produces thyroid hormone, which is important to the normal regulation of the metabolism of the body. There are four major types of cancer of the thyroid gland. Persons who received radiation to the head or neck in childhood should be examined by a doctor every one to two years. The most common symptom of thyroid cancer is a lump, or nodule, that can be felt in the neck. The only certain way to tell whether a thyroid lump is cancer is by examining thyroid tissue obtained by using a needle or surgery for biopsy.

**cancer, uterine**   A malignant tumor of the uterus (womb), which occurs most often in women between the ages of 55 and 70. Abnormal bleeding after menopause is the most common symptom. Cancer of the uterus is diagnosed based on the results of a pelvic examination, Pap smear, biopsy of the uterus, and/or dilation and curettage (D and C).

**Candida albicans**   A yeast-like fungal organism found in small amounts in the normal human intestinal tract. Normally kept in check by the body's own helpful bacteria, C. albicans can increase in numbers when this balance is disturbed to cause candidiasis of the intestinal tract, or yeast infections of other parts of the body. See also *candidiasis.*

**candidiasis**   Overgrowth of C. albicans in the gastrointestinal tract, or infection of other body areas with this yeast. Vaginal yeast infections; some forms of diaper rash, and other skin rashes that emerge in moist, warm areas of skin; and thrush (a condition characterized by patches of white inside the mouth and/or throat) are all forms of yeast infection. Candidiasis tends to develop when the normal balance of intestinal bacteria (flora) is upset, as sometimes occurs with antibiotic use. Prevention measures include the use of probiotics, and in some cases, dietary changes. Treatment is via antifungal medications. Candidiasis is usually a minor and easily addressed problem, but can take on greater importance for those with immune-system disorders, such as AIDS. See also *probiotics*.

**canker sores**   Also known as aphthous ulcers, these are small, frequently painful and sensitive craters in the lining of the mouth. About 20 percent of the population have canker sores at any one time. Sores typically last for 10 to 14 days, and should heal without scarring.

**cannabis**   Marijuana (Cannibis sativa), a drug derived from the family of plants that includes hemp. Use of cannabis produces a mild sense of euphoria, as well as impairments in judgment and lengthened response time. Cannabis may be smoked or eaten. Although cannabis use is illegal in most parts of the world, the plant appears to have some potential for medical use, particularly as a palliative for glaucoma and disease-related loss of appetite and wasting, as is often seen in cancer, AIDS, and other illnesses. Some compounds in cannabis have an antiseizure effect. In some areas of the US, individuals whose physicians recommend the medical use of cannabis can obtain special permission.

**cannula**   A hollow tube with sharp, retractable inner core that can be inserted into a vein, artery, or other body cavity.

**CAPD**   Central auditory processing disorder.

**capillaries**   The smallest of blood vessels, capillaries distribute oxygenated blood from arteries to the tissues of the body, and feed deoxygenated blood from the tissues back into the veins. The capillaries are thus a central component of the circulatory system. When pink areas of light-colored skin are compressed, blanching occurs because blood is pressed out of the capillaries.

**capitation**   In US health services, capitation refers to a fixed "per capita" amount that is paid to a hospital, clinic, or doctor for each person served. If that person uses few services, the excess amount paid is potential profit for the payee. If the person uses many services, the payee may lose money.

**caps**   Abbreviation for capsules.

**carbohydrate**   One of the three nutrient compounds used as energy sources (calories) by the body (the others are fats and proteins). Carbohydrates come in the form of simple sugars or in more complex forms, such as starches and fiber. Complex carbohydrates come naturally from plants. Intake of complex carbohydrates can lower blood cholesterol when they are substituted for saturated fat. Carbohydrates produce four calories of energy per gram. When eaten, all carbohydrates are broken down into the sugar glucose.

**carbon monoxide poisoning**   A potentially deadly condition caused by breathing carbon monoxide gas, which prevents oxygenation of the blood. Common causes of carbon monoxide poisoning include malfunctioning furnaces, and the use of kerosene heaters or similar devices in unventilated indoor spaces. Carbon monoxide is also emitted by automobile and other engines, so these should not be run in an unventilated space, such as a closed garage. Inexpensive alarms are available that can detect a dangerous buildup of carbon monoxide. Treatment is via immediate reoxygenation of the blood in a hospital.

**carbuncles**   A collection of skin abscesses (boils), accompanied by profuse drainage in several areas, and loss of skin. Usually caused by local infection with the bacteria Staphylococcus aureus. Treatment is via antibiotics (usually in the form of topical creams), and in severe cases, surgery. See also *abscess*.

**carcinoembryonic antigen test**   A blood test to detect carcinoembryonic antigen (CEA), a protein found in many types of cells but primarily associated with tumors of the developing fetus. The normal range is under 2.5 ng/ml in an adult nonsmoker, and under 5.0 ng/ml in a smoker. Benign conditions that can increase CEA include smoking, infection, inflammatory bowel disease, pancreatitis, cirrhosis of the liver, and some benign tumors (in the same organs that produce cancers accompanied by increased CEA). Benign disease does not usually cause a CEA increase over 10 ng/ml. The main medical use of CEA testing is as a tumor marker, especially for intestinal cancer. The most common cancers that elevate CEA are in the colon and rectum. Others include cancer of the pancreas, stomach, breast, or lung, and certain types of thyroid and ovarian cancer. Levels over 20 ng/ml before therapy are associated with cancer that has already spread. CEA is useful in monitoring the treatment of CEA-rich tumors. If the CEA is high before treatment, it should fall to normal after successful therapy. A rising CEA level indicates progression or recurrence of the cancer. Chemotherapy and radiation therapy can themselves cause a rise in CEA, due to death of tumor cells and release of CEA into the bloodstream, but that rise is typically temporary.

**carcinogen** A substance or agent that is known to cause cancer. A suspected carcinogen is a substance or agent for which there is some evidence of a link to cancer, but no definitive proof.

**carcinogenic** Having a cancer-causing action.

**carcinoma** Cancer that begins in the tissues lining or covering an organ (the epithelium), including the skin.

**carcinoma in situ** Cancer that stays in the place where it began, and has not spread. For example, squamous cell carcinoma in situ is an early cancer of the skin. It develops from squamous cells, which are flat, scale-like cells in the outer layer of the skin. Carcinoma in situ is an early-stage tumor, and is usually curable via chemotherapy, radiation, surgery, or other means.

**carcinoma in situ, squamous cell** An early stage of skin cancer, this is a tumor that develops from the flat, scale-like cells in the outer layer of the skin. The hallmark of squamous cell carcinoma in situ is a persistent, progressive, slightly raised, red, scaly or crusted plaque. It may occur anywhere on the skin surface or on mucosal surfaces, such as the mouth. Under the microscope, atypical squamous cells are seen to have proliferated through the whole thickness of the epidermis (the outer layer of the skin), but no further. The classical cause was prolonged exposure to arsenic. Today, squamous cell carcinoma occurs most often in the sun-exposed areas of the skin in older white males. Treatment options include freezing the affected area with liquid nitrogen, cauterization (burning), surgical removal, and chemosurgery. Also known as Bowen disease.

**carcinoma of the breast, infiltrating ductal** One of several recognized specific patterns of cancer of the breast, so named because it begins in the cells forming the ducts of the breast. It is the most common form of breast cancer, comprising 65 to 85 percent of all cases. On a mammogram, invasive ductal carcinoma is usually visualized as a mass with fine spikes radiating from the edges (spiculation). It may also appear as a smooth-edged lump in the breast. On physical examination, this lump usually feels much harder or firmer than benign lumps (whether natural structures or cysts) in the breast. On microscopic examination, the cancerous cells are found to have invaded and replaced the normal breast tissue. Treatment may include radiation, chemotherapy, or surgery.

**carcinoma of the breast, infiltrating lobular** Infiltrating lobular carcinoma is the second most common type of invasive breast cancer, accounting for 5 to 10 percent of breast cancer. Infiltrating lobular carcinoma starts in the glands that secrete milk (lobules), and then invades surrounding tissue. On mammography, a lobular carcinoma can look similar to a ductal carcinoma, appearing as a mass with fine spikes radiating from the edges (spiculation). However, on physical examination of the breast, a lobular carcinoma is usually not a hard mass like a ductal carcinoma, but rather a vague thickening of the breast tissue. Lobular carcinoma can occur in more than one site in the breast (as a multicentric tumor) or in both breasts at the same time (as bilateral lobular carcinoma). Treatment may include radiation, chemotherapy, or surgery.

**carcinoma, squamous cell** Cancer that begins in squamous cells, which are thin, flat cells resembling fish scales. Squamous cells are found in the tissue that forms the surface of the skin, the lining of the hollow organs of the body, and the passages of the respiratory and digestive tracts. See also *carcinoma in situ, squamous cell*.

**carcinoma, transitional cell** Cancer that develops in the lining of the renal pelvis. This type of cancer also occurs in the ureter and the bladder.

**cardiac** Having to do with the heart.

**cardiac aneurysm** See *aneurysm, cardiac*.

**cardiac arrest** A heart attack, in which the heart suddenly stops pumping sufficient blood. See also *myocardial infarction, acute*.

**cardiac conduction system** The electrical conduction system that controls the heart rate. This system generates electrical impulses and conducts them throughout the muscle of the heart, stimulating the heart to contract and pump blood. Among the major elements in the cardiac conduction system are the sinus node, the atrioventricular (AV) node, and the autonomic nervous system. The sinus node generates impulses; the AV node slows down current to contract the atria of the heart, and then stimulates the ventricles; and the autonomic nervous system transmits control messages to start or speed up the cycle in response to physical exertion and other circumstances. See also *atrioventricular node, autonomic nervous system, sinoatrial node*.

**cardiac defibrillator, implantable** A device put within the body that is designed to recognize certain types of abnormal heart rhythms (arrhythmias) and correct them by delivering precisely calibrated and timed electrical shocks to restore a normal heartbeat. Defibrillators continuously monitor the heart rhythm in order to detect overly rapid arrhythmias, such as ventricular tachycardia (rapid regular beating of the ventricles, the bottom chambers of the heart) or ventricular fibrillation (rapid irregular beating of the ventricles). These ventricular arrhythmias impair the pumping efficiency of the heart, raising the risks of fainting (syncope) and sudden cardiac arrest. They tend to develop in people with coronary artery disease or heart-muscle diseases (cardiomyopathies), and are life-threatening. Today's implantable defibrillators are about the size of a minicassette, and can be implanted with less invasive surgical techniques than were used in the past.

**cardiac muscle**   A type of muscle tissue with unique features. It is found only in the heart.

**cardiac output**   The amount of blood the heart pumps through the circulatory system in a minute. The amount of blood put out by the left ventricle of the heart in one contraction is called the stroke volume. The stroke volume and the heart rate determine the cardiac output. A normal adult's heart can easily pump five quarts (4.7 liters) of blood a minute; that is the cardiac output.

**cardiac septum**   The dividing wall between the right and left sides of the heart. That portion of the septum that separates the two upper chambers (the right and left atria) of the heart is termed the atrial (or interatrial) septum; the portion that lies between the two lower chambers (the right and left ventricles) of the heart is called the ventricular (or interventricular) septum.

**cardiac tamponade**   A life-threatening situation in which there is such a large amount of fluid (usually blood) inside the pericardial sac around the heart that it interferes with the performance of the heart. If left untreated, the end result is dangerously low blood pressure, shock, and death. The excess fluid in the pericardial sac acts to compress and constrict the heart. Cardiac tamponade can be due to excessive pericardial fluid, a wound to the heart, or rupture of the heart. Also known as pericardial tamponade.

**cardiac ventricle**   One of the two lower chambers of the heart. The right ventricle is the chamber that receives blood from the right atrium and pumps it into the lungs via the pulmonary artery. The left ventricle is the chamber that receives blood from the left atrium and pumps it into the circulatory system via the aorta.

**cardiologist**   A doctor who specializes in treating heart disorders.

**cardiology**   The study and treatment of heart disorders.

**cardiomyopathy, hypertrophic**   A heart defect characterized by increased thickness (hypertrophy) of the wall of the left ventricle, the largest of the four chambers of the heart. Abbreviated as HCM, it can surface at any time in life. It may, in a worst-case scenario, lead to death.

**cardiopulmonary**   Having to do with both the heart and lungs.

**cardiopulmonary bypass**   Bypass of the heart and lungs as, for example, in open-heart surgery. Blood returning to the heart is diverted through a heart-lung machine (a pump-oxygenator) before it is returned to the arterial circulation. The machine does the work both of the heart and the lungs, by pumping blood and supplying oxygen to red blood cells.

**cardiopulmonary resuscitation**   Better known as CPR, this life-saving emergency procedure involves breathing for the victim and applying external chest compression to make the heart pump. In the case of an early heart attack, death can often be avoided if a bystander starts CPR within five minutes of the onset of ventricular fibrillation. When paramedics arrive, medications and/or electrical shock (cardioversion) to the heart can be administered to convert ventricular fibrillation to a normal heart rhythm. Therefore, prompt CPR and rapid paramedic response can improve the chances of survival from a heart attack.

**cardiovascular system**   The circulatory system, comprising the heart, lungs, and blood vessels.

**cardioversion**   The conversion of one cardiac rhythm or electrical pattern to another, almost always from an abnormal to a normal one. This conversion can be accomplished by using medications or by electrical cardioversion with a special defibrillator. Also known as countershock.

**cardioverter**   Although cardioversion (the conversion of one cardiac rhythm to another) may sometimes be done with medications, a cardioverter is now synonymous with a defibrillator. See *cardiac defibrillator, implantable.*

**carditis**   Inflammation of the heart.

**care proxy, health**   See *health care proxy*. See also *advance directives.*

**care, ambulatory**   See *ambulatory care.*

**care, managed**   See *managed care.*

**care, nail**   See *nail care.*

**caries**   Dental cavities in the two outer layers of a tooth (the enamel and the dentin). Small cavities may not cause pain, and may not be noticed by the patient. Larger cavities can collect food, and the inner pulp of the affected tooth can become irritated by bacterial toxins or by foods that are cold, hot, sour, or sweet. The result can be a toothache. Caries is believed to be caused by the Streptococcus bacteria, which produces an enamel-dissolving acid as it devours carbohydrate deposits (plaque) on the teeth. To prevent caries, brush and floss the teeth daily, use a bacteriocidal mouthwash, and have regular dental cleanings by a professional. If caries does occur, the eroded area can be cleaned and filled by a dentist to prevent further damage.

**carotene, beta** See *beta carotene.* See also *Appendix C, "Vitamins."*

**carotenemia** Temporary yellowing of the skin due to excessive carotene in the diet. Carotenemia is most commonly seen in infants fed too much mashed carrots, or adults consuming high quantities of carrots, carrot juice, or beta carotene in supplement form.

**carotid** Pertaining to the carotid artery and the area near that key artery, which is located in the front of the neck.

**carotid arteries** Either of two key arteries located in the front of the neck, through which blood from the heart goes to the brain. The right and left common carotid arteries are located on each side of the neck. Together, these arteries provide the principal blood supply to the head and neck. The left common carotid arises directly from the aorta. The right common carotid artery arises from the brachiocephalic artery which, in turn, comes off the aorta. Each of the two divides to form external and internal carotid arteries. The external carotids are closer to the surface than the internal carotids, which run deep within the neck. Cholesterol plaques on the inner wall of the carotid artery can lead to strokes.

**carpal tunnel** A bony canal in the palm side of the wrist that provides passage for the median nerve to the hand.

**carpal tunnel release** A surgical procedure to relieve pressure exerted on the median nerve within the carpal tunnel (carpal tunnel syndrome). Surgical release is performed via a small incision, using conventional surgery techniques or a fiberoptic scope (endoscopic carpal tunnel repair).

**carpal tunnel syndrome** A type of compression neuropathy caused by compression and irritation of the median nerve in the wrist. The nerve is compressed and irritated within the carpal tunnel, due to pressure from the transverse carpal ligament. Abbreviated as CTS, carpal tunnel syndrome can be due to trauma from repetitive work, such as that of retail checkers and cashiers, assembly line workers, meat packers, typists, writers, accountants, and so on. Other factors predisposing individuals to CTS include obesity, pregnancy, hypothyroidism, arthritis, and diabetes. The symptoms of CTS include numbness and tingling of the hand, wrist pain, a "pins and needles" feeling at night, weakness in the grip, and a feeling of

incoordination. In some cases the pain seems to migrate up from the wrist and into the arm, shoulder, and neck. This occurs when the affected person tries to reduce wrist pain by changing posture, stressing new sets of muscles in turn. The diagnosis is suspected based on symptoms, supported by signs on physical examination, and confirmed by nerve conduction testing. Treatment depends on the severity of symptoms and the underlying cause. Early CTS is usually treated by modification of activities, a removable wrist brace, exercises and/or manipulation (massage), and anti-inflammatory medicines. Caught early, CTS is reversible. If numbness and pain continue in the wrist and hand, a cortisone injection into the carpal tunnel can help. Surgery is indicated only when other treatments have failed. In advanced CTS, particularly if there is profound weakness and muscle atrophy (wasting), surgery is done to avoid permanent nerve damage.

**carrier test** A test designed to detect carriers of a gene for recessive genetic disorder. For example, carrier testing is done for sickle cell trait, thalassemia trait, and the Tay-Sachs gene.

**cartilage** Firm, rubbery tissue that cushions bones at joints. A more flexible kind of cartilage connects muscles with bones and makes up other parts of the body, such as the larynx and the outside parts of the ears.

**casein** The main protein found in milk and other dairy products.

**cast** **1** A protective shell of plaster and bandage molded to protect a broken or fractured limb as it heals. **2** An abnormal mass of dead cells that forms in a body cavity.

**casting** The use of successive casts to reshape deformed or spastic limbs.

**castration** Removal of the sex glands. The term is ordinarily used to indicate removal of the male testicles.

**CAT scan** Computerized axial tomography (CAT) scanning uses a computer to generate cross-section views of a patient's anatomy. It can identify normal and abnormal structures, and can be used to guide procedures. CAT scanning is painless. Iodine-containing contrast material is sometimes used in CAT scanning. If you are allergic to iodine or contrast materials and are scheduled to have a CAT scan, you should notify your physician and the radiology staff of your allergy.

**cat scratch disease** See *benign lymphoreticulosis.*

**cat scratch fever** An infection caused by the Bartonella henslae bacteria. This bacteria is carried by almost half of all domestic cats, who can transmit it to humans through a scratch or bite. It causes swelling of the lymph nodes, which usually does not require treatment. In people with suppressed immune systems, cat scratch fever can progress to bacillary angiomatosis, a bacterial skin infection that can be treated with the antibiotics rifampin, ciprofloxacin, trimethoprim-sulfamethoxazole, and gentamicin.

**catabolism** See *metabolism*.

**catalepsy** The state of persisting in unusual postures or facial expressions, regardless of outside stimuli, as is seen in schizophrenia and some other diseases of the nervous system.

**catalyst** A substance that speeds up a chemical reaction but is not consumed or altered in the process. Catalysts are of immense importance in chemistry and biology. All enzymes are catalysts that expedite the biochemical reactions necessary for life. The enzymes in saliva, for example, accelerate the conversion of starch to glucose, doing in minutes what would otherwise take weeks.

**catamenia** See *menstruation*.

**cataract** A clouding or loss of transparency of the eye lens. There are many causes of cataracts, including aging, cortisone medication, trauma, diabetes, and other diseases. Cataracts will affect most people who live into old age. Symptoms include double or blurred vision, and sensitivity to light and glare. Cataracts can be diagnosed when the doctor examines the eyes with a viewing instrument. The ideal treatment for cataracts is surgical implantation of a new lens. Sunglasses can help to prevent cataracts.

**cataract surgery** Removal of the clouded (cataractous) lens in its entirety by surgery, and replacement of the lens with an intraocular lens (IOL) made of plastic. The typical cataract operation takes about an hour, requires local anesthesia only, and usually does not need hospitalization.

**cataract with poikiloderma atrophicans** See *Rothmund-Thomson syndrome*.

**catatonic** In a state of catalepsy. See *catalepsy*.

**cath** Medical shorthand for catheter.

**cathartic** A laxative.

**catheter** A thin, flexible tube.

**catheter, Foley** A flexible plastic tube inserted into the bladder to provide continuous urinary drainage. The Foley has a balloon on the bladder end. After the catheter is inserted in the bladder, the balloon is inflated with air or fluid so that the catheter cannot pull out, but is retained in the bladder as an indwelling catheter. Removal

is accomplished simply by deflating the balloon and slipping the catheter out.

**catheter, indwelling bladder** Any catheter inserted into the bladder that remains there to provide continuous urinary drainage. The principal type is the Foley catheter. See *catheter, Foley*.

**catheter, IV** A catheter placed in a vein to provide a pathway for drugs, nutrients, fluids, or blood products. Blood samples can also be withdrawn through the catheter.

**catheter, oximetry** A catheter used with monitoring equipment that can measure the amount of oxygenated hemoglobin in the bloodstream. See also *catheter, Swan-Ganz*.

**catheter, PA** A catheter that is inserted into the pulmonary artery.

**catheter, Swan-Ganz** A style of oximetry catheter that is inserted into a major vein under the collarbone or in the neck, threaded through the right side of the heart, and then threaded into the pulmonary artery. Doctors can use monitoring equipment with a Swan-Ganz catheter to measure blood pressure inside the heart, and to find out how much blood the heart is pumping.

**cauda equina** A bundle of spinal nerve roots that arise from the end of the spinal cord. The cauda equina comprises the roots of all the spinal nerves below the first lumbar (L1) vertebra in the lower back.

**cauda equina syndrome** Impairment of the nerves in the cauda equina, characterized by dull pain in the lower back and upper buttocks and lack of feeling (analgesia) in the buttocks, genitalia, and thigh, together with disturbances of bowel and bladder function.

**caudad** Toward the feet (or tail, in embryology), as opposed to cranial. See also *Appendix B, "Anatomic Orientation Terms."*

**caudal regression syndrome** A disorder characterized by dysfunction of the bowels, bladder, and legs. Infants with caudal regression syndrome are missing all or part of the sacrum, and may also have underdeveloped legs. About 20 percent are born to mothers with diabetes. Treatment is usually with surgery to correct these defects, as possible.

**caul** Folk term for the membranes that surround the fetus in the womb, and particularly for the presence of these membranes over the newborn infant's face or head at birth, a relatively common and usually harmless occurrence. In some cultures, the presence of a caul at birth is considered spiritually significant.

**cauliflower ear**   An acquired deformity of the external ear to which wrestlers and boxers are particularly vulnerable. The cause is damage from trauma. When trauma causes a blood clot (hematoma) under the skin of the ear, the clot disrupts the connection of the skin to the ear cartilage. The cartilage has no other blood supply except for the overlying skin, so if the skin is separated from the cartilage it is deprived of nutrients and dies. The ear cartilage then shrivels up to form the classic cauliflower ear, so named because the tissue resembles that lumpy vegetable's surface. Treatment for cauliflower ear begins by draining the blood clot through an incision in the ear. Then a compressive dressing is applied, to sandwich the two sides of the skin against the cartilage. When ear damage is treated promptly and aggressively, the cauliflower-ear deformity is unlikely. Delay in diagnosis leads to more difficulty in managing this problem, and can leave greater ear deformity.

**cauliflower-ear deformity**   Destruction of the underlying cartilage framework of the outer ear (pinnae), usually caused by either infection or trauma, resulting in a thickening of the ear. Classically, blood collects (hematoma) between the ear cartilage and the skin. There is a marked thickening of the entire ear, which may be so extensive that the shape of the ear becomes unrecognizable. The ear is said to look like a piece of cauliflower. See also *cauliflower ear*.

**causes of cancer**   See *cancer, causes*.

**cauterization**   The use of heat to destroy abnormal cells. Also called diathermy or electrodiathermy.

**cavernous sinus**   A large channel of venous blood creating a cavity (sinus) that is bordered by the sphenoid bone and the temporal bone of the skull. The cavernous sinus is an important structure because of its location and its contents, which include the third cranial (oculomotor) nerve, the fourth cranial (trochlear) nerve, parts 1 (the ophthalmic nerve) and 2 (the maxillary nerve) of the fifth cranial (trigeminal) nerve, and the sixth cranial (abducens) nerve.

**cavernous sinus syndrome**   A condition characterized by edema (swelling) of the eyelids and the conjunctivae of the eyes, and paralysis of the cranial nerves which course through the cavernous sinus. It is caused by a cavernous sinus thrombosis.

**cavernous sinus thrombosis**   A blood clot within the cavernous sinus A thrombosis in this key crossroads causes the cavernous sinus syndrome.

**cavities**   See *caries*.

**cavity, abdominal**   The cavity within the abdomen, the space between the abdominal wall and the spine. The abdominal cavity is hardly an empty space. It contains a number of crucial organs, including the lower part of the esophagus, the stomach, small intestine, colon, rectum, liver, gallbladder, pancreas, spleen, kidneys, and bladder.

**CBC**   Complete blood count. See *blood count, complete*.

**CBT**   Cognitive behavior therapy.

**CCD**   **1** Central core disease of muscle. **2** Cleidocranial dysostosis.

**CD4**   Transmembrane glycoprotein, which is expressed by T-4 cells (also known simply as T cells). See also *T cells, T-4 cells*.

**CD4 count, absolute**   See *T-4 count*.

**CD8**   Transmembrane glycoprotein expressed by T-4 cells. See also *T lymphocytes, cytotoxic; T-suppressor cells*.

**CDC**   The Centers for Disease Control and Prevention, the US agency charged with tracking and investigating public health trends. A part of the US Public Health Services (PHS) under the Department of Health and Human Services (HHS), the CDC is based in Atlanta, GA. It publishes key health information, including weekly data on all deaths and diseases reported in the United States ("Morbidity and Mortality Weekly Report") and travelers' health advisories. The CDC also fields special rapid-response teams to halt epidemic diseases.

**CDH**   Congenital dislocation of the hip. See *congenital hip dislocation*.

**cDNA**   Complementary DNA.

**CEA**   Carcinoembryonic antigen.

**CEA assay**   Blood test for heightened levels of carcinoembryonic antigen protein. See *carcinoembryonic antigen test*.

**cecal**   See *caecal*.

**Ceclor**   See *cefaclor*.

**cecum**   See *caecum*.

**Cedax**   See *ceftibutin*.

**cefaclor**   An antibiotic medication (brand name: Ceclor). Take on an empty stomach to ensure absorption. See also *cephalosporin antibiotics*.

**cefadroxil**   An antibiotic medication (brand name: Duricef). See also *cephalosporin antibiotics*.

**cefixime**  An antibiotic medication (brand name: Suprax). See also *cephalosporin antibiotics*.

**cefpodoxime proxetil**  An antibiotic medication (brand name: Vantin). Take with food for best results. See also *cephalosporin antibiotics*.

**cefprozil**  An antibiotic medication (brand name: Cefzil). See also *cephalosporin antibiotics*.

**ceftibutin**  An antibiotic medication (brand name: Cedax). Take on an empty stomach to ensure absorption. See also *cephalosporin antibiotics*.

**Ceftin**  See *cefuroxime axetil*.

**cefuroxime axetil**  An antibiotic medication (brand name: Ceftin). Take with food for best results. This drug can cause a false positive result on blood-sugar tests. See also *cephalosporin antibiotics*.

**Cefzil**  See *cefprozil*.

**celiac disease, adult**  See *celiac sprue*.

**celiac sprue**  An immune-system reaction to gluten, a protein found in wheat and related grains. Celiac sprue causes impaired absorption and digestion of nutrients through the small intestine. Symptoms include frequent diarrhea and weight loss. A skin condition called dermatitis herpetiformis can be associated with celiac sprue. The most accurate test for celiac sprue is a biopsy of the involved small bowel. Treatment is to avoid gluten in the diet; some people must also avoid milk products, which contain a similar protein. Medications are used for refractory (stubborn) sprue.

**cell**  The basic structural and functional unit in all living things. Each cell is a small container of chemicals and water wrapped in a membrane. There are 100 trillion cells in a human being, and each contains the entire human genome, all the genetic information necessary to build a human being. This information is encoded within the cell nucleus in 6 billion subunits of DNA called base pairs. These base pairs are packaged in 23 pairs of chromosomes, with 1 chromosome in each pair coming from each parent. Each of the 46 human chromosomes contains the DNA for thousands of individual genes, the units of heredity.

**cell cloning**  The process of producing a group of cells that are genetically identical (clones) to a single ancestral cell.

**cell cycle**  The sequence of events within the cell between mitotic (cell) divisions. The cell cycle is conventionally divided into five phases: G0 (G zero, the G standing for gap); G1, (G one, the first gap); S (synthesis phase, during which the DNA is synthesized, replicated); G2 (G two, the second gap); and M (mitosis). Cells that are not destined to divide again are considered to be in the G0 phase. The transition from G0 to G1 is thought to commit the cell to completing the cell cycle by dividing.

**cell, alpha**  See *alpha cell, pancreatic*.

**cell, beta**  See *beta cell, pancreatic*.

**cell, delta**  See *delta cell, pancreatic*.

**cells, germ**  The eggs and sperm, which are the reproductive cells. Each mature germ cell is haploid, in that it has a single set of 23 chromosomes containing half the usual amount of DNA and half the usual number of genes. This makes them notable exceptions to the usual rules governing chromosomes, genes, and DNA.

**cells, reproductive**  See *cells, germ*.

**cellulite**  Popular term for deposits of fat that have a cottage cheese–like texture. Medically, cellulite is not considered abnormal.

**Center for Information Technology**  See *National Institutes of Health*.

**Center for Scientific Review**  See *National Institutes of Health*.

**Centers for Disease Control and Prevention**  See *CDC*.

**centimorgan**  A unit of measure of genetic recombination frequency. One centimorgan is equal to a 1 percent chance that a marker at one genetic locus will be separated from a marker at another locus due to crossing over in a single generation. In humans, 1 centimorgan is equivalent, on average, to 1 million base pairs. Abbreviated as cM.

**central**  At or near the center.

**central auditory processing disorder**  A neurological disorder that makes it difficult to properly interpret sounds received by the ears, particularly the phonemes of speech. It can result in difficulties with attention, speech production, and reading. Abbreviated as CAPD.

**central core disease of muscle**  One of the conditions that produces "floppy baby" syndrome. Central core disease of muscle causes hypotonia (low muscle tone) in the newborn baby, slowly progressive muscle weakness, and muscle cramps after exercise. Muscle biopsy shows a key diagnostic finding of absent mitochondria in the center of many type I muscle fibers. It is caused by a gene on chromosome 19, involves ryanodine receptor-1, and is inherited as a dominant trait. Abbreviated as CCD.

**central line** An infusion tube located in or near the heart, which is at the center of the circulatory system. For example, a Swan-Ganz catheter with its tip in the right atrium and ventricle of the heart is a central line.

**central nervous system** That part of the nervous system that consists of the brain and spinal cord. Abbreviated as CNS, it is one of the two major divisions of the nervous system. The other is the peripheral nervous system (PNS), which is outside the brain and spinal cord. The peripheral nervous system connects the central nervous system to sensory organs, such as the eye and ear, and to other organs of the body, muscles, blood vessels, and glands.

**central nervous system, spongy degeneration of the** See *Canavan disease*.

**central vision** As a person reads, light is focused onto the macula in the center of his or her retina, the light-sensitive layer of tissue at the back of the eye. In this process of central vision, millions of cells change the light into nerve signals that tell the brain what the person is seeing. Thanks to this ability, humans are able to read, drive, and perform other activities that require fine, sharp, straight-ahead vision.

**centromere** The "waist" of the chromosome, which is essential for the division and retention of the chromosome in the cell. The centromere is a uniquely specialized region of the chromosome to which spindle fibers attach during cell division.

**CEPH** The Centre d'Etudes du Polymorphisme Humain, an internationally renowned research laboratory in Paris that provides the scientific community with resources for human genome mapping. Also known as the Fondation Jean Dausset-CEPH.

**cephal-** Prefix indicating the head.

**cephalexin** An antibiotic medication (brand name: Keflex). Take on an empty stomach to ensure absorption. See also *cephalosporin antibiotics*.

**cephalgia** Headache.

**cephalgia, histamine** See *cluster headache*.

**cephalosporin antibiotics** A group of over 20 antibiotic drugs (brand names include: Ceclor, Cedax, Ceftin, Cefzil, Duricef, Keflex, Keftab, Lorabid, Suprax, Vantin, Velosef) that are based on compounds originally isolated from the fungus Cephalosporium acremonium. They are given in pill, capsule, liquid, or injectable forms to treat bacterial infections. As with all antibiotics, cephalosporin antibiotics can affect gastrointestinal-tract function and can cause allergic reactions in some people. They may

interact with other antibiotics and with anticoagulant medications. See also *antibiotic*.

**cephalothoracic lipodystrophy** A disorder characterized by painless symmetrical diffuse deposits of fat beneath the skin of the neck, upper trunk, arms, and legs. The condition is thought to be genetic, although its exact mode of inheritance is uncertain—it may be a mitochondrial DNA disease. It frequently appears in association with alcoholic liver disease, macrocytic anemia ("low blood" with big red blood cells), and peripheral neuropathy (disease of the peripheral nervous system, as opposed to the brain and spinal cord). The peripheral neuropathy has often been laid to alcoholism, but the neuropathy is likely an integral part of the syndrome. This disorder affects mainly men, and is more frequent in the Mediterranean area than elsewhere. Also known as multiple symmetrical lipomatosis, Launois-Bensaude syndrome, and Madelung disease.

**cerclage** Encirclement with a ring, loop, wire, or ligature. Cerclage can be done around bone fragments to hold them together, but it usually refers to an operation performed on the cervix.

**cerebellum** The portion of the brain in the back of the head, between the cerebrum and the brain stem. It is involved in the control of voluntary and involuntary movement.

**cerebral** Of or pertaining to the brain or skull cavity.

**cerebral aneurysm** See *aneurysm, brain*.

**cerebral calcification, nonarteriosclerotic** A genetic, inherited neurological disorder characterized by abnormal deposits of calcium in certain of areas of the brain, including the basal ganglia and the cerebral cortex. Symptoms may include motor function deterioration, dementia, mental retardation, spastic paralysis, dyspraxia of speech (poorly articulated speech), spasticity (stiffness of the limbs), eye problems, and athetosis (involuntary, writhing movements). Features of Parkinson disease, such as tremors, rigidity, a mask-like facial appearance, shuffling gait, and a "pill-rolling" motion of the fingers may also occur in individuals with this syndrome. Other symptoms may include dystonia (disordered muscle tone), chorea (involuntary, rapid, jerky movements), and seizures. Onset of the disorder may occur at any time from childhood to adulthood. The syndrome thus involves abnormalities of the neurological system; skull (microcephaly); eyes (glaucoma, optic nerve atrophy retinitis pigmentosa); and a significant hormone problem, hypoparathyroidism (underactivity of the parathyroid gland, which regulates calcium). The disease is inherited as an autosomal recessive trait, in which both parents carry the gene and each of their children stands a one in four risk of receiving both genes and therefore having the disease. There is no cure for nonarteriosclerotic cerebral calcification, nor is there a standard course of treatment. Treatment is directed toward minimizing symptoms. The prognosis for patients is poor. Progressive neurological deterioration generally results in disability and death. Also known as Fahr syndrome, Fahr disease, striopallidodentate calcinosis, SPD calcinosis, and cerebrovascular ferrocalcinosis.

**cerebral fornix**  An arching fibrous band in the brain, connecting the two lobes of the cerebrum. There are two such bands, each of which is an arched tract of nerves.

**cerebral hemispheres**  The two halves of the cerebrum, the largest part of the brain.

**cerebral palsy**  A syndrome of weakness, spasticity, poor coordination of the limbs and other muscles, impaired sensory perception, and sometimes impaired intelligence. The cause of cerebral palsy is not always known, although many cases are linked with lack of oxygen during birth. Treatment may include casting and braces to prevent further loss of limb function, speech therapy, physical therapy, occupational therapy, the use of augmentative communication devices, and the use of medications or botulism toxin (botox) injections to treat spasticity.

**cerebral ventricle**  One of a system of four communicating cavities within the brain that are continuous with the central canal of the spinal cord. They include two lateral ventricles in the cerebral hemispheres, each consisting of a triangular central body and four horns. The lateral ventricles communicate with the third ventricle through an opening called the interventricular foramen. The third ventricle, a median (midline) cavity in the brain, is bounded by the thalamus and hypothalamus on either side. In front, the third ventricle communicates with the lateral ventricles, and in back it communicates with the aqueduct of the midbrain, also called the aqueduct of Sylvius. The fourth ventricle, which is the lowest of the four ventricles of the brain, extends from the aqueduct of the midbrain to the central canal of the upper end of the spinal cord, with which it communicates by the two foramina of Luschka and the foramen of Magendie. The ventricles are filled with cerebrospinal fluid.

**cerebritis**  Inflammation of the brain.

**cerebrospinal fluid**  A watery fluid, continuously produced and absorbed, which flows in the ventricles within the brain and around the surface of the brain and spinal cord. Abbreviated as CSF, this fluid is produced by the choroid plexus, a series of infolded blood vessels

projecting into the cerebral ventricles, and it is absorbed into the venous system. If production exceeds absorption, CSF pressure rises and the result is hydrocephalus. This can also occur if the CSF pathways are obstructed, causing the fluid to accumulate.

**cerebrovascular accident**  A stroke: the sudden death of brain cells due to lack of oxygen, caused by blockage of blood flow or rupture of an artery to the brain. Sudden weakness or paralysis of one side of the body can be a symptom. A suspected stroke can be confirmed by scanning the brain with special X-ray tests, such as CAT scanning. Prevention involves minimizing risk factors, such as by controlling high blood pressure and diabetes.

**cerebrovascular accident prevention**  See *stroke prevention*.

**cerebrovascular ferrocalcinosis**  See *cerebral calcification, nonarteriosclerotic*.

**cerebrum**  The largest part of the brain, it is divided into two hemispheres, or halves. The left and right hemispheres are connected by two arching bands of nerves. See also *cerebral fornix*.

**cervical**  Having to do with any kind of neck, including the neck upon which the head is perched and the neck of the uterus.

**cervical cancer**  See *cancer, cervical*.

**cervical cap**  A specially fitted contraceptive device that bars the entry of sperm into the cervix. For best results, the cervical cap customarily is used with spermicidal gel or cream. See also *birth control, contraceptive*.

**cervical cerclage**  Encircling a cervix that is abnormally liable to dilate (an incompetent cervix) with a ring or loop to prevent a miscarriage.

**cervical dystocia**  Difficult labor and delivery caused by mechanical obstruction at the cervix.

**cervical intraepithelial neoplasia**  A general term for the growth of abnormal cells on the surface of the cervix. Numbers from one to three may be used to describe how much of the cervix contains abnormal cells. Abbreviated as CIN.

**cervical rib**  See *rib, cervical*.

**cervical vertebra, first**  See *atlas, C1*.

**cervical vertebra, second**  See *axis, C2*.

**cervical vertebrae**  The upper seven vertebrae in the spinal column, which make up the neck. They are designated C1 through C7, from the top down. See *C1 through C7*.

**cervicitis** Inflammation of the cervix.

**cervix** The lower, narrow part of the uterus. The cervix forms a canal that opens from the uterus into the vagina. Its inner surface is covered with mucus. During ovulation, this mucus is specially adapted to speed sperm to the egg. Normally very small, the cervix dilates during birth to permit the newborn's head to emerge.

**cervix, incompetent** A cervix that is abnormally liable to dilate, and so may not be able to keep the fetus from being spontaneously aborted (miscarried).

**Cesarian section** See *Caesarian section*.

**Chagas disease** A disease caused by the parasite Trypanosoma cruzi. The parasite can be transmitted through bites from bugs that carry it, via blood transfusion, or by crossing the placenta during pregnancy to affect the fetus. Also known as American trypanosomiasis. See also *kissing bugs*.

**chalazion** See *cyst, Meibomian*.

**CHAMPUS** Civilian Health and Medical Program of the Uniformed Services. CHAMPUS is a federally funded health program that provides beneficiaries with medical care supplemental to that available in US military and Public Health Service facilities. All CHAMPUS beneficiaries move over to Medicare at age 65. CHAMPUS is like Medicare in that the government contracts with private parties to administer the program. Recently revamped as a managed-care system and renamed TRICARE, but still widely known under its old moniker.

**chancre** The classic nonpainful ulcer of syphilis. The chancre forms in the first (primary) stage of syphilis, is highly contagious, and can last from one to five weeks. The disease can be transmitted from any contact with a chancre, which is teeming with spirochetes. If the ulcer is outside of the vagina or on the scrotum of the male, the use of condoms may not help in preventing transmission of the disease. Likewise, if the ulcer is in the mouth, merely kissing the infected individual can spread syphilis. See also *syphilis*.

**change of life** See *menopause*.

**charbon** See *anthrax*.

**Charcot-Marie-Tooth disease** An inherited neurological disease characterized by increasing and debilitating weakness, including that of the limbs and hands. Physical therapy can help to prevent the wasting of limbs often seen in Charcot-Marie-Tooth. Abbreviated as CMT.

**chart, Snellen's** The familiar eye chart used to measure how well you see at various distances. Snellen's chart is imprinted with block letters that decrease in size line by line, corresponding to the distance at which that line of letters is normally visible. The letters on Snellen's chart are, not surprisingly, called Snellen's test type. Each block letter is quite scientific in design, so that at the appropriate distance the letter subtends a visual angle of 5 degrees, and each component part subtends an angle of 1 minute.

**chemical menopause** See *menopause, induced*.

**chemical reaction** A process in which one substance is transformed into another.

**chemokine** One of a big group of proteins that act as lures, and were first found attracting white blood cells. The chemokines are involved in several forms of acute and chronic inflammation, infectious diseases, and cancer.

**chemokine receptor** A molecule that receives a chemokine and a chemokine dock. Several chemokine receptors are essential coreceptors for the HIV virus.

**chemoprevention** The use of natural or laboratory-made substances to prevent cancer.

**chemotherapy** Treatment with drugs to kill cancer cells. Most anticancer drugs are injected into a vein or a muscle. Some are given by mouth. Chemotherapy is systemic treatment, meaning that the drugs flow through the bloodstream to nearly every part of the body. Often, patients who need many doses of IV chemotherapy receive the drugs through a catheter. One end of the catheter is placed in a large vein in the chest, while the other end is outside the body or attached to a small device just under the skin. This can make chemotherapy more comfortable for the patient. Patients and their families are shown how to care for the catheter and keep it clean. For some types of cancer, doctors are studying whether it helps to put anticancer drugs directly into the affected area. Chemotherapy is generally given in cycles: a treatment period is followed by a recovery period, then another treatment period, and so on. Usually a patient has chemotherapy as an outpatient at the hospital, at the doctor's office, or at home. However, depending on which drugs are given and the patient's general health, the patient may need to stay in the hospital for a short time. The side effects of chemotherapy depend mainly on the drugs and doses the patient receives. Generally, anticancer drugs affect cells that divide rapidly, including blood cells, which fight infection, help the blood to clot, and carry oxygen to all parts of the body. When blood cells are affected by anticancer drugs, patients are more likely to develop infections, may bruise or bleed easily, and may have less energy. Cells that line the digestive tract also divide rapidly. As a result of chemotherapy, patients can have such side effects as loss of appetite, nausea and vomiting, hair loss, or mouth sores. For some patients, medicines can be prescribed to help with side effects, especially with nausea and vomiting. Usually these side effects gradually go away during the recovery period or after treatment stops. Hair loss, another side effect of chemotherapy, is a concern for many patients. Some chemotherapy drugs only cause the hair to thin out, while others may result in the loss of all body hair. Patients may feel better if they decide, before starting treatment, how to handle hair loss. In some men and women, chemotherapy drugs may result in a loss of the ability to have children. Loss of fertility can be temporary or permanent, depending on the drugs used and the patient's age. For men, sperm banking before treatment may be a choice; women may choose to have eggs extracted and stored. Women's menstrual periods may stop, and they may have hot flashes and vaginal dryness due to induced menopause. Periods are more likely to return in young women. In some cases, bone-marrow transplantation and peripheral stem-cell support are used to replace tissue that forms blood cells, when that tissue has been destroyed by the effects of chemotherapy or radiation therapy. See also *adjuvant chemotherapy, cancer.*

**chemotherapy, adjuvant** See *adjuvant chemotherapy.*

**cherubism** A familial (genetic) disorder of childhood that leads to prominence of the lower face and an appearance reminiscent of the cherubs portrayed in Renaissance art. Cherubism is due to a problem in bone formation that is largely limited to the upper and lower jaws (the maxilla and mandible), with loss of bone in the jaws and its replacement by excessive amounts of fibrous tissue. These abnormalities often resolve after puberty. Cherubism is inherited as an autosomal dominant condition. Most boys and girls with it have a parent who had cherubism; the few children with cherubism without a family history are thought to have a new mutation for cherubism. The gene responsible for cherubism has been localized to chromosome 4, specifically in band 4p16.

**chest film** See *chest X-ray.*

**chest pain** The many causes for chest pain include angina, heart attack (coronary occlusion), and other important diseases. Do not try to ignore chest pain and "work through it." Chest pain is a warning to seek medical attention.

**chest X-ray** A type of X-ray commonly used to detect abnormalities in the lungs. It can also detect abnormalities in the heart, aorta, and the bones of the thoracic area. Metallic objects, such as jewelry, are removed from the chest and neck areas for a chest X-ray to avoid interference with X-ray penetration and improve accuracy of the interpretation.

**chicken pox** A highly infectious viral disease, chicken pox is known medically as varicella. It is caused by herpes zoster, a member of the herpes family of viruses. Chicken pox has nothing to do with chicken: the name originated to distinguish this mild pox from smallpox (chicken being used, as in chickenhearted, to mean weak or timid). Chicken pox is no major matter unless it occurs in an immunodeficient person or the pox become infected with bacteria through scratching. Treatment, other than the use of calamine lotion or other topical solutions to diminish itching, is not normally necessary. However, adults (and sometimes children) can have major problems from chicken pox, including pneumonia and encephalitis (inflammation of the brain) leading to difficulty with balance and coordination (cerebellar ataxia). Other serious complications can include ear infections, damaged nerves (palsies), and Reye syndrome, a potentially fatal complication. In such cases, antiviral medications may be tried. Reactivation of the chicken pox virus is responsible for shingles. The current aim in the US is to achieve universal immunization of children with the chicken pox vaccine. See also *chicken pox immunization; herpes zoster; neuralgia, postherpetic; shingles.*

**chicken pox immunization** This vaccine prevents the common disease known as chicken pox. The vaccination requires only one shot, given at about one year of age. If an older person has not had chicken pox, the shot may be given at any time. There have been few significant reactions to the chicken pox vaccine. All children, except those with a compromised immune system or a known neurological condition, should have the vaccination. See also *chicken pox.*

**chicken pox rash** The rash that characterizes chicken pox, which develops in crops. Raised red spots arrive first, progressing to blisters that burst to create open sores before crusting over. This process usually starts on the scalp, then the trunk (its area of greatest concentration), and finally the arms and legs. Any area of skin that is irritated (by diaper rash, eczema, sunburn, and so on) is likely to be hard-hit by the rash. The rash is typically very itchy. In rare cases, a person may have chicken pox without the rash. See also *chicken pox.*

**chilblains** A form of cold injuries that may go along with trench foot and frostbite. Cold injuries occur with and without freezing of body tissues. The young and the elderly are especially prone to cold injuries, and alcohol use increases their risk. It is important not to thaw an extremity if there is a risk of it refreezing. Chilblains can lead to loss of body parts, and even to death.

**child abuse** A complex set of behaviors that include child neglect and the physical, emotional, and sexual abuse of children. Although most people think first of physical abuse when they hear the term, physical abuse makes up only 25 percent of reported cases. It is defined as physical injury inflicted upon the child with cruel and/or malicious intent, although the law recognizes that in some cases the parent or caretaker may not have intended to hurt the child; rather, the injury may have resulted from excess discipline or physical punishment. Physical abuse includes punching, beating, kicking, biting, burning, shaking, or otherwise harming a child. Fatal injuries from maltreatment can result from many different acts. Such injuries include severe head trauma, shaken baby syndrome, trauma to the abdomen or chest, scalding, burns, drowning, suffocation, poisoning, and so on. Many physically abused children suffer multiple injuries over the years; they may go untreated to cover up for the abuse. Factors that may predispose a caregiver to child abuse include:

- The abuser's childhood. Child abusers often were abused as children.

- Substance abuse. At least half of all child-abuse cases involve some degree of alcohol or drug abuse by the caregiver.

- Family stress, particularly if it erupts in spousal abuse. Stress is exacerbated if caregivers do not have outside resources to turn to for help.

- The child. Children at higher risk for child abuse include infants who are felt to be overly fussy, handicapped children, and children with chronic diseases.

- Specific trigger events. Events that occur just before many fatal parental assaults on infants and young children include an infant's inconsolable crying, feeding difficulties, a toddler's failed toilet training, and exaggerated parental perceptions of acts of "disobedience" by the child.

- Social forces. Experts debate whether a postulated reduction in religious/moral values coupled with an increase in the depiction of violence by the entertainment and informational media may increase child abuse. Statistically, this seems unlikely, as acts now generally thought of as child abuse were both legal and accepted in past times.

Child abuse should always be reported, investigated, and stopped. Along with medical care for any physical injury, treatment possibilities include parenting classes; helping caregivers access support from professionals and the community; home visits from a nurse, social worker, or other professional to reinforce good parenting skills and monitor the child's well-being; and in cases where these measures fail, temporary or permanent removal of the child from the home. Education is key, because many

incidents of physical abuse are accidental, or occur because parents have not learned effective nonphysical methods of discipline. The best strategy is to prevent child abuse. It's important to note that children were not even granted the same legal status as domesticated animals in regards to protection against cruelty and neglect until the 19th century. In 1962 the term "battered child syndrome" entered medicine. By 1976 all states in the US had adopted laws mandating the reporting of suspected instances of child abuse by health professionals, teachers, and others. See also *child abuse, emotional; child abuse, sexual; child neglect*.

**child abuse, emotional** The third most frequently reported form of child abuse, accounting for 17 percent of reported cases. It is likely that emotional child abuse is greatly underreported, since it can be difficult to detect and document. It includes acts or omissions by the parents or other caregivers that could cause serious behavioral or emotional disorders. In some instances of emotional child abuse, these acts alone, without any harm yet evident in the child's behavior or condition, are sufficient to warrant the intervention of child protective services. For example, the parents/caregivers may use extreme or bizarre forms of punishment, such as confinement of a child in a dark closet. Emotional child abuse is also sometimes termed psychological child abuse, verbal child abuse, or mental injury of a child.

**child abuse, psychological** See *child abuse, emotional*.

**child abuse, sexual** The least frequently reported form of child abuse, sexual abuse is believed to be the most underreported type of child maltreatment. Sexual abuse includes fondling a child's genitals, intercourse, incest, rape, sodomy, exhibitionism, and commercial exploitation through prostitution or the production of pornographic materials. Most cases of child sexual abuse involve parents, relatives, or other adults that the child knows well. Sexual abuse committed by strangers, in daycare centers, or in schools is comparatively rare. Diagnosis and treatment of sexual child abuse is complex. Diagnosis involves a thorough, nonjudgmental history of the immediate events, as well as a review of potential similar experiences. This history is often independently done by a physician, a social worker, and the police department to ensure accuracy. A complete physical exam of the child may include taking photographs to document sexual abuse, X-rays, and laboratory tests. Treatment of offenders depends on the situation. In most proven cases, conviction results in imprisonment. Psychiatric treatment, counseling, and reeducation should be provided to all offenders, whether in or out of prison. Pedophiles (people who prefer sex with children) require intense psychological and pharmacological therapy prior to release into the community, because of the high rate of repeat offenders. Although some offenders can be successfully treated, truly effective treatment has not yet been found for pedophilia. As with all forms of child abuse, prevention is the best policy. Home and school programs that teach recognition of "good touch" and "bad touch" can provide a forum for helping children avoid potentially harmful scenarios. Parents should also be aware of the behavior of other adults in their children's lives, and choose licensed day-care centers and schools that have an open-door policy regarding parental visitation. See also *pedophilia.*

**child abuse, verbal**   See *child abuse, emotional.*

**child health**   Child health is the purview of pediatrics, which became a medical specialty in the mid-19th century. Before that time the care and treatment of childhood diseases were included within such areas as general medicine, obstetrics, and midwifery.

**Child Health and Human Development, National Institute of**   See *National Institutes of Health.*

**child injury, mental**   See *child abuse, emotional.*

**child neglect**   The most frequently reported form of child abuse, child neglect is defined as the failure to provide for the shelter, safety, supervision, and/or nutritional needs of a child. Child neglect can include physical, educational, or emotional neglect. Physical neglect includes refusal of or delay in seeking health care, abandonment, expulsion from the home or refusal to allow a runaway to return home, and inadequate supervision. Educational neglect includes the allowance of chronic truancy, failure to enroll a child of mandatory school age in school, and failure to attend to a special educational need. Emotional neglect includes such actions as marked inattention to the child's needs for affection, refusal of or failure to provide needed psychological care, spouse abuse in the child's presence, and permitting drug or alcohol use by the child.

**childbed fever**   Fever due to an infection after childbirth, usually of the placental site within the uterus. If the infection involves the bloodstream, it constitutes puerperal sepsis. Childbed fever was once a common cause of death for women of childbearing age, but is now comparatively rare in the developed world due to improved sanitary practices in midwifery and obstetrics. Also known as childbirth fever or puerperal fever.

**childbirth**   See *labor.*

**childbirth fever**   See *childbed fever.*

**childhood disintegrative disorder**   A late-onset and particularly virulent form of autism, marked by loss of normal childhood skills and a rapidly declining prognosis. The cause is unknown, but seizure activity has been suspected. In some cases, the use of antiepileptic medications halts or slows the progress of symptoms. See also *autism, developmental disorder.*

**childhood schizophrenia**   See *schizophrenia, childhood.* See also *autism.*

**children's immunizations**   In the US, it is currently recommended that all children receive vaccination against:

Hepatitis B

Diphtheria, tetanus, pertussis (as separate vaccinations, or in combination as the DPT)

Haemophilus influenzae type B (HIB)

Poliovirus

Measles, mumps, rubella (as separate vaccination or in combination as the MMR)

Varicella zoster virus (chicken pox)

Every child in the US should have these vaccinations except when there are special circumstances, such as a compromised immune system or a neurological disorder.

**chimera**   1 An imaginary monster made up of incongruous parts. 2 In medicine, a person composed of two genetically distinct types of cells. This may be due to the fusion of two embryos at a very early (blastula) stage. More commonly today, the formation of a chimera is due to transplantation. When bone marrow from one person is used to reconstitute the bone marrow of an irradiated recipient, the recipient becomes a chimera. 3 A viral, bacterial, or other cell that seems to be composed of two genetically distinct strains, as might be seen when genetic engineering techniques are used to enclose therapeutic properties from one cell in another type of cell for delivery.

**chiropractic**   A system of diagnosis and treatment based on the concept that the nervous system coordinates all of the body's functions, and that disease results from a lack of normal nerve function. Chiropractic employs manipulation and adjustment of body structures, such as the spinal column, so that pressure on nerves coming from the spinal cord due to displacement (subluxation) of a vertebral body may be relieved. Practitioners believe that misalignment and nerve pressure can cause problems not only in the local area, but also at some distance from it. Chiropractic treatment appears to be effective for muscle spasms of the back and neck, tension headaches, and some sorts of leg pain. It may or may not be useful for other ailments. Some chiropractors also recommend other forms of treatment, such as massage, diet changes, vitamins and minerals, or herbal supplements. See also *chiropractor.*

**chiropractor** Someone who practices chiropractic treatment. Becoming a doctor of chiropractic (DC) requires a minimum of two years of college and four years in a school of chiropractic medicine. Some chiropractors also earn a traditional medical degree (MD) or other additional qualifications. Not all chiropractors are alike in their practice. The International Chiropractors Association believes that patients should be treated by spinal manipulation alone, whereas the American Chiropractors Association advocates a multidisciplinary approach that combines spinal adjustment with other modalities, such as physical therapy, psychological counseling, and dietary measures.

**chlamydia** An infectious type of bacteria that may be found in the cervix, urethra, throat, or rectum. It is destructive to the Fallopian tubes that transport eggs from a woman's ovary to the womb, and can cause infertility, tubal pregnancy, and severe pelvic infection. Because it is common for infected women to have no symptoms, chlamydia is often untreated. Chlamydia is also associated with an increased incidence of preterm births. The infant can also acquire the disease during passage through the birth canal, leading to eye involvement or pneumonia. For this reason, almost all newborns in the US are treated with antibiotic eye drops after birth.

**chloroform** A clear, volatile liquid with a strong smell similar to that of ether, chloroform was once administered by inhalation to produce anesthesia, given to relieve pain, and used as a remedy for cough. It is quite toxic to the kidney and the liver.

**choking** Partial or complete obstruction of the airway, usually due to the presence of food, a bead, a toy, or another foreign body in the upper throat or trachea. See also *airway obstruction.*

**cholangitis, primary sclerosing** See *primary sclerosing cholangitis.*

**cholangitis, sclerosing** See *primary sclerosing cholangitis.*

**cholecystitis** Inflammation of the gallbladder, a complication that can occur when gallstones are formed by the combination of cholesterol and the bilirubin pigment found in bile. Cholecystitis is frequently associated with infection in the gallbladder. The most common symptom is pain in the upper abdomen, although some patients have no symptoms. Diagnosis is usually made with ultrasound of the abdomen. Surgery (standard or laparoscopic) is considered for patients with cholecystitis,

although in some cases medication may be used instead to treat the infection and/or inflammation, and to dissolve the gallstones.

**cholera** A devastating disease characterized by intense vomiting and profuse watery diarrhea, rapidly leading to dehydration and often death. Cholera is caused by infection with the bacteria *Vibrio cholerae,* which may be transmitted via infected fecal matter, food, or water. Thanks to modern sanitary practices it is no longer as common as it once was, but epidemics of cholera still occur whenever people must live in crowded and unsanitary conditions, such as in refugee camps. The disease is treated by IV administration of saline solution, with antibiotics to kill the bacteria. Cholera has also been known as Asian cholera, due to its one-time prevalence in that area of the world.

**cholescintigraphy** A diagnostic test in which a twodimensional picture of a radiation source in the biliary system is obtained by the use of radioisotopes. Cholescintigraphy is done by nuclear medicine physicians to examine the biliary system and diagnose obstruction of the bile ducts (for example, by a gallstone or a tumor), disease of the gallbladder, and bile leaks. For cholescintigraphy, a radioactive chemical is injected intravenously. The chemical is removed from the blood by the liver, and secreted into the bile that the liver makes. The chemical then goes everywhere the bile goes—into the bile ducts, the gallbladder, and the intestine. By placing a radiation-sensitive camera over the patient's abdomen, a "picture" of the liver, bile ducts, and gallbladder may be obtained that corresponds to where the radioactive bile has migrated.

**cholestasis with peripheral pulmonary stenosis** See *Alagille syndrome.*

**cholesterol** The most common type of steroid in the body, cholesterol has gotten something of a bad name. However, this critically important molecule is essential to the formation of bile acids, which aid in the digestion of fats; vitamin D; progesterone; estrogens (estradiol, estrone, estriol); androgens (androsterone, testosterone); mineralocorticoid hormones (aldosterone, corticosterone); and glucocorticoid hormones (cortisol). Cholesterol is also necessary to the normal permeability and function of the membranes that surround cells. Cholesterol is carried in the bloodstream as lipoproteins. A diet high in saturated fats tends to increase blood cholesterol levels, whereas a diet high in unsaturated fats tends to lower blood cholesterol levels. Although some cholesterol is obtained from the diet, most cholesterol is made in the liver and other tissues. The treatment of elevated cholesterol therefore involves not only diet but also weight loss, regular exercise, and occasionally medications. After the age of 20, cholesterol testing is recommended every five years.

**cholesterol, "bad"** See *cholesterol, low-density lipoprotein.*

**cholesterol, "good"** See *cholesterol, high-density lipoprotein.*

**cholesterol, HDL** See *cholesterol, high-density lipoprotein.*

**cholesterol, high-density lipoprotein** Abbreviated as HDL, high-density lipoprotein cholesterol is the "good" cholesterol, since high HDL levels are associated with less coronary disease. Lipoproteins, which are combinations of fats (lipids) and proteins, are the form in which lipids are transported in the blood. The high-density lipoproteins transport cholesterol from the tissues of the body to the liver, so it can be gotten rid of in the bile.

**cholesterol, LDL** See *cholesterol, low-density lipoprotein.*

**cholesterol, low-density lipoprotein** Abbreviated as LDL, low-density lipoprotein cholesterol is called the "bad" cholesterol, because elevated LDL levels are associated with an increased risk of heart disease. Lipoproteins, which are combinations of fats (lipids) and proteins, are the form in which lipids are transported in the blood. The low-density lipoproteins transport cholesterol from the liver to the tissues of the body.

**cholesterol, lowering with fibrates** The fibrates are cholesterol-lowering drugs that are primarily effective in lowering triglycerides and, to a lesser extent, in increasing HDL-cholesterol levels. Gemfibrozil (brand name: Lopid), the fibrate most widely used in the US, can be very effective for patients with high triglyceride levels. However, it is not particularly effective for lowering LDL cholesterol. As a result, it is used less often than other drugs in patients with heart disease for whom LDL-cholesterol lowering is the main goal of treatment. The FDA does not recommend gemfibrozil therapy by itself for patients with heart disease. Fibrates are usually given in two daily doses, 30 minutes before the morning and evening meals. If treatment is successful, reductions in triglycerides will be in the range of 20 to 50 percent, with increases in HDL cholesterol of 10 to 15 percent. Fibrates are well tolerated by most patients. Gastrointestinal complaints are the most common side effect, and fibrates appear to increase the likelihood of a patient's developing cholesterol gallstones. Fibrates can increase the effect of medications that thin the blood; this increased effectiveness should be monitored by your physician.

**cholesterol, lowering with niacin** Niacin, also known as nicotinic acid, is a water-soluble B vitamin that improves levels of all lipoproteins when given in doses well above the vitamin requirement. Niacin lowers the total cholesterol, LDL cholesterol, and triglyceride levels, while raising the HDL cholesterol level. Niacin can reduce LDL levels by 10 to 20 percent, lower triglyceride levels by 20 to 50 percent, and raise HDL levels by 15 to 35 percent. Most experts recommend starting with the immediate-release form of niacin, which is also available in a timed-release formulation. Discuss with your doctor which type is best for you. Niacin is inexpensive and widely accessible to patients without a prescription, but because of potential side effects must not be used for cholesterol-lowering without being monitored by a physician. Patients are usually started on a low daily dose, which gradually is increased to an average daily dose of 1.5 to 3 grams. A common and troublesome side effect of niacin is flushing or hot flashes, which are the result of the widening of blood vessels. Most patients develop a tolerance for flushing, and in some patients it can be decreased by taking the drug during or after meals, or by the use of aspirin or other similar medications prescribed by your doctor. "No-flush" niacin formulations are also available. The effect of high blood–pressure medicines may also be increased while you are on niacin. If you are taking high blood–pressure medication, it is important to set up a blood pressure monitoring system while you are getting used to your new niacin regimen. A variety of gastrointestinal symptoms, including nausea, indigestion, gas, vomiting, diarrhea, and the activation of peptic ulcers have been seen in some patients who use niacin. Three other major adverse effects include liver problems, gout, and high blood sugar. Risk of these complications increases as the dose of niacin increases. Your doctor will probably not prescribe this medicine for you if you have diabetes, because of its effect on blood sugar. Nicotinamide, another form of niacin, does not lower cholesterol levels.

**chondromalacia patella** See *patellofemoral syndrome.*

**chondroplasia** The formation of cartilage by specialized cells called chondrocytes.

**chondrosarcoma** A cancer that forms in cartilage. See also *sarcoma.*

**chorda tympani** A branch of the facial nerve (the seventh cranial nerve) that serves the taste buds in the front of the tongue, runs through the middle ear, and carries taste messages to the brain. The chorda tympani is part of one of three cranial nerves involved in taste. The taste system involves a complicated feedback loop, with each nerve acting to inhibit the signals of others. The chorda tympani appears to exert a particularly strong inhibitory influence on other taste nerves, as well as on pain fibers in the tongue. When the chorda tympani is damaged, its inhibitory function is disrupted, leading to less inhibited activity in the other nerves.

**chordae tendineae**   Thread-like bands of fibrous tissue that attach on one end to the edges of the tricuspid and mitral valves of the heart, and on the other end to the papillary muscles within the heart that serve to anchor the valves.

**chordoma**   A form of bone cancer that usually starts in the lower spinal column. See also *sarcoma*.

**chorea**   Restless, wiggling, turning movements, often of the feet and hands only, although they can extend to other parts of the body. See also *Huntington disease, Sydenham chorea*.

**chorea, Huntington**   See *Huntington disease*.

**chorea, Sydenham**   See *Sydenham chorea*.

**choreaform movements**   Movements like those seen in chorea disorders.

**chorioangioma, placental**   A benign tumor of a blood vessel in the placenta (afterbirth). Large chorioangiomas can cause complications, including excess amniotic fluid (polyhydramnios), maternal and fetal clotting problems (coagulopathies), premature delivery, toxemia, fetal heart failure, and hydrops (excess fluid) affecting the fetus. Chorioangiomas probably act as peripheral shunts between arteries and veins (arteriovenous shunts), leading to progressive heart failure of the fetus. Labor is usually induced once the fetus is viable. Fetal blood transfusion has also been used in fetuses found to be anemic. Alcohol injection into the placental chorioangioma is being tried as a new method of treatment.

**chorion**   The outermost of the two fetal membranes (the amnion is the innermost) that surround the embryo. The chorion develops villi (vascular fingers) and give rise to the placenta.

**chorionic gonadotropin, human**   See *human chorionic gonadotropin*.

**chorionic villus sampling**   A procedure used between the eighth and tenth weeks of pregnancy to diagnose conditions present in the fetus before birth. Tissue is withdrawn from the villi of the chorion, a part of the placenta. Abbreviated as CVS.

**choroiditis**   An inflammation of the layer of the eye behind the retina, either in its entirely (multifocal choroiditis) or in patches (focal choroiditis). Usually the only symptom is blurred vision. See also *uveitis*.

**chromatids**   The daughter strands of a duplicated chromosome joined together by a centromere.

**chromatography, gas**   An automated technique for separating mixtures of substances in which the mixture to be analyzed is vaporized and carried by an inert gas through a special column, and thence to a detection device. The special column can contain an inert porous solid (gas-solid chromatography) or a liquid coated on a solid support (gas-liquid chromatography). The basic aim is to separate each component that was in the mixture so that it produces a different peak in the detection device output, which is graphed on a chart recorder. Gas chromotography is a valuable tool in biochemistry. Abbreviated as GC.

**chromosome**   One of the microscopic, thread-like structures found within every cell nucleus. Chromosomes carry all of an individual's genetic material. All human chromosomes have two arms, the p (short) arm and the q (long) arm. They are separated from each other only by a primary constriction, the centromere, the point at which the chromosome is attached to the spindle during cell division. Each chromosome has a helix structure made of a double strand of DNA and protein, with the genes that carry the genetic code arranged in order along its length. The genes provide instructions for building new individuals, including coding for everything from organ formation to gender to hair color.

**chromosome complement**   The whole set of chromosomes for the species. In humans, the chromosome complement (also called the karyotype) consists of 46 chromosomes, including the two sex chromosomes.

**chromosome disorder**   An abnormal condition due to a difference in the individual's chromosomes. For example, Down syndrome is a chromosome disorder caused by the presence of three copies of chromosome 21 instead of two.

**chromosome inversion**   A condition in which a chromosome segment is clipped out, turned upside down, and reinserted back into the chromosome. A chromosome inversion can be inherited from one or both parents, or may be a mutation that appears for the first time in a child. An inversion can be "balanced," meaning that it has all the genes present in the normal, uninverted chromosome; or it can be "unbalanced," meaning that genes have been deleted (lost) or duplicated. A balanced inversion causes no problems. An unbalanced inversion is often associated with problems such as development delay, mental retardation, and multiple birth defects. Inversions can also be acquired in a body cell, and in such cases may be a step toward involving that cell in a precancerous process.

**chromosome inversion, paracentric**   A basic type of chromosome rearrangement. A segment that does not include the centromere (and so is paracentric) has been snipped out of a chromosome, inverted, and inserted right back into its original location in the chromosome. The feature that makes it paracentic is that both breaks are on the same side of the centromere, so that the centromere is not affected.

**chromosome inversion, pericentric**   A basic type of chromosome rearrangement in which a segment that includes the centromere (and so is pericentric) has been snipped out of a chromosome, inverted, and inserted back into its original location in the chromosome. The feature that makes it pericentric is that both breaks are on either side of the centromere.

**chromosome map**   The chart of the linear array of genes on a chromosome. The Human Genome Project aims to map all the human chromosomes. See also *Human Genome Project*.

**chromosome, acentric**   A fragment of a chromosome that lacks a centromere, and so is lost when the cell divides.

**chromosome, acrocentric**   A chromosome with its centromere located quite near one end of the chromosome. Humans have five pairs of acrocentric chromosomes. Down syndrome is due to an extra acrocentric chromosome, namely chromosome 21.

**chromosome, dicentric**   An abnormal chromosome with two centromeres rather than the normal one. Since the centromere is essential for chromosome division, a dicentric chromosome is pulled in opposite directions when the cell divides. This causes the chromosome to form a bridge and then break. Dicentric chromosomes are a cause of chromosome instability.

**chromosome, marker**   An abnormal chromosome that is distinctive in appearance but not fully identified. A marker chromosome is not necessarily a "marker" for a specific disease or abnormality, but is one merely in the sense that it can be distinguished under the microscope from all of the normal human chromosomes. For example, the Fragile X (FRAXA) chromosome was once called the marker X.

**chromosome, X**   The sex chromosome found twice in normal females and singly, along with a Y chromosome, in normal males. The complete chromosome complement (consisting of 46 chromosomes, including the two sex chromosomes) is thus conventionally written as 46,XX for chromosomally normal females and 46,XY for chromosomally normal males. The X chromosome not only determines gender, but also carries the genetic code for many essential functions in both males and females.

**chromosome, Y**   The sex chromosome found in normal males, together with an X chromosome. Once thought to be a genetic wasteland, the Y now is known to contain at least 20 genes, some of them unique to the Y. These include the male-determining gene and male fitness genes that are active only in the testis, and that are thought to be responsible for the formation of sperm. Other genes on the Y have counterparts on the X chromosome, are active in many body tissues, and play crucial "housekeeping" roles within the cell.

**chromosomes in multiple miscarriages**   Couples who have had more than one miscarriage have about a 5 percent chance that one member of the couple is carrying a chromosome translocation responsible for the miscarriages.

**chromosomes, metaphase**   The stage in the cell life cycle of a chromosome in which it is most condensed, easiest to see separately, and therefore easiest to study. Metaphase chromosomes are often chosen for karyotyping and chromosome analysis.

**chronic**   A medical term for "lasting a long time." A chronic condition is one that lasts three months or more. Chronic diseases are in contrast to those that are acute (abrupt, sharp, and brief) or subacute (within the midground between acute and chronic).

**chronic arthritis, systemic-onset juvenile**   See *Still disease*.

**chronic bronchitis**   See *bronchitis, chronic*.

**chronic fatigue syndrome**   A debilitating medical condition, chronic in nature, with unknown causes. Diagnosis of CFS is usually done by exclusion. When patients report severe fatigue, doctors should check for common infectious diseases, autoimmune conditions, and other health problems known to cause this symptom. Fatigue is not the only symptom associated with CFS: many patients also report memory loss, thought disturbance, depression, pain in diverse areas of the body, and unusual muscle weakness. In some cases "hot spots" are visible in brain images, such as SPECT scans, of CFS patients. This constellation of symptoms, along with signs of heightened immune-system activity and the effectiveness of antiviral medication for many patients, indicates that some sort of unknown infectious process is involved in many, if not most, cases of CFS. Although there is no specific test for CFS, treatment is often possible via lifestyle changes, rest, and sometimes medication (particularly antiviral drugs). Also known as chronic fatigue and immune dysfunction syndrome (CFIDS) and myalgic encephalomyelitis (ME).

**chronic illness**   An illness that has persisted for a long period of time.

**chronic leukemia**   Cancer of the blood cells that progresses slowly. See also *leukemia, chronic phase of*.

**chronic obstructive lung disease**  Any disorder that persistently obstructs bronchial airflow. Abbreviated as COLD, this disorder mainly involves two related diseases: chronic bronchitis and emphysema. Both cause chronic obstruction of air flowing through the airways and in and out of the lungs. The obstruction is generally permanent, and becomes worse over time. In asthma there is also obstruction of airflow out of the lungs, but the obstruction is usually reversible. Between asthma attacks the flow of air through the airways is generally good. Also known as chronic obstructive pulmonary disease.

**chronic obstructive pulmonary disease**  See *chronic obstructive lung disease*.

**chronic phase**  See *leukemia, chronic phase of*.

**chronic tamponade**  A situation in which a long-standing excess of fluid inside the pericardial sac combines with thickening of the pericardial sac to progressively compress the heart and impair its performance.

**chronicity**  Characterized by long duration. The state of being chronic.

**Churg-Strauss syndrome**  A disease characterized by inflammation of the blood vessels in persons with a history of asthma or allergy. The symptoms of Churg-Strauss syndrome include fatigue, weight loss, inflammation of the nasal passages, numbness, and weakness. The ultimate test for the diagnosis of Churg-Strauss syndrome is a biopsy of involved tissue. Treatment involves stopping inflammation and suppressing the immune system. Also known as allergic granulomatosis, allergic granulomatous angiitis.

**chyme**  A predigested, acidified mass of food that passes from the stomach into the small intestine.

**Ci**  The abbreviation for a Curie, a unit of radioactivity. See also *Curie*.

**-cide**  Suffix indicating killing or killer, as in bactericide (a solution capable of killing bacteria).

**ciliary neuralgia**  See *cluster headache*.

**cilostazol**  A medication (brand name: Pletal) prescribed to treat intermittent claudication and other peripheral artery problems.

**circadian**  Refers to events occurring within the span of a full, 24-hour day, as in a circadian rhythm.

**circadian clock**  An internal time-keeping system. Circadian rhythmicity is a fundamental property of all organisms. Changes in the external environment, particularly in the light-dark cycle, train this biologic clock. When environmental conditions are constant, rhythms driven by the circadian clock follow a near-perfect 24-hour pattern. The human circadian clock regulates many daily activities, such as sleep and waking. When we don't follow these natural rhythms, or when the external environment strays from its usual rhythm (as occurs in the long nights and short days of deep winter), the circadian clock must readjust. Rapid environmental changes and circadian clock–adjustment problems are among the causes of jet lag, problems affecting shift workers, some types of sleep disorders, and bipolar disorders, particularly seasonal affective disorder. Genetic researchers have recently identified some of the physical structures and genes that serve to set and control the circadian clock. See also *bipolar disorders, jet lag, seasonal affective disorder, sleep disorders*.

**circinate balanitis**  See *balanitis, circinate*. See also *Reiter syndrome*.

**circle of Willis**  An arterial circle at the base of the brain that is of critical importance. The circle of Willis receives all of the blood pumped up the two internal carotid arteries that come up the front of the neck, and from the basilar artery formed by the union of the two vertebral arteries that come up the back of the neck. All of the principal arteries supplying cerebral hemispheres of the brain branch off from the circle of Willis.

**circulation**  The movement of fluid in a regular or circuitous course. Although circulation does not necessarily refer to the circulation of the blood, that is the most common way this word is used in medicine. Heart failure is an example of a problem with the circulation.

**circulation, fetal**  The blood circulation in an unborn baby. Before birth, blood from the fetal heart that is destined for the lungs is shunted away from the lungs through a short vessel called the ductus arteriosus, and returned to the aorta. When this shunt is open, it is said to be a patent ductus arteriosus (PDA). The PDA usually closes at or shortly after birth, allowing blood to course freely to the lungs.

**circulatory**  Having to do with the circulation, the movement of fluid in a regular or circuitous course.

**circulatory system**  The system that moves blood through the body. The circulatory system is composed of the heart, arteries, capillaries, and veins. It transports blood that has been depleted of oxygen by the body to the lungs and heart via the veins, and transports oxygenated blood from the lungs and heart throughout the body via the arteries. See also *arteries; blood; heart; lungs; respiratory system; vein*.

**circumcision, female**  The excision (removal) of part or all of the external female genitalia, including the clitoris, and sometimes extending to the labia. Female circumcision is traditionally practiced in some parts of the Middle East and Africa, particularly Sudan. Also known as female genital mutilation. See also *clitoridectomy*.

**circumcision, male** Surgery that removes the protective ring of loose skin (foreskin) that normally covers the glans of the penis. Circumcision dates back to prehistoric times. It may be performed for religious or cultural reasons, or to promote cleanliness.

**cirrhosis** An abnormal liver condition characterized by irreversible scarring of the liver. Alcohol and viral hepatitis B and C are among the many causes of cirrhosis. Cirrhosis can cause yellowing of the skin (jaundice), itching, and fatigue. Diagnosis is suggested by physical examination and blood tests, and can be confirmed by liver biopsy in some patients. Complications of cirrhosis include mental confusion, coma, fluid accumulation (ascites), internal bleeding, and kidney failure. Treatment is designed to limit any further damage to the liver and to prevent complications. Liver transplantation is becoming an important option for patients with advanced cirrhosis.

**cirrhosis with diffuse degeneration of cerebral gray matter, Alpers** See *Alpers disease*.

**cirrhosis, primary biliary** A liver disease caused by an abnormality of the immune system. Small bile ducts within the liver become inflamed and obliterated. Backup of bile causes intense skin itching and yellowing of the skin (jaundice). Lack of bile decreases absorption of calcium and vitamin D, leading to osteoporosis. Cirrhosis (scarring of the liver) develops over time. See also *cirrhosis*.

**Civilian Health and Medical Program of the Uniformed Services** See *CHAMPUS*.

**Cl** The chemical symbol for chloride.

**clap** Slang term for gonorrhea. See *gonorrhea*.

**clarithromycin** A macrolide antibiotic (brand name: Biaxin) that kills bacteria or inhibits bacterial growth. It is usually prescribed to treat respiratory tract infections, ulcers, and infections of the skin or body membranes. Clarithromycin interacts with a number of other medications, sometimes dangerously so, so be sure to tell your doctor about anything else you are taking. Typical side effects include nausea and upset stomach.

**clasped thumbs and mental retardation** See *adducted thumbs, Gareis-Mason syndrome, MASA syndrome*.

**claudication** Limping.

**claudication, intermittent** Pain in the calf that comes and goes, typically felt while walking, and subsiding with rest. Intermittent claudication can be due to temporary artery narrowing due to vasospasm, permanent artery narrowing due to atherosclerosis, or complete occlusion of an artery to the leg. It is more common in men than women. It affects 1 to 2 percent of the population under 60 years of age, but increases to affect over 5 percent of those over 70. The prognosis is generally favorable because the condition often stabilizes or improves in time. Conservative therapy is advisable. Walking often helps increase the distance that the patient can walk without symptoms. Two drugs that may be prescribed for management of intermittent claudication are pentoxifylline (brand name: Trental) and cilostazol (brand name: Pletal). If conservative therapy is inadequate and claudication is severe and persistent, correction of the narrowing in the affected artery might be suggested, depending on the location and severity of the narrowing in the artery and the underlying medical condition of the patient. Procedures used to correct the narrowing of arteries include surgery, such as bypass grafting; and interventional radiology, such as balloon angioplasty.

**claudication, venous** Limping and/or pain resulting from inadequate venous drainage.

**clavicle** The bone extending from the breastbone (sternum) at the base of the front of the neck to the shoulder.

**clavus** See *corn*.

**clay-shoveler's fracture** See *fracture, clay-shoveler's*.

**cleft lip** A fissure in the upper lip due to failure of the left and right sides of the fetal lip tissue to fuse, an event that should take place by 35 days of uterine age. Cleft lip can be on one side only (unilateral) or on both sides (bilateral). Since failure of lip fusion can impair the subsequent closure of the palatal shelves, cleft lip often occurs in association with cleft palate. It is one of the most common physical birth defects, and can be easily corrected with surgery.

**cleft palate** An opening in the roof of the mouth due to a failure of the palatal shelves to come fully together from either side of the mouth and fuse during embryonic development. The opening in the palate permits communication between the nasal passages and the mouth. Surgery is needed to close the palate. Cleft palate can occur alone or in association with cleft lip.

**cleft uvula** A common minor anomaly, occurring in about 1 percent of Europeans and 10 percent of Native Americans, in which the uvula at the back of the soft palate is cleft. Persons with a cleft uvula should not have their adenoids removed, because without the adenoids they cannot achieve proper closure between the soft palate and pharynx while speaking, and will develop hypernasal speech. Also known as bifid uvula.

**cleidocranial dysostosis** A genetic (inherited) disorder of bone development characterized by absent or incompletely formed collarbones (the child with this disorder can bring its shoulders together, or nearly so), and cranial and facial abnormalities that may include square skull, late closure of the sutures of the skull, late closure of the fontanels, low nasal bridge, delayed eruption of the teeth, and abnormal permanent teeth. The gene for cleidocranial dysostosis has been found on chromosome 6 in band p21 and is for the transcription factor core-binding factor alpha subunit 1 (CBFA1). Mutations of CBFA1 cause this disorder. Also known as cleidocranial dysplasia.

**cleidocranial dysplasia** See *cleidocranial dysostosis*.

**click-murmur syndrome** See *mitral valve prolapse*.

**clinical cytogenetics** The application of chromosome studies to clinical medicine. For example, clinical cytogenetic testing is done to look for an extra chromosome 21 in a child with possible Down syndrome. Clinical cytogenetics is a specialty certified by the American Board Of Medical Genetics.

**clinical depression** Depressed mood that meets the DSM-IV criteria for a depressive disorder. The term is commonly used to describe depression that is not a normal, temporary mood caused by life events or grieving.

**clinical disease** A disease with recognizable clinical signs and symptoms, as distinct from a subclinical illness, which does not have obvious symptoms. Diabetes, for example, can be subclinical for some years before emerging as a clinical disease.

**clinical research trials** Studies intended to evaluate the safety and effectiveness of medications or medical devices by monitoring their effects on large groups of people. Studies may be conducted by government health agencies (such as NIH and NIMH), researchers affiliated with a hospital or university medical program, independent researchers, or private industry. Usually volunteers are recruited, although in some cases research subjects may be paid. Subjects are generally divided into two or more groups, including a control group that does not receive the experimental treatment, receives a placebo (inactive substance) instead, or receives a tried-and-true therapy for comparison purposes. Typically, government agencies approve or disapprove new treatments based on clinical trial results. Although they are important and highly effective in preventing obviously harmful treatments

from coming to market, clinical research trials are not always perfect for discovering all side effects, particularly effects associated with long-term use and interactions between experimental drugs and other medications. For some patients, clinical research trials represent an avenue for receiving promising new therapies that would not otherwise be available. Patients with difficult to treat or "incurable" diseases, such as AIDS or certain types of cancer, may want to pursue participation in clinical research trials if standard therapies are not effective.

**clinical trials** See *clinical research trials*.

**clitoridectomy** The surgical excision (removal) of the clitoris to reduce a woman's ability to be sexually stimulated during intercourse. Also known as female circumcision and female genital mutilation. See also *circumcision, female*.

**clitoris** A small mass of erectile tissue situated at the anterior apex of the female vulva, near the meeting of the lower vulvar lips. Like the penis, whose tissue it resembles, the clitoris is highly sensitive to stimulation during sex.

**Clomid** See *clomiphene*.

**clomiphene** A medication (brand name: Clomid) used to induce ovulation in women.

**Clonazepam** An antispasmodic medication (brand name: Klonopin) prescribed to treat seizure disorders, panic disorders, restless leg syndrome, and other conditions. It is in the benzodiazepine family, so it may interact with a wide variety of medications, particularly other central nervous system depressants. It can be habit-forming. See also *benzodiazepine tranquilizer*.

**clone** **1** A group of cells derived from a single ancestral cell; for example, a group of bacteria or a macromolecule such as DNA. **2** An individual developed from a single somatic (nongerm) cell from a parent, representing an exact replica of that parent.

**clone bank** Synonym for genomic library.

**clones, recombinant** Clones containing recombinant DNA molecules.

**cloning** The process by which a genetically identical copy is made.

**cloning, cell** The process of producing a group of cells (clones), all genetically identical, from a single ancestor.

**cloning, DNA** The use of DNA manipulation procedures to produce multiple copies of a single gene or segment of DNA.

**Clostridium**   A genus of oxygen-avoiding (anaerobic) bacteria. The Clostridium genus contains over 100 species.

**Clostridium difficile**   A bacterium that is one of the most common causes of infection of the colon in the US. Patients taking antibiotics are at risk of becoming infected with C. difficile. Antibiotics disrupt the normal bacteria of the bowel, allowing C. difficile bacteria to become established in the colon. Many persons infected with C. difficile bacteria have no symptoms. These people become carriers of the bacteria, and can infect others. In other people, a toxin produced by C. difficile causes diarrhea, abdominal pain, severe inflammation of the colon (colitis), fever, an elevated white blood count, vomiting, and dehydration. In severely affected patients, the inner lining of the colon becomes severely inflamed (a condition called pseudomembranous colitis). Rarely, the walls of the colon wear away and holes develop (colon perforation), which can lead to a life-threatening infection of the abdomen. Abbreviated as C. difficile.

**Clostridium perfrigens**   See *Clostridium welchii*.

**Clostridium welchii**   A bacterium that is the most common agent of gas gangrene. Abbreviated as C.welchii, it also causes food poisoning and a fulminant form of bowel disease called necrotizing colitis. Also known as C. perfrigens.

**clot-dissolving medications**   Agents such as plasminogen-activator (t-PA) and streptokinase that are effective in dissolving clots and reopening arteries. They may be used in the treatment of heart attacks. Also known as thrombolytic agents.

**clubfoot**   A common malformation of the foot that is evident at birth. The foot is turned in sharply so that the person seems to be walking on his or her ankle. The medical term for the common ("classic") type of clubfoot is talipes equinovarus. Clubfoot can sometimes, but not always, be corrected with a combination of surgery, bracing, and physical therapy. When it cannot be fully corrected, special shoes and braces are available to help the person achieve a more comfortable gait and avoid stressing and deforming other muscles and bones.

**cluster headache**   A distinctive syndrome of headaches. The most common cluster headache pattern, acute cluster headache, is characterized by one to three short attacks of pain each day around the eyes, clustered over a stretch of one to two months, and followed by a pain-free period that averages a year. The other main pattern of cluster headaches, chronic or episodic cluster headache, is characterized by the absence of sustained periods of remission, with pain occurring out of the blue or emerging several years after an episodic pattern. The

episodic and acute forms of cluster headache may transform into one another, so it seems they are merely different-appearing patterns of one and the same disease. Cluster headache looks different and distinct from migraine. For example, propranolol is effective for migraine but not for cluster headache, whereas lithium benefits cluster headache syndrome but not migraine, although the mechanisms underlying cluster headache and migraine may have a degree of commonality. Cluster headache has gone by a bevy of other names including ciliary neuralgia, erythroprosopalgia, histamine cephalgia, migrainous neuralgia, Raeder syndrome, spenopalatine neuralgia, and vidian neuralgia.

**cluttering**   A speech disorder characterized by the unwanted repetition of entire words. It resembles stuttering, in which only sounds or parts of words are repeated. See also *speech disorders*.

**cM**   Abbreviation for centimorgan, a unit of measure of genetic recombination frequency.

**CME**   Continuing Medical Education. Doctors are required to earn CME credits to retain their medical licenses. They may do so by taking courses, attending medical conferences where they learn about new developments, or in some cases by reading and taking a test.

**CNS**   Central nervous system.

**CNS prophylaxis**   Chemotherapy or radiation therapy to the central nervous system (CNS) as a preventative treatment. It is given to kill cancer cells that may be in the brain and spinal cord, even though no cancer has been detected there.

**coagulation, blood**   See *blood coagulation*.

**coarctation**   A narrowing, stricture, or constriction. Although the best known coarctation is of the aorta, any artery can have a coarctation. The sides of the vessel at the point of a coarctation appear to be pressed together.

**coarctation of the aorta**   Pinching or constriction of the aorta, impeding the flow of blood below the level of the constriction and increasing blood pressure above the constriction. Symptoms may not be evident at birth, but develop as soon as the first week after birth with congestive heart failure or high blood pressure that call for early surgery. The surgery otherwise can be delayed. The outlook after surgery is favorable. Some cases have been treated by balloon angioplasty.

**cocaine**   A substance derived from the leaves of the coca plant. Cocaine is a bitter, addictive anesthetic (pain-blocking) substance. Safer anesthetics were developed in the 20th century, and cocaine fell into disuse in medicine, although it is still used as an injectable anesthetic by some dentists. Synthetic alternatives, such as procaine, are used far more widely. Tragically, cocaine continues in use as a highly addictive and destructive street drug, an inadvertent contribution by medicine to the contemporary drug culture.

**cocci**   Plural form of coccus.

**coccus**   A bacterial cell in the shape of a sphere.

**coccygeal vertebrae**   The three to five (the average number is four) rudimentary vertebrae that make up the coccyx.

**coccyx**   The small tail-like bone at the bottom of the spine, very near the anus. It is the lowest part of the spinal column. Also known as the tailbone.

**cochlear implant**   A device that is surgically placed (implanted) within the inner ear to help selected persons with certain forms of deafness to hear. Cochlear implants rarely cure severe or profound deafness, but they can unquestionably help some hearing-impaired people to distinguish the sounds of language clearly enough to participate in a verbal environment. For children who are congenitally deaf (that is, born deaf), a cochlear implant can markedly increase a preschool child's chances of being able to function effectively in mainstream school classes. Although cochlear implant surgery is expensive, it may be amortized over time by reduced reliance on costly support services, such as speech therapy and tutoring, and particularly by the lower cost of mainstreaming compared to special classes for the deaf. However, cochlear implants are controversial in the deaf community, which relies on highly expressive sign language and other forms of communication that deaf people do not consider to be inferior to verbal speech.

**cockroach allergy**   A condition that manifests as an allergic reaction when one is exposed to tiny protein particles shed or excreted by cockroaches. Asthma can be due to exposure to cockroach allergens. See also *allergy*.

**code, genetic**   The correspondence between the triplet of bases in DNA with the amino acids. The discovery of the genetic code clearly ranks as one of the premiere events of what has been called the Golden Age of biology (and medicine).

**codon**   A triplet of any three chemical components in the genetic material called bases.

**coefficient of inbreeding**   A measure of how close two people are genetically to each another. The coefficient of inbreeding, symbolized by the letter F, is the probability that a person with two identical genes received both genes from one ancestor.

**Cogan corneal dystrophy**   A disorder in which the cornea shows grayish fingerprint lines, geographic map-like lines, and dots (or microcysts). These can be seen on examination with a slit-lamp, which focuses a high intensity light beam through a slit while the examiner uses a magnifying scope to look at the front of the eye. The disorder is usually without symptoms. However, about one patient in 10 has recurrent erosion of the cornea that generally begins after age 30. Conversely, half of patients with recurrent corneal erosions of unknown origin have this disorder. Under the microscope, a structure called the epithelial basement membrane is abnormal, so the disorder is sometimes called epithelial basement corneal dystrophy. Also known as map-dot-fingerprint type corneal dystrophy and microcystic corneal dystrophy.

**Cogan syndrome**   Arteritis (also referred to as vasculitis) that involves the ear. Cogan syndrome features not only problems of the hearing and balance portions of the ear, but also inflammation of the cornea, and often fever, fatigue, and weight loss. Joint and muscle pains can also be present. Less frequently, the arteritis can involve blood vessels elsewhere in the body, as in the skin, kidneys, nerves, and other tissues and organs. Cogan syndrome can lead to deafness or blindness. Treatment is directed toward stopping the inflammation of the blood vessels. Cortisone-related medications, such as prednisone, are often used. Some patients with severe disease can require immune suppression medications, such as cyclophosphamide (brand name: Cytoxan). Cogan syndrome is extremely rare, and its cause is not known.

**cognition**   The process of knowing. Cognition includes both awareness and judgment.

**cognitive**   Having to do with thought, judgment, or knowledge.

**cognitive behavior therapy**   A therapeutic practice that helps patients recognize and remedy dysfunctional thought patterns. One characteristic technique is exposure and response prevention, in which a patient with a phobia deliberately exposes him- or herself to the feared situation, gradually decreasing the panic response. Cognitive behavior therapy is used to treat obsessive-compulsive disorder, panic disorders, and other biologically based psychiatric illnesses, often in combination with medication. Evidence gathered from brain scans indicates that over time this therapy can sometimes create actual changes in brain and neurotransmitter function. Abbreviated as CBT.

**cognitive disability**   A broad term used to describe such diverse conditions as mental retardation, thought disturbances, or neurological conditions that affect a certain type of perception or mental ability.

**cognitive disturbance**   Disruption of one's ability to think logically.

**cognitive dulling**   Loss of mental faculties; difficulty in thinking logically or quickly. Cognitive dulling can occur due to a medical condition or as a side effect of medication.

**cognitive science**   The study of the mind. It is an interdisciplinary science that draws upon many fields, including neuroscience, psychology, philosophy, computer science, artificial intelligence, and linguistics. The purpose of cognitive science is to develop models that help explain human perception, thinking, and learning. Its central tenet is that the mind is an information processor. This processor receives, stores, retrieves, transforms, and transmits information. The information and the corresponding information processes can be studied as patterns.

**cohort**   In a clinical research trial, a group of study subjects or patients.

**coinsurance**   See *copayment*.

**coitus**   Sexual intercourse.

**coitus interruptus**   Sexual intercourse in which, as a birth-control measure, the male attempts to withdraw the penis before ejaculation. It is not usually an effective means of birth control, as sperm are present in preejaculate fluid produced during intercourse. See also *birth control*.

**colchicine**   A substance found in a plant that is used in clinical medicine for the treatment of gouty arthritis, and in the laboratory to arrest cells during cell division by disrupting the spindle so that their chromosomes can be visualized.

**COLD**   Chronic obstructive lung disease.

**cold injury**   Injuries caused by exposure to extreme cold, including chilblains, trench foot, and frostbite.

**cold, common**   A viral upper respiratory tract infection. This contagious illness can be caused by many different types of viruses, and the body can never build up resistance to all of them. For this reason, colds are a frequent and recurring problem. In fact, kindergarten children average 12 colds per year, while adolescents and adults typically have around 7 colds per year. Going out into the cold weather has no effect on the spread of a cold, and antibiotics do not cure or shorten the common cold.

**cold, June**   Another term for hay fever, an allergic disorder.

**cold, summer**   Another term for hay fever, an allergic disorder.

**colectomy**   An operation to remove all or part of the colon. In a partial colectomy, the surgeon removes only the cancerous part of the colon and a small amount (called a margin) of surrounding healthy tissue.

**colic**   An attack of irritability, crying, and apparent abdominal pain in early infancy. This is a common condition, occurring in about 1 in 10 babies. An infant with colic often has a rigid abdomen and draws up its legs. Overfeeding, undiluted juices, food allergies, and stress can aggravate colic. Colic usually lasts from early infancy to the third or fourth month of age. Although some experts say it is not harmful to the baby, it is extremely wearing on parents. Other experts note that very little is known about colic, and feel that all efforts should be made to relieve the infant's distress. Treatment can include dietary changes, carefully measured feedings, and extra burping. Parents should not chalk up new abdominal pain and loud crying in their baby to colic. It is important for the baby to be seen by a doctor to rule out more serious conditions.

**colitis**   Inflammation of the colon (large intestine). There are many forms of colitis, including amebic, Crohn, infectious, pseudomembranous, spastic, and ulcerative.

**colitis, amebic**   Inflammation of the intestine, with ulcers in the colon, due to infection with an ameba called Entamoeba histolytic. This single-celled parasite can be transmitted to humans via contaminated water and food. Symptoms, which include diarrhea, indigestion, nausea, and weight loss, can begin shortly after infection, or the ameba may live in the GI tract for months or years before symptoms erupt. Amebic colitis can be treated with medication, including injections of emetine and oral antibiotics. Also known as amebic dysentery or amebiasis.

**colitis, Crohn**   Crohn disease affecting only the colon. Also called granulomatous colitis. See also *Crohn disease*.

**colitis, granulomatous**   Crohn disease affecting only the colon. See also *Crohn disease*.

**colitis, pseudomembranous**   Severe inflammation of the inner lining of the colon, usually due to the clostridium difficile (C. difficile) bacterium. Patients taking antibiotics are at particular risk of becoming infected with C. difficile, as the natural bacteria of the bowel can usually keep C. difficile at bay but are disrupted by antibiotics. A toxin produced by C. difficile causes colitis symptoms, including diarrhea, abdominal pain, and severe inflammation. Rarely, the walls of the colon wear away and holes develop (colon perforation), which can lead to a life-threatening infection of the abdomen. See also *Clostridium difficile*.

**colitis, spastic**   See *irritable bowel syndrome*.

**colitis, ulcerative**   A common form of inflammatory bowel disease that is similar to a related disorder, Crohn disease. Its cause is unknown. The end of the colon (the rectum) is always involved in ulcerative colitis. When the inflammation is limited to the rectum, it is called ulcerative proctitis. The inflammation may extend to varying degrees into the upper parts of the colon. When the entire colon is involved, the terms pancolitis or universal colitis are used. Intermittent rectal bleeding, crampy abdominal pain, and diarrhea can be symptoms of ulcerative colitis. Ulcerative colitis characteristically waxes and wanes. Many patients experience long remissions, even without medication. Ulcerative colitis may mysteriously resolve after a long history of symptoms. Direct visualization (sigmoidoscopy or colonoscopy) with sampling of the lining of the bowel is the most accurate diagnostic test. Especially in new cases, infections and other diseases that can mimic ulcerative colitis have to be considered and excluded. Long-standing ulcerative colitis increases the risk for colon cancer. Ulcerative colitis can also be associated with inflammation in joints, spine, skin, eyes, liver, and bile ducts. Treatment of ulcerative colitis involves medications and/or surgery; changes in diet can sometimes help.

**colitis, universal**   Ulcerative colitis that involves the entire colon (the large intestine).

**collagen**   The principal protein of the skin, tendons, cartilage, bone, and connective tissue.

**collagen disease**   See *connective tissue disease*.

**collagen injection**   The practice of injecting collagen into a part of the face or body to make it larger, most often performed on the lips. The effects are long-lasting but not permanent. Collagen injections are normally done by a plastic surgeon.

**collapsed lung**   Failure of full expansion of a once fully expanded lung. Medically called atelectasis.

**collarbone**   A horizontal bone above the first rib that makes up the front part of the shoulder. Also called the clavicle, the collarbone links the sternum (breastbone) with the scapula, a triangular bone in the back of the shoulder. The collarbone ends at the sternum, forming one side of the sternoclavicular joint. It ends at the shoulder, there forming one side of the acromioclavicular joint.

**collateral**   In anatomy, a subordinate or accessory part. A collateral is also a side branch, as of a blood vessel or

nerve. After a coronary artery occlusion, collateral vessels often develop to shunt blood around the blockage.

**collateral knee ligament, lateral**   The knee joint is surrounded by a joint capsule, with ligaments strapping the inside and outside of the joint (collateral ligaments) as well as crossing within the joint (cruciate ligaments). These ligaments provide stability and strength to the knee joint. The lateral collateral ligament of the knee is on the outside of the joint.

**collateral knee ligament, medial**   The medial collateral ligament of the knee is on the inner side of the joint, and adds stability and strength to the knee joint.

**colon**   The long, coiled, tubelike organ that removes water from digested food. The remaining material, solid waste called stool, moves through the colon to the rectum and leaves the body through the anus. The colon is sometimes called the large bowel or the large intestine.

**colon cancer**   See *cancer, colon*.

**colon cancer prevention**   Colorectal cancer can run in families. The colon cancer risk is higher if an immediate family member (parent, sibling, or child) had colorectal cancer, and even higher if more than one such relative had colorectal cancer or if a family member developed the cancer when younger than 55 years of age. Individuals to whom any of these circumstances apply should undergo a colonoscopy every three years, starting at an age that is 7 to 10 years younger than when the youngest family member with the cancer was diagnosed.

**colon polyps**   Benign tumors of the large intestine are called polyps. Benign polyps do not invade nearby tissue or spread to other parts of the body. Benign polyps can be easily removed during colonoscopy, and are not life threatening. If benign polyps are not removed from the large intestine, they can become malignant (cancerous) over time. Most cancers of the large intestine are believed to have developed from polyps.

**colonoscope**   A flexible, lighted instrument used to view the inside of the colon.

**colonoscopy**   A procedure whereby a doctor inserts a viewing tube (colonoscope) into the rectum for the purpose of inspecting the colon. Upon detecting abnormal areas of the colon, a biopsy can be performed.

**colony-stimulating factors**   Laboratory-made agents similar to substances in the body that stimulate the production of blood cells. Treatment with colony-stimulating factors (CSFs) can help the blood-forming tissue recover from the effects of chemotherapy and radiation therapy.

**colorblindness**  Conditions that cause colors to be misperceived. The most common is red-green color-blindness (also known as deuteranomaly, deuteranopia, or Daltonism), in which red and green are perceived as identical. It is thought to be caused by aberrant functioning of the retina. Total inability to perceive color (monochromatism) is very rare. See also *monochromatism*.

**colorectal**  Related to the colon and/or rectum.

**colorectal cancer**  See *cancer, colon*.

**colostomy**  Creating an alternative exit from the colon by diverting waste through a hole in the colon and through the wall of the abdomen. A colostomy is commonly performed by severing the colon, and then attaching the end leading to the stomach to the skin, through the wall of the abdomen. At the exterior opening (stoma), a bag can be attached for waste removal. The end of the colon that leads to the rectum is closed off and becomes dormant. This is known as a Hartmann colostomy. There are other types of colostomy procedures. Usually a colostomy is performed because of infection, blockage, cancer, or in rare instances, severe trauma of the colon. This is not an operation to be taken lightly. It demands the close attention of both patient and doctor. A colostomy is often performed so that an infection can be stopped and/or the affected colon tissues can heal.

**colostomy bag**  A removable, disposable bag that attaches to the exterior opening of a colostomy (stoma) to permit sanitary collection and disposal of bodily wastes.

**colostomy, iliac**  A colostomy in which the exterior opening (stoma) is located on the lower left side of the abdomen.

**colostomy, transverse**  A colostomy in which the exterior opening (stoma) is located on the upper abdomen.

**colostrum**  A sticky white or yellow fluid secreted by the breasts during the second half of pregnancy, and for a few days after birth before the breast milk comes in. It is high in protective antibodies, giving the newborn's immune system a jump-start.

**colpo-**  Prefix referring to the vagina.

**colpopexy**  The use of surgical-quality stitches to bring a displaced vagina back into position against the abdominal wall.

**colpoptosis**  A condition in which the vagina has dropped from its normal position against the abdominal wall.

**colporrhaphy**  Surgical repair of the vagina.

**colposcopy**  A procedure in which a lighted magnifying instrument called a colposcope is used to examine the vagina and cervix. Also called a vaginoscope.

**colpotomy**  A surgical incision in the vagina.

**coma**  A state of deep, unarousable unconsciousness, a coma may occur as the result of head trauma, disease, poisoning, or numerous other causes. Coma states may be graded based on the absence or presence of reflexive responses to stimuli.

**comminuted fracture**  See *fracture, comminuted*.

**common bile duct**  The duct formed by the junction of the cystic duct from the gallbladder and the common hepatic duct from the liver. It carries bile to the duodenum.

**common cold**  See *cold, common*.

**communicable disease**  A disease caused by an infectious organism.

**communication disorders**  Disorders of the speech apparatus, and/or of the mental faculties used to speak or communicate by other means. Treatment is with speech therapy, and other interventions as appropriate for the underlying condition. See *aphasia, apraxia of speech, articulation disorder, autism, cluttering, speech disorders, stuttering*.

**comorbid**  Occurring together. For example, if a person has both Crohn disease and stomach ulcers, these are comorbid conditions.

**complementary DNA**  DNA made from a messenger RNA template. The single-stranded form is often used as a probe in physical mapping. Abbreviated as cDNA.

**complementary sequence**  Nucleic acid sequence of bases that can form a double-stranded structure by matching base pairs. For example, the complementary sequence to C-A-T-G (where each letter stands for one of the bases in DNA) is G-T-A-C.

**complete blood count**  See *blood count, complete*.

**complete hysterectomy**  See *hysterectomy, total*.

**complete syndactyly**  See *syndactyly, complete*.

**compound fracture**  See *fracture, compound*.

**compound microscope**  A microscope that actually consists of two microscopes in series, the first serving as the ocular lens (close to the eye) and the second serving as the objective lens (close to the object to be viewed).

**compress** Cloth or another material applied under pressure to an area of the skin and held in place for a period of time. A compress can be any temperature, and it can be dry or wet. It may also be impregnated with medication or, in traditional medicine, an herbal remedy. Most compresses are used to relieve inflammation.

**compression fracture** See *fracture, compression.*

**computed tomography** See *CAT scan.*

**computerized axial tomography** See *CAT scan.*

**conception** The union of a sperm and an egg to create the first cell of a new organism. See also *pregnancy.*

**concussion** A traumatic injury to soft tissue, usually the brain, as a result of a violent blow or shaking. A brain concussion can cause immediate but temporary impairment of brain functions, such as thinking, vision, equilibrium, and consciousness.

**conditioning** Exercise and practice to build up the body for either improved normal performance, as in physical therapy, or in preparation for sports performance.

**conditioning, Pavlovian** Use of a system of rewards and punishments to influence behavior. Named after the Russian physiologist Ivan Petrovich Pavlov, who conditioned dogs to respond in what proved to be a predictable manner by giving them rewards.

**condom** A sheath made of latex, lambskin, or other material that covers the penis during sexual intercourse. It collects the semen, preventing it from reaching the female partner's cervix, and thereby preventing conception. When used consistently, especially if combined with spermicide or a female barrier method, condoms are a reasonably reliable contraceptive method. Latex (but not lambskin) condoms also provide some protection against venereal diseases, including the HIV virus. See also *barrier method, birth control.*

**condom, female** A sheath made of plastic or latex that is anchored outside the vagina and lines the interior of the vagina. It collects semen, preventing it from reaching the cervix, and thereby preventing conception. It also provides some protection against venereal diseases, including the HIV virus. See also *barrier method, birth control.*

**conduction system, cardiac** See *cardiac conduction system.*

**condyloma** Wartlike growths around the anus, vulva, or glans penis. There are three major types of condyloma, each of which is sexually transmitted. These include condyloma acuminatum or genital warts; condyloma latum, a form of secondary syphilis; and condyloma subcutaneum or molluscum contagiosum.

**condyloma acuminatum** See *genital warts.*

**condyloma latum** A form of the secondary stage of syphilis manifest by wartlike growths around the anus.

**condyloma subcutaneum** Molluscum contagiosum. Wartlike growths around the anus and genitals caused by a virus.

**cone** Light-sensitive cells in the retina of the eye. Cone cells absorb light, and are essential for distinguishing colors.

**congenital** Present at birth.

**congenital aganglionic megacolon** See *Hirschsprung disease.*

**congenital clasped thumb with mental retardation** See *adducted thumbs, Gareis-Mason syndrome, MASA syndrome.*

**congenital defect** A birth defect.

**congenital dislocation of the hip** See *congenital hip dislocation.*

**congenital heart disease** A birth defect of the heart, or of the aorta or other large blood vessels.

**congenital hemolytic jaundice** See *spherocytosis, hereditary.*

**congenital hip dislocation** A birth defect in which the hip joint is malformed or does not rotate properly due to muscle problems. Treatment can include splinting, physical therapy, and in some cases, surgery. Also known as infantile hip dislocation, congenital dislocation of the hip (CDH), developmental dysplasia of the hip (DDH).

**congenital hypothyroidism** See *cretinism.*

**congenital malformation** Abnormal formation of a structure, which is evident at birth.

**congenital neutropenia, severe** See *severe congenital neutropenia.*

**congenital ptosis of the eyelids** Drooping of the upper eyelids at birth. The lids may droop only slightly or they may cover the pupils and restrict or even block vision. Moderate or severe ptosis calls for treatment to permit normal vision development. If not corrected, amblyopia (lazy eye) may develop, which can lead to permanently poor vision. Ptosis at birth is often caused by poor development of the levator muscle, which lifts the eyelid. Children with ptosis may tip their heads back into a chin-up position to see underneath the eyelids, or raise their eyebrows in an attempt to lift up the lids. Congenital ptosis rarely improves with time. Mild or moderate ptosis usually does not require surgery early in life. Treatment is usually surgery to tighten the eyelid-lifting muscles (levators). If the levator is very weak, the lid can be attached or suspended from under the eyebrow so that the forehead muscles can do the lifting. Even after surgery, focusing problems can develop as the eyes grow and change shape. All children with ptosis, whether they have had surgery or not, should therefore be followed by an ophthalmologist.

**congenital torticollis**  A deformity of the neck, evident at birth, and due to shortening of the neck muscles. Congenital torticollis tilts the head to the side on which the neck muscles are shortened, so that the chin points to the other side. The shortened neck muscles are principally supplied by the spinal accessory nerve. Also called wry neck.

**congestive heart failure**  Inability of the heart to keep up with the demands on it and, specifically, failure of the heart to pump blood with normal efficiency. When this occurs, the heart is unable to provide adequate blood flow to other organs, such as the brain, liver, and kidneys. Heart failure may be due to failure of the right or left ventricle, or both. The signs and symptoms depend on which side of the heart is failing. They can include shortness of breath (dyspnea), asthma due to the heart (cardiac asthma), pooling of blood (stasis) in the general body (systemic) circulation or in the liver's (portal) circulation, swelling (edema), blueness or duskiness (cyanosis), and enlargement (hypertrophy) of the heart. The many causes of congestive heart failure include coronary artery disease leading to heart attacks and heart muscle weakness; primary heart muscle weakness from viral infections or toxins, such as prolonged alcohol exposure; heart valve disease causing heart muscle weakness due to too much leaking of blood, or heart muscle stiffness from a blocked valve; and hypertension (high blood pressure). Rarer causes include hyperthyroidism (high thyroid hormone), vitamin deficiency, and excess use of amphetamines. The aim of therapy is to improve the pumping function of the heart. General treatment includes salt restriction, diuretics to get rid of excess fluid, digoxin to strengthen the heart, and other medications. Specific treatment of congestive heart failure needs to be directed also at underlying causes.

**conization**  Surgery to remove a cone-shaped piece of tissue from the cervix and cervical canal. Conization may be used to diagnose or treat a cervical condition. Also known as cone biopsy.

**conjunctivitis**  Inflammation of the membrane covering the surface of the eyeball. It can be a result of infection or irritation, or related to systemic diseases, such as Reiter syndrome. Also known as pinkeye.

**conjunctivitis arida**  See *xerophthalmia*.

**conjunctivitis, allergic**  Inflammation of the whites of the eyes (the conjunctivae), with itching, redness of the eyes, and tearing. Caused by an allergic reaction, and frequently accompanied by hay fever.

**Conn syndrome**  Overproduction of the hormone aldosterone by a tumor containing tissue like that in the outer portion (cortex) of the adrenal gland. The excessive aldosterone results in low potassium levels (hypokalemia), underacidity of the body (alkalosis), muscle weakness, excessive thirst (polydipsia), excessive urination (polyuria), and high blood pressure (hypertension). Also known as primary aldosteronism and hyperaldosteronism.

**connectionism**  A theory of information-processing within cognitive science, connectionism is based on the known neurophysiology of the brain. The basic tenets of connectionism are that signals are processed by elementary units (in this case, neurons), processing units are connected in parallel to other processing units, and connections between processing units are weighted. The weights may be hardwired, learned, or both. The weights represent the strength of connection (either excitatory or inhibitory) between two units. These basic concepts have permitted the development of a spectrum of models in connectionist research.

**connective tissue**  A material consisting of fibers that form a framework which provides support structure for body tissues. See also *collagen*.

**connective tissue disease**  A disease (autoimmune or otherwise) that attacks the collagen or other components of connective tissue; lupus is such a disease.

**Conor and Bruch disease**  See *typhus, African tick*. See also *rickettsial diseases*.

**consanguinity**  Close blood relationship; sometimes used to denote human inbreeding. There are always added risks from the mating of closely related persons, and those risks are not negligible. Everyone carries rare recessive genes that, in the company of another gene of the same type, are capable of causing an autosomal recessive disease. First cousins share a set of grandparents, so for any particular gene in the father, the chance that the mother inherited the same allele from the same source is one in eight. For this reason, marriage between first cousins (not to mention closer relatives) is generally frowned upon, and in many areas is illegal. Marriage between more distant relatives carries lesser risks. In families where a recessive genetic disorder is known or suspected to be present, genetic testing and counseling is advised, even if the level of consanguinity is very low (as, for example, in marriages between third or fourth cousins).

**conserved sequence**   A base sequence in a DNA molecule, or in an amino acid sequence in a protein, that has remained essentially unchanged (conserved) throughout evolution.

**constipation**   Infrequent (and frequently incomplete) bowel movements. The opposite of diarrhea, constipation is commonly caused by irritable bowel syndrome, diverticulosis, or medications. Paradoxically, constipation can be caused by overuse of laxatives. Colon cancer can also narrow the colon and thereby cause constipation. Barring a condition such as cancer, a high-fiber diet can frequently relieve constipation.

**contig**   Group of clones representing overlapping regions of the genome.

**contig map**   A map depicting the relative order of a linked library of small overlapping clones, representing a complete chromosome segment.

**continuous positive airway pressure**   A treatment for sleep apnea that involves wearing over the face a breathing mask that forces air through the nasal passages at a steady rate, preventing the airway from collapsing during sleep. Abbreviated as CPAP. See also *sleep apnea.*

**contraceptive**   Something capable of preventing conception from taking place. See also *barrier method; birth control; cervical cap; condom; condom, female; contraceptive, emergency; contraceptive, implanted; Depo-Provera; diaphragm; intrauterine device; Norplant; oral contraceptive.*

**contraceptive device, intrauterine**   See *intrauterine device.*

**contraceptive, emergency**   An oral contraceptive that can be taken after unprotected intercourse. For example, emergency contraceptives may be given to victims of rape as part of after-care procedures. Also known as the morning-after pill.

**contraceptive, implanted**   A time-release contraceptive that is surgically implanted under the skin. At this time, Norplant is the only implantable contraceptive approved for use in the US. See *Norplant.*

**contraction**   The tightening and shortening of a muscle.

**contraction, uterine**   The tightening and shortening of the uterine muscles. During labor, contractions cause the cervix to thin and dilate, and aid the baby in its entry into and progress through the birth canal.

**contralateral**   On the other side. The opposite of iposilateral (the same side). For example, a stroke involving the right side of the brain may cause contralateral paralysis of the left leg.

**control**   In research, control subjects are those who do not receive the treatment under investigation. They may be given a placebo treatment, or receive a treatment with known results to permit comparison with experimental results. In lab research that does not use live subjects (in vitro research rather than in vivo research), control procedures serve the same purpose.

**contusion**   See *bruise.*

**copayment**   A payment made by an individual who has health insurance, usually at the time a service is received, to offset some of the cost of care. Copayments are a common feature of HMO (Health Maintenance Organization) and PPO (Preferred Provider Organization) health plans in the US. Copayment size may vary depending on the service, generally with low copayments required for visits to a regular medical provider and higher payments for services received in the emergency room, the latter intended to discourage insured persons from using the emergency room unless it is absolutely necessary. Also known as coinsurance.

**COPD**   Chronic obstructive pulmonary disease. See *chronic obstructive lung disease.*

**coprolalia**   The involuntary uttering of obscene, derogatory, or embarrassing words or phrases. Coprolalia is a symptom experienced by about 10 percent of patients with Tourette syndrome, a tic disorder. Like other tics, it tends to appear and disappear, and responds to medication. See also *tic, tic disorder, Tourette syndrome.*

**cords, vocal**   See *vocal cords.*

**corn**   A small callused area of skin caused by local pressure irritating tissue over a bony prominence. Although the surface area of a corn may be small, the area of hardening actually extends into the deeper layers of skin and flesh. It is the inside projection of the corn that causes discomfort. Corns most commonly occur over a toe, where they form what is referred to as a hard corn. Between the toes, pressure can form a soft corn of macerated skin, which often yellows. Corns can be softened by soaking in hot water, with or without softening agents available over the counter or by prescription. In some cases, minor, outpatient surgery may be used to remove excess tissue. Prevention of corns is easier: Simply choose properly fitted footwear, and use commercially available corn pads to prevent further irritation and growth of any corn that may begin to emerge. A corn on the toe may also be called a clavus.

**cornea** The clear front window of the eye. The cornea transmits and focuses light into the eye. The cornea is more than a protective film; it is a fairly complex structure with five layers.

**cornea, conical** See *keratoconus*.

**corneal dystrophy, Cogan** See *Cogan corneal dystrophy*.

**corneal dystrophy, epithelial basement** See *Cogan corneal dystrophy*.

**corneal dystrophy, map-dot-fingerprint type** See *Cogan corneal dystrophy*.

**corneal dystrophy, microcystic** See *Cogan corneal dystrophy*.

**corneal ring, intrastromal** A plastic ring designed to be implanted in the cornea in order to flatten the cornea and thereby correct, or reduce the degree of, nearsightedness (myopia). The ring is placed in the corneal stroma, the middle of the five layers of the cornea.

**coronal** A coronal plane through the body is a vertical plane from head to foot, and parallel to the shoulders.

**coronary arteries** The vessels that supply the heart muscle with blood rich in oxygen. They are called the coronary arteries because they encircle the heart in the manner of a crown (in Latin, *corona*). Like other arteries, the coronaries may be subject to arteriosclerosis (hardening of the arteries). See also *arteries*.

**coronary artery bypass graft** See *bypass, coronary*.

**coronary artery disease** The coronary arteries can fall victim to arteriosclerosis (hardening of the arteries), with hardened plaques on the artery walls impeding or blocking the flow of blood to the heart. This condition may be treated by bypass surgery, balloon angioplasty, stents, or other techniques.

**coronary artery spasm** A sudden constriction of a coronary artery, depriving the heart muscle (myocardium) of blood and oxygen. This can cause a type of sudden chest pain referred to as variant angina or Printzmetal angina. Coronary artery spasm can be triggered by emotional stress, medicines, street drugs (particularly cocaine), or exposure to extreme cold. Treatments include beta-blocker medications and, classi-

cally, nitroglycerin to permit the coronary arteries to open up.

**coronary occlusion** See *cardiac arrest*. See also *myocardial infarction, acute*.

**corpora cavernosa** Two chambers in the penis, which run the length of the organ and are filled with spongy tissue. Blood flows in and fills the open spaces in the spongy tissue to create an erection.

**corpus** The body of the uterus.

**Corrigan pulse** A pulse that is full and then suddenly collapses. It is usually found in patients with aortic regurgitation, a condition caused by a leaky aortic value in the heart. The left ventricle of the heart ejects blood under high pressure into the aorta. Then the aortic valve normally shuts tight so that blood cannot return to the ventricle. If, however, the aortic valve cannot close completely, the blood in the aorta comes sloshing back into the ventricle and the pressure and the pulse collapse. Also known as a water-hammer pulse.

**cortex** The outer layer of any organ.

**cortex, cerebral** The gray outer portion of the cerebrum, the main part of the brain. As it is structured with thousands of complex folds, the cerebral cortex has a much larger surface area than one might think. Areas of this structure appear to govern sensory perception, voluntary response to stimuli, thought, memory, and the unique human capability of consciousness. The white matter of the brain lies within the cerebral cortex, and carries instructions arising within the cortex to all other parts of the brain and body through an intricate network of nerve fibers.

**cortical** Having to do with the cortex, the outer layer of an organ.

**cortical desmoid** See *desmoid, cortical*.

**corticosteroid** Any of the steroid hormones made by the cortex of the adrenal gland. There are two sets of these hormones: the glucocorticoids, which are produced in reaction to stress and also help in the metabolization of fats, carbohydrates, and proteins; and the mineralocorticoids, which regulate the balance of salt and water within the body.

**cortisol** A metabolite of the primary stress hormone cortisone, and an essential factor in the proper metabolism of starches, cortisol is the major natural glucocorticoid (GC) in humans.

**cortisone** A naturally occurring hormone produced in minute amounts by the adrenal gland and, hence, an adrenocorticoid hormone. Synthetic cortisone is also available; it is metabolized by the body into cortisol. Uses for synthetic cortisone medications include treatment of adrenocortical deficiency and of conditions associated with inflammation. Also called hydrocortisone.

**coryza** A head cold with a runny nose.

**cosmid** An artificially constructed vector (carrier) used in cloning pieces of DNA. On a technical level, a cosmid contains the cos gene of phage lambda, and can be packaged in a lambda phage particle for infection into the common bacteria E. coli. This permits cloning of larger DNA fragments that can be introduced into bacterial hosts in plasmid vectors.

**costal margin** The lower edge of the chest (thorax) formed by the bottom edge of the rib cage.

**costochondritis** Inflammation and swelling of the cartilage of the chest wall, usually involving the cartilage that surrounds the breast bone (sternum) but sometimes including a rib. Costochondritis causes local pain and tenderness of the chest around the sternum. It is sometimes associated with allergies or asthma. Treatment options include anti-inflammatory medications, and in severe cases, corticosteroid injections. Also known as Tietze syndrome.

**cough** A rapid expulsion of air from the lungs, typically in order to clear the lung airways of fluids, mucus, or material. Also known as tussis.

**cough suppressant** A drug used to control coughing, particularly with a dry, nagging, unproductive cough.

**coughing syncope** See *syncope, coughing*. See also *syncope*.

**Coulter test** A blood test that measures the level of P-24 antigen in the blood of patients infected with the HIV virus. See *P-24 antigen*.

**Coumadin** See *warfarin*.

**counseling** The therapeutic practice of using discussion to help patients understand and better cope with life's problems. Areas in which counseling may be used in medicine include genetic counseling and family counseling (particularly to help the family cope with a member's illness or death). Counselors may also see individuals or married couples, or may work with students in a school setting. Counseling is not applicable to treatment of psychiatric disorders.

**counseling, genetic** See *genetic counseling*.

**counselor** A person who practices counseling. Depending on state laws, counselors may or may not be required to hold a particular license. Credentials used by counselors include MFC (marriage and family counselor) and LMFC (licensed marriage and family counselor).

**cousin marriage** See *consanguinity*.

**cox-1** Cyclooxygenase-1, a protein that acts as an enzyme to speed up the production of certain chemical messengers, called prostaglandins, within the stomach. The prostaglandins work within certain cells responsible for inflammation and other functions. For example, they promote the production of the natural mucus lining that protects the inner stomach. The cox-1 enzyme is normally present in a variety of areas of the body, including not only the stomach but also any site of inflammation.

**cox-1 inhibitor** Common anti-inflammatory drugs like aspirin, ibuprofen, and naproxen block the action of both cox-1 and cox-2. They thereby can reduce inflammation, but may also decrease the natural protective mucus lining of the stomach. That's why these medications can cause stomach upset, intestinal bleeding, and ulcers. In some cases, using a buffered form can eliminate or reduce these adverse effects.

**cox-2** Cyclooxygenase-2, another protein that acts as an enzyme to speed up the production of certain chemical messengers called prostaglandins. Some of these messengers are responsible for promoting inflammation. When cox-2 activity is blocked, inflammation is reduced. Unlike the cox-1 enzyme, cox-2 is active only at the site of inflammation, not in the stomach.

**cox-2 inhibitor** A class of drugs that selectively blocks the cox-2 enzyme. Blocking this enzyme impedes the production of the chemical messengers that cause the pain and swelling of arthritis inflammation. Unlike the cox-1 enzyme, cox-2 does not play a role in the normal function of the stomach or intestinal tract. Therefore, medications that selectively block cox-2 do not present the risk of injuring the stomach or intestines. These drugs pose a significant advantage over previous anti-inflammatory drugs. Cox-2 inhibitors now on the market include celecoxib (brand name: Celebrex).

**CPAP** Continuous positive airway pressure.

**CPR** Cardiopulmonary resuscitation.

**cracked-tooth syndrome** A toothache caused by a broken tooth (tooth fracture) without associated caries (cavities) or advanced gum disease. Biting on the area of tooth fracture can cause severe, sharp pains. These fractures are usually caused by chewing or biting hard objects, such as hard candies, pencils, nuts, or ice. Sometimes a near-invisible fracture can be exposed by painting a special dye onto the tooth. Treatment usually involves protecting the tooth with a crown. However, if placing a crown does not relieve pain symptoms, a root canal may be necessary.

**cradle cap**   A form of seborrheic dermatitis of the scalp, usually seen in infants but sometimes found in older children. It is characterized by flaking or scaling of the skin, which may also be reddened. Although cradle cap is on the scalp, the same process can involve the skin on the nose, eyebrows, scalp, ears, and trunk, particularly within skin folds. Seborrheic dermatitis is an inflammatory skin rash due to overactivity of the sebaceous glands in the skin.

**cramp, writer's**   A dystonia that affects the muscles of the hand and sometimes the forearm, and that only occurs during handwriting. Similar focal dystonias have been called typist's cramp, pianist's cramp, musician's cramp, and golfer's cramp.

**cranial**   Toward the head. See also *Appendix B, "Anatomic Orientation Terms."*

**cranial arteritis**   See *arteritis, cranial.*

**cranial dystonia**   See *dystonia, cranial.*

**cranial nerves**   The nerves of the brain, which emerge from or enter the skull (the cranium), as opposed to the spinal nerves, which emerge from the vertebral column. Cranial nerves come directly from the brain through the skull. There are 12 cranial nerves, each of which is accorded a Roman numeral and a name:

Cranial nerve I: the olfactory nerve

Cranial nerve II: the optic nerve

Cranial nerve III: the occulomotor nerve

Cranial nerve IV: the trochlear nerve

Cranial nerve V: the trigeminal nerve

Cranial nerve VI: the abducent nerve

Cranial nerve VII: the facial nerve

Cranial nerve VIII: the vestibulocochlear nerve

Cranial nerve IX: the glossopharyngeal nerve

Cranial nerve X: the vagus nerve

Cranial nerve XI: the accessory nerve

Cranial nerve XII: the hypoglossal nerve

**craniocleidodysostosis**   See *cleidocranial dysostosis.*

**craniofacial disorders**   Disorders that affect the structure of the skull and face.

**craniopharyngioma**   A type of brain tumor that emerges from embryonic tissue that also forms part of the pituitary gland. Pressure on the pituitary reduces the availability of the hormone vasopressin, raising the pressure within the cranium. A craniopharyngioma usually includes hard, calcified components within the tumor itself, and disrupts normal skull development in its vicinity. Treatment is usually via surgery.

**craniosacral therapy**   An alternative therapy in which practitioners attempt to create positive effects by manipulating the bones of the skull and spine, and the fascia that underlies muscle tissue.

**craniosynostosis**   Premature fusion of the growth plates in a child's skull, preventing normal skull expansion. Craniosynostosis can cause hydrocephalus and behavior problems, as well as disrupting normal growth of the skull and face. Treatment is via surgery.

**craniotomy**   An operation in which an opening is made in the skull so the doctor can reach the brain.

**cranium**   The top portion of the skull, which protects the brain. The cranium includes the frontal, parietal, occipital, temporal, sphenoid, and ethmoid bones.

**cretinism**   Congenital hypothyroidism (underactivity of the thyroid gland at birth), resulting in growth retardation, developmental delay, and other abnormal features. Can be due to deficiency of iodine in the mother's diet during pregnancy.

**Creutzfeldt-Jakob disease**   A degenerative disease of the brain that causes dementia and, eventually, death. It is believed to be caused by an unconventional transmissible agent called a prion, rather than by bacteria or virus. Symptoms of CJD include forgetfulness, nervousness, trembling hand movements, unsteady gait, muscle spasms, chronic dementia, balance disorder, and loss of facial expression. CJD is classified as a spongiform encephalopathy, and has some relationship to animal diseases in that category, most notably bovine spongiform encephalopathy (mad cow disease). Most cases occur as a result of a random mutation, but inherited forms also exist. In the 1990s, an epidemic of a transmissible CJD variant broke out in Britain, leading to wholesale destruction of English cattle to prevent further cases. In the US, several lots of blood and blood products had to be destroyed when donors later developed CJD. There is neither treatment nor cure for CJD. Also known as Creutzfeldt-Jakob syndrome, Jakob-Creutzfeldt disease, and spastic pseudoparalysis.

**crib death**   See *SIDS.*

**crippled**  A medically outmoded and politically incorrect term that implies a serious loss of normal function through damage or loss of an essential part or element.

**Crohn colitis**  Crohn disease involving only the large intestine (colon). See also *Crohn disease*.

**Crohn disease**  A chronic inflammatory disease that primarily involves the small and/or large intestine, but which can affect other parts of the digestive system as well. Crohn disease is usually diagnosed in persons in their teens or twenties, but can occur at any point in life. It can be a chronic, recurrent condition, or it can cause minimal symptoms—with, or even without, medical treatment. In mild forms, Crohn disease causes scattered, shallow, crater-like areas (erosions) called apthous ulcers in the inner surface of the bowel. In more serious cases, deeper and larger ulcers can develop, causing scarring, stiffness, and possibly narrowing of the bowel, sometimes leading to obstruction. Deep ulcers can puncture holes in the bowel's wall, leading to infection in the abdominal cavity (peritonitis) and in adjacent organs. Abdominal pain, diarrhea, vomiting, fever, and weight loss can be symptoms. Crohn disease can also be associated with reddish, tender skin nodules, as well as inflammation of the joints, spine, eyes, and liver. Diagnosis is commonly made by X-ray or colonoscopy. Helpful medications may include anti-inflammatories, immune suppressors, or antibiotics. Dietary changes can reduce symptoms and increase the patient's comfort level. Surgery can be necessary in severe cases. Also known as regional enteritis.

**Crohn enteritis**  Crohn disease involving only the small intestine.

**Crohn enterocolitis**  Crohn disease involving both the small and large intestines.

**Crohn ileitis**  Inflammation of the ileum (the lowest part of the small intestine) due to Crohn disease. See also *Crohn disease*.

**Crohn ileocolitis**  Crohn disease involving the ileum (the lowest portion of the small intestine) and the colon (the large intestine).

**crossed embolism**  Passage of a clot (thrombus) from a vein to an artery. When clots in veins break off (embolize), they travel first to the right side of the heart and, normally, then to the lungs, where they lodge. The lungs act as a filter to prevent the clots from entering the arterial circulation. However, when there is a hole in the wall between the two upper chambers of the heart (an atrial septal defect), a clot can cross from the right to the left side of the heart, and then pass into the arteries. Once in the arterial circulation, a clot can travel to the brain, block a vessel there, and cause a stroke (cerebrovascular accident). Because of the risk of stroke from crossed embolism, it is usually recommended that even small atrial septal defects be closed. Also known as paradoxical embolism.

**crossing over**  The exchange of genetic material between two paired chromosomes. Crossing over is a way to recombine the genetic material so that each person (except for identical twins) is genetically unique.

**crossover study**  A type of clinical trial in which the study subjects receive each treatment in a random order. With this type of study, every patient serves as his or her own control. Crossover studies are often used when researchers feel it would be difficult to recruit subjects willing to risk going without a promising new treatment.

**cross-section**  In anatomy, a cross-section is a transverse cut through a structure or tissue. The opposite of a cross-section is a longitudinal section. By analogy, a research study may be cross-sectional or longitudinal.

**cross-sectional study**  A study done at one time, not over the course of time. A cross-sectional study might be of a disease such as AIDS at one point in time to learn its prevalence and distribution within the population. Also known as a synchronic study.

**croup**  An infection of the larynx, trachea, and bronchial tubes that occurs mainly in children. It is usually caused by viruses, less often by bacteria. Symptoms include a cough that sounds like a barking seal, and a harsh crowing sound during inhaling. A low-grade fever (around 100° to 101°F) is common. The child may become very frightened. The major concern in croup is breathing difficulty as the air passages narrow. Treatment may include moist air (as from a humidifier), saltwater nose drops, decongestants and cough suppressants, pain medication, fluids, and if the infection is bacterial, antibiotics. The breathing of a child with croup should be closely monitored, especially at night, when croup usually gets worse due to prone body position while sleeping. Although most children recover from croup without hospitalization, some may develop life-threatening breathing difficulties. Therefore, close contact with the doctor during this illness is especially important.

**Crouzon syndrome**  A hereditary craniofacial disorder characterized by craniosynostosis, small eye sockets that cause the eyes to protrude, a large jaw, and a beaked nose with narrowed breathing passages. Some people with Crouzon syndrome also have sleep apnea, hearing loss, and other difficulties. Treatment is by surgery. The gene for Crouzon syndrome has not been found, but it is believed to be on chromosome 10. Also known as craniofacial dysostosis. See also *craniosynostosis*.

**CRP**   C-reactive protein.

**cruciate**   Cross-shaped.

**cruciate ligament, anterior**   See *anterior cruciate ligament*. See also *knee*.

**cruciate ligament, posterior**   See *posterior cruciate ligament*. See also *knee*.

**cruciate ligaments**   Ligaments, such as those in the knee, that cross each other. See *anterior cruciate ligament, posterior cruciate ligament*.

**cryopreservation**   The process of cooling and storing cells, tissues, or organs at very low temperatures to maintain viability. For example, the technology of cooling and storing cells at a temperature below the freezing point (−196° C) permits high rates of survivability upon thawing.

**cryoprotectant**   A chemical component of a freezing solution used in cryopreservation to help protect what is being frozen from freeze damage. The chemical glycerol, for example, is commonly used as a cryoprotectant to protect frozen red blood cells.

**cryosurgery**   Treatment performed with an instrument that freezes and destroys abnormal tissue.

**crypt**   In anatomy, a crypt is variously a blind alley, a tube with no exit, a depression, or a pit in an otherwise fairly flat surface. For example, the tonsillar crypts are little, pitlike depressions in the tonsils.

**cryptorchidism**   A condition in which one or both testicles fail to move from the abdomen, where they develop before birth, into the scrotum. Boys who have had cryptorchidism that was not corrected in early childhood are at increased risk for developing cancer of the testicles. Also called undescended testicles.

**Crystodigin**   See *digitoxin*.

**CSF**   Cerebrospinal fluid.

**CT scan**   See *CAT scan*.

**CTL**   Cytotoxic T lymphocytes. See *T lymphocytes, cytotoxic*.

**CTS**   Carpal tunnel syndrome.

**cuboid bone**   The cube-shaped outer bone in the instep of the foot. The cuboid bone has a joint in back, allowing it to articulate posteriorly with the calcaneus (the heel bone). It also has a joint in the front, permitting it to articulate anteriorly with the fourth and fifth metatarsals (the bones just behind the fourth and fifth toes).

**cul-de-sac**   In anatomy, a blind pouch or cavity that is closed at one end. Examples include a colonic diverticulum, a small bulging sac that pushes outward from the colon wall, as is seen in diverticulosis; and the cecum, the first part of the colon, to which the appendix is attached. Cul-de-sac is also used specifically to refer to the rectouterine pouch (the pouch of Douglas), an extension of the peritoneal cavity between the rectum and back wall of the uterus.

**culdocentesis**   The puncture and aspiration (withdrawal) of fluid from the rectouterine pouch (the pouch of Douglas), an extension of the peritoneal cavity between the rectum and back wall of the uterus.

**culdoscope**   The viewing tube (endoscope) introduced through the end of the vagina into the rectouterine pouch (the pouch of Douglas) in a culdoscopy.

**culdoscopy**   The introduction of a viewing tube (called an endoscope or culdoscope) through the end of the vagina into the rectouterine pouch (the pouch of Douglas), an extension of the peritoneal cavity between the rectum and back wall of the uterus.

**cultural evolution**   By contrast with biologic evolution, cultural or social evolution is mediated by ideas, shows a rapid (exponential) rate of change, is usually purposeful and often beneficial, is widely disseminated by diverse means, is frequently transmitted in complex ways, and is enriched by the frequent formation of new ideas and new technologies. Cultural evolution is unique to humans among all forms of life. See also *biologic evolution*.

**culture**   The propagation of microorganisms in a growth media. Any body tissue or fluid can be evaluated in the laboratory by culture techniques to detect and identify infectious processes. Culture techniques also be used to determine sensitivity to antibiotics.

**curettage**   Removal of tissue with a curette.

**curette**   A spoon-shaped instrument with a sharp edge.

**curettement**   See *curettage*.

**Curie**   A unit of radioactivity. Specifically, the quantity of any radioactive nuclide in which the number of disintegrations per second is $3.7 \yen 10$ to the 10th power.

**Cushing syndrome**   A constellation of symptoms and signs caused by an excess of cortisol hormone. Cushing syndrome is an extremely complex hormonal condition that involves many areas of the body. Common symptoms are thinning of the skin; weakness; weight gain; bruising; hypertension; diabetes; thin, weak bones (osteoporosis); facial puffiness; and, in women, cessation of menstrual periods. Ironically, one of the most common causes of Cushing syndrome is the administration of cortisol-like medications for the treatment of diverse diseases. All other cases of Cushing syndrome are due to the excess production of cortisol by the adrenal gland. This may be caused by an abnormal growth of the pituitary gland, which can stimulate the adrenal gland; a benign or malignant growth within the adrenal gland itself, which produces cortisol; or production within another part of the body (ectopic production) of a hormone that directly or indirectly stimulates the adrenal gland to make cortisol.

**Cushingoid**   Having the constellation of symptoms and signs caused by an excess of cortisol hormone, particularly facial puffiness and unexplained weight gain. See *Cushing syndrome*.

**cusp**   **1** In reference to heart valves, one of the triangular segments of the valve, which opens and closes with the flow of blood. **2** In reference to teeth, a raised area of the biting surface.

**cut**   An area of severed skin. Wash a cut with soap and water, and keep it clean and dry. Avoid putting alcohol, hydrogen peroxide, or iodine into a wound; all can delay healing. Seek medical care if you think you might need stitches, as delay can increase the rate of wound infection. If the cut results from a puncture wound through the shoe, there is a high risk of infection, and you should see your health-care professional. Redness, swelling, increased pain, and pus draining from the wound also indicate an infection that requires professional care.

**cutaneous**   Related to the skin.

**cutaneous papilloma**   See *skin tag*.

**cutaneous syndactyly**   See *syndactyly, cutaneous*.

**cutis anserina**   See *goose bumps*.

**CVS**   Chorionic villus sampling.

**cyanosis**   Blueness or duskiness of the skin, caused by a lack of oxygen in the blood, including at birth. An infant with cyanosis is sometimes called a "blue baby."

**cycle, cell**   See *cell cycle*.

**cycle, menstrual**   The monthly progression of changes in the endometrium (the lining of the uterus), which ends with the shedding of part of the endometrium, and menstruation (monthly vaginal bleeding). This cycle is governed by a complex sequence of hormones, which influence fertility and may impact mood and a variety of physical functions as well. By convention, the menstrual cycle is considered to begin again on the first day of menstrual bleeding. See also *menstruation*.

**cyclooxygenase-1**   See *cox-1*.

**cyclooxygenase-2**   See *cox-2*.

**cyclooxygenase-2 inhibitor**   See *cox-2 inhibitor*.

**cyclophosphamide**   A medication (brand name: Cytoxan) prescribed primarily to people with autoimmune disorders and certain types of cancer. It has immunosuppressive and cytotoxic qualities.

**cyclosporine**   An immune-suppressant medication (brand names: Neoral, Sandimmune) prescribed chiefly for organ transplant recipients and people with autoimmune disorders. The two formulations work differently, and they may be prescribed together. Cyclosporine has many major potential side effects. Always work closely with your physician when taking this medication.

**cyclothymia**   A form of bipolar disorder in which the mood swings are less severe. See also *bipolar disorders*.

**cyst**   A closed sac or capsule, usually filled with fluid or semisolid material.

**cyst of the ovary, follicular**   A fluid-filled sac in the ovary, the most common type of ovarian cyst. It results from the overgrowth of a follicle, the fluid-filled cyst that contains an egg, which does not rupture to release the egg. Normally ovarian cysts resolve with no intervention over the course of days to months. See also *cyst, ovarian*.

**cyst, Baker**   A swelling in the space behind the knee (the popliteal space), composed of a membrane-lined sac filled with synovial fluid that has escaped from the joint. Also known as a synovial cyst of the popliteal space.

**cyst, Meibomian**   An inflammation of the oil gland of the eyelid. Also called a chalazion or a tarsal cyst.

**cyst, ovarian**   A fluid-filled sac in the ovary. The most common type is called a follicular cyst. Other cysts can contain blood; these are called hemorrhagic or endometriod cysts. Still other types of ovarian cysts are called dermoid cysts, or ovarian teratomas. These bizarre but usually benign tumors can contain many different body tissues, such as hair, teeth, bone, or cartilage. Most ovarian cysts are never noticed. When a cyst causes symptoms, pain is by far the most common presentation. Pain from an ovarian cyst can be caused by rupture of the cyst; rapid growth of the cyst; and stretching, bleeding into the cyst; or the cyst twisting around its blood supply. Diagnosis is usually made by ultrasound imaging. Blood tests, such as a CA-125 to help evaluate the growth for the potential of cancer, may also be ordered. It should be noted that interpretation of the CA-125 blood test has limitations: Women without cancer may have an elevated blood level, and those with cancer may have a negative blood test. Treatment of ovarian cysts depends on the woman's age, the size and type of the cyst, and its appearance on ultrasound. If it is causing severe pain, is not resolving, or is suspicious in any way, then it can be removed through laparoscopy or, if necessary, through an open laparotomy (bikini incision). After a cyst is removed, it should be sent to a pathologist for microscopic examination. For benign cysts, the outcome is usually excellent. See also *cyst of the ovary, follicular; ovarian teratoma.*

**cyst, pilonidal**   A special kind of abscess that occurs in the cleft between the buttocks. Forms frequently in adolescence after long trips that involve sitting.

**cyst, sebaceous**   A rounded, swollen area of the skin formed by an abnormal sac of retained oily excretion (sebum) from the sebaceous glands. See also *glands, sebaceous.*

**cyst, synovial, of the popliteal space**   See *cyst, Baker.*

**cyst, tarsal**   See *cyst, Meibomian.*

**cyst, thyroglossal**   A fluid-filled sac present at birth, and located in the midline of the neck. A thyroglossal cyst results from incomplete closure of a segment of the thyroglossal duct, a tube-like structure that normally closes as the embryo develops. Also known as a thyrolingual cyst.

**cyst, thyrolingual**   See *cyst, thyroglossal.*

**cystectomy**   Surgery to remove the bladder.

**cystic acne**   A localized infection (abscess) formed when oil ducts become clogged and infected. Cystic acne is most common in the teenage years. Treatment includes avoiding irritants on the face, including many cleansers and cosmetics; and in some severe cases, steroid or antibiotic medication. Cystic acne can cause permanent scarring in severe cases and in those who are prone to forming keloids.

**cystic fibrosis**   One of the most common serious genetic (inherited) diseases. Cystic fibrosis affects the exocrine glands, and is characterized by the production of abnormal secretions, leading to mucus build-up. This accumulation of mucus can impair the pancreas and, secondarily, the intestine. Mucus build-up in lungs can impair respiration. Without treatment, CF results in death for 95 percent of affected children before age five; however, a few long-lived CF patients have survived past age 60. Early diagnosis is of great importance. Early and continuing treatment of CF is valuable. Treatment includes physical therapy to loosen the mucus in the lungs, pancreatic enzymes, and medications to fight dangerous infections of the lungs. One in 400 couples is at risk for having children with CF. About 70 percent of CF cases are caused by a deletion on chromosome 7. Genetic testing can be done, and effective gene therapy may soon be commercially available.

**cystine**   A sulpherous amino acid, cystine is particularly notable because it is the least soluble of all naturally occurring amino acids, and because it precipitates out of solution in the heritable disease cystinuria. See also *cystinuria.*

**cystine kidney stones**   Kidney stones formed due to an excess of cystine in the urine. Small stones are passed in the urine. However, big stones remain in the kidney (nephrolithiasis), impairing the outflow of urine. Medium-size stones can make their way from the kidney into the ureter and lodge there, further blocking the flow of urine. Cystine kidney stones are responsible for all the signs and symptoms of cystinuria. See *cystinuria.*

**cystine transport disease**   See *cystinuria.*

**cystinuria**   An inherited (genetic) disorder of the transport of an amino acid called cystine, resulting in an excess of cystine in the urine and the formation of cystine stones. Cystinuria is the most common defect in the transport of an amino acid. Although cystine is not the only overly excreted amino acid in cystinuria, it is the least soluble of all naturally occurring amino acids. Cystine tends to precipitate out of urine and form stones (calculi) in the urinary tract, which can obstruct the flow of urine. This obstruction puts pressure back up on the ureter and kidney, causing the ureter to widen (dilate) and the kidney to be compressed. Obstruction also causes the urine to be stagnant, an open invitation to repeated urinary tract infection. Together, pressure on the kidneys and urinary infections result in damage to the kidneys. This damage can progress to renal insufficiency and end-stage kidney disease, requiring renal dialysis or a transplant. Signs and symptoms of cystinuria include blood in the urine (hematuria); pain in the side (flank), due to kidney pain; intense, cramping pain due to stones in the urinary tract (renal colic); urinary tract disease due to obstruction (obstructive uropathy); and urinary tract infections (UTIs). See also *cystine kidney stones.*

**cystitis**   Inflammation of the bladder. Cystitis can be due to infection from bacteria that ascend the urethra to the bladder. Symptoms include a frequent need to urinate, often accompanied by a burning sensation. As cystitis progresses, blood may be observed in the urine and the patient may suffer cramps after urination. In young children, attempts to avoid the pain of cystitis can be a cause for daytime wetting (enuresis). Treatment includes avoiding irritants, such as perfumed soaps, near the urethral opening; increased fluid intake; and antibiotics. Untreated cystitis can lead to scarring and the formation of stones when urine is retained for long periods of time to avoid painful urination.

**cystitis, interstitial**   Cystitis that involves inflammation or irritation of the bladder wall. This inflammation can lead to scarring and stiffening of the bladder, and even to ulcerations and bleeding. Diagnosis is based on symptoms, findings on cystoscopy and biopsy, and elimination of other treatable causes, such as infection. Because doctors do not know what causes interstitial cystitis, treatments are aimed at relieving symptoms. Most people are helped for variable periods of time by one or a combination of treatments. Abbreviated as IC.

**cystoscope**   An optical instrument that is inserted through the urethra into the bladder. A cystoscope has two ports: an optical port that permits one to see inside the bladder, and an additional port for insertion of various instruments designed for biopsy (removal of tissue samples), treatment of small bladder tumors, removal of stones from the bladder, and removal of the prostate (prostatectomy).

**cystoscopy**   A procedure in which the doctor inserts a lighted instrument into the urethra to look at the bladder.

**cytogenetics**   The study of the chromosomes, the visible carriers of the hereditary material. Cytogenetics is a fusion science, joining cytology (the study of cells) with genetics (the study of inherited variation).

**cytogenetics, clinical**   The application of cytogenetics to clinical medicine. For example, clinical cytogenetic studies might be done to determine whether a child with possible Down syndrome has an extra chromosome 21.

**cytomegalovirus**   A DNA-containing virus from the herpesvirus family. Infection with human cytomegalovirus causes mononucleosis. It can also cause viral hepatitis and viral pneumonia. Also known as human herpesvirus 5, abbreviated as HHV-5. See also *mononucleosis*.

**cytometry, flow**   See *flow cytometry*.

**cytoplasm**   The substance of the cell that lies outside the nucleus.

**cytosine**   One member of the G-C (guanine-cytosine) pair of bases in DNA.

**Cytoxan**   See *cyclophosphamide*.

**cytotoxic T lymphocytes**   See *T lymphocytes, cytotoxic*.

# Dd

**D & C**   Dilatation and curettage. See also *abortion*.

**D.O.**   Doctor of Osteopathy, an osteopathic physician. See *osteopath, osteopathy*.

**da Vinci, Leonardo**   The father of anatomic art, as well as accomplished architect, scientist, engineer, inventor, poet, sculptor, and painter, Leonardo da Vinci dissected and drew more than 10 human bodies in the cathedral cellar of the mortuary of Santa Spirito under the secrecy of candlelight, necessitated by the Church's belief in the sanctity of the human body and a papal decree that forbade human dissection. Leonardo recognized that a scientific knowledge of human anatomy could only be gained by dissecting the human body. This was in striking contrast to the pronouncements of Galen and other anatomists. Da Vinci injected the blood vessels and cerebral ventricles with wax for preservation, an anatomical technique still used today. His drawings of the human anatomy have long been considered to be unrivaled.

**dactyl-, -dactyl**   Prefix or suffix denoting involvement of the digits (fingers or toes).

**dactyledema**   Swelling of the fingers or toes.

**dactylitis**   Inflammation of a finger or toe.

**dactylomegaly**   Enlargement of the fingers or toes.

**dactylospasm**   A cramp of the fingers or toes.

**Daily Prayer of a Physician**   Said to have been written by the 12th-century physician-philosopher Moses Maimonides (but possibly penned by German physician Marcus Herz), the prayer of Maimonides is often recited by new medical graduates.

**Daltonism**   See *colorblindness*.

**dander**   Tiny scales shed from human or animal skin or hair. Dander floats in the air, settles on surfaces, and makes up much household dust. Cat dander is a classic cause of allergic reactions.

**dandy fever**   See *dengue fever*.

**Danlos syndrome**   See *Ehlers-Danlos syndrome*.

**Darier disease**   See *keratosis follicularis*.

**daw**   Abbreviation meaning "dispense as written."

**day sight**   Night blindness. See *nyctanopia*.

**DDH**   Developmental dysplasia of the hip. See *congenital hip dislocation*.

**DDX**   Abbreviation for differential diagnosis.

**DEA**   The Drug Enforcement Administration of the US Department of Justice, which regulates interstate commerce in prescription drugs to prevent them from being used as drugs of abuse. The DEA has established five schedules (categories) that classify controlled substances—including many prescription drugs, such as narcotics, barbituates, and stimulants—according to how dangerous they are, how great their potential for abuse, and whether they have any legitimate medical value. Every prescription written in the United States bears the DEA number of the prescribing doctor.

**deafness**   Partial or complete hearing loss, due to genetic causes, which may be structural (physical) or neurological; or to accidental, environmental, or acquired illness.

**deafness with goiter**   See *Pendred syndrome*.

**deafness, ichthyosis-keratitis**   See *keratitis-ichthyosis-deafness syndrome*.

**death rate**   The number of deaths in the population divided by the average population (or the population at midyear) is the crude death rate. In 1994, for example, the crude death rate per 1,000 population was 8.8 in the United States, 7.1 in Australia, and so on. A death rate can also be tabulated according to age or cause.

**death, black**   See *bubonic plague*.

**debilitate**   To impair the strength or to enfeeble. A chronic progressive disease may debilitate a patient. So may, temporarily, a major surgical procedure. In both cases the weakness is pervasive. Weakness in an arm or leg following the removal of a cast is not debility, but rather the temporary result of muscle atrophy from disuse.

**debrillator**   A device used to defibrillate the heart.

**decongestants**   Drugs that shrink the swollen membranes in the nose and make it easier to breath. Decongestants can be taken orally or by nasal spray. Decongestant nasal spray should not be used for more than five days without a doctor's recommendation, in which case it will usually be accompanied by a nasal steroid. Many decongestant nasal sprays cause a worsening of symptoms (a rebound effect) when they are taken for too long and then discontinued. This is a result of a tissue dependence on the medication. Decongestants should not be used by patients with high blood pressure (hypertension) unless they are under doctor's supervision.

**decubitous sore**   See *bedsore.*

**decubitous ulcer**   See *bedsore.*

**deep**   Away from the exterior surface or farther into the body, as opposed to superficial. The bones are deep to the skin. See also *Appendix B, "Anatomic Orientation Terms."*

**deep vein thrombosis**   Blood clotting in the veins of the inner thigh or leg. A blood clot (thrombus) can break off as an embolism and make its way to the lung, where it can cause respiratory distress and respiratory failure. Deep vein thrombosis is sometimes called "economy-class syndrome." Even in young, healthy travelers, long stretches of time spent immobilized in the cramped seat of an aircraft with very low humidity sets the stage for formation of a blood clot in the lower leg. Abbreviated as DVT.

**defecation syncope**   See *vasovagal syncope.*

**defect, atrial septal**   See *atrial septal defect.*

**defect, enzyme**   See *enzyme defect.* See also *deficiency, glucose-6-phosphate dehydrogenase; galactosemia; phenylketonuria.*

**defect, ventricular septal**   See *ventricular septal defect.*

**defibrillation**   The use of a carefully controlled electric shock, administered either through a device on the exterior of the chest wall or directly to the exposed heart muscle, to restart or normalize heart rhythms.

**defibrillator, implantable cardiac**   See *cardiac defibrillator, implantable.*

**deficiency, adenosine deaminase**   See *adenosine deanimase deficiency.*

**deficiency, alpha-1 antitrypsin**   See *alpha-1 antitrypsin deficiency.*

**deficiency, ankyrin**   See *spherocytosis, hereditary.*

**deficiency, calcium**   See *calcium deficiency.* See also *calcium.*

**deficency, FALDH**   See *Sjogren-Larsson syndrome.*

**deficency, FAO**   See *Sjogren-Larsson syndrome.*

**deficency, fatty alcohol: NAD+ oxidoreductase**   See *Sjogren-Larsson syndrome.*

**deficency, fatty aldehyde dehydrogenase**   See *Sjogren-Larsson syndrome.*

**deficency, glucocerebrosidase**   See *Gaucher disease.*

**deficency, glucose-6-phosphate dehydrogenase**   The most common disease-causing enzyme defect in humans, affecting an estimated 400 million people. The gene for producing glucose-6-phosphate dehydrogenase (G6PD) is on the X chromosome. Males with genetic coding for this enzyme deficiency develop anemia due to breakup of their red blood cells when they are exposed to oxidant drugs, such as the antimalarial primaquine, the sulfonamide antibiotics or sulfones, naphthalene moth balls, or fava beans.

**deficency, hex-A**   See *Tay-Sachs disease.*

**deficency, hexosaminidase A**   See *Tay-Sachs disease.*

**deficency, iron**   A lack of iron, which results in anemia. Iron is necessary to make hemoglobin, the key molecule in red blood cells responsible for the transport of oxygen. In iron deficiency anemia, the red cells are unusually small (microcytic) and pale (hypochromic). Characteristic features of iron deficiency anemia in children include failure to thrive (grow) and increased infections. The treatment of iron deficiency anemia, whether it be in children or adults, is to add iron supplements and iron-containing foods to the diet. Food sources of iron include meat, poultry, eggs, vegetables, and cereals (especially those fortified with iron). According to the National Academy of Sciences, the recommended dietary allowances of iron are 15 mg per day for women and 10 mg per day for men. Do not give iron supplements to children unless a doctor recommends it, however.

**deficency, lactase**   Lack of an enzyme called lactase in the small intestine; it is needed to digest lactose, a sugar found in milk and most other dairy products. Lactose is sometimes also used as an ingredient in other foods, so those with a lactase deficiency should check labels carefully. Although most people are born with the ability to make adequate amounts of lactase, production normally decreases with age, and there are significant differences in lactase production among ethnic groups. People of African or Asian descent are highly likely to have some degree of difficulty digesting products that contain lactose. The most common symptoms of lactase deficiency are diarrhea, bloating, and gas. Diagnosis may be made by a trial of a lactose-free diet or by special testing. In some cases, other diseases of the intestine may need to be excluded by further medical evaluation. Treatment is usually by avoiding lactose in the diet, although many people with a lactase deficiency can find relief with over-the-counter lactase supplements taken before eating such foods.

**deficiency, LCHAD** Acute fatty liver of pregnancy (AFLP) has been found to be associated in some cases with an abnormality of fatty-acid metabolism. This abnormality is a deficiency of the enzyme long-chain-3-hydroxyacyl-CoA dehydrogenease (LCHAD). In such cases, both parents have LCHAD activity at half of normal levels, but the fetus has none. The metabolic disease in the baby's liver apparently causes the fatty liver disease in the mother. In cases of AFLP due to LCHAD deficiency, there is a 25 percent or greater risk of AFLP in each pregnancy. See also *acute fatty liver of pregnancy*.

**deficiency, long-chain-3-hydroxyacyl-CoA dehydrogenease** See *deficiency, LCHAD*.

**deficiency, magnesium** Can occur because of inadequate intake or impaired intestinal absorption of magnesium. Low magnesium (hypomagnesemia) is often associated with low calcium (hypocalcemia) and potassium (hypokalemia) levels, because these nutrients interact with each other. Magnesium deficiency causes increased irritability of the nervous system, as evidenced by spasms of the hands and feet (tetany), muscular twitching and cramps, spasms of the larynx, and other symptoms. Treatment is by ensuring intake and absorption of the recommended dietary allowances of magnesium, currently 420 mg per day for men and 320 mg per day for women. One should not take more than 350 mg per day in supplement form, however.

**deficiency, niacin** See *pellagra*. See also *Appendix C, "Vitamins."*

**deficiency, protein C** Lack of protein C, a protein in plasma that enters into the cascade of biochemical events that leads to the formation of a clot. Deficiency of protein C results in thrombotic (clotting) disease.

**deficiency, selenium** Lack of the essential mineral selenium, which can cause Keshan disease, a fatal form of cardiomyopathy (disease of the heart muscle) that was first observed in Keshan province in China and has since been found elsewhere. Treatment is by ensuring intake of the recommended dietary allowance of selenium, currently 70 mg per day for men and 55 mg per day for

women. Food sources of selenium include seafoods; some meats, such as kidney and liver; and some grains and seeds.

**deficiency, UDP-glucuronosyltransferase** Underactivity of a liver enzyme, UDP-glucuronosyltransferase, which is essential to the disposal of bilirubin (the chemical that results from the normal breakdown of hemoglobin from red blood cells). This deficiency results in a condition called Gilbert disease, in which there are mild elevations of bilirubin pigment in the blood. The elevated bilirubin pigment can sometimes cause mild yellowing (jaundice) of the eyes. There is no need for treatment, and the prognosis is excellent. See also *Gilbert syndrome*.

**deficiency, zinc** Deficiency of zinc is associated with short stature, anemia, increased pigmentation of skin (hyperpigmentation), enlarged liver and spleen (hepatosplenomegaly), impaired gonadal function (hypogonadism), impaired wound healing, and immune deficiency. The key laboratory finding is an abnormally low blood zinc level, reflecting the impaired zinc uptake. Treatment with zinc is curative. One form of zinc deficiency is the hereditary disease acrodermatitis enteropathica. The current recommended dietary allowance of zinc is 12 mg per day for women and 10 mg per day for men. Food sources of zinc include meat, eggs, seafood, nuts, and cereals. See also *acrodermatitis enteropathica*.

**deformation** A change from the normal size or shape. A deformation can be present at birth (congenital) or develop after birth (acquired). Also known as deformity, malformation.

**deformity, cauliflower ear** See *cauliflower ear*.

**degenerative arthritis** See *arthritis, degenerative*.

**degenerative joint disease** See *arthritis, degenerative*.

**dehydration** Excessive loss of body water. Diseases of the gastrointestinal tract may lead to dehydration. One clue to dehydration is a rapid drop in weight. A loss of over 10 percent (15 pounds in a person weighing 150 pounds) in a short period of time is considered severe. Symptoms include increasing thirst, dry mouth, weakness or lightheadedness (particularly when it worsens on standing), or a darkening/decrease in urination. Severe dehydration can lead to changes in the body's chemistry, kidney failure, and death. The best way to treat dehydration is to prevent it from occurring. If one suspects fluid loss is excessive, notify a physician. Intravenous or oral fluid replacement may be needed.

**déjà vu**   A disquieting feeling of having been somewhere or done something before, even though one has not. Although most people have experienced this feeling at one time or another, in some people sensations of déjà vu are part of a seizure or migraine aura; in others, they themselves are a seizure phenomenon. See also *jamais vu, seizure disorders.*

**delay, developmental**   See *developmental delay.*

**deletion**   Loss of a segment of DNA from a chromosome, which can result in genetic disorders. An example is cri du chat syndrome, which is due to loss of part of chromosome 5. A deletion is the opposite of a duplication.

**delirium tremens**   A neurological symptom of alcohol withdrawal seen in chronic alcoholism, with symptoms of psychosis. These may include uncontrollable trembling, hallucinations, severe anxiety, sweating, and sudden feelings of terror. Delirium tremens can be both frightening and, in severe cases, deadly. Treatment includes observation, comfort care, and in some cases medication.

**delivery, breech**   A buttocks-first birth.

**delivery, footling**   A foot- or feet-first birth. A footling birth is called single-footling or double-footling, depending on whether the presenting part of the baby at delivery is just one foot or both feet.

**delivery, vertex**   A head-first birth, which is the usual pattern.

**delta cell, pancreatic**   A type of cell located in areas called the islets of Langerhans in the pancreas. The delta cells make somatostatin, a hormone that inhibits the release of numerous hormones in the body.

**delta-storage pool disease**   See *Hermansky-Pudlak syndrome.*

**deltoid**   The muscle, roughly triangluar in shape, that stretches from the clavicle (collarbone) to the humerus, the upper bone of the arm. It is flexed to move the arm up and down from the side.

**dementia**   Significant loss of intellectual abilities, such as memory capacity, severe enough to interfere with social or occupational functioning. Criteria for the diagnosis of dementia include impairment of attention, orientation, memory, judgment, language, motor and spatial skills, and function. By definition, dementia is not due to major depression or schizophrenia. Dementia is reported in as many as 1 percent of adults 60 years of age. It has been estimated that the frequency of dementia doubles every five years after the age of 60. Alzheimer disease is the

most common cause of dementia. Other causes include AIDS, alcoholism (the dementia is due to thiamine deficiency), brain injury, brain tumors, drug toxicity, encephalitis (infection of brain), hydrocephalus, meningitis, multiple sclerosis, Pick disease, syphilis, and thyroid disease.

**dementia complex, AIDS**   See *AIDS dementia complex.*

**dementia, MELAS**   See *MELAS syndrome.*

**demulcent**   Any agent that tends to form a soothing, protective film when administered onto a mucous membrane surface.

**demyelination**   A degenerative process that erodes away the myelin sheath that normally protects nerve fibers. Demyelination exposes these fibers and appears to cause problems in nerve impulse conduction that may affect many physical systems. Demyelination is seen in a number of diseases, particularly multiple sclerosis. Diagnosis is by functional observation and by testing for myelin protein in the blood.

**dendrite**   A short, arm-like protuberance from a nerve cell (neuron). Dendrites from juxtaposed neurons are tipped by synapses, tiny transmitters and receivers for chemical messages between the cells. See also *neuron, axon.*

**dengue**   See *dengue fever.*

**dengue fever**   An acute mosquito-borne viral illness of sudden onset that usually follows a benign course, with headache, fever, prostration, severe joint and muscle pain, swollen glands (lymphadenopathy), and rash. The presence of fever, rash, and headache (the "dengue triad") is particularly characteristic of dengue. Dengue fever is endemic throughout the tropics and subtropics. Also called breakbone fever, dandy fever, dengue. Victims of dengue often have contortions due to the intense joint and muscle pain.

**dengue hemorrhagic fever**   A syndrome caused by the dengue virus, which tends to affect children under age 10, causing abdominal pain, hemorrhage (bleeding), and circulatory collapse (shock). DHF starts abruptly with high continuous fever and headache, plus respiratory and intestinal symptoms with sore throat, cough, nausea, vomiting, and abdominal pain. Shock occurs after 2 to 6 days with sudden collapse; cool, clammy extremities; weak, thready pulse; and blueness around the mouth (circumoral cyanosis). There is bleeding with easy bruising, blood spots in the skin (petechiae), spitting up blood (hematemesis), blood in the stool (melena), bleeding gums and nosebleeds (epistaxis). Pneumonia and heart inflammation (myocarditis) may be present. Mortality ranges from 6 to 30 percent. Most deaths occur in children, with infants at particular risk. DHF is also called Philippine, Thai, or Southeast Asian hemorrhagic fever, or dengue shock syndrome. Abbreviated as DHF.

**dengue shock syndrome** See *dengue hemorrhagic fever*.

**Dental Association, American** See *American Dental Association*.

**dental braces** Devices used by orthodontists to move teeth or adjust underlying bone. The ideal age for starting orthodontic treatment is between ages 3 to 12 years. Temporomandibular joint (TMJ) problems also can sometimes be corrected with dental braces. Teeth can be moved by removable appliances or by fixed braces. If there is crowding of teeth, some teeth may need to be extracted before braces are applied. Retainers may be necessary long after dental braces are placed, especially in orthodontic treatment of adults.

**dental impaction** Teeth pressing together. For example, molar teeth (the large teeth in the back of the jaw) can be impacted; cause pain; and require pain medication, antibiotics, and surgical removal.

**dental pain** The most common cause of toothache is a dental cavity. The second most common is gum disease. Toothache can be caused by a problem that does not originate from a tooth or the jaw.

**Dental Research, National Institute of** See *National Institutes of Health*.

**dentin** The hard tissue of the tooth surrounding the central core of nerves and blood vessels (pulp).

**deoxyribonucleic acid** See *DNA*.

**Depo-Provera** A contraceptive that is injected, and lasts three months between doses. Depo-Provera is also used to regulate the menstrual cycle in women with uneven or painful menses. It contains the hormonal compound medroxyprogesterone acetate.

**depression** Low spirits; dejection. Symptoms of depression include apathy, changes in eating habits, lack of emotional expression (flat affect), social withdrawal, and fatigue. The most common type is situational depression: the normal feelings of extreme sadness that accompany the grieving process. Situational depression usually resolves within three months, although cultural and personal issues can have an impact on its length and severity. Clinical depression can begin with situational depression that does not resolve, or it can have no relationship at all

to life events. It is believed to be caused by a chemical imbalance in the brain, which may be inherited. Major forms include unipolar depression (chronic depressed mood), dysthymia (chronic but milder depressed mood), and bipolar disorders (alternating depressed and hypomanic or manic moods). Depression may also be a symptom of physical illnesses, such as diabetes and lupus, that affect neurotransmitter production and use. The first step in getting appropriate treatment is a complete physical and psychological evaluation. Effective treatment is available, including antidepressant drugs and therapy. Outcome is best if both medication and therapy are used.

**depression, bipolar** See *bipolar disorders*.

**depression, dysthmia** A less severe type of depression, dysthymia involves long-term chronic symptoms that do not disable, but keep one from functioning at "full steam" or from feeling good. Sometimes people with dysthymia also experience major depressive episodes.

**depression, major** Major depression is manifested by a combination of symptoms that interfere with the ability to work, sleep, eat, and enjoy once-pleasurable activities. These disabling episodes of depression can occur once, twice, or several times in a lifetime. See also *depression*.

**depression, manic** See *bipolar disorders*.

**depression, unipolar** See *depression*.

**depression, winter** See *seasonal affective disorder*. See also *bipolar disorders*.

**Dercum disease** A condition characterized by fatty tumors beneath the skin. Also called adiposis dolorosa.

**dermabrasion** A surgical procedure that involves the controlled scraping away of the upper layers of the skin with sandpaper or some other mechanical means. The purpose of dermabrasion is to smoothe the skin and, in the process, remove small scars (as from acne), moles (nevi), tattoos, or fine wrinkles. Dermabrasion is performed by a dermatologist. Chemical skin peels are an alternative to dermabrasion.

**dermatitis** Inflammation of the skin, either due to direct contact with an irritating substance, or to an allergic reaction. Symptoms of dermatitis include redness, itching, and in some cases blistering. There are two types of dermatitis: eczematous (eczema) and noneczematous (also called occupational). Eczema can be particularly severe and difficult to treat once it is established. It can be caused by direct contact, or it may emerge when an allergen is breathed in, injected, or ingested. Noneczematous dermatitis is usually caused by direct contact with an irritant. Frequent offenders include detergents, especially those with perfumes; chemicals used in photo development; and some types of solvents. Treatment is twofold: People who suffer from dermatitis must identify and avoid substances that cause attacks; during attacks they may use topical treatments, such as steroid creams. See also *eczema*.

**dermatitis and diarrhea, zinc deficiency** Among the consequences of zinc deficiency, dermatitis (skin inflammation) and diarrhea are particularly prominent features. See also *acrodermatitis enteropathica*.

**dermatologic** Having to do with the skin.

**dermatologist** A doctor who specializes in the diagnosis and treatment of skin problems.

**dermatome** 1 A localized area of skin that receives its sensations via a single nerve from a single nerve root of the spinal cord. Shingles (herpes zoster) typically affects one or several isolated dermatomes. 2 A cutting instrument used for skin grafting or for slicing thin pieces of skin.

**dermatomyositis** A chronic inflammatory disease of muscle, which is associated with patches of slightly raised reddish or scaly rash. The rash can be on the bridge of the nose, around the eyes, or on sun-exposed areas of the neck and chest. Classically, however, it is over the knuckles. See *polymyositis*.

**dermatopathy** Any disease of the skin. Synonymous with dermopathy.

**dermatophytic onychomycosis** Ringworm of the nail (onychomycosis), the most common fungus infection of the nails. Onychomycosis makes the nails look white and opaque, thickened, and brittle. Older women (perhaps because estrogen deficiency may increase the risk of infection), and men and women with diabetes or disease of the small blood vessels (peripheral vascular disease) are at increased risk. Artificial nails (acrylic nails or "wraps") increase the risk, because the nail surface is usually abraded when an artificial nail is applied. If the emery board carries infection, and water collects under the nail, it creates a moist, warm environment for fungal growth. Also known as nail fungus or tinea unguium. Treatment includes avoiding artificial nails, using safer application techniques and only new artificial nails and emery boards for each customer, and topical antifungal medication.

**dermis** The lower or inner layer of the two main layers of cells that make up the skin.

**dermoid** See *dermoid cyst of the ovary*.

**dermoid cyst of the ovary** A bizarre, usually benign, tumor in the ovary, which typically contains a diversity of tissues including hair, teeth, bone, thyroid, and so on. A dermoid cyst develops from a totipotential germ cell (a primary oocyte) that is retained within the ovary. Being totipotential, that cell can give rise to all orders of cells necessary to form mature tissues and often recognizable structures such as hair, bone and sebaceous (oily) material, neural tissue, and teeth. Dermoid cysts may occur at any age, but the prime age of detection is in the childbearing years. The average age is 30. Up to 15 percent of women with dermoid cysts have them in both ovaries. Dermoid cysts can range in size from less than a half inch up to about 17 inches in diameter. These cysts can cause the ovary to twist (torsion) and imperil its blood supply. The larger the dermoid cyst, the greater the risk of rupture with spillage of the greasy contents, which can create problems with adhesions, pain, and so on. Although about 98 percent of these tumors are benign, the remaining fraction become cancerous (malignant). Removal of the dermoid cyst is usually the treatment of choice. This can be done by laparotomy (open surgery) or laparoscopy (with a scope). Torsion (twisting) of the ovary by the cyst is an emergency and calls for urgent surgery. Also known as dermoids, ovarian teratomas.

**dermopathy** See *dermatopathy*.

**descending aorta** The part of the aorta that runs down through the chest and the abdomen. The descending aorta starts after the arch of the aorta, and ends by splitting into the common iliac arteries. The descending aorta, by convention, is subdivided into the thoracic aorta and the abdominal aorta. Also known as the aorta descendens and the pars descendens aortae. See also *aorta*.

**desensitization, allergy** See *allergy desensitization*.

**"designer estrogen"** An engineered drug that possesses some, but not all, of the actions of estrogen. Designer estrogens are also called selective estrogen-receptor modulators (SERMs). For example, raloxifene (trade name: Evista) is classified as a SERM because, like estrogen, it prevents bone loss and lowers serum cholesterol, but it does not stimulate the endometrial lining of the uterus.

**desmoid tumor** Benign soft-tissue tumors (sarcomas) that occur most often in young adults. They usually involve the limbs or trunk, but can also arise in the abdomen or thorax. Desmoid tumors never spread to other parts of the body. However, they are very difficult to remove because they intertwine extensively with the surrounding tissues. These tumors look like dense scar tissue, and adhere tenaciously to surrounding structures and organs. Surgery has been the traditional main mode of therapy for desmoid tumors, but up to 70 percent recur after surgery. Radiation therapy has also been used, although it exposes the patient to significant radiation with damage to surrounding tissues, and puts the patient at risk for a cancer caused by the radiation (a secondary malignancy). Radiation also is hampered by a moderate recurrence rate. The combination of surgery and radiation has also been used to treat these stubborn tumors. While somewhat successful, the combination of wide-resection surgery and high-dose radiation represents very aggressive treatment for a benign condition. Limited (low-dose) chemotherapy emerged in 1989 as a less aggressive treatment for desmoid tumors. The antitumor drugs are given in low doses, so there are minimal short-term (and usually no long-term) side effects. Limited chemotherapy causes one-third of desmoid tumors to vanish and one-third to shrink. The remaining third appear not to change, but they rarely progress and usually stop hurting. Desmoid tumors are also called aggressive fibromatosis, because they are locally aggressive and fibrous like scar tissue.

**desmoid, cortical**   A tumor that arises in embryonic tissue.

**desmoplasia**   The growth of fibrous or connective tissue.

**desmoplastic reaction**   A type of reaction associated with some tumors, characterized by the pervasive growth of dense fibrous tissue around the tumor. Scar tissue (adhesion) within the abdomen after abdominal surgery is another type of desmoplastic reaction.

**desquamate**   To shed the outer layers of the skin.

**desquamation**   The shedding of the outer layers of the skin. For example, once the rash of measles fades, there is desquamation.

**deuteranomaly**   See *colorblindness.*

**deuteranopia**   See *colorblindness.*

**development**   The process of growth and differentiation. The most important stage of human development occurs before birth, as tissues and organs arise from differentiation of cells in the embryo. This process continues until birth, and interuptions result in the most serious types of birth defects, such as anencephaly and spina bifida. The developmental process continues after birth as the infant and child grows physically, develops basic brain-based abilities such as speech and hand-eye coordination, and learns. Interruptions in any of these processes can result in developmental delay.

**developmental delay**   Behind schedule in reaching milestones of early childhood development. Unfortunately, this term is often used as a euphemism for mental retardation, which can be less a delay than a permanent limitation of the child's ability to progress.

**developmental disorder**   One of several disorders that interrupt normal development in childhood. They may affect a single area of development (specific developmental disorders) or several areas (pervasive developmental disorders). With early intervention, most specific developmental disorders can be accommodated and overcome. Early intervention is absolutely essential for pervasive developmental disorders, many of which will respond to an aggressive approach that may combine speech therapy, occupational therapy, physical therapy, behavior modification techniques, play therapy, and in some cases medication. See also *autism, cerebral palsy, developmental dyspraxia, dysarthria, dyscalculia, dyslexia, specific developmental disorders.*

**developmental dysplasia of the hip**   See *congenital hip dislocation.*

**developmental dyspraxia**   A pattern of delayed, uneven, or aberrant development of physical (gross and/or fine motor) abilities. Developmental dyspraxia may be seen alone or in combination with other developmental problems, particularly apraxia or dyspraxia of speech. Treatment is via early intervention, using physical therapy to improve gross motor skills, and occupational therapy to assist in fine motor development and sensory integration.

**device, assistive**   Any device that is designed, made, and/or adapted to help a person perform a particular task which might otherwise be difficult. For example, canes, crutches, walkers, wheelchairs, and shower chairs are all assistive devices. See also *assistive technology, augmentative communication device.*

**device, intrauterine**   See *intrauterine device.*

**device, medical**   Broadly defined, any physical item used in medical treatment, from a heart pacemaker to a wheelchair. In insurance parlance, "medical device" is usually synonymous with assistive device, although it may include items more frequently thought of as medical supplies, such as dressings needed for wound care at home or syringes for self-administration of insulin. Medical devices are not covered by most insurance policies, although they may be available through supplemental insurance or, in some cases, on an inexpensive rental basis through local hospitals, clinics, or pharmacies. See *assistive device.*

**dextro-**   Prefix from the Latin word *dexter,* meaning on the right side. For example, a molecule that shows dextrorotation is turning or twisting to the right. The opposite of dextro- is levo-, from the Latin *laevus.*

**dextrocardia**   In this condition, the heart's location is actually reversed anatomically, placing it in the right side of the chest rather than in its normal location on the left. This is a true anatomic reversal: The apex (tip) of the heart points to the right instead of the left. Dextrocardia occurs in an abnormal condition present at birth, called Kartagener syndrome. See also *dextroposition of the heart.*

**dextroposition**   Move to the right.

**dextroposition of the heart**   A condition in which the heart is displaced to the right side of the chest, but without any anatomic alteration in the heart itself. Dextroposition occurs when the contents of the left side of the chest shove the heart to the right, or when the contents of the right chest are reduced (for example, by collapse of the right lung) and the heart moves toward the sparsely occupied space on the right. See also *dextrocardia.*

**dextrose**   Glucose, a simple sugar.

**DHF**   Dengue hemorrhagic fever.

**Di Ferrante syndrome**   A rare form of mucopolysaccharidosis (MPS). It is an autosomal recessive genetic disorder. Also known as mucopolysaccharidosis Type IX. See also *mucopolysaccharidosis.*

**dia-**   Prefix meaning through, throughout, or completely, as in diachronic, diagnosis, and dialysis.

**Diabetes and Digestive and Kidney Diseases, National Institute of**   See *National Institutes of Health.*

**diabetes**   See *diabetes mellitus.*

**diabetes and diet**   Dietary control is the primary method for treating all forms of diabetes. The goal of these changes is to minimize the chance of overloading the patient's system glucose. Patients with diabetes benefit from eating carefully controlled amounts and types of food at regular intervals throughout the day, rather than at two or three large meals. Soluble fibers, such as oat bran, apples, citrus, pears, peas and beans, and psyllium, slow down the digestion of carbohydrates (sugars), which results in better glucose metabolism. Of course, patients should avoid consumption of sugary foods, and moderate their intake of starches that convert quickly to glucose.

Some patients with adult-onset diabetes may be successfully treated with diet alone, and those on insulin can often reduce their insulin requirements by adhering to an appropriate diet. Learning proper eating habits is especially important for children with diabetes, as they run the highest long-term risk of severe symptoms.

**Diabetes Association, American**   The nation's leading nonprofit health organization providing diabetes research, information, and advocacy.

**diabetes insipidus**   A metabolic disorder that mimics symptoms of diabetes, including increased output of urine and increased thirst. It is caused by a malfunction in the pituitary gland, and can be treated by administering vasopressin, a pituitary hormone.

**diabetes mellitus**   A chronic condition associated with abnormally high levels of sugar (glucose) in the blood. Absence of, insufficient production of, or autoimmune resistance to the pancreatic hormone insulin causes diabetes. Insulin provides the body with a natural method for oxidizing glucose to provide energy; without enough insulin, glucose builds up in the bloodstream to dangerous levels. The tendency to develop diabetes runs in families, but not all patients have such a family history. Symptoms of diabetes include increased urine output, increased appetite and thirst, unexplained weight loss or fluctuation, and fatigue. Diabetes mellitus is diagnosed by blood sugar testing. Major complications include dangerously elevated blood sugar, abnormally low blood sugar due to incorrect dosing of diabetes medications, and disease of the blood vessels, which can damage the eyes, kidneys, nerves, and heart. Circulation problems due to blood-vessel damage may also endanger the patient's feet and legs, leading in some cases to amputation. When the body cannot use glucose for energy, it turns to burning fat as energy. This process creates compounds called ketones. If the blood level of ketones gets too high, the result is a dangerous condition called ketosis that, if unchecked, can cause convulsions, coma, and death. Treatment depends on the type of the diabetes. Diet is always the primary treatment. Many patients take medications that help to regulate their production and use of insulin. Others may need insulin injections. Insulin can be self-administered via syringe or, more recently, via an almost-painless "gun" device, an external insulin pump, or an internally implanted insulin pump. See also *diabetes, insulin-dependent; diabetes, non-insulin-dependent.*

**diabetes, adult-onset**   Diabetes that begins in adulthood, usually after age 40 or, more characteristically, in old age. Also known as type 2 diabetes.

**diabetes, brittle**   See *diabetes, labile.*

**diabetes, bronze** Diabetes mellitus that occurs as a result of damage to the pancreas from iron deposition of hemochromatosis. See also *diabetes mellitus, hemochromatosis.*

**diabetes, childhood** When diabetes starts in childhood, the likelihood of serious complications, including dependence on insulin injections and/or medication, is greater than with adult-onset diabetes. It is more likely to be caused by an autoimmune reaction to the body's own insulin than by other factors. Also known as type 1 diabetes.

**diabetes, gestational** A diabetic condition that appears during pregnancy, and usually goes away after the birth of the baby. Gestational diabetes is best controlled via diet. Because a woman's dietary needs increase and change during pregnancy, the services of a professional dietitian, and careful monitoring by a midwife, obstetrician, and/or physician with expertise in gestational diabetes are necessary. Gestational diabetes can cause birth complications, as one of the side effects is increased fetal size.

**diabetes, insulin-dependent** A form of diabetes that is more likely to develop in childhood or early adulthood. Administration of insulin or drugs that increase the body's own production of insulin is necessary. Insulin-dependent diabetes is a chronic disorder that requires life-long dietary restrictions and medical treatment. Also known as type 1 diabetes. See also *diabetes, non-insulin-dependent.*

**diabetes, insulin-resistent** An autoimmune form of diabetes, in which the body develops an immune response to its own insulin hormone. This form of diabetes is probably the most difficult type to treat, but it can be done. Treatment includes very careful diet, medication, and in experimental cases, immunology treatment.

**diabetes, labile** A form of diabetes in which the blood glucose level tends to swing quickly and widely from high to low, and from low to high. Labile diabetes occurs in Type 1 diabetes that is untreated, poorly controlled, or resistant to treatment. Also called brittle diabetes or unstable diabetes.

**diabetes, non-insulin-dependent** This form of diabetes, also called type 2 diabetes, is more likely to emerge in middle or old age. It can usually be treated via diet alone, sometimes in combination with medication to control glucose levels. Although this chronic condition is very treatable, it carries the same serious risks as insulin-dependent diabetes—and if left untreated, can develop into insulin-dependent diabetes. Therefore, consistent treatment with diet is essential, as is medication, when warranted.

**diabetes, type 1** Insulin-dependent diabetes, or juvenile diabetes.

**diabetes, type 2** Non-insulin-dependent diabetes, adult-onset diabetes, or insulin-resistant diabetes.

**diabetes, unstable** See *diabetes, labile.*

**diabetic coma** Coma due to the buildup of ketones in the bloodstream. Ketones are a product of the body's metabolizing fats for energy rather than glucose. The best treatment is prevention. Careful diet, medication, and insulin dosing as needed should prevent ketone buildup. Patients with diabetes and their family members should be aware of the early signs of ketone buildup. These include weight loss; nausea; confusion; gasping for breath; and a characteristically sweet, chemical odor, similar to that of acetone or alcohol ("acetone breath"), to the patient's breath, and sometimes sweat. Diabetic coma may be presaged by confusion and convulsions. Immediate emergency medical treatment is needed in a hospital setting for patients who show the early signs of incipient diabetic coma.

**diabetic nephropathy** Kidney disease associated with long-standing diabetes. It affects the network of tiny blood vessels (the microvasculature) in the glomerulus, a key structure in the kidney that is composed of capillary blood vessels. This structure is critical for blood filtration. Features of diabetic nephropathy include the nephrotic syndrome, which is characterized by excessive filtration of protein into the urine (proteinuria), high blood pressure (hypertension), and progressively impaired kidney function. When severe, kidney failure, end-stage renal disease, and the need for chronic kidney dialysis or a kidney transplant may result. Also known as intercapillary glomerulonephritis, Kimmelstiel-Wilson disease, Kimmelstiel-Wilson syndrome.

**diabetic neuropathy** Pain, weakness, or lack of sensation in a body part, that is associated with nerve damage from diabetes. Typically, diabetic neuropathy affects the feet, legs, hands, or arms. Treatment can include physical therapy, medication, and improved treatment of the underlying diabetes.

**diabetic retinopathy** A disorder of the retina, associated with diabetes. It is caused by thickening of the arteries and high blood pressure. It may cause sight impairment or blindness.

**diabetic shock** Hypoglycemia (low blood sugar) associated with diabetes. Symptoms include a sweet, chemical odor on the patient's breath that is similar to that of acetone or alcohol ("acetone breath"), fatigue, lightheadedness or fainting, and often reddening of the skin if the patient is Caucasian, or darkening of the skin in patients with darker skin. Immediate treatment is administration of glucose in a prescription sublingual form, or even in the form of hard candy if nothing else is available. Patients with diabetes and their families should learn the early warning signs of hypoglycemia, and carry glucose tablets for emergency use. Patients in a state of diabetic shock should also be evaluated medically immediately after emergency treatment. Changes in diet, medication, or insulin administration can then be made, to prevent future episodes.

**diachronic** Over a period of time, as opposed to synchronic, which means at one point in time.

**diachronic study** A study done over the course of time. For example, a diachronic study of children with Down syndrome might involve the study of 100 children with this condition from birth to 10 years of age. Also known as a longitudinal study.

**diagnosis** Knowledge of the nature of a disease. Patients who speak of "getting a diagnosis" mean learning the medical name for what ails them, and gaining an understanding of their condition. Abbreviated as dx, DX. See also *differential diagnosis*.

**diagnosis, differential** See *differential diagnosis*.

**dialysis** The process of cleansing the blood by passing it through a special machine. Dialysis is necessary when the kidneys are not able to filter the blood. It gives patients with kidney failure a chance to live productive lives. There are two types of dialysis: hemodialysis and peritoneal dialysis. Each type of dialysis has advantages and disadvantages. Patients can often choose the type of long-term dialysis that best matches their needs. Also known as hemodialysis. See also *dialysis, peritoneal*.

**dialysis machine** A machine that filters a patient's blood to remove excess water and waste products when the kidneys are damaged, dysfunctional, or missing. Blood is drawn through a specially created vein in the forearm, which is called an arteriovenous (AV) fistula. From the AV fistula, blood is taken to the dialysis machine through plastic tubing. The dialysis machine itself can be thought of as an artificial kidney. Inside, it consists of more plastic tubing that carries the removed blood to the dialyser, a bundle of hollow fibers that forms a semipermeable membrane for filtering out impurities. In the dialyser, blood is diffused with a saline solution called dialysate, and the dialysate is in turn diffused with blood. Once the filtration process is complete, the cleansed blood is returned to the patient. Most patients who undergo dialysis because of kidney impairment or failure use a dialysis machine at a special dialysis clinic. Most sessions take about four hours, and typical patients visit the clinic one to three times per week.

**dialysis, peritoneal** A dialysis technique that uses the patient's own body tissues inside the belly (abdominal cavity) as a filter. The intestines lie in the abdominal cavity, the space between the abdominal wall and the spine. A plastic tube called a dialysis catheter is placed through the abdominal wall and into the abdominal cavity. A special fluid called dialysate is then flushed into the abdominal cavity and washes around the intestines. The intestinal walls act as a filter between this fluid and the bloodstream. By using different types of solutions, waste products and excess water can be removed from the body through this process.

**diaper rash** Also called "diaper dermatitis," diaper rash is an inflammatory reaction localized to the area of skin usually covered by the diaper. It can have many causes, including infections (yeast, bacterial, or viral), friction irritation, chemical allergies (perfumes, soaps), sweat, and plugged sweat glands. Most diaper rash problems are solved by cleansing the skin with nonperfumed, gentle products; frequent diaper changes; and exposing the affected skin area to air. Commercially available diaper rash ointments may be helpful for prevention, but may actually cause further irritation if used on the inflamed areas.

**diaphragm** **1** The muscle that separates the chest (thoracic) cavity from the abdomen. Contraction of the diaphragm muscle helps to expand the lungs when one breathes in air. **2** A specially fitted contraceptive device that covers the cervix to prevent the entry of sperm. For greatest effectiveness, a diaphragm is used with spermicidal gel or cream. See also *birth control, contraceptive*.

**diaphragmatic hernia** Passage of a loop of bowel through the diaphragm muscle. This type of hernia occurs as the bowel from the abdomen "herniates" upward through the diaphragm into the chest (thoracic) cavity.

**diarrhea** A familiar phenomenon with unusually frequent or unusually liquid bowel movements, excessive watery evacuations of fecal material. The opposite of constipation. There are myriad infectious and noninfectious causes of diarrhea. Persistent diarrhea is both uncomfortable and dangerous to the health, as it can indicate an underlying infection. It may also mean that the body is not able to absorb some nutrients due to a problem in the bowels. Treatment includes drinking plenty of fluids to prevent dehydration, over-the-counter remedies in most cases, and medical examination if diarrhea persists for more than a couple of days, particularly in small children or elderly people.

**diarrhea and dermatitis, zinc deficiency** See *deficiency, zinc*.

**diarrhea, antibiotic-induced**   Diarrhea caused by the bacterium Clostridium difficile (C. difficile), one of the most common causes of infection of the large bowel (colon). Patients taking antibiotics are at particular risk of becoming infected with C. difficile. Antibiotics disrupt the normal bacteria of the bowel, allowing C. difficile and other bacteria to become established and overgrow inside the colon. Many infected persons have no symptoms, but can become carriers of the bacteria and infect others. In others, a toxin produced by C. difficile causes diarrhea, abdominal pain, severe inflammation of the colon (colitis), fever, an elevated white blood count, vomiting, and dehydration. In severely affected patients, the inner lining of the colon becomes severely inflamed (a condition called pseudomembranous colitis). Rarely, the walls of the colon wear away and holes develop (colon perforation), which can lead to a life-threatening infection of the abdomen.

**diarrhea, rotavirus**   A leading cause of severe winter diarrhea in infants and young children, often accompanied by fever and dyhydration. Treatment includes frequent administration of fluids to prevent dehydration, rest, good nutrition, and in some cases medication. A preventative vaccine has recently been developed. See also *rotavirus*.

**diarrhea, travelers'**   Illness, including diarrhea, that is associated with travel to a foreign country. Among the causes of travelers' diarrhea are viruses and enterotoxigenic E. coli (ETEC), which may be transmitted via food or water. Prevention is the best policy, including drinking bottled water; filtering tap water or, if camping, water from natural sources; washing fruits and vegetables purchased in local markets with a solution of water and a few drops of bleach; and whenever possible, choosing restaurants with high standards of sanitation. Treatment is replacement of fluids and electrolytes (sodium and other ions) lost via diarrhea. In serious cases of persistent travelers' diarrhea, medical care should be sought.

**diathermy**   The use of heat to destroy abnormal cells. Also called cauterization or electrodiathermy.

**diathesis**   In medicine, diathesis is an elegant term for predisposition or tendency. Thus, a hemorrhagic diathesis is nothing more than a tendency to bleed.

**diazepam**   A medication (brand name: Valium) used as a tranquilizer and sedative. See also *benzodiazepine tranquilizer*.

**dicentric chromosome**   See *chromosome, dicentric*.

**dietary supplement**   A substance that may be added to the diet, usually in pill, liquid, or powder form, ostensibly to promote health. Dietary supplements range from natural (nonsteroidal) weight-gain concoctions used by body-builders, to vitamins, herbs, minerals, and salts that claim health benefits. Many dietary supplements are harmless when taken as directed, and the health benefits of some have been substantiated. Always tell a doctor what supplements are being taken, however, because they can interact with prescription medications, and some are not suitable for people with certain medical conditions.

**diethylstilbestrol**   A drug (brand name: Stilphostrol), based on synthetic estrogen, that was once widely prescribed to prevent miscarriage. Women whose mothers were given diethylstilbestrol (DES) during pregnancy to prevent miscarriage are at increased risk for developing cancer of the cervix.

**differential diagnosis**   The process of weighing the probability of one disease versus that of other diseases that might account for a patient's symptoms. Abbreviated as DDX. See also *diagnosis*.

**differentiation**   The process of change during development that leads to the progressive diversity in structure and function of cells.

**diffuse degeneration of cerebral gray matter with hepatic cirrhosis, Alpers**   See *Alpers disease*.

**diffuse idiopathic skeletal hyperostosis**   A form of degenerative arthritis characteristically associated with flowing calcification along the sides of the vertebrae of the spine. It commonly includes inflammation (tendinitis) and calcification of the tendons at their attachment points to bone. Because areas of the spine and tendons can become inflamed, anti-inflammatory medications (NSAIDs), such as ibuprofen, can be helpful in relieving both pain and inflammation. Also called Forestier disease. Abbreviated as DISH.

**DiGeorge syndrome**   A disorder characterized by low blood-calcium levels (hypocalcemia) due to underdevelopment (hypoplasia) of the parathyroid glands needed to control calcium; underdevelopment (hypoplasia) of the thymus, an organ behind the breastbone in which lymphocytes mature and multiply; and defects involving the outflow tracts from the heart. Most cases of DiGeorge syndrome are due to a very small deletion (microdeletion) in chromosome band 22q11.2. A small number of patients have defects in other chromosomes, notably 10p13. Abbreviated as DGS. Also known as hypoplasia of the thymus and parathyroids, third and fourth pharyngeal pouch syndrome.

**Digestive and Kidney Diseases, National Institute of Diabetes and**   See *National Institutes of Health*.

**digestive system** The organs responsible for getting food into and out of the body, and for making use of food to keep the body healthy. These include the mouth, esophagus, stomach, liver, gallbladder, pancreas, small intestine, colon, and rectum.

**digit** A finger or toe.

**digit, supernumerary** An extra finger or toe.

**digital rectal exam** An exam to detect rectal cancer. The doctor inserts a lubricated, gloved finger into the rectum and feels for abnormal areas. It is also an important screening test for detection of prostate abnormalities, including cancer.

**digitalis glycosides** See *digitoxin*.

**digitoxin** A medication (brand name: Crystodigin) prescribed to improve heart function in cases of congestive heart failure and tachycardia (overly rapid heartbeat).

**digoxin** A medication (brand names: Lanoxin, Lanoxicaps) prescribed to improve heart function in cases of congestive heart failure and tachycardia (overly rapid heartbeat).

**Dilantin** See *phenytoin*.

**dilatate** In medicine, "dilatate" means the same thing as "dilate," namely to enlarge or expand.

**dilatation** The process of enlargement or expansion. The word "dilation" means the same thing.

**dilatation and curettage** A minor operation in which the cervix is expanded (dilated) enough to permit the cervical canal and uterine lining to be scraped with a spoon-shaped instrument called a curette (curettage). Dilatation and curettage is normally used to remove abnormal material from the uterus, such as unexpelled placental material after birth. In some cases (as in areas where abortion is illegal) this procedure is used to perform an abortion. Also called a "D and C."

**dilate** To stretch or enlarge.

**dilating** Usually used to describe the widening and opening of the cervix caused by uterine contractions. Traditionally, the amount of widening was described in terms of the number of fingers that could fit in the cervical opening. Today most midwives and doctors use more precise measurements in centimeters, although the traditional method is equally useful.

**dilation** The process of enlargment or expansion.

**dilation, pupil** A type of eye examination that enables an eye-care professional to see more of the retina, the light-sensitive layer of tissue at the back of the eye. Dilating (widening) the pupil permits the retina to be examined for signs of disease. To dilate the pupil, drops are placed into the eye. After the examination, the patient's vision may remain blurred for awhile, and the brightness of the sun may be bothersome for several hours.

**dilator** A device used to stretch or enlarge an opening. Patients with scarring of the muscular tube through which food passes from the throat to the stomach (esophagus) can require a dilator procedure to open the esophagus for adequate passage of food and fluids.

**dimethylglycine** A dietary supplement, related to the B vitamins, believed to affect the serotonin system. Also known as pangamic acid; once known as vitamin B15, but no longer considered a vitamin per se.

**diphtheria** An acute infectious disease that typically strikes the upper respiratory tract, including the throat. It is caused by infection with the bacteria Corynebacterium diphtheriae. Symptoms include sore throat and mild fever at first. As the disease progresses, a membranous substance forms in the throat that makes it difficult to breathe and swallow. Diphtheria can be deadly. It is one of the diseases that the DTP (Diphtheria-Tetanus-Pertussis) and DTaP (Diphtheria-Tetanus-acellular-Pertussis) vaccines are designed to prevent.

**diploid** The number of chromosomes in most cells of the body. This number is 46 in humans. It is naturally twice the haploid number of 23 chromosomes contained in human eggs (ova) and sperm.

**diplopia** A condition in which a single object appears as two objects. Also called double vision.

**directives, advance** See *advance directives, durable power of attorney, health care proxy, living will*.

**directives, advance medical** See *advance directives, durable power of attorney, health care proxy, living will*.

**directly observed therapy** The practice of giving medication under supervision. Directly observed therapy is used in cases where the medication is essential, and compliance may be a problem. The most common uses for directly observed therapy in the US are tuberculosis treatment and the administration of methadone for heroin addiction.

**dirithromycin** An antibiotic medication (brand name: Dynabac). See also *macrolide antibiotic*.

**disaster supplies**   Items stored in case of emergency, such as a prolonged power outage, earthquake, or flood. Recommended disaster supplies include the following:

- Water. Store at least three gallons of water per person (two quarts for drinking, two quarts for food preparation/sanitation times three days). Store it in plastic containers, such as soft drink bottles.

- Food. Store at least a three-day supply of foods that require no refrigeration, preparation, or cooking (and little or no water). If you must heat food, see a camping goods store for options that do not require electricity or natural gas. Good choices include ready-to-eat canned meats, fruits, and vegetables; canned juices, milk, and soup (if powdered, store extra water); staples, particularly sugar, salt, and pepper; high-energy foods like peanut butter, granola bars, and trail mix; vitamin pills; special foods for infants, elderly persons, or persons on special diets; and "comfort foods" like cookies, hard candy, sweetened cereals, lollipops, instant coffee, and tea.

- First aid kit. Assemble a first aid kit for your home and one for each car. A first aid kit should include: sterile adhesive bandages in assorted sizes, four to six two-inch sterile gauze pads, four to six four-inch sterile gauze pads, hypoallergenic adhesive tape, three triangular bandages, three rolls of two-inch sterile roller bandages, three rolls of three-inch sterile roller bandages, scissors, tweezers, needle, moistened towelettes, antiseptic (cream and/or liquid), thermometer, two tongue depressors, a tube of petroleum jelly or other lubricant, assorted sizes of safety pins, cleansing agent and/or soap, a medicine dropper, two pairs of latex gloves, and sunscreen. Contact your local American Red Cross chapter to obtain a basic first aid manual.

- Nonprescription drugs. Over-the-counter drugs that you might need in an emergency include aspirin or nonaspirin pain relievers, antidiarrhea medication, antacid for stomach upset, syrup of ipecac and activated charcoal (use if advised by the Poison Control Center), laxatives.

- Tools and supplies. Keep the items you would most likely need during an evacuation in an easy-to-carry container, such as a large, covered trash container, camping backpack, or duffle bag. These emergency items include: mess kits (or paper cups, plates, and plastic utensils), an emergency-preparedness manual, a battery-operated radio with extra batteries, a flashlight with extra batteries, cash or traveler's checks, change, a nonelectric can opener, a utility knife, a small canister fire extinguisher of the ABC type, a tube tent, pliers, tape, compass, matches in a waterproof container, aluminum foil, plastic storage containers, a signal flare, paper and pencil, needles and thread, a shut-off wrench for turning off household gas and water, a whistle, plastic sheeting, and a map of the area for locating shelters. A map showing the precise location of local shelters may be available in advance from your local emergency-preparedness office.

- Sanitation. Have on hand an adequate supply of toilet paper and/or towelettes, soap, liquid detergent, feminine supplies, personal hygiene items, plastic garbage bags with ties for personal sanitation uses, a plastic bucket with a tight lid, disinfectant, and household chlorine bleach.

- Clothing and bedding. At least one complete change of clothing and footwear per person, preferably items that are easy to clean. Depending on your location, you may also need to include sturdy shoes or work boots, hats and gloves, coats and/or rain gear, thermal underwear, blankets or sleeping bags, and sunglasses.

- Special items. Remember family members with special needs, such as infants and elderly or disabled persons. For babies, store an adequate supply of formula, diapers, bottles, powdered milk, and medications. For older children and adults, remember essentials such as heart and high blood pressure medication, insulin and syringes, prescription drugs, denture needs, contact lenses and supplies, extra eyeglasses, and games and books for entertainment. Ask your physician or pharmacist about how to store prescription medications.

- Important documents. Keep these records in a waterproof, portable container: wills, insurance policies, contracts, deeds, stocks and bonds, passports, Social Security cards, immunization records, bank account numbers, credit card account numbers and companies, an inventory of valuable household goods, important telephone numbers, and family records (such as birth, marriage, and death certificates).

Store your kit in a convenient place known to all family members. Keep a smaller version in the trunk of your car. Keep items in air-tight plastic bags, and change your stored water supply every six months so it stays fresh. Rotate your stored food every six months. Rethink your kit and family needs at least once a year. Replace batteries, update clothes, and so on.

**discharge**   The flow of fluid from part of the body, such as the nose or vagina.

**discoid lupus**   See *lupus, discoid.*

**disease**   Illness or sickness, often characterized by typical patient problems (symptoms) and physical findings (signs). For a specific disease, see its alphabetical listing.

**diseases, inherited metabolic**   See *metabolic disorders, inherited*.

**diseases, Musculoskeletal and Skin, National Institute of Arthritis and**   See *National Institutes of Health*.

**Diseases, National Institute of Allergy and Infectious**   See *National Institutes of Health*.

**diseases, obesity-related**   Obesity increases the risk of developing a number of diseases, including type 2 (adult-onset) diabetes; high blood pressure (hypertension); stroke (cerebrovascular accident, or CVA); heart attack (myocardial infarction, or MI); congestive heart failure; certain forms of cancer, such as prostate and colon cancer; gallstones and gall bladder disease (cholecystitis); gout and gouty arthritis; osteoarthritis (degenerative arthritis) of the knees, hips, and lower back; sleep apnea (failure to breath normally during sleep, thus lowering blood oxygen); and Pickwickian syndrome (obesity, red face, underventilation, and drowsiness).

**diseases, polygenic**   Genetic disorders caused by the combined action of more than one gene. Examples of polygenic conditions include some forms of coronary heart disease, autism, and diabetes. Because such disorders depend on the simultaneous presence of several genes, they are not inherited as simply as single-gene diseases.

**diseases, rickettsial**   See *rickettsial diseases*.

**diseases, single-gene**   Hereditary disorders caused by a change (mutation) in a single gene. There are thousands of single-gene diseases, including achondroplastic dwarfism, Huntington disease, cystic fibrosis, sickle cell anemia, Duchenne muscular dystrophy, and hemophilia. Single-gene diseases typically describe classic simple Mendelian patterns of inheritance (as autosomal dominant, autosomal recessive, and X-linked traits), compared to polygenic diseases, which follow a more complex pattern of inheritance.

**DISH**   See *Forestier disease*.

**disinsection**   The procedure of spraying aircraft for insects. Some countries in Africa, Latin America, the Caribbean, Australia, and the South Pacific require that the aircraft passenger compartment be sprayed with insecticide while passengers are present. This is done to prevent the importation of insects, such as mosquitos, from one country to another. Disinsection procedures have been determined to be safe by the World Health Organization (WHO), but they may aggravate allergies.

**diskitis**   Inflammation of the disks between the vertebrae in the spinal column.

**diskitis, tuberculous**   See *tuberculous diskitis*.

**disorder, attention deficit**   See *attention deficit disorder*.

**disorder, seasonal affective**   See *seasonal affective disorder*. See also *bipolar disorders*.

**disorders, lymphoproliferative**   Malignant diseases of the lymphoid cells, and of cells from the reticuloendothelial system that take up and sequester inert particles.

**disorders, myeloproliferative**   Malignant diseases of certain bone-marrow cells, including those that give rise to the red blood cells, the granulocytes (types of white blood cells), and the platelets (crucial to blood clotting).

**disruption sequence**   The events that occur when a fetus that is developing normally is subjected to a destructive agent, such as the rubella (German measles) virus.

**dissecting aneurysm**   See *aneurysm, dissecting*. See also *Marfan syndrome*.

**dissociation**   The act of temporarily disconnecting from reality. A person who is dissociating may believe him- or herself to be someone else, or may simply experience unusual sensory experiences unrelated to the actual environment. See also *dissociative disorder*.

**dissociative disorder**   A psychiatric disorder characterized by the ability to temporarily disconnect from reality. Multiple personality disorder is a type of dissociative disorder in which, while dissociating, the person believes him- or herself to be another person.

**distal**   Farther from the beginning, as opposed to proximal. The lungs are distal to the mouth. See also *Appendix B, "Anatomic Orientation Terms."*

**diuretic**   Anything that promotes the formation of urine by the kidney. All diuretic drugs cause a person to "lose water," but they do so by diverse means, including inhibiting the kidney's ability to reabsorb sodium, thus enhancing the loss of sodium and consequently water in the urine (a high-ceiling or loop diuretic); enhancing the excretion of both sodium and chloride in the urine so that water is excreted with them (a thiazide diuretic); or blocking the exchange of sodium for potassium, resulting in excretion of sodium and potassium but relatively little loss of potassium (a potassium-sparing diuretic). Some diuretics work by still other mechanisms, and some have other effects and uses, such as in treating hypertension. Also known as a water pill.

**diuretic, loop**   A diuretic that works by encouraging the loss of sodium (salt) and water by affecting sodium transport at the loop area of the kidneys. As the sodium is removed, it takes water with it. Loop diuretics are very strong, and should be used only under constant medical supervision. They can deplete the electrolyte balance, cause dehydration, reduce blood volume, and worsen certain medical conditions. See also *diuretic*.

**diuretic, potassium-sparing**  A diuretic that blocks the exchange of sodium (salt) for potassium, encouraging the excretion of sodium and therefore of water, but generally retaining potassium. See also *diuretic*.

**diuretic, thiazide**  A diuretic that works by encouraging excretion of both sodium (salt) and chloride. See also *diuretic*.

**diurnal**  Occurring in the daytime. A patient may have a diurnal fever rather than a nocturnal one. Diurnal also can refer to something that recurs every day.

**diverticula**  The plural of diverticulum. As a person ages, pressure within the large intestine (colon) causes pockets of tissue (sacs) that push out from the colon walls. A small bulging sac pushing outward from the colon wall is a diverticulum. Diverticula can occur throughout the colon, but are most common near the end of the left side of the colon (the sigmoid colon).

**diverticulitis**  Inflammation of diverticula along the wall of the colon, the large intestine. For diverticulitis to occur, there must be diverticulosis: the presence of diverticula. Diverticulosis can occur anywhere in the colon, but is most typical in the sigmoid colon, the S-shaped segment of the colon located in the lower-left part of the abdomen. Diverticulitis can be diagnosed with barium X-rays of the colon or with sigmoidoscopy or colonoscopy. Treatment of diverticulitis is designed to combat the inflammation and infection. See also *diverticulosis*.

**diverticulitis, bleeding from**  Bleeding caused by diverticulitis, which typically occurs intermittently over several days. Colonoscopy is usually performed to confirm the diagnosis and exclude bleeding from other causes. Thermal probes cannot be employed to stop active diverticular bleeding. Therefore, surgical removal of the bleeding diverticula is necessary for those with persistent bleeding.

**diverticulitis, treatment of acute**  Antibiotics are usually needed to treat acute diverticulitis. Oral antibiotics are sufficient when symptoms are mild. Liquid or low-fiber foods are advised during acute diverticulitis attacks. In severe diverticulitis, with high fever and pain, patients are hospitalized and given intravenous antibiotics. Surgery is necessary for persistent bowel obstruction and for abscesses that do not respond to antibiotics.

**diverticulosis**  The condition of having diverticula, small outpouchings from the large intestine (the colon). Diverticulosis can occur anywhere in the colon, but is most typical in the sigmoid colon, the S-shaped segment of the colon located in the lower-left part of the abdomen. The incidence of diverticulosis increases with age. Age causes a weakening of the walls of the colon, and this weakening permits the formation of diverticula. By age 80, most people have diverticulosis. A key factor promoting the formation of diverticulosis is elevated pressure within the colon. Pressure within the colon is raised when a person is constipated and has to push down to pass small, hard bits of stool. Most patients with diverticulosis have few or no symptoms, although some have mild symptoms, such as abdominal cramping and bloating. Diverticulosis sets the stage for inflammation and infection of the outpouching, a condition called diverticulitis. The best way to avoid developing diverticulosis in the first place (aside from the impossibility of staying young) is to eat a proper healthy diet with plenty of fiber. A diet high in fiber keeps the bowels moving, keeps the pressure in the colon within normal limits, and slows or stops the formation of diverticula. See also *diverticulitis*.

**diverticulosis/diverticulitis and fiber**  High-fiber diets help delay the progression of diverticulosis, and may prevent or reduce bouts of diverticulitis.

**diverticulum**  A small bulging sac pushing outward from the colon wall. The plural is diverticula.

**diverticulum, Meckel**  An outpouching of the small bowel. About 1 in every 50 people has a Meckel diverticulum. It is usually located about two feet before the junction of the small bowel with the colon (the large intestine) in the lower-right abdomen. Meckel diverticulum can become inflamed, ulcerate, and perforate (break open or rupture). This can cause obstruction of the small bowel. If it is inflamed or perforated, Meckel diverticulum is usually removed by surgery.

**dizziness**  Painless head discomfort with many possible causes, including disturbances of vision, the brain, the balance (vestibular) system of the inner ear, or the gastrointestinal system. Dizziness is a medically indistinct term. Laypersons use it to describe a variety of conditions, ranging from lightheadedness or unsteadiness to vertigo. See also *lightheadedness, unsteadiness, vertigo*.

**dizziness, anxiety as a cause of**  One cause of dizziness is overbreathing (hyperventilation) due to anxiety. The overbreathing also causes lightheadedness, a sense of unsteadiness, and tingling around the mouth and fingertips. Relief can be had by breathing in and out of a paper bag to increase the level of carbon dioxide in the blood. In persistent cases, as in repeated panic attacks, antianxiety medication can be very helpful.

**dizziness, presyncopal** Dizziness before fainting. Some symptoms of dizziness, such as "wooziness," feeling as though one is about to black out, and tunnel vision may be presyncopal, and are due to insufficient blood flow to the brain. These symptoms are typically worse when standing, improve with lying down, and may be experienced by healthy individuals who rise quickly from a chair (often after a meal), and have a few seconds of disorientation. See also *syncope.*

**DMD** Dystonia musculorum deformans.

**DMG** Dimethylglycine.

**DNA** **1** Deoxyribonucleic acid, the molecule that encodes genetic information. DNA is a double-stranded molecule held together by weak bonds between base pairs of nucleotides to form a double helix. The four nucleotides in DNA contain the bases adenine (A), guanine (G), cytosine (C), and thymine (T). Base pairs form naturally only between A and T and between G and C, so the base sequence of each single strand of DNA can be simply deduced from that of its partner strand. The code is in triplets, such as ATG (the base sequence of ATG's partner strand would be TAC). **2** In the UK, an abbreviation for "did not attend" (in the US, the term used for a patient who missed an appointment is "no-show").

**DNA cloning** The use of DNA-manipulation procedures to produce multiple copies of a single gene or segment of DNA.

**DNA molecules, recombinant** A combination of DNA molecules of different origin, joined by using recombinant DNA technology. See also *DNA technology, recombinant.*

**DNA polymerase** An enzyme that catalyzes (speeds) the polymerization of DNA. DNA polymerase uses preexisting nucleic acid templates, and assembles the DNA from deoxyribonucleotides.

**DNA repair** The cell has a series of special enzymes to repair mutations (changes) in the DNA and restore the DNA to its original state.

**DNA repair gene** A gene engaged in DNA repair. When a DNA repair gene is altered, mutations pile up throughout the DNA.

**DNA repair pathway** The sequence of steps in the repair of DNA. Each step is governed by an enzyme.

**DNA replication** A wondrous and complex process whereby the "parent" strands of DNA in the double helix are separated, and each one is copied to produce a new (daughter) strand. This process is said to be "semicon-

servative," since one of each parent strand is conserved and remains intact after replication has taken place.

**DNA sequence** The precise ordering of the bases (A, T, G, C) from which the DNA is composed.

**DNA technology, recombinant** A series of procedures used to join together (recombine) DNA segments. A recombinant DNA molecule is constructed from segments of two or more different DNA molecules. Under certain conditions, a recombinant DNA molecule can enter a cell and replicate there, either on its own or after it has become integrated into a chromosome.

**DNA, mitochondrial** Mitochondrial DNA (mtDNA) is the DNA of the mitochondrion, a structure situated in the cytoplasm of the cell rather than in the nucleus, where all the other chromosomes are located. All mtDNA is inherited from the mother. There are 2 to 10 copies of the mtDNA genome in each mitochondrion. mtDNA is a double-stranded, circular molecule. It is very small relative to the chromosomes in the nucleus, and so contains only a limited number of genes. It is specialized in the information it carries, and encodes a number of the subunits in the mitochondrial respiratory-chain complex that the cell needs to respire. (It also contains genes for some ribosomal RNAs and transfer RNAs.) Mutations (changes) in mtDNA can cause disease. These point mutations often impair the function of oxidative-phosphorylation enzymes in the respiratory chain. This is especially manifest in tissues with a high energy expenditure, such as brain and muscle tissues. All mtDNA at fertilization comes from the oocyte, so inherited mtDNA mutations are transmitted from the mother to all offspring, male and female alike. The higher the level of mutant mtDNA in the mother's blood, the higher the frequency of clinically affected offspring, and the more severely those children tend to be affected. Each cell in the body contains different mtDNA populations. Due to the presence of multiple mitochondria in cells, each cell contains several mtDNA copies. This produces tissue variation, so that a mutation in mtDNA versus normal mtDNA can vary widely among tissues in an individual. There is thus a threshold effect. The percent of mutant mtDNAs must be above a certain threshold to produce clinical disease. This threshold varies from tissue to tissue because the percent of mutant mDNAs needed to cause cell dysfunction varies according to the oxidative requirements of the tissue. See also *mitochondrial diseases.*

**DNA, repetitive** DNA sequences that are repeated in the genome.

**DNA, satellite** DNA that contains many tandem (not inverted) repeats of a short basic repeating unit. Satellite DNA is located at very specific spots in the genome: It is found only on chromosomes 1, 9, and 16; on the Y chromosome; on the tiny short arms of chromosomes 13, 14, 15, 21, and 22; and near the centromeres of chromosomes.

**DNR**   Do not resuscitate.

**do not resuscitate**   On a medical chart, a directive to not attempt mechanical or manual resuscitation should the patient stop breathing. Abbreviated as DNR. See also *advance directives*.

**DOB**   Abbreviation for date of birth, frequently used in medical charting.

**doctor**   In a medical context, the word "doctor" is quite unspecific. It can refer to any medical professional with an MD, a PhD, or any other doctoral degree. A doctor may, for example, be a physician, psychologist, biomedical scientist, dentist, or veterinarian. In a nonmedical context, a professor of history might be addressed as doctor; an eminent theologian might be named a doctor of a church; and a person awarded an honorary doctorate by a college or university might also be called a doctor.

**doctors' symbol**   See *Aesculapius*.

**DOE**   Department of Energy, one of the US agencies contributing to the Human Genome Project.

**domain**   In biomedicine, a domain is a discrete portion of a protein with its own function. The combination of domains in a single protein determines its overall function.

**dominant**   A genetic trait is considered dominant if it is expressed in a person who has only one copy of that gene. (In genetic terms, a dominant trait is one that is phenotypically expressed in heterozygotes.) A dominant trait is the opposite of a recessive trait, which is expressed only when two copies of the gene are present. (In genetic terms, a recessive trait is one that is phenotypically expressed only in homozygotes.) Examples of dominant disorders include achondroplasia (a common form of dwarfism with short arms and legs), Huntington disease (a form of progressive dementia, from which the folksinger Woody Guthrie suffered), and neurofibromatosis (NF1, a neurologic disorder with an increased risk of malignant tumors). Most dominant traits are due to genes located on the autosomes (the non-sex chromosomes). An autosomal dominant trait typically affects males and females with equal likelihood, and with similar severity. The gene responsible for the trait can be transmitted from generation to generation, and each child born to someone with the gene has a fifty-fifty chance of receiving the gene and manifesting the disease.

**donor**   The giver of a tissue or organ: for example, a blood donor or kidney donor.

**donor insemination**   See *artificial insemination by donor*.

**dopa-responsive dystonia**   Characterized by progressive difficulty in walking, and in some cases by spasticity, DRD begins in childhood or adolescence. It can be successfully treated with drugs. Segawa dystonia is an important variant of DRD. Some scientists feel that DRD is not only rare but also rarely diagnosed, since it mimics many of the symptoms of cerebral palsy. See also *dystonia; dystonia, Segawa*.

**dorsal**   Pertaining to the back or posterior side of a structure, as opposed to the ventral or front side. Some of the dorsal surfaces of the body are the back, buttocks, calves, and the knuckle side of the hand (the palm is ventral). See also *Appendix B, "Anatomic Orientation Terms."*

**dorsum**   The back or posterior side of a structure. Something that pertains to the dorsum is dorsal.

**DOT**   Directly observed therapy.

**double helix**   The structure of DNA, with the two strands of DNA spiraling about each other.

**double-blinded study**   A medical study in which at least two separate groups receive the experimental medication or procedure at different times, with neither group being made aware of when the experimental medication or procedure has been given. Double-blinded studies are often chosen when a treatment shows particular promise and the illness involved is serious. It can be difficult to recruit human subjects for a blinded study of a promising treatment when one group will receive only a placebo or an existing medicine.

**douche**   A stream of water applied to the vagina for cleansing purposes. A douche can also be with a solution, such as vinegar and water, and it can be directed at any body cavity or part.

**douching**   Using water or a medicated solution to clean the vagina and cervix.

**Douglas, pouch of**   See *pouch of Douglas*.

**Down syndrome**   A common chromosome disorder due to an extra chromosome 21 (trisomy 21). Down syndrome causes mental retardation, a characteristic facial structure with a small mouth, and multiple malformations. It is somewhat more common in children born to mothers over the age of 30. It is associated with a major risk for heart problems, a lesser risk of duodenal atresia (partialy undeveloped intestines), and a minor but still significant risk of acute leukemia. Treatment for Down syndrome includes early intervention to develop the mental and physical capacities to their utmost, speech therapy to offset the difficulties presented by a smaller mouth and somewhat protruding tongue, surgery to repair problems in internal organs, and in some cases special nutritional support because of problems with nutrient absorption. With appropriate intervention, most children with Down syndrome will live active, productive lives into at least middle age. Most will be only mildly retarded, and some will have IQs in the low-normal range. Unfortunately, most adults with Down syndrome eventually develop Alzheimer disease as they grow older. Down syndrome was also once called mongolism, a term now considered out of date, as the disorder has no relationship to Mongolian or Asian heritage. It can occur in any racial or ethnic group.

**DPT** Diphtheria-Pertussis-Tetanus vaccine. Today the more frequent abbreviation is DTP, for Diphtheria-Tetanus-Pertussis vaccine.

**DPT immunization** DPT immunization protects from diphtheria, pertussis (whooping cough), and tetanus, and is given in a series of five shots at 2, 4, 6, and 18 months of age, and again at 4 to 6 years of age. Thanks to vaccination programs, these diseases have become less common. However, there are still unvaccinated individuals capable of carrying and passing diphtheria and pertussis to others who are not vaccinated. Tetanus bacteria are prevalent in natural surroundings, such as contaminated soil. Children with compromised immune systems or known neurological disorders generally should not receive the DPT immunization, particularly during infancy. See also *DTaP immunization*.

**dreams** Thoughts, visions, and other sensations that occupy the mind in sleep. Dreams occur during that part of sleep when there are rapid eye movements (REM sleep). Humans have three to five periods of REM sleep per night, which usually come at intervals of one to two hours, and are quite variable in length. An episode of REM sleep may be brief and last but five minutes, or it may be much longer. Dreams are penetrable: It has been found experimentally that one can communicate with a person who is dreaming. Dreaming is not uniquely human. Cats and dogs dream, judging from the physiologic features. So, apparently, do many other animals. The content of dreams is sometimes the topic of psychoanalysis. While this method of therapy is less common than it once was, some doctors still look at dreams as a diagnostic clue to medical disorders. For example, children with bipolar disorders have been found to frequently have a particular type of nightmares, and especially lucid dreams are a side effect of certain medications. These clues indicate that chemicals in the brain, as well as life events and our own preoccupations, influence our dreams. See also *REM sleep*.

**drip** In medical usage, a device for administering a fluid drop-by-drop into a vein via an intravenous (IV) fluid drip.

**drug activity** A measure of the physiological response a drug produces. A less active drug produces less response (and vice versa).

**Drug Enforcement Administration** The Drug Enforcement Administration of the US Department of Justice. See also *DEA*.

**drug resistance** The ability of bacteria and other microorganisms to withstand a drug that once stalled them or killed them outright.

**drug, ACE-inhibitor** See *ACE inhibitors*.

**drug, antihypertensive** See *antihypertensive*.

**drug, anti-infective** See *agent, anti-infective*.

**drug, antiviral** See *antiviral agent*.

**drug, over-the-counter** A drug for which a prescription is not needed.

**drug, prescription** A drug you can purchase only with a physician's order (prescription). See also *prescription*.

**drugs during pregnancy, dangerous** See *teratogen*.

**drugs, anti-angiogenesis** See *anti-angiogenesis drugs*.

**drugs, teratogenic** See *teratogen*.

**dry eyes** See *xerophthalmia*.

**dry mouth** See *xerostomia*.

**dry skin** See *xeroderma*.

**DT immunization** A vaccination against diphtheria and tetanus, which does not protect from pertussis as the DPT or DTaP immunizations do. It is usually reserved for individuals who have had a significant adverse reaction to a DPT shot, or who have a personal or family history of a seizure disorder or brain disease. See also *diphtheria, tetanus*.

**DTaP immunization** Like DPT, DTaP protects from diphtheria, pertussis (whooping cough), and tetanus.

DTaP is the same as DTP, except that it contains only acellular pertussis vaccine, which is thought to cause fewer of the minor reactions associated with immunization. Acellular pertussis vaccine is also probably less likely to cause the more severe reactions occasionally seen following pertussis vaccination. DTaP is currently recommended only for the shots given at 18 months and 4 to 6 years of age. See also *diphtheria, pertussis, tetanus.*

**DTP** Diphtheria-Tetanus-Pertussis vaccine.

**dual diagnosis** Diagnosed with both a mental illness and a substance abuse disorder.

**duct** A walled passageway, such as a lymph duct, that carries fluid from one place to another. Also known as a ductus.

**duct, thoracic** See *thoracic duct.*

**ductal carcinoma of the breast, infiltrating** See *carcinoma of the breast, infiltrating ductal.*

**ductular hypoplasia, syndromatic hepatic** See *Alagille syndrome.*

**ductus** See *duct.*

**ductus arteriosus** Before birth, the blood headed from the heart via the pulmonary artery to the lungs is shunted away from the lungs, and returned to the aorta. The shunt is through a short vessel called the ductus arteriosus. When the shunt is open, it is said to be patent. The patent ductus arteriosus (PDA) usually closes at or shortly after birth, and blood is permitted from that moment on to course freely to the lungs. If the ductus stays open, flow reverses, and blood from the aorta is shunted into the pulmonary artery and recirculated through the lungs. The PDA may close later spontaneously (on its own) or need to be ligated (tied off) surgically.

**due date** The estimated calendar date when a baby is due to be born. Also called the estimated date of confinement (EDC).

**dumping syndrome** A group of symptoms that occur when food or liquid enters the small intestine too rapidly. These symptoms include cramps, nausea, diarrhea, and dizziness.

**duodenal ulcer** A hole (ulcer) in the lining of the first portion of the small intestine (duodenum). Ulcer formation is related to H. pyloridus bacteria, anti-inflammatory medications, and smoking cigarettes. Ulcer pain may not correlate with the presence or severity of ulceration. Diagnosis is made with barium X-ray or endoscopy. Complications of ulcers include bleeding, perforation, and blockage. Treatment involves antibiotics to eradicate H. pyloridus, elimination of risk factors, and prevention of complications.

**duodenitis** Inflammation of the first part of the small intestine (duodenum).

**duodenum** The first part of the small intestine. The duodenum is a common site for peptic ulcer formation.

**duplication** Part of a chromosome in duplicate. The opposite of a deletion.

**durable power of attorney** A type of advance medical directive in which legal documents provide the power of attorney to another person in the case of an incapacitating medical condition. The durable power of attorney allows another person to make bank transactions, sign Social Security checks, apply for disability, or simply write checks to pay the utility bill while an individual is medically incapacitated. Such documents are recommended for any patient who may be unable to make his or her wishes known during a long medical confinement.

**Duricef** See *cefadroxil.*

**DVT** Deep vein thrombosis.

**dwarfism** Abnormally short stature, which may be due to a variety of causes. Some forms are hereditary. See also *achondroplasia; dwarfism, hypochondroplastic; dwarfism, pituitary; Seckel syndrome.*

**dwarfism, achondroplastic** See *achondroplasia.*

**dwarfism, hypochondroplastic** A form of dwarfism in which the short stature and limb shortening can be mild, especially as compared to achrondroplastic dwarfism. A child with hypochondroplastic dwarfism usually has a prominent forehead, mildly shortened extremities and digits, limited range of motion at the elbows, and inward curvature of the lower back (lumbar lordosis). Diagnosis is by exam and X-rays. Hypochondroplasia is an autosomal dominant condition, so each child born to a person with hypochondroplasia has a 50 percent chance of inheriting the condition. It can also occur spontaneously. The gene for hypochondroplasia is the same gene that causes achondroplastic dwarfism: the fibroblast growth factor receptor 3 (FGFR3). However, the two forms of dwarfism are apparently caused by different mutations.

**dwarfism, microcephalic primordial** See *Seckel syndrome.* See also *dwarfism.*

**dwarfism, nanocephalic** See *Seckel syndrome.* See also *dwarfism.*

**dwarfism, pituitary** Dwarfism caused by a lack of growth hormone, usually due to malfunction of the anterior pituitary gland. Pituitary dwarves are proportioned like nondwarves, but are abnormally short. This condition can be treated with growth hormones given in childhood.

**dwarfism, rhizomelic** Dwarfism with shortening especially of the ends of the limbs. See *dwarfism, hypochondroplastic.* See also *dwarfism.*

**dwarfism, Seckel-type** See *Seckel syndrome.* See also *dwarfism.*

**dwarfism, thanatophoric** An inherited form of dwarfism that includes severe lung deformities. Patients always die in infancy. See also *dwarfism.*

**dx, DX** Abbreviation for diagnosis.

**Dynabac** See *dirithromycin.*

**dys-** Prefix denoting an inability or lack of function, as in dyspraxia (lack of ability to adequately control muscle movements).

**dysarthria** One of several speech problems caused by paralysis, weakness, or inability to coordinate the muscles of the mouth. Speech is characteristically slurred, slow, and difficult to produce, and the person with a dysarthria may also have problems controlling the pitch, loudness, rhythm, and voice qualities of his or her speech. Dysarthria can occur as a developmental disability, or as a symptom or result of a neuromuscular disorder, such as cerebral palsy. It may also be caused by a stroke, brain injury, or brain tumor. Treatment is via intensive speech therapy, with the focus on oral-motor skill development.

**dyscalculia** A specific developmental disability affecting a person's ability to conceptualize and perform mathematics. Mild cases can often be compensated for with use of a calculator, but those with severe dyscalculia will need special education services.

**dysentery** Inflammation of the intestine, with pain, diarrhea, bloody stools, and often a fever above 101°F. It is usually caused by infestation of the bowel by an ameba. Dysentery can be fatal, usually because of severe dehydration. Treatment includes rapid rehydration, sometimes via IV, and medication.

**dysentery, amebic** See *amebic dysentery.*

**dysfunction, erectile** A consistent inability to sustain an erection sufficient for sexual intercourse, commonly known as impotence. Medically, the term erectile dysfunction is used to differentiate this form of impotence from other problems that interfere with sexual intercourse, such as lack of sexual desire, and problems with ejaculation and orgasm. Impotence usually has a physical cause, such as disease, injury, drug side effects, or a disorder that impairs blood flow in the penis. Impotence is treatable in all age groups by medication, implants, or other methods.

**dysgraphia** A specific developmental disability that affects the person's ability to write. Problems may include fine-motor-muscle control of the hands, and/or processing difficulties. Sometimes occupational therapy is helpful. Most successful students with dysgraphia that does not respond to occupational therapy or extra writing help choose to use a typewriter, computer, or verbal communication.

**dyskinesia** The presence of involuntary movements, such as the choreaform movements seen in some cases of rheumatic fever, or the characteristic movements of tardive dyskinesia. Some forms of dyskinesia are a side effect of certain medications, particularly L-dopa and, in the case of tardive dyskinesia, the antipsychotics.

**dyslexia** Dyslexia is a specific developmental disability that alters the way the brain processes written material. Dyslexia, because it is due to a defect in the brain's processing of graphic symbols, is thought of primarily as a learning disability. The effects of dyslexia vary from person to person. The only common trait among people with dyslexia is that they read at levels significantly lower than are typical for people of their age and intelligence. Dyslexia is different from reading retardation which may, for example, reflect mental retardation or cultural deprivation. Treatment of dyslexia should be directed to the specific learning problems of affected individuals. The usual course is to modify teaching methods and the educational environment to meet the specific needs of the individual with dyslexia. The outlook for people with dyslexia is mixed. The disability affects such a wide range of people, producing different symptoms and varying degrees of severity, that predictions are hard to make. The prognosis is generally good, however, for individuals whose dyslexia is identified early, who have supportive family and friends and a strong self-image, and who are involved in a proper remediation program.

**dysmorphic feature** A body characteristic that is abnormally formed. A malformed ear, for example, is a dysmorphic feature.

**dysmorphology** A term describing the study of human congenital malformations (birth defects), particularly those affecting the anatomy (morphology) of the individual.

**dysostosis, cleidocranial** See *cleidocranial dysostosis.*

**dyspareunia** Pain during sexual intercourse.

**dyspepsia** Upper abdominal symptoms, which may include pain or discomfort, bloating, feeling of fullness with very little intake of food (early satiety), a feeling of unusual fullness following meals (postprandial fullness), nausea, loss of appetite, heartburn, regurgitation of food or acid, and belching. The term dyspepsia is often used for these symptoms when they are not typical of a well-described disease (for example, gastrointestinal reflux), and the cause is not clear. Once a cause for the symptoms has been determined, the term dyspepsia usually is dropped for a more specific diagnosis.

**dysphagia** Difficulty in swallowing due to problems in muscle control.

**dysphonia, spasmodic** Involves the muscles of the throat that control speech. Also called spastic dysphonia or laryngeal dystonia, it causes strained and difficult speaking, or breathy and effortful speech.

**dysphoria** Anxiety.

**dysplasia** Abnormality in form or development. For example, retinal dysplasia is abnormal formation of the retina during embryonic development.

**dysplasia, arteriohepatic** See *Alagille syndrome*.

**dysplasia, bronchopulmonary** Chronic lung disease in infants who have received mechanical respiratory support with high oxygenation in the neonatal period.

**dysplasia, cleidocranial** See *cleidocranial dysostosis*.

**dysplastic nevi** Moles whose appearance is different from that of common moles. Dysplastic nevi are generally larger than ordinary moles, and have irregular borders. Their color often is not uniform. They usually are flat, but parts may be raised above the skin surface. Dysplastic nevi can be cancerous. See *cancer, skin*.

**dyspraxia** See *developmental dyspraxia*.

**dyspnea** Difficult or labored breathing; shortness of breath. Dyspnea is a sign of serious disease of the airway, lungs, or heart. The onset of dyspnea should not be ignored—it is reason to seek medical attention.

**dyspnoea** See *dyspnea*.

**dyspraxia** Impaired or painful function of any organ of the body.

**dyspraxia of speech** A developmental disability characterized by difficulty in muscle control, specifically of the muscles involved in producing speech. It is caused by a neurological difference that has not yet been pinpointed. Treatment is via intensive speech therapy concentrating on oral-motor skills.

**dyspraxia, developmental** A developmental disability characterized by difficulty in muscle control. It is caused by a neurological difference that has not yet been pinpointed. Treatment includes physical therapy and occupational therapy.

**dysthymia** A type of depression involving long-term, chronic symptoms that do not disable you, but keep you from functioning at "full steam" or from feeling good. Dysthymia is a less severe type of depression than what is considered a major depression. However, people with dysthymia may also sometimes experience major depressive episodes.

**dystocia** Difficult or abnormal labor or delivery.

**dystocia, cervical** Dystocia caused by mechanical obstruction at the cervix.

**dystocia, fetal** Dystocia caused by the fetus, due to its size (too big), shape, or position in the uterus.

**dystocia, placental** Trouble delivering the placenta (afterbirth).

**dystonia** Involuntary movements and prolonged muscle contraction, resulting in twisting body motions, tremors, and abnormal posture. These movements may involve the entire body or only an isolated area. Dystonia can be inherited, may occur sporadically without any genetic pattern, may be associated with medications (particularly antipsychotic drugs), or may be a symptom of certain diseases (for example, a specific form of lung cancer). The gene responsible for at least one form of dystonia has recently been identified. Some types of dystonia respond to dopamine. It can sometimes be controlled also with sedative-type medications or surgery.

**dystonia musculorum deformans** See *dystonia, torsion*.

**dystonia, cranial** A form of dystonia that affects the muscles of the head, face, and neck. Meige syndrome is the combination of blepharospasm, oromandibular dystonia, and sometimes spasmodic dysphonia. Spasmodic torticollis can be classified as a type of cranial dystonia.

**dystonia, dopa-responsive** See *dopa-responsive dystonia*.

**dystonia, focal** A form of dystonia that affects only one muscle group. Common focal dystonias that affect the muscles of the hand and sometimes the forearm have been called typist's cramp, pianist's cramp, musician's cramp, and golfer's cramp, and include so-called writer's cramp.

**dystonia, focal, due to blepharospasm** The second most common focal dystonia, this is the involuntary, forcible closure of the eyelids. The first symptoms may be uncontrollable blinking. Only one eye may be affected initially, but eventually both eyes are usually involved. The spasms may leave the eyelids completely closed, causing functional blindness even though the eyes and vision are normal. Uncontrollable blinking may also be caused by tic disorders, including Tourette syndrome.

**dystonia, focal, due to torticollis** See *torticollis*.

**dystonia, generalized torsion** See *dystonia, torsion; dystonia, idiopathic torsion*.

**dystonia, idiopathic torsion** A form of torsion dystonia that begins in childhood around the age of 12. Symptoms typically start in one part of the body, usually in an arm or leg, and eventually spread to the rest of the body within about five years. Early-onset torsion dystonia is not fatal, but it can be severely debilitating. Also known as generalized torsion dystonia. See also *dystonia, torsion*.

**dystonia, laryngeal** Dystonia that involves the muscles of the throat that control speech, causing strained or breathy speech that is difficult to produce. Also known as spasmodic or spastic dysphonia.

**dystonia, oromandibular** Dystonia that affects the muscles of the jaw, lips, and tongue. The jaw may be pulled either open or shut, and speech and swallowing can be difficult.

**dystonia, Segawa** See *dopa-responsive dystonia*.

**dystonia, torsion** A type of dystonia in which symptoms typically start in one part of the body, usually in an arm or leg, and eventually spread to the rest of the body. A form that strikes in childhood is known as early-onset torsion dystonia or generalized torsion dystonia. See also *dystonia, idiopathic torsion*.

**dystonia, writer's cramp** See *dystonia, focal*.

**dystrophy, muscular** See *muscular dystrophy*.

**dystrophy, myotonic** Inherited disease with myotonia (irritability and prolonged contraction of muscles), mask-like face, premature balding, cataracts, and cardiac disease. It is due to a trinucleotide repeat (a stuttering sequence of three bases) in the DNA.

**dysuria** Pain on urination, or difficulty urinating.

# Ee

**E. coli**   Short for Escherichia coli, a bacterium that normally resides in the human colon. E. coli has been studied intensively in genetics, and in molecular and cell biology, because of its availability, its small genome size, its normal lack of disease-causing ability, and its ease of growth in the laboratory. In the future, the E. coli bacteria may be used as a host cell for delivering gene therapies. Although E. coli is normally present in the human colon with no harmful consequences, it can cause disease when transmitted from human to human via water, food, or feces. Infants, young children, the elderly, and people with compromised immune systems are especially at risk for E. coli infection.

**Eagle syndrome**   Inflammation of the styloid process. The styloid process is a spike-like growth that projects out from the base of the skull. If the styloid process is oversized or projects too far, the tissues in the throat can rub on it during the act of swallowing, causing pain. Diagnosis of Eagle syndrome is made by history and an X-ray showing an abnormal styloid process. Anti-inflammatory drugs are the first line of treatment, although surgical removal of the styloid process may be necessary.

**ear**   The hearing organ. There are three sections of the ear: outer, middle, and inner. The external ear helps concentrate the vibrations of air created by sound (sound waves) onto the eardrum, causing it to vibrate in turn. These vibrations are transmitted by a chain of little bones in the middle ear to the inner ear. There they stimulate the fibers of the auditory nerve to transmit impulses to the brain. One should also think of the brain as part of the ear, because the auditory cortex of the brain interprets speech and other sounds as information we can use. See also *ear, inner; ear, middle; ear, outer.*

**ear canal, self-cleaning**   Most of the time the ear canals are self-cleaning, meaning that there is a slow and orderly migration of ear-canal skin from the eardrum to the outer opening. Old earwax is constantly being transported from the deeper areas of the ear canal to the opening, where it usually dries, flakes, and falls out.

**ear cleaning by a doctor**   When so much wax accumulates that it blocks the ear canal (and hearing), a physician may have to wash it out, vacuum it, or remove it with special instruments. Alternatively, a physician may prescribe ear drops designed to soften the wax.

**ear cleaning by oneself**   Never put anything smaller than one's elbow in one's ear! Wax is not formed in the deep part of the ear canal near the eardrum, but only in the outer part of the canal. So when a patient has wax pushed up against the eardrum, it is often because he or she has been probing the ear with such things as cotton-tipped swabs, bobby pins, or twisted napkin corners. Such objects only serve as ramrods to push the wax in deeper. Also, the skin of the ear canal and the eardrum is very thin, fragile, and easily injured. The ear canal is more prone to infection after it has been wiped clean of its wax coating. In addition, many perforated eardrums occur as a result of self-cleaning.

**ear infection**   What most people think of as an ear infection is inflammation of the middle ear, medically known as acute otitis media. Acute otitis media typically causes fluid in the middle ear, accompanied by signs or symptoms of ear infection: a bulging eardrum, usually accompanied by pain; or a perforated eardrum, often with drainage of pus. Middle ear infections are the most frequent diagnosis in sick children in the US, especially affecting infants and preschoolers. Almost all children have one or more bouts of otitis media before age six. The Eustachian tube is shorter in children, allowing easy entry of bacteria and viruses into the middle ear. Bacteria such as Streptococcus pneumoniae (strep) and Hemophilus influenzae (H. flu) account for about 85 percent of cases, with viruses causing the remaining 15 percent. Babies under six weeks of age tend to have infections from different bacteria in the middle ear. Bottle-feeding is a risk factor for ear infections. Breast-feeding passes immunity to the baby that helps prevent them. The position of the breast-feeding child is better than that of the bottle-feeding child for Eustachian tube function. If a child needs to be bottle-fed, holding the infant rather than allowing the child to lie down with the bottle is best. A child should not take the bottle to bed. Upper respiratory infections are a prominent risk factor, so exposure to other children results in more frequent colds, and therefore more earaches. Irritants, such as tobacco smoke in the air, also increase the chance of ear infections. Children with cleft palate or Down syndrome are predisposed to ear infections. Children who have acute otitis media before six months of age have more frequent later ear infections. Young children with otitis media may be irritable, fussy, or have problems feeding or sleeping. Older children may complain about pain and fullness in the ear. Fever may be present in a child of any age. These symptoms are often associated with signs of upper respiratory infection, such as a runny or stuffy nose or a cough. The buildup of pus within the middle ear causes pain and dampens the vibrations of the eardrum, so there is usually transient hearing loss during the infection. Severe ear infections may cause the eardrum to rupture. The pus then drains from the middle ear into the ear canal. The hole in the eardrum from the rupture usually heals without medical treatment. The treatment for acute otitis media is antibiotics, usually for 7 to 10 days. About 10 percent of children do not respond within the first 48 hours of treatment. Even after antibiotic treatment, 40 percent are left with some fluid in the middle ear, which can cause temporary hearing loss, lasting for up to 3 to 6 weeks. In most children, the fluid eventually disappears (resorbs) spontaneously (on its own). Children who have recurring bouts of otitis media may have a tympanostomy tube (ear tube) placed into the ear during surgery to permit fluid to drain from the middle ear. If a child has a bulging eardrum and is experiencing severe pain, a myringotomy (surgical incision of the eardrum) to release the pus may be done. The eardrum usually heals within a week. Ear infections are not contagious, but the bacteria or viruses that cause them may be. A child with an ear infection can travel by airplane, but if the Eustachian tube is not functioning well, changes in pressure can cause discomfort. A child with a draining ear should not fly or swim. The inner and outer parts of the ear can also become inflamed and infected, but this is much rarer.

**ear piercing**    The practice of using a needle or needle gun to make holes through the ear lobe or other parts of the ear for wearing jewelry. When done under hygenic conditions, there is little danger from ear piercing, other than localized and transitory inflammation. Unhygenic conditions, handling the new piercing with unwashed hands, or the use of irritating jewelry can result in inflammation and/or infection. Infected ear piercings should be washed and then treated with antibiotic cream. One may choose either to allow the piercing to close or to use only nonirritating jewelry (usually gold or hypoallergenic plastic). The likelihood of inflammation and infection is greater for piercings that go through hard cartilage, as found on the side and top of the outer ear, than for the soft bottom lobe of the ear.

**ear pit**    A tiny pit in front of the ear, also called a preauricular pit. This minor anomaly is of no consequence in and of itself. It is more common in blacks than in whites, and in females than males. It can recur in families. However, the presence of two or more minor anomalies in a child increases the probability that the child has a major malformation.

**ear puncture**    Puncture of the eardrum may be due to an accident: for example, when something is stuck into the ear. Eardrums may also be punctured due to fluid pressure in the middle ear. Today the eardrum is occasionally punctured on purpose with surgery. A tiny incision (a myringotomy) is made in the eardrum to allow fluid trapped behind the eardrum, usually thickened secretions, to be removed. An ear tube may be inserted after draining.

**ear ringing**    See *tinnitus*.

**ear tag**    A rudimentary tag of ear tissue, often containing a core of cartilage, usually located just in front of the ear (auricle). This minor anomaly is common and harmless. However, the presence of two or more minor anomalies in a child increases the probability that the child has a major malformation. Also known as a preauricular tag.

**ear tubes**    Formally known as tympanostomy tubes, these small plastic tubes are inserted into the eardrum (the tympanum) to keep the middle ear aerated for a prolonged period of time. To put the tubes in place, a tiny surgical incision in the eardrum is done. Any fluid present is removed. The ear tubes remain in place from six months to several years. Water should not be allowed to enter the ear canal while the tubes are in place. Eventually, they will move out of the eardrum (extrude) and fall into the ear canal. The doctor may remove the tube during a routine office visit, or it may simply fall out of the ear without the patient realizing it.

**ear tumor**    Benign (noncancerous) bumps on the external ear or within the external ear canal. Most of these lumps and bumps are just harmless sebaceous cysts. However, some are bony overgrowths known as exostoses or osteomas. If they are large and interfere with hearing, they can be surgically removed with comparative ease.

**ear wax**    A natural wax-like substance secreted by special glands in the skin on the outer part of the ear canal. It repels water, and traps dust and sand particles. Usually a small amount of wax accumulates, and then dries up and falls out of the ear canal, carrying with it unwanted particles. Ear wax is helpful in normal amounts. The absence of ear wax may result in dry, itchy ears, and even infection.

**ear, cauliflower**    See *cauliflower ear*.

**ear, external**    See *ear, outer*.

**ear, inner**    A highly complex structure whose essential component for hearing is the membranous labyrinth, where the fibers of the nerve connecting the ear to the brain (the auditory nerve) end. The membranous labyrinth is a system of communicating sacs and ducts (tubes) filled with fluid (the endolymph). The membranous labyrinth is lodged within a cavity called the bony labyrinth. At some points the membranous labyrinth is attached to the bony labyrinth, and at other points the membraneous labyrinth is suspended within the bony labyrinth in a fluid called the perilymph. The bony labyrinth has three parts: a central cavity (the vestibule); semicircular canals, which open into the vestibule; and the cochlea, a spiraling tube. The membranous labyrinth also has a vestibule, which consists of two sacs (called the utriculus and sacculus) that are connected by a narrow tube. The larger of the two sacs, the utriculus, is the principal organ of the vestibular system or system of balance. This system informs one about the position and movement of the head. The smaller of the two sacs, the sacculus, is also connected by a membranous tube to the cochlea that contains the organ of Corti. The hair cells, which are the special sensory receptors for hearing, are found within the organ of Corti.

**ear, internal**   See *ear, inner.*

**ear, low-set**   A minor anomaly involving an ear that is situated below the normal location. Technically, the ear is low-set when the helix of the ear meets the cranium at a level below that of a horizontal plane through both inner canthi (the inside corners of the eyes). The presence of two or more minor anomalies in a child increases the probability that the child has a major malformation.

**ear, malrotated**   See *ear, slanted.*

**ear, middle**   This part of the ear consists of the eardrum (also called the tympanum, or tympanic membrane) and, beyond it, a cavity. This cavity is connected to the pharynx (the nasopharynx) via a canal known as the Eustachian tube. The Eustachian tube permits the gas pressure in the middle ear cavity to adjust to external air pressure. As you're descending in a plane, it's the Eustachian tube that opens when your ears "pop." The middle ear cavity also contains a chain of three little bones, the ossicles, that connect the eardrum to the internal ear. The ossicles are the malleus, incus, and stapes. In sum, the middle ear communicates with the pharynx, equilibrates with external pressure, and transmits the eardrum vibrations to the inner ear.

**ear, outer**   The part of the ear that's visible along the sides of the human head, behind the temples. The outer ear looks complicated, but is actually the simplest part of the ear. It consists of the pinna or auricle (the visible projecting portion of the ear), the external acoustic meatus (the outside opening to the ear canal), and the external ear canal that leads to the eardrum. The external ear has only to concentrate air vibrations on the eardrum and make the drum vibrate.

**ear, "railroad track"**   See *ear, slanted.*

**ear, slanted**   An ear that is slanted more than usual. Technically, an ear is slanted when the angle of the slope of the auricle is more than 15 degrees from the perpendicular. Considered a minor anomaly. The presence of two or more minor anomalies in a child increases the probability that the child has a major malformation. Slanted (or "railroad track") ears are a common sign of fetal alcohol syndrome and fetal alcohol effect. Both of these conditions also feature a very high rate of sensorineural hearing loss and ear infections. Also known as a malrotated ear. See also *fetal alcohol effect, fetal alcohol syndrome.*

**eardrum**   The tympanic membrane of the ear.

**earthquake supplies kit**   See *disaster supplies.*

**Ebola virus**   A virus that causes a deadly form of hemorrhagic fever: a rise in temperature, together with bleeding problems (hemorrhaging). Epidemics have occurred mainly in Sudan and Zaire. The initial symptoms are fever and headache, followed by vomiting and diarrhea, muscle pain, rash, and bloody nose (epistaxis), spitting up blood from the lungs (hemoptysis) and stomach (hematemesis), and bloody eyes (conjunctival hemorrhages). Transmitted by contact with blood, feces, or body fluids from an infected person. The incubation period ranges from 2 to 21 days. There is no specific treatment for the disease. Death can occur within 10 days.

**EBV**   Epstein-Barr virus.

**ecchymosis**   The skin discoloration caused by a bruise (contusion).

**ecchymotic**   Characterized by ecchymosis.

**ECG**   Abbreviation for electrocardiogram.

**echocardiography**   A diagnostic test that uses ultrasound waves to make images of the heart chambers, valves, and surrounding structures. It can measure cardiac output, and is a sensitive test for detecting inflammation around the heart (pericarditis). It can also be used to detect abnormal anatomy or infections of the heart valves.

**echolalia**   Persistent repetition (echoing) of heard speech. In response to the question, "Do you want milk?" a child with the symptom of echolalia might answer, "Milk?" Echolalia is most commonly seen in autism, but is also found in some children with Tourette syndrome.

**echovirus**   One of a group of viruses that researchers think may be associated with some types of meningitis, stomach ailments, and the common cold. The "echo" part of the name stands for enteric cytopathic human orphan viruses.

**eclampsia**   The presence of one or more convulsions in a pregnant woman who has preeclampsia. Eclampsia is a frequent cause of maternal death outside the developed world, and a serious problem everywhere. Treatment is with antispasmodic medication, notably magnesium sulfate. See also *preeclampsia, HELLP syndrome.*

**ecogenetics** The interaction of genetics with the environment. The genetic disease phenylketonuria (PKU) provides an illustration of ecogenetics. Persons with PKU lack an enzyme to process the amino acid phenylalanine, and so require a special environment: a diet low in phenylalanine.

**economy-class syndrome** See *deep vein thrombosis*.

**ECT** Electroconvulsive therapy.

**ectoderm** In a developing fetus, the outer layer of the organism. This layer differentiates to give rise to many important structures, including the sweat glands, hair, nails, teeth, the lens of the eye, parts of the inner ear, and perhaps most importantly, the nerves, brain, and spinal cord.

**ectodermal dysplasia** A group of over 150 disorders characterized by malfunction or absence of at least two derivatives of ectodermal tissue.

**-ectomy** The surgical removal of something. For example, a lumpectomy is the surgical excision of a lump, a tonsillectomy is the removal of the tonsils, and an appendectomy is removal of the appendix.

**ectopia cordis** A birth defect that results in an abnormal location of the heart. Most often, the heart protrudes outside the chest.

**ectopic** In the wrong place, out of place. An ectopic kidney, for example, is one that is not in the usual location.

**ectopic pregnancy** A pregnancy that is located outside the inner lining of the uterus. In 95 percent of ectopic pregnancies, a fertilized egg settles and grows in the Fallopian tube. However, ectopic pregnancies can occur in other locations, such as the ovary, cervix, and abdominal cavity. An ectopic pregnancy occurs in about 1 in 60 pregnancies. Most occur in women 35 to 44 years of age. Ectopic pregnancies are frequently due to an inability of the fertilized egg to make its way through a Fallopian tube into the uterus. Risk factors predisposing to an ectopic pregnancy include pelvic inflammatory disease (PID), which can damage the tube's functioning or leave it partly or completely blocked; surgery on or near a Fallopian tube, which can leave adhesions (bands of tissue that bind together surfaces); endometriosis, a condition in which tissue like that normally lining the uterus is found outside the uterus; a prior ectopic pregnancy; a history of repeated induced abortions; a history of infertility problems or use of medications to stimulate ovulation; and an abnormality in the shape of the Fallopian tube, as with a birth defect. A major concern with an ectopic pregnancy is internal bleeding. If there is any doubt, seek medical attention promptly. Pain is usually the first symptom of an ectopic pregnancy. The pain, often one-sided, may be in the pelvis, abdomen, or even in the shoulder or neck (due to blood from a ruptured ectopic pregnancy building up under the diaphragm and the pain being "referred" up to the shoulder or neck). The pain is usually sharp and stabbing. Weakness, dizziness or lightheadedness, and a sense of passing out upon standing can represent serious internal bleeding, requiring immediate medical attention. Diagnosis of an ectopic pregnancy includes a pelvic exam to test for pain, tenderness, or a mass in the abdomen. The most useful laboratory test is the measurement of the hormone hCG (human chorionic gonadotropin). In a normal pregnancy, the level of hCG doubles about every 2 days during the first 10 weeks, whereas in an ectopic pregnancy, the hCG rise is usually slower and lower than normal. Ultrasound can also help determine whether a pregnancy is ectopic, as may sometimes culdocentesis, the insertion of a needle through the vagina into the space behind the uterus to see whether there is blood there from a ruptured Fallopian tube. Treatment of an ectopic pregnancy is surgery, often by laparoscopy today, to remove the ill-fated pregnancy. A ruptured tube usually has to be removed. If the tube has not yet burst, it may be possible to repair it. The outlook for future pregnancies depends on the extent of the surgery. If the Fallopian tube has been spared, the chance of a successful pregnancy is usually better than 50 percent. If a Fallopian tube has been removed, an egg can be fertilized in the other tube, and the chance of a successful pregnancy drops somewhat below 50 percent.

**eczema** A particular reaction pattern of the skin, the most common type in children being atopic (allergic) dermatitis. See also *dermatitis*.

**EDC** Estimated date of confinement.

**edema** The swelling of soft tissues as a result of excess water accumulation. It is often more prominent in the lower legs and feet toward the end of the day, because fluid pools while people maintain an upright position.

**edema, hereditary angioneurotic** A genetic form of angioedema. Persons with it are born lacking an inhibitor protein called C1 esterase inhibitor. This protein normally prevents activation of a cascade of proteins that leads to the swelling of angioedema. Patients can develop recurrent attacks of swollen tissues, pain in the abdomen, and swelling of the voice box (larynx), which can compromise breathing. The diagnosis is suspected with a history of recurrent angioedema. It is confirmed by finding abnormally low levels of C1 esterase inhibitor in the blood. Treatment options include antihistamines and male steroids (androgens) that can also prevent the recurrent attacks. Also called hereditary angioedema.

**edema, periorbital**   Swelling around the eyes due to excess water accumulation.

**Edwards syndrome**   Trisomy 18 syndrome, in which there are three copies of chromosome 18 instead of the normal two. Children with this condition have multiple malformations and mental retardation. They characteristically have low birth weight, small head (microcephaly), small jaw (micrognathia), malformations of the heart and kidneys, clenched fists with abnormal finger positioning, and malformed feet. The mental retardation is profound, with the IQ too low to even test. Nineteen out of twenty of these children die before their first birthday.

**EEG**   Electroencephalogram.

**effacement**   Thinning of the cervix, which occurs before and while it dilates.

**effect, founder**   See *founder effect*.

**efferent**   Carrying away. An artery is an efferent vessel carrying blood away from the heart. An efferent nerve carries impulses away from the central nervous system. The opposite of efferent is afferent.

**efferent nerve**   A nerve that carries impulses away from the central nervous system.

**efferent vessel**   A vessel carrying blood away from the heart: an artery or arteriole.

**Effexor**   See *venlafaxine*.

**effusion**   Too much fluid, an outpouring of fluid. A hemorrhagic effusion is one with blood in the fluid.

**effusion, pericardial**   Too much fluid within the fibrous sac (pericardium) that surrounds the heart. The inner surface of the pericardium is lined by a layer of flat cells (mesothelial cells) that normally secrete a small amount of fluid, which acts as a lubricant to allow normal heart movement within the chest. A pericardial effusion involves the presence of an excessive amount of pericardial fluid, a pale yellow serous fluid, within the pericardium.

**effusion, pleural**   Outpouring of fluid between the two layers of the pleural membranes that cover the lungs.

**EFAs**   Essential fatty acids.

**EGD**   Esophagogastroduodenoscopy. See *endoscopy, upper*.

**egg**   See *ovum*.

**egg sac**   See *ovary*.

**Ehlers-Danlos syndrome**   An inherited disorder characterized by easy bruising, joint hypermobility (loose joints), skin laxity, and weakness of tissues. There are nine different Ehlers-Danlos syndromes, each of which share these features. Abbreviated as EDS.

**Ehlers-Danlos syndrome, Type I**   The "gravis" form of EDS, EDS Type I is characterized by marked joint hypermobility, skin hyperextensibility (laxity) and fragility, joint dislocations, and scoliosis (curvature of the spine). It is inherited as an autosomal (non-sex-linked) dominant genetic trait. Dominant means that a single gene is capable of producing the disease.

**Ehlers-Danlos syndrome, Type II**   The "mitis" form of EDS, EDS Type II is similar to but less severe than Type I EDS. It, too, is inherited as an autosomal dominant genetic trait.

**Ehlers-Danlos syndrome, Type III**   In this, the benign hypermobility form of EDS, joint hypermobility is the major manifestation. It is inherited as an autosomal dominant genetic trait.

**Ehlers-Danlos syndrome, Type IV**   The arterial form, Type IV EDS, can cause spontaneous rupture of arteries and the bowel: a serious manifestation. Skin laxity is variable. It is inherited as an autosomal dominant and recessive genetic trait.

**Ehlers-Danlos syndrome, Type V**   This type of EDS is clinically similar to type II, but is X-linked (the gene responsible is carried on the X chromosome). If a woman is carrying the gene, each of her children has a 50 percent chance of receiving the gene. A son with the gene is affected with the disease, while a daughter with the gene is merely a carrier, like her mother.

**Ehlers-Danlos syndrome, Type VI**   The ocular-scoliotic form of EDS, Type VI EDS is characterized by a fragile globe of the eyes, significant skin and joint laxity, and severe curvature of the spine (scoliosis). It is inherited as an autosomal recessive genetic trait. Recessive means that two copies of the gene are required to produce the disease.

**Ehlers-Danlos syndrome, Type VII**   Patients with arthrochalasis multiplex congenita, or Type VII EDS, are short in height and severely affected by joint laxity and dislocations. Skin involvement is variable. Both autosomal dominance and recessive inheritance are possible.

**Ehlers-Danlos syndrome, Type VIII**   Patients with Type VIII EDS have different degrees of joint hypermobility, as well as inflammation of the gums and bone adjacent to the teeth (periodontitis).

**Ehlers-Danlos syndrome, Type IX** In this form of EDS, patients have mildly hypermobile joints and can have mitral valve prolapse. It is inherited as an autosomal dominant trait.

**Ehrlichiosis** An acute (abrupt-onset) disease first reported in humans in 1986, Erlichiosis is due to infection by the rickettsial agent Ehrlichia canis. The brown dog tick is the common vector (carrier). The disease is similar to Rocky Mountain spotted fever, with high fever, headache, malaise, and muscle pain but no rash. See also *rickettsial diseases*.

**eight-day measles** See *measles*.

**eighth cranial nerve** See *vestibulocochlear nerve*. See also *cranial nerves*.

**ejaculation** Ejection of sperm and seminal fluid.

**ejection fraction** The percentage of blood that is pumped out of a filled ventricle as a result of a heartbeat. The heart does not eject all of the blood in the ventricle. Only about two-thirds of the blood is normally pumped out with each beat. That fraction is referred to the ejection fraction. The ejection fraction is an indicator of the heart's health. If the heart is diseased from a heart attack or another cardiac condition, the ejection fraction may fall, for example, to one-third.

**elbow** The juncture of long bones in the middle portion of the arm. The bone of the upper arm (humerus) meets both the ulna (the inner bone of the forearm) and radius (the outer bone of the forearm) to form a hinge joint at the elbow. The radius and ulna also meet one another in the elbow to permit a small amount of rotation of the forearm. The elbow therefore functions to move the arm like a hinge (forward and backward) and in rotation (outward and inward). The biceps muscle is the major muscle that flexes the elbow hinge, whereas the triceps muscle is the major muscle that extends it. The primary stability of the elbow is provided by the ulnar collateral ligament, located on the medial (inner) side of the elbow. The outer bony prominence of the elbow is the lateral epicondyle, a part of the humerus bone. Tendons attached to this area can be injured, causing inflammation or tendinitis: lateral epicondylitis, or "tennis elbow." The inner portion of the elbow is a bony prominence called the medial epicondyle of the humerus. Additional tendons from muscles attach here and can be injured, likewise causing inflammation or tendinitis: medial epicondylitis, or "golfer's elbow."

**elbow bursitis** At the tip of the elbow (the olecranon area) is the olecranon bursa, a fluid-filled sac that functions as a gliding surface to reduce friction with motion. Because of its location, the olecranon bursa is subject to trauma, ranging from simple repetitive weight-bearing while leaning, to banging in a fall. This trauma can cause olecranon bursitis, a common, aseptic form of bursitis that includes varying degrees of swelling, warmth, tenderness, and redness in the area overlying the point of the elbow. If the condition is not caused by infection, treatment includes rest, ice, and medications for inflammation and pain. Infectious bursitis is treated with antibiotics, aspiration, and surgery.

**elbow joint** See *elbow*.

**elbow pain** The elbow joint is quite complex because it is the area of union of three long bones. Elbow pain can have many causes, including arthritis and bursitis. Tendinitis can affect the inner or outer elbow; the treatment includes ice, rest, and medication for inflammation. Bacteria can also infect the skin of the scraped (abraded) elbow. The "funny bone" nerve can be irritated at the elbow to cause numbness and tingling of the little and ring fingers.

**elbow, arthritis of the** Inflammation (arthritis) of the elbow joint can be due to many systemic forms of arthritis, including rheumatoid arthritis, gouty arthritis, psoriatic arthritis, ankylosing spondylitis, and Reiter disease. Generally, arthritis is associated with signs of inflammation of the elbow joint, including heat, warmth, swelling, pain, tenderness, and decreased range of motion. Range of motion of the elbow, impeded by the swollen joint, is decreased.

**elbow, cellulitis of the** Inflammation of the skin around the elbow, due to infection (cellulitis), commonly occurs as a result of abrasions or puncture wounds that permit bacteria on the surface of the skin to invade the deeper layers of the skin. This causes inflamed skin characterized by heat, redness, and swelling. The most common bacteria that cause cellulitis are staphylococcus (Staph) and streptococcus (Strep). Patients may have an associated low-grade fever. Cellulitis generally requires antibiotic treatment, either orally or intravenously. Heat application can help in the healing process.

**elbow, golfer's** The inner portion of the elbow is a bony prominence called the medial epicondyle. Tendons from the muscles attach here, and can be injured, causing medial epicondylitis. To those who play the ancient Scottish sport, this is "golfer's elbow."

**elbow, tennis** The outer bone of the elbow is the lateral epicondyle and is a part of the humerus bone. Tendons attached to this area can be injured, causing inflammation or tendinitis (lateral epicondylitis), known to tennis players as "tennis elbow."

**elbow, tip of the** The bony tip of the elbow is called the olecranon. It is formed by the near end of the ulna, one of the two long bones in the forearm (the other is the radius). The triceps muscle tendon of the back of the arm attaches to the olecranon. Diseases can affect the olecranon. For example, inflammation of the tiny fluid-filled sac (bursa) at the tip of the elbow can occur; this is referred to as olecranon bursitis. Also, a firm nodule can form at the tip of the elbow; this is referred to as an olecranon nodule, and may be due to gout or rheumatoid arthritis. The olecranon is also called the olecranon process of the ulna.

**elder abuse** The physical, sexual, or emotional abuse of an elderly person, usually one who is disabled or frail. Like child abuse, elder abuse is a crime that all health and social services professionals are mandated to report.

**elective mutism** Complete lack of speech, believed to be volitional on the part of the patient. True elective mutism may be a reaction to a traumatic event, the aftermath of damage to or pain in the mouth or throat, or a symptom of extreme shyness. In other cases, the lack of speech is eventually found not to be volitional, but rather a symptom of damage or deformity of the speech apparatus, or of autism. See also *selective mutism*.

**electric shock** Contact with electrical current can cause unconsciousness, burning at the site of entry, and death. While waiting for emergency treatment, try to ensure that the source of the shock is turned off, keep the victim warm, and use CPR if necessary.

**electric shock therapy** See *electroconvulsive therapy*.

**electrocardiogram** A recording of the electrical activity of the heart. An electrocardiogram is a simple, noninvasive procedure. Electrodes are placed on the skin of the chest and connected in a specific order to a machine that, when turned on, measures electrical activity all over the heart. Output is usually in the form of a long scroll of paper displaying a printed graph of activity. Newer models output the data directly to a computer and screen, although a printout may still be made. The initial diagnosis of a heart attack is usually made by a combination of clinical symptoms and characteristic electrocardiogram changes. The electrocardiogram can detect areas of muscle ischemia (muscle deprived of oxygen) and/or dead tissue in the heart. If a medication is known to sometimes adversely affect heart function, a baseline electrocardiogram may be ordered before the patient starts taking the medicine, with follow-up testing at regular intervals to detect any changes. Abbreviated as either EKG or ECG.

**electroconvulsive therapy** The use of controlled, measured doses of electric shock to induce a convulsion. Convulsions so induced can sometimes treat clinical depression that is unresponsive to medication.

**electrodesiccation** Use of an electric current to destroy cancerous tissue and control bleeding.

**electroencephalogram** A study of electrical current within the brain. Electrodes are attached to the scalp. Wires attach these electrodes to a machine, which records the electrical impulses. The results are either printed out or displayed on a computer screen. Different patterns of electrical impulses can denote various forms of epilepsy. Most EEGs see only a moment in time within the brain, and can catch only gross abnormalities in function. An overnight EEG is designed to check the electrical activity in the brain of a sleep-deprived patient, increasing the chance that seizure activity will be revealed. Also available are 24- or 48-hour EEGs, which measure electrical activity over one or two days, ordinarily using mobile EEG units.

**electrogastrogram** A study in which the electrical current generated by the muscle of the stomach is sensed and recorded in a manner very similar to an electrocardiogram of the heart. The electrogastrogram is performed by taping electrodes to the skin on the upper abdomen over the stomach. Recordings from the muscle are stored and analyzed by a computer. The electrogastrogram is performed to diagnose motility disorders of the stomach, conditions that prevent the muscles of the stomach from working normally.

**electrolarynx** A battery-operated instrument that makes a humming sound to help people who have lost their larynx talk.

**electrolysis** Permanent removal of body hair, including the hair root, with an electronic device. Although it is billed as a permanent process, many people find that hair does grow back (albeit slowly) after electrolysis. Electrolysis may be done by a dermatologist, by an electrolysis technician, or in some cases by a facial technologist or esthetician.

**electrolyte** A substance that will dissociate into ions in solution, acquiring the capacity to conduct electricity. The electrolytes include sodium, potassium, chloride, calcium, and phosphate. Electrolyte replacement is called for when a patient has prolonged vomiting or diarrhea, and as a response to strenuous athletic activity. Commercial solutions are available, particularly for sick children (solutions like Pedialyte) and athletes (sports drinks, such as Gatorade). Electrolyte-monitoring is important in treatment of anorexia and bulimia. Informally known as lytes.

**electron microscope** A microscope in which an electron beam replaces light to form the image. It permits greater magnification and resolution than optical microscopes, but you see the electron densities of objects rather than their actual image, and artifacts may abound. Abbreviated as EM.

**electron microscopy**   See *electron microscope*.

**electrophoresis**   Method used in clinical and research laboratories for separating molecules according their size and electrical charge. Electrophoresis is used to separate large molecules (such as DNA fragments or proteins) from a mixture of molecules. An electric current is passed through a medium containing the mixture of molecules. Each kind of molecule travels through the medium at a different rate, depending on its electrical charge and molecular size. Separation of the molecules is based on these differences. Although many substances, including starch gels and paper, have historically served as media for electrophoresis, agarose and acrylamide gels are the most commonly used media for electrophoresis of proteins and nucleic acids.

**electroretinography**   A test in which the electrical potentials generated by the retina of the eye are measured when it is stimulated by light. In an ERG, an electrode is placed on the cornea at the front of the eye. The electrode measures the electrical response of the rods and cones, the visual cells in the retina at the back of the eye. An ERG may be useful in the evaluation of hereditary and acquired disorders of the retina. A normal ERG shows the appropriate responses with increased light intensity. An abnormal ERG is found in conditions such as arteriosclerosis of the retina, detachment of the retina, and temporal arteritis with eye involvement. The instrument used to do electroretinography is an electroretinograph, and the resultant recording is called an electroretinogram.

**electroshock therapy**   See *electroconvulsive therapy*.

**elephant nails**   See *Jadassohn-Lewandowski syndrome*.

**eleventh cranial nerve**   See *accessory nerve*. See also *accessory neuropathy, cranial nerves*.

**ELISA**   Acronym for enzyme-linked immunosorbent assay, this is a rapid immunochemical test that involves an enzyme (a protein that catalyzes a biochemical reaction). It also involves an antibody or antigen (immunologic molecules). ELISA tests detect substances that have antigenic properties, primarily proteins rather than small molecules and ions, such as glucose and potassium. Some of these substances include hormones, bacterial antigens, and antibodies. There are variations of this test, but the most basic consists of an antibody attached to a solid surface. This antibody will latch onto the substance of interest: for example, human chorionic gonadotropin (HGC), the commonly measured protein that indicates pregnancy.

A mixture of purified HCG linked (coupled) to an enzyme and the test sample (blood, urine, etc.) are added to the test system. If no HCG is present in the test sample, then only the HCG with the linked enzyme will bind. The more HCG present in the test sample, the less enzyme-linked HCG will bind. The substance the enzyme acts on is then added, and the amount of product is measured in some way, such as by a change in color of the solution. ELISA tests are generally highly sensitive and specific, and compare favorably with radioimmune assay (RIA) tests. They have the added advantage of not requiring the use of radioisotopes or a radiation-counting apparatus.

**elliptocytosis**   A blood disorder characterized by elliptically shaped red blood cells (elliptocytosis) with variable breakup of red cells (hemolysis) and varying degrees of anemia. Inherited as a dominant trait, this disorder is due to the mutation of one of the genes that encodes proteins of the red cell membrane skeleton. There are at least two forms of elliptocytosis, one form not linked to the Rh blood group, and another form linked to Rh and now known to be on chromosome 1. The Rh-linked form in chromosome region 1p34.2-p33, called EL1, is due to a mutation in erythrocyte membrane protein 4.1. Forms of elliptocytosis not linked to Rh are due to mutations in the alpha-spectrin gene, the beta-spectrin gene, or the band 3 gene.

**Eltroxin**   See *levothyroxine sodium*.

**EM**   Electron microscope or electron microscopy.

**embolism, crossed**   See *embolism, paradoxical*.

**embolism, paradoxical**   Passage of a clot (thrombus) from a vein to an artery. When clots in veins break off (embolize), they travel first to the right side of the heart and, normally, then to the lungs, where they lodge. The lungs act as a filter to prevent the clots from entering the arterial circulation. However, when there is a hole in the wall between the two upper chambers of the heart (an atrial septal defect), a clot can cross from the right to the left side of the heart, then pass into the arteries as a paradoxical embolism. Once in the arterial circulation, a clot can travel to the brain, block a vessel there, and cause a stroke (cerebrovascular accident). Because of the risk of stroke from paradoxical embolism, it is usually recommended that even small atrial septal defects be repaired. Also called crossed embolism.

**embolization**   A treatment that clogs small blood vessels and blocks the flow of blood, such as to a tumor.

**embolus**   A blockage or plug that is obstructing a blood vessel. Examples of emboli are a detached blood clot, a clump of bacteria, or other foreign material, such as air.

**embryo**   The nascent living organism from fertilization to, in humans, the beginning of the third month of pregnancy. After that point in time, it is termed a fetus.

**emergency contraceptive**   See *contraceptive, emergency*.

**emergency medical technician**   A person trained in the performance of the procedures required in emergency medical care. One is most likely to find an EMT working with a mobile emergency response team, such as an ambulance or fire and rescue team. Some EMTs are employed in emergency rooms, or are hired to be present at sporting events, camps, or other locations where emergency response might be needed.

**emergency supplies kit**   See *disaster supplies.*

**emesis**   Vomiting.

**emetic**   Something that causes vomiting. A common emetic is syrup of ipecac.

**EMLA**   An anesthetic cream that can be spread on the skin to numb it. EMLA cream has many medical uses, including reducing the pain associated with slow injections, repeated injections, IV insertion, debridement of veinous leg ulcers, and more.

**emotional child abuse**   See *child abuse, emotional.*

**emphysema**   **1** A lung condition featuring an abnormal accumulation of air in the lung's many tiny air sacs, a tissue called alveoli. As air continues to collect in these sacs, they become enlarged, and may break, or be damaged and form scar tissue. Emphysema is strongly associated with smoking cigarettes, a practice that causes lung irritation. It can also be associated with or worsened by repeated infection of the lungs, such as is seen in chronic bronchitis. The best response to the early warning signs of emphysema is prevention: Stop smoking and get immediate treatment for incipient lung infections. Curing established emphysema is not yet possible. Because patients don't have an adequate amount of space in the lungs to breathe, they gasp for breath, and may not be able to obtain enough oxygen. Those with severe emphysema usually end up using an oxygen machine to breathe. In some cases, medication may be helpful to ease symptoms or to treat infection in already-damaged lungs. **2** The escape of air into other body tissues, as may occur during surgery. This is called surgical emphysema.

**empiric risk**   The chance that a disease will occur in a family, based upon the doctor's experience with this diagnosis, past history, and medical records rather than theory.

**empirical**   Based on experience and observation, rather than systematic logic. Experienced physicians often use empirical reasoning to make diagnoses, based on having seen many cases over the years. Less-experienced physicians are more likely to use diagnostic guides and manuals. In practice, both approaches (if properly applied) will usually come up with the same diagnosis.

**empyema**   Pus in the pleural space between the outer surface of the lung and the chest wall. Empyema typically is a result of a serious bacterial infection.

**EMT**   Emergency medical technician.

**enathem**   A rash inside the body. For example, the measles spots inside the mouth. Called Koplik spots, these look like tiny grains of white sand surrounded by a red ring.

**encapsulated**   Confined to a specific area. An encapsulated tumor remains in a compact form.

**encephalitis**   Inflammation of the brain, which may be caused by a bacteria, a virus (such as one of the human herpes viruses or the viruses that cause mumps and measles), or an allergic reaction to a virus or vaccination. Some forms of viral encephalitis are contagious. For example, encephalitis occurs in 1 in 1,000 cases of measles. It may start up to three weeks after onset of the measles rash, and presents with high fever, convulsions, and coma. It usually runs a blessedly short course, with full recovery within a week. Encephalitis can cause brain damage, which may result in or exacerbate the symptoms of a developmental disorder or mental illness. The form called encephalitis lethargica ("sleeping sickness") results in a set of Parkinson disease–like symptoms called postencephalitic parkinsonianism. In some cases encephalitis causes death. Treatment of encephalitis must begin as early as possible to avoid potentially serious and lifelong effects. Depending on the cause of the inflammation, this may include antibiotics, antiviral medications, and anti-inflammatory drugs. If brain damage results from encephalitis, therapy (such as physical therapy or cognitive restoration therapy) may help patients regain lost functions.

**encephalomyelitis**   Inflammation of both the brain and the spinal cord. Encephalomyelitis can be caused by a variety of conditions, including viruses that infect the nervous system. One type of encephalomyelitis, acute disseminated encephalomyelitis, occurs most commonly after an acute viral infection, such as measles (rubeola). It is due to be an autoimmune attack upon the the nervous system, meaning that the immune system mistakenly attacks body tissue that it believes is the measles virus. Also called myeloencephalitis.

**encephalopathic syndrome** A dangerous condition with symptoms similar to those of neuroleptic malignant syndrome (NMS), of which it may be a variant. It is associated with lithium toxicity.

**encephalopathy, mitochondrial** See *MELAS syndrome*.

**encephelotrigeminal angiomatosi** See *Sturge-Weber syndrome*.

**enchondroma** A benign tumor of the bone that resembles cartilage. Enchondromas are most frequently seen on the bones of a child's hands or feet, and can be a side effect of a poorly healed fracture. Rarely, an enchondroma will become malignant in adulthood, turning into a chondrosarcoma. Treatment, if warranted, is by surgical removal.

**enchondromatosis** A condition characterized by multiple enchondromas, affecting not only the hands and feet but the long bones of the limbs as well. Enchondromatosis can cause deformity and pain. Also known as Ollier disease.

**encopresis** Inability to control the elimination of stool. Encopresis can have a variety of causes, including inability to control the anal sphincter muscle or gastrointestinal problems, particularly chronic diarrhea and Crohn disease. Several neurological disorders, including Tourette syndrome and obsessive-compulsive disorder, are also occasionally associated with the symptom of encopresis, particularly in children. Preventive care for encopresis includes frequent scheduled toileting, and pads or diapers to prevent embarassing soiling. Careful cleaning is important to prevent skin breakdown. Treatment of encopresis usually involves treatment of the underlying disorder; cognitive behavioral therapy or behavior modification is also sometimes helpful. Also known as fecal incontinence.

**endemic** Present in a community at all times, but occurring in low frequency. For example, malaria is endemic in some areas of the world, such as parts of India. The opposite of epidemic, which denotes a sudden outbreak, or pandemic, which denotes an epidemic that has spread across a whole region.

**endemic typhus** See *typhus, murine*.

**endocardium** The lining of the interior surface of the heart chambers. The endocardium consists of a layer of endothelial cells and an underlying layer of connective tissue.

**endocervical curettage** The removal of tissue from the inside of the cervix, using a spoon-shaped instrument called a curette.

**endocrinology** The study of the medical aspects of hormones, including diseases and conditions associated with hormonal imbalance, damage to the glands that make hormones, or the use of synthetic or natural hormonal drugs. An endocrinologist is a doctor who specializes in the management of hormone conditions.

**endocrinopathy** Literally, a disease of an endocrine gland, commonly used as a medical term for a hormone problem. Common endocrinopathies include hyperthyroidism and hypothyroidism.

**endogenous** Inside. For example, endogenous cholesterol is cholesterol that is made inside the body, not derived from the diet.

**endometrial biopsy** A common and medically valuable procedure for sampling the lining of the uterus (the endometrium). Endometrial biopsy is usually done to learn the cause of abnormal uterine bleeding, although it may be used to determine the cause of infertility, test for uterine infections, and even monitor the response to certain medications. The procedure can be done in the doctor's office. There are few risks, the leading one being cramping and pain. Oral pain medications taken beforehand may help reduce cramping and pain. Vaginal bleeding, infection and, very rarely, perforation of the uterus can also occur.

**endometrial hyperplasia** A condition characterized by overgrowth of the lining of the uterus.

**endometriosis** A noncancerous condition in which tissue that looks like endometrial tissue grows in abnormal places, most often in the abdomen. Although most women with endometriosis have no symptoms, pelvic pain during menstruation or ovulation can be a symptom of endometriosis. Endometriosis can also be suspected by a doctor during a physical examination and confirmed by surgery, usually laparoscopy. Treatment options include medication for pain, hormone therapy, and laparoscopic surgery to remove the growths (hysterectomy was once done, but is usually ineffective). Most women with endometriosis are completely unaware of these growths, and are not harmed by their presence. However, endometriosis can increase the risk of ectopic pregnancy, a potentially life-threatening condition that can cause infertility.

**endometriosis interna** See *adenomyosis*.

**endometriosis uterina** See *adenomyosis*.

**endometritis** Inflammation of the endometrium, the inner layer of the uterus.

**endometrium** The inner layer of the uterus.

**endonuclease**   An enzyme that leaves a nucleic acid (DNA or RNA) at specific internal sites in the nucleotide base sequence.

**endorphins**   Hormonal compounds made by the body in response to pain or extreme physical exertion. They are similar in structure and effect to opiate drugs. Endorphins are responsible for the so-called "runner's high," and release of these essential compounds permits humans to endure childbirth, accidents, and strenuous everyday activities.

**endoscope**   A lighted optical instrument used to get a deep look inside the body. An endoscope, which may be rigid or flexible, can be used to examine organs, such as the throat or esophagus. Specialized endoscopes are named for where they are intended to look. Examples include the cystoscope (bladder), nephroscope (kidney), bronchoscope (bronchi), laryngoscope (larynx), otoscope (ear), arthroscope (joint), laparoscope (abdomen), and gastrointestinal endoscopes.

**endoscopic gastrostomy, percutaneous**   See *gastrostomy, percutaneous endoscopic*.

**Endoscopic Retrograde Cholangio-Pancreatography**
A diagnostic procedure to examine diseases of the liver, bile ducts, and pancreas. ERCP is uncomfortable, but not painful. It is usually performed under intravenous sedation rather than general anesthesia, and has a low incidence of complications. ERCP provides important information unobtainable by other diagnostic means. Therapeutic measures can often be taken at the time of ERCP to remove stones in the bile ducts, or to relieve obstructions of the bile ducts.

**endoscopy**   A procedure in which the doctor looks inside the body through a lighted tube called an endoscope. Endoscopy is frequently used to examine the intestines for evidence of gastrointestinal disease or malfunction. Hormones, particularly the pancreatic hormone secretin, may be administered to enable the examiner to check various functions within the digestive system. The process of endoscopy is rather uncomfortable, and patients are sedated in advance.

**endoscopy, upper**   A procedure that enables the examiner (usually a gastroenterologist) to examine the esophagus, stomach, and the first portion of small bowel (duodenum) by using a thin, flexible tube that can be looked through or seen on a TV monitor. Also known as esophagogastroduodenoscopy or EGD.

**endostatin**   A fragment of a protein, collagen 18, found in all blood vessels. This fragment is normally secreted by tumors. It appears to halt the process of developing new blood vessels (angiogenesis), which is necessary to tumor development. It is hoped that endostatin represents a prototype for a new class of agents for treating cancer.

**endothelium**   The layer of cells lining the closed internal spaces of the body, such as the blood vessels and lymph nodes. See also *epithelium*.

**endotracheal tube**   A flexible plastic tube that is put in the mouth and then down into the trachea (airway). The doctor inserts the tube under direct vision with the help of a laryngoscope, in a procedure called endotracheal intubation. The purpose is to ventilate the lungs.

**endourologist**   A urologist with special expertise in navigating inside the kidney, ureter, and bladder, using endoscopic optical instruments and other tools. Endourologists are specialists in diagnosing and treating diseases of these organs.

**engagement**   In obstetrics, this term refers to the sensation that a pregnant woman feels when the presenting (lowermost) part of the fetus descends and is engaged in the mother's pelvis, an event that classically occurs two to three weeks before labor begins. Women who have had two or more prior viable pregnancies (multiparas) may not experience engagement until labor actually begins. When engagement occurs, there is a visible change in the shape of the woman's stomach due to the baby dropping lower in the abdomen. Engagement is also called "lightening" because the pregnant woman feels lighter after this event. Most women feel more comfortable after engagement, but some may experience lower back pain as the fetus presses close to the tailbone and the sciatic nerve. Others may find movement more difficult due to the lower center of gravity caused by engagement.

**ENGERIX-B**   A vaccine against hepatitis B that stimulates the body's immune system to produce antibodies against the virus.

**engram**   An enduring change in the brain postulated to account for the persistence of memory.

**enophthalmos**   Sunken eyeball.

**enoxaparin**   A low-molecular-weight version of heparin, enoxaparin acts like heparin as an anticoagulant medication. It is used to prevent thromboembolic complications (blood clots that travel from their site of origin through the bloodstream to clog another vessel) and in the early treatment of blood clots in the lungs (pulmonary embolisms).

**ENT**   Ear, nose, and throat. An ENT physician is a specialist in the diagnosis and treatment of disorders of the head and neck, particularly those of the ears, nose, and throat. ENT doctors are also called otolaryngologists.

**Entamoeba histolytica**   The agent that causes amebic dysentery, Entamoeba histolytica is a single-celled parasite that is transmitted to humans via contaminated water and food. It can also infect the liver and other organs. See also *amebiasis, amebic colitis, amebic dysentery*.

**enteric**   Of or relating to the small intestine.

**enteric-coated**   Coated with a material that permits transit through the stomach to the small intestine before the medication is released. Aspirin, which commonly causes stomach irritation and upset, is among the medications that may have an enteric coating.

**enteritis, Crohn**   See *Crohn enteritis*.

**enteritis, regional**   See *Crohn disease*.

**entero-**   Prefix referring to the intestine.

**enterobiasis**   An infection caused by a small, white intestinal worm known as the pinworm or, more formally, Enterobius vermicularis. See *pinworm infestation*.

**enterocentesis**   The use of a hollow needle inserted through the wall of the stomach or intestine to relieve pressure from gas or fluid buildup.

**enterocolitis, Crohn**   See *Crohn enterocolitis*.

**enterogenous**   Carried within the intestine, as in an enterogenous bacterial infection.

**enteropathy**   Any disease of the intestine.

**enteropathy, gluten**   A condition in which the absorption of food nutrients through the small intestine is impaired because of an allergic reaction to gluten, a protein found in wheat, related grains, and many other foods. Frequent diarrhea and weight loss can be symptoms. A skin condition called dermatitis herpetiformis can be associated with gluten enteropathy. The most accurate test is a biopsy of the small bowel. Treatment is avoidance of gluten in the diet, and—in some cases—medications. See also *celiac sprue*.

**enteropathy, protein-losing**   A condition in which an excessive amount of plasma protein is lost into the intestine. It can be due to diverse causes, including gluten enteropathy, extensive ulceration of the intestine, intestinal lymphatic blockage, and infiltration of leukemic cells into the intestinal wall.

**enterospasm**   A painful, intense contraction of the intestine.

**enterostomal therapist**   A health care specialist trained to help patients care for and adjust to their colostomy.

**enterostomy**   An operation that opens the small intestine and brings it through the abdominal wall. An external shunt (stoma) is attached to the new opening to permit intestinal draining. See also *colostomy*.

**enterovirus**   A virus that comes into the body through the gastrointestinal tract and thrives there, often moving on to attack the nervous system. Enteroviruses include the polioviruses, rhinoviruses, and echoviruses.

**enuresis**   Involuntary urination, which may be caused by a variety of factors. These include disorders of the kidneys, bladder, or ureter, and poor control of the muscles that control release of urine. Enuresis is also occasionally associated with neurological disorders, such as Tourette syndrome, particularly in children. Nighttime (nocturnal) enuresis may be related to any of the above, or may be a symptom of a sleep disorder. Palliative treatment options include regularly scheduled toileting, increasing awareness of the need to urinate, exercises intended to strengthen the muscles that control release of urine (see *Kegel exercises*), pads or diapers to prevent embarassing and uncomfortable wetness, and in some cases special devices that alert the patient to initial signs of wetness. Treatment of enuresis usually involves treatment of the underlying disorder. Cognitive behavioral therapy or behavior modification techniques may also prove helpful. See also *bedwetting*.

**environmental tobacco smoke**   Smoke that comes from the burning end of a cigarette or that is exhaled by smokers. Also called ETS, or secondhand smoke. Inhalation of environmental tobacco smoke is called involuntary or passive smoking. It can cause the same illnesses that actually smoking cigarettes causes.

**enzyme**   A protein that acts as a catalyst to mediate and speed a specific chemical reaction.

**enzyme defect**   A disorder resulting from a deficiency (or functional abnormality) of an enzyme. Today, newborns are routinely screened for certain enzyme defects, such as phenylketonuria (PKU), and galactosemia, an error in the metabolism of the sugar galactose.

**enzyme, Warburg yellow**   A key respiratory enzyme. Warburg yellow enzyme is a flavoprotein that catalyzes an oxidation-reduction reaction that is necessary for cells to breathe normally. See also *enzymes, yellow*.

**enzyme-linked immunosorbent assay**   See *ELISA*.

**enzymes, yellow**   A group of respiratory enzymes that catalyze reactions in the body, permitting cells to respire or breathe. These biochemical reactions are termed oxidation-reduction reactions. All yellow enzymes are flavoproteins. See also *enzyme, Warburg's yellow*.

**eosinophil**   A type of white blood cell that has coarse granules within its cytoplasm. The numbers of eosinophils in blood often rise when an allergic reaction is in progress.

**eosinophilic fasciitis**   A disease that leads to inflammation and thickening of the skin, and of the lining tissue under the skin that covers the surface of underlying tissues (fascia). In eosinophilic fasciitis, the involved fascia is inflamed with the eosinophil white blood cells. There is progressive thickening, and often redness, warmth, and hardness of the skin surface. Also known as Shulman syndrome.

**eosinophilic granuloma**   See *histiocytosis X*.

**ependymoma**   A type of brain tumor, ependymomas derive from the glial cells that line the cavities within the brain's ventricles. Because cerebrospinal fluid normally flows through these ventricles, blockage due to an ependymoma can cause buildup of fluid, pressure on the brain, and hydrocephalus.

**ephedrine**   A vasoconstricting, bronchodilating drug used to treat asthma. Also found in over-the-counter remedies for cold and flu symptoms and, in the form of the ephedrine-containing herbs ephedra or Ma Huang, in some herbal remedies. Side effects of ephedrine can include jitteriness, racing heartbeat, nausea, sleeplessness, and headache. Ephedrine misuse or abuse can be dangerous, even life-threatening, especially for people with underlying heart conditions.

**epicanthal fold**   A fold of skin that comes down across the inner angle of the eye. The epicanthal fold is more common in children with Down syndrome and other birth defects than in normal children, and so is of value in diagnosis. To the untrained eye, the epicanthal fold may look similar to the eye fold found in peoples of Asian origin, but the normal Asian eye fold is actually quite distinct. The epicanthal fold is instead continuous with the lower edge of the upper eyelid.

**epicardium**   The inner layer of the pericardium, a conical sac of fibrous tissue that surrounds the heart and the roots of the great blood vessels. It consists of a layer of mesothelial cells and underlying stromal layer. Also called the visceral pericardium.

**epidemic**   The occurrence of more cases of a disease than would be expected to occur in a community or region during a given time period. A sudden outbreak (as, for example, of cholera). The opposite of endemic. When an epidemic becomes widespread, affecting a whole region, a continent, or the world, it is called a pandemic.

**epidemic hemorrhagic fever**   A number of diseases characterized by abrupt onset of high fever and chills,

headache, cold, cough; and pain in the muscles, joints, and abdomen, with nausea and vomiting. These symptoms are followed by bleeding into the kidneys and elsewhere. Many arboviruses (including those in the families Togaviridae, Flaviviridae, Filoviridae, and Bunyaviridae) and the hantaviruses, which are spread by rodents or biting insects, can cause epidemic hemorrhagic fever. The Ebola virus is a notorious cause of epidemic hemorrhagic fever. Also known as hemorrhagic fever with renal syndrome.

**epidemic myalgia**   See *Bornholm disease*.

**epidemic typhus**   See *typhus, epidemic*.

**epidemiologist**   A person engaged in epidemiology. Epidemiologists can be people with an MD, PhD, DPH (Doctor of Public Health), MPH (Master of Public Health), RN, or other degrees.

**epidemiology, classical**   The study of populations in order to determine the frequency and distribution of disease, and then to measure the risk of disease.

**epidemiology, clinical**   Epidemiology focused specifically on patients.

**epidermis**   The upper or outer layer of the two main layers of cells in the skin. The epidermis is mostly made up of flat, scale-like cells called squamous cells. Under the squamous cells are round cells called basal cells. The deepest part of the epidermis also contains melanocytes, cells that produce the substance melanin, which gives skin its color. See also *dermis*.

**epidermoid carcinoma**   A type of lung cancer in which the cells are flat and look like fish scales. Also known as squamous cell carcinoma.

**epididymis**   A structure within the scrotum that is attached to the back side of the testis. The epididymis is a coiled segment of the spermatic ducts. It serves to store, mature, and transport spermatozoa between the testis and the vas deferens.

**epididymitis**   Inflammation of the epididymis. Epididymitis can be caused by sexually acquired bacteria, such as gonorrhea and chlamydia; or by bacteria that come from somewhere else, such as E. coli from the bowel. Sometimes no bacteria are found associated with inflammation of the epididymis. Epididymitis from bacteria is treated with antibiotics. If gonorrhea or chlamydia are suspected, both ceftriaxone and doxycycline are often used. If bowel microbes are suspected, ofloxacin is used.

**epidural anesthetic**   An anesthetic injected into the epidural space surrounding the fluid-filled sac (the dura) around the spine, partially numbing the abdomen and legs. An epidural is used fairly commonly in childbirth, if anesthesia is requested, and during birth by Caesarian section.

**epigastrium**   The part of the abdominal wall above the umbilicus (belly button).

**epiglottis**   The flap that covers the trachea during swallowing, so that food does not enter the lungs.

**epilation**   Removal of body hair, including the hair root, by means of electrical device, tweezer, or wax. Epilation may be performed by a dermatologist, but is more commonly done for cosmetic purposes by a facial technologist or esthetician. After epilation the skin may be particularly sensitive. Also known as depilation.

**epilepsy**   A seizure disorder. When nerve cells in the brain fire electrical impulses at a rate up to four times higher than normal, this causes a sort of electrical storm in the brain, known as a seizure. A pattern of repeated seizures is referred to as epilepsy. Known causes of epilepsy include head injuries, brain tumors, lead poisoning, maldevelopment of the brain, and genetic and infectious illnesses. However, in fully half of cases, no cause can be found. Medication can control seizures for the majority of patients. In cases of epilepsy that cannot be managed with drugs, the ketogenic diet or brain surgery may be considered. See also specific types of seizures, such as *seizure, tonic-clonic;* and the specific seizure disorders *Aicardis syndrome, Landau-Kleffner syndrome, Lennox-Gastaut syndrome, Otabara syndrome, Ramsey Hunt syndrome, Rasmussen syndrome, Rett syndrome, Sturge-Weber syndrome, Tassinari syndrome*. See also *seizure, seizure disorders*.

**epilepsy, akinetic**   A seizure disorder characterized by drop seizures, in which the patient experiences a temporary loss of consciousness and lack of movement (akinesia).

**epilepsy, benign rolandic**   The most common partial seizure disorder. It is usually characterized by partial seizures during sleep, whose only outward sign may be movements of the face and mouth, and/or staring spells. It begins between the ages of 2 and 13, and remits on its own by adulthood as the nervous system matures. The proper clinical definition states that it occurs in children with no other neurological or intellectual deficit, but similar symptoms may occur in children who do have other impairments. Diagnosis is by observation and by sleep-deprived or 24-hour EEG. On the EEG, blunted, high-voltage central temporal ("rolandic") spiking is seen, followed by slow waves, and activated by sleep. These spikes tend to spread or to shift from side to side. Most children diagnosed with benign rolandic epilepsy are not treated with antiseizure medications, due to the high

side-effect profile of these medications compared with the minor nature of these seizures. However, 30 percent will need medication due to repeated and more difficult-to-handle episodes. Also known as benign rolandic epilepsy of childhood (BREC), and benign partial epilepsy with centrotemporal spikes. See also *seizure, partial*.

**epilepsy, grand mal**   Epilepsy that includes tonic-clonic (grand mal) seizures. See *seizure, tonic-clonic*.

**epilepsy, Jacksonian**   A seizure disorder characterized by partial seizures: brief alterations in movement, sensation, or nerve function, which are caused by abnormal electrical activity in a localized area of the brain. Diagnosis is by observation and EEG. Treatment, if necessary, is with antiseizure medications. See also *seizure, partial*.

**epilepsy, juvenile myoclonic**   A form of epilepsy that occurs between the ages of 8 and 26, most commonly in the teenage years. It is characterized by jerking (myoclonic) movements of the arms and upper torso, without loss of consciousness. Seizures are most likely to occur while awakening from sleep. Many children with this disorder are sensitive to light (photosensitive), and may have myoclonic jerks or seizures when exposed to bright light. Diagnosis is by observation and by EEG. During a myoclonic seizure, polyspike-wave discharges over a normal EEG background are seen. Juvenile myoclonic epilepsy appears to be an inheritable genetic disorder, with the gene located on chromosome 6. Treatment is with antiseizure medications.

**epilepsy, Landau-Kleffner**   See *Landau-Kleffner syndrome*. See also *autism*.

**epilepsy, partial**   Any of several forms of epilepsy that do not cause grand mal seizures. See also *seizure, seizure disorders*.

**epilepsy, petit mal**   A form of epilepsy in which only absence (petit mal, minor) seizures are seen. See also *seizure, absence*.

**epilepsy, temporal lobe**   Epilepsy characterized by abnormal electrical activity in the temporal lobe of the brain. This activity does not cause grand mal seizures, but rather causes unusual behaviors and patterns of cognition. Temporal lobe epilepsy may, for example, cause sudden outburts of unexpected aggression or agitation, or it may be characterized by aura-like phenomena. It is difficult to diagnose, because temporal lobe seizures may not show up on an EEG. Diagnosis may instead be by observation of symptoms, or through the use of brain imaging technology. Temporal lobe epilepsy can often be treated with the same antiseizure medications used for other forms of epilepsy. See also *seizure, seizure disorders*.

**epileptic aura**   See *aura*.

**epileptic regression**   See *Landau-Kleffner syndrome*. See also *autism*.

**epilepticus, status**   See *status epilepticus*.

**epinephrine**   A substance produced by the interior (medulla) of the adrenal gland. Technically speaking, epinephrine is a sympathomimetic catcholamine. It causes quickening of the heartbeat, strengthens the force of the heart's contraction, opens up the airways (bronchioles) in the lungs, and has numerous other effects. The secretion of epinephrine is part of the fight-or-flight reaction. Adrenaline is a synonym of epinephrine, and is its official name in the British Pharmacopoeia.

**epiphyseal plate fracture**   See *fracture, Salter-Harris*.

**epiphysis**   The growth area near the end of a bone.

**episiotomy**   A surgical procedure for widening the outlet of the birth canal to facilitate delivery of the baby, and to avoid a jagged rip of the area between the anus and the vulva (perineum). During an episiotomy, an incision is made between the vagina and the rectum. The usual cut goes straight down, and does not involve the muscles around the rectum or the rectum itself. An episiotomy can decrease the amount of maternal pushing, but may also decrease trauma to the vaginal tissues and expedite delivery of the baby when delivery is necessary quickly. However, episiotomy is associated with a higher incidence of extensions or tears into the muscle of the rectum, or even the rectum itself. This is more difficult to repair, and more painful for the mother. In fact, current obstetrical opinion holds that jagged tears of the periteum that occur naturally are less likely to affect muscle, and more likely to heal quickly and cleanly than a surgical episiotomy. Episiotomy and natural tearing can often be avoided by the use of perineal massage during delivery. Repair of the episiotomy is by simple stitching. The typical healing time for an episiotomy is about four to six weeks, depending on the size of the incision and the type of suture material used to close the episiotomy.

**epispadias**   A congenital malformation in which the opening of the urethra is on the top side of the penis. Hypospadias is the corresponding malformation, in which the opening of the urethra is on the underside of the penis. Surgical repair is possible.

**epistaxis**   See *nosebleed*.

**epistaxis, treatment of**   See *nosebleed, treatment of*.

**epithelial basement corneal dystrophy**   See *Cogan corneal dystrophy*. See also *Cogan syndrome*.

**epithelial carcinoma**   Cancer that begins in the cells that line an organ.

**epithelium**   The outside layer of cells that covers all free, open surfaces of the body, including the skin and the mucous membranes that communicate with the outside of the body. By contrast, the endothelium is the layer of cells lining the closed internal spaces of the body, such as the blood vessels and lymphatic vessels.

**EPO**   1 See *erythropoietin*. 2 Evening primrose oil.

**EPO test**   A test of the hormone erythropoietin (EPO) in blood. The EPO level can indicate bone marrow disorders, kidney disease, or EPO abuse. Testing EPO blood levels is of value, as too little EPO might be responsible for too few red blood cells (such as in evaluating anemia); too much EPO can cause too many red blood cells (polycythemia), might be evidence for a kidney tumor, and in an athlete suggests EPO abuse. The patient is usually asked to fast for 8 to 10 hours (overnight), and may be asked to lie quietly and relax for 20 or 30 minutes before the test. The test requires a routine sample of blood. Normal levels of EPO are 0 to 19 (some say up to 24) milliunits per milliliter (mU/ml). Subnormal values of EPO are sometimes found, for example, in anemia due to chronic kidney failure. Elevated EPO levels are found, for example, in polycythemia rubra vera, a disorder characterized by an excess of red blood cells. The correct interpretation of an abnormal EPO level depends on the patient's particular picture.

**eponym**   Something named after someone. For example, a condition called Shiel syndrome might be named after someone named Shiel who discovered it, or who was the first to describe and clearly delineate it.

**EPS**   Extrapyramidal side effects.

**Epstein-Barr virus**   A double-stranded DNA virus in the herpes family, EBV is best known as the cause of infectious mononucleosis ("mono," also called glandular fever). EBV infection is characterized by fatigue and general malaise. It was at one time believed to be the cause of chronic fatigue syndrome, but chronic infection with this virus is actually a separate (if similar) disorder. Infection with EBV is fairly common, and is normally a transient and minor thing. However, in some individuals EBV can trigger chronic illness, including immune and lymphoproliferative syndromes. It is a particular danger to people with compromised immune systems, including those with AIDS. Treatment is with antiviral medication and rest. Also known as human herpesvirus 4, abbreviated HHV-4.

**ERCP**   Endoscopic Retrograde Cholangio-Pancreatography.

**erectile dysfunction**    A consistent inability to sustain an erection sufficient for sexual intercourse. While commonly known as impotence, erectile dysfunction is properly described as impotence due to a physical cause, such as disease, injury, drug side effects, or a disorder that impairs blood flow in the penis. Other forms of impotence include lack of sexual desire and problems with ejaculation and orgasm. Erectile dysfunction is treatable in all age groups. Typical treatments include medication (notably Viagra) and penile implants.

**erection, penile**    The state of the penis when it is filled with blood and becomes rigid. The penis contains two chambers called the corpora cavernosa, which run the length of the organ, are filled with spongy tissue, and are surrounded by a membrane called the tunica albuginea. The spongy tissue contains smooth muscles, fibrous tissues, spaces, veins, and arteries. The urethra, which is the channel for urine and ejaculate, runs along the underside of the corpora cavernosa. Erection begins with sensory and mental stimulation. Impulses from the brain and local nerves cause the muscles of the corpora cavernosa to relax, allowing blood to flow in and fill the open spaces. The blood creates pressure in the corpora cavernosa, making the penis expand. The tunica albuginea helps to trap the blood in the corpora cavernosa, thereby sustaining erection. Erection is reversed when muscles in the penis contract, stopping the inflow of blood and opening outflow channels.

**ERG**    **1** Electroretinography. **2** Electroretinograph, the instrument used to perform electroretinography. **3** An electroretinogram, the recording produced by an electroretinograph.

**ergonomics**    The science of making things fit people, instead of asking people to fit things. Ergonomics uses knowledge from anatomy, mechanics, physiology, and psychology to utilize human energy most effectively. Something that is ergonomic is designed for safe, comfortable, and efficient use. For example, a computer keyboard with an ergonomic design is intended to help the user avoid carpal tunnel syndrome and wrist pain.

**ergot**    Ergot could be called a "cereal killer," for it comes from cereals such as rye and wheat, and is quite capable of killing someone. A fungus (Claviceps purpurea) that contaminates rye and wheat produces substances (alkaloids) termed ergotamines. Ergotamines constrict blood vessels, and cause the muscle of the uterus to contract. They have been much used—and are very useful—for the treatment of migraine. They have also been used and misused as abortifacients. In excess, however, ergotamines can cause symptoms such as hallucinations, severe gastrointestinal upset, a type of dry gangrene, and a painful burning sensation in the limbs and extremities. Chronic ergot poisoning (ergotism) was rife during the Middle Ages due to the consumption of contaminated rye. Because of the burning pain, it was known as *ignis sacer* (holy fire), *ignis infernalis* (hell's fire), and St. Anthony's fire. A form of ergot was also the original basis for the illicit drug lysergic acid diethylamide (LSD).

**erotomania**    The false yet persistent belief that one is loved by a person (often a famous or prominent person), or the pathologically obsessive pursuit of a disinterested object of love. Erotomania can be a symptom of schizophrenia or other psychiatric disorders that are characterized by delusional symptoms.

**error of the first kind**    See *alpha error*.

**error of the second kind**    See *beta error*.

**error, alpha**    See *alpha error*.

**error, beta**    See *beta error*.

**error, type I**    See *alpha error*.

**error, type II**    See *beta error*.

**errors of metabolism, inborn**    See *metabolism, inborn errors of*.

**ERT**    Estrogen replacement therapy.

**erythem**    A redness of the skin resulting from inflammation, as caused, for example, by sunburn.

**erythema chronicum migran**    The classic initial rash of Lyme disease. In the early phase of the illness, within hours to weeks of the tick bite, the local skin develops an expanding ring of unraised redness. There may be an outer ring of brighter redness and a central area of clearing. See also *Lyme disease*.

**erythema infectiosum**    See *fifth disease*.

**erythroblastosis**    See *hemolytic disease of the newborn*.

**erythrocyanosis**    Discoloration on the legs that takes on a bluish or purple hue.

**erythrocyte**    A blood cell containing hemoglobin to carry oxygen to all parts of the body. Erythrocytes are made in the bone marrow. Also called a red blood cell (RBC). See also *blood cell*.

**erythrocyte membrane protein band 4.1**    See *elliptocytosis*.

**erythroleukemia**    Leukemia that develops in erythrocytes. In this rare disease, the body produces large numbers of abnormal red blood cells.

**erythromycin** An antibiotic medication (brand names include Benzamycin, E-Mycin, Eygel, Ilotycin, Theramycin) prescribed to treat bacterial infection. See also *macrolide antibiotic*.

**erythroplakia** A reddened patch with a velvety surface, found in the mouth.

**erythropoietin** Abbreviated as EPO, erythropoietin is a hormone, produced by the kidney, that leads to the formation of red blood cells in the bone marrow. Human EPO is a glycoprotein (a protein with an attached sugar) with a molecular weight of 34,000. The kidney cells that make EPO are specialized, and are sensitive to low oxygen levels in the blood that comes into the kidney. These cells release erythropoietin when the oxygen level is low in the kidney. Erythropoietin stimulates the bone marrow to produce more red blood cells, which in turn increases the oxygen-carrying capacity of the blood. EPO is produced not only in the kidney but also, to a lesser extent, in the liver. The amount of EPO in the blood can indicate bone marrow disorders or kidney disease. Normal levels of EPO are 0 to 19 milliunits per milliliter (mU/ml). Elevated levels can be seen in polycythemia rubra vera, a disorder characterized by an excess of red blood cells. Lower than normal values of EPO are seen in chronic renal failure. Using recombinant DNA technology, EPO has been synthetically produced for use in persons with anemia due to kidney failure, anemia secondary to AZT treatment of AIDS, and anemia associated with cancer. EPO has been much misused as a performance-enhancing drug in endurance athletes, reportedly including cyclists in the Tour de France, long-distance runners, speed skaters, and Nordic (cross-country) skiers. When misused in such situations, EPO is thought to be especially dangerous, perhaps because dehydration can further increase the viscosity of the blood, increasing the risk for heart attacks and strokes. EPO has been banned by the Tour de France, the Olympic committee, and other sports organizations.

**erythropoietin test** See *EPO test*.

**erythroprosopalgia** See *cluster headache*.

**eschar** The scab formed when a wound or skin is sealed by the heat of cautery or burning. Also the dark crusted ulcer (*tache noire*) at the site of the chigger (mite larva) bite in scrub typhus.

**Escherichia coli** Full term for E. coli, the colon bacillus. See *E.coli*.

**esophageal** Related to the esophagus.

**esophageal cancer** A malignant tumor of the esophagus. Cancer of the esophagus can cause difficulty and pain with swallowing solid food, and of course can spread (metastasize) to other parts of the body. The risk of cancer of the esophagus is increased by long-term irritation of the esophagus, such as with smoking, heavy alcohol intake, and Barrett esophagitis. Diagnosis of esophageal cancer can be made by barium X-ray of the esophagus, and confirmed by endoscopy with biopsy of the cancer tissue. Treatment is by chemotherapy, and sometimes surgery.

**esophageal reflux** See *gastroesophageal reflux*.

**esophageal speech** Speech produced with air trapped in the esophagus and forced out again.

**esophageal stricture, acute** A narrowing or closure of the normal opening of the swallowing tube leading to the stomach, usually caused by scarring from acid irritation. Acute, complete obstruction of the esophagus occurs when food (usually meat) is lodged in the esophageal stricture. Patients experience chest pain, and are unable to swallow saliva. Attempts to relieve the obstruction by inducing vomiting at home are usually unsuccessful. Patients with complete esophageal obstruction can breathe, and are not at any risk of suffocation. Endoscopy is usually employed to retrieve the obstruction and relieve the condition.

**esophageal stricture, chronic** A long-standing narrowing or closure of the normal opening of the swallowing tube leading to the stomach, usually caused by scarring by acid irritation. It is a common complication of chronic gastroesophageal reflux disease (GERD). Several procedures are available for stretching (dilating) the strictures without having to resort to surgery. One procedure involves placing a deflated balloon across the stricture at the time of endoscopy. The balloon is then inflated, thereby opening the narrowing caused by the stricture. Another method involves inserting tapered dilators of different sizes through the mouth and into the esophagus to dilate the stricture.

**esophageal ulcer** A hole in the lining of the esophagus corroded by the acidic digestive juices secreted by the stomach cells. Ulcer formation is related to H. pylori bacteria in the stomach, anti-inflammatory medications, and the smoking of cigarettes. Ulcer pain may not correlate with the presence or severity of ulceration. Diagnosis is made with barium X-ray or endoscopy. Complications of ulcers include bleeding and perforation. Treatment involves antibiotics to eradicate H. pylori, eliminating risk factors, and preventing complications.

**esophagectomy** An operation to remove a portion of the esophagus.

**esophagitis** Inflammation of the esophagus.

**esophagogastric tamponade** See *balloon tamponade*.

**esophagogastroduodenoscopy** Abbreviated as EGD. See *endoscopy, upper*.

**esophagoscopy** Examination of the esophagus by using a thin, lighted instrument.

**esophagram** A series of X-rays of the esophagus. The X-ray pictures are taken after the patient drinks a barium solution that coats and outlines the walls of the esophagus. See also *barium swallow*.

**esophagus** Part of the digestive tract, the esophogus is a tube that connects the throat with the stomach. It lies between the trachea (windpipe) and the spine. In an adult, the esophagus is about 10 inches long. When a person swallows, the muscular walls of the esophagus contract to push food down into the stomach. Glands in the lining of the esophagus produce mucus, which keeps the passageway moist and makes swallowing easier. Commonly referred to as the gullet.

**esotropia** Cross-eyed or, in medical terms, convergent or internal strabismus.

**essential** A hallowed term meaning "We don't know the cause," as in essential hypertension. Synonymous with idiopathic.

**essential fatty acids** A group of unsaturated fatty acids that are essential to human health but cannot be manufactured in the body. There are three types of EFOs: arachnoidic acid, linoleic acid, and linolenic acid. When obtained in the diet, linoleic acid can be converted to both arachnoidic and linolenic acid. It is commonly found in cold-pressed oils, and is particularly high in oils extracted from cold-water fish and certain seeds. Recent research has explored the role of EFOs in the health of the nervous system. Supplementation with certain EFOs appears to be useful as a treatment for certain neurological disorders, including multiple sclerosis and bipolar disorders, indicating that low dietary levels or poor metabolism of these substances may be involved in causing these illnesses. However, arachnoidic acid may lower the seizure threshold. For that reason (and because careful treatment of these disorders is of great importance) always consult a knowledgeable physician before starting a program of EFO supplementation.

**essential oil** An oil derived from a natural substance, usually either for its healing properties or as a perfume. Some pharmaceuticals, and many over-the-counter or "holistic" remedies, are based on or contain essential oils. Examples include products containing camphor or eucalyptus that help relieve congestive coughs, and the essential oils used in the practice of aromatherapy.

**EST** Expressed sequence tag.

**estimated date of confinement** The due date or estimated calendar date when a baby will be born. Abbreviated as EDC.

**estrogen** Estrogen is a female steroid hormone produced by the ovaries and, in lesser amounts, by the adrenal cortex, placenta, and male testes. It helps to control and guide sexual development, including the physical changes associated with puberty. It also influences the course of ovulation in the monthly menstrual cycle, lactation after pregnancy, aspects of mood, and the aging process. Production of estrogen changes naturally over the female lifespan, reaching adult levels with the onset of puberty (menarche), and decreasing in middle age until the onset of the menopause. Estrogen deficiency can lead to lack of menstruation (amenorrhea), persistent difficulties associated with menopause (such as mood swings and vaginal dryness), and osteoporosis in older age. In cases of estrogen deficiency, natural and synthetic estrogen preparations may be prescribed. These include estradiol (brand names: Climara, Estrace, Estroderm), estrafied estrogens (brand names: Estratab, Memest), estropipate (brand name: Ogen), and conjugated estrogens (brand name: Premarin), among others. Estrogen is also a component of many oral contraceptives. An overabundance of estrogen in men causes development of female secondary sexual characteristics (feminization), such as enlargement of breast tissue. Estrogen supplements are therefore taken as a part of the male-to-female sex-reassignment process, usually before surgery.

**estrogen replacement therapy** The use of natural or synthetic estrogen to treat short-term changes associated with menopause, such as hot flashes, disturbed sleep, and vaginal dryness, that are associated with lower estrogen levels. ERT can also prevent osteoporosis, which can be a consequence of lowered estrogen levels. ERT also reduces the risk of heart disease by up to 50 percent. Vaginal ERT products help with vaginal dryness, more severe vaginal changes, and bladder effects. The use of unopposed ERT (ERT alone) is associated with an increase in the risk of endometrial cancer (cancer of the lining of the uterus). However, by taking the hormone progestogen along with estrogen, the risk of endometrial cancer is reduced substantially. Progestogen protects the uterus by keeping the endometrium from thickening (an effect caused by estrogen). The combination therapy of estrogen plus progestogen is called hormone replacement therapy (HRT).

**estrogen, designer** See *designer estrogen*.

**estrogen-associated blood clots** See *estrogen-associated hypercoagulability*.

**estrogen-associated hypercoagulability** Hypercoagulability (a supranormal tendency for blood to clot) occurs as an occasional but serious side effect of estrogen therapy. The blood clots in this situation are dose-related; that is, they occur more frequently with higher doses of estrogen. All estrogen therapy preparations carry this risk. Cigarette smokers on estrogen therapy are at a higher risk than nonsmokers for blood clots. Therefore, patients requiring estrogen therapy are strongly encouraged to quit smoking.

**ESWL** A brand name for extracorporeal shock wave lithotripsy, registered by lithotriptor developer Dornier Medical Systems.

**ethosuximide** A succinimide antispasmodic (brand name: Zarontin), ethosuximide helps to control seizures but can paradoxically increase seizures in some patients. Side effects can include nausea, abdominal pain, changes in appetite, weight loss, drowsiness, headache, dizziness, irritability, and insomnia. Ethosuximide is also associated with a chemically induced form of lupus, an autoimmune disorder.

**ethotoin** Hydantoin antispasmodic (brand name: Peganone) that inhibits activity in the part of the brain where local-focal (grand mal) seizures begin. Side effects can be serious, including gum growth, twitching, depression, and irritability. See *phenytoin*.

**etiology** The study of causes: for example, the causes of a disease. The form "aetiology" is generally used in the UK.

**etodolac** A nonsteroidal anti-inflammatory drug (brand name: Lodine) used to treat rheumatoid arthritis and other conditions that cause joint pain. See also *NSAID*.

**eugenics** Literally meaning "normal genes," eugenics is a pseudoscience with the stated aim of improving the genetic constitution of the human species by selective breeding. The use of Albert Einstein's sperm to conceive a child by artificial insemination would represent an attempt at positive eugenics. The Nazis notoriously engaged in negative eugenics by genocide. The practice of eugenics was first legally mandated in the US state of Indiana, resulting in the forcible sterilization, incarceration, and occasionally euthanasia of the mentally or physically handicapped, the mentally ill, and ethnic minorities (particularly people of mixed racial heritage), and the adopting out of their children to nondisabled, Caucasian parents. Similar programs spread widely in the early part of the 20th century, and still exist in some parts of the world. It is important to note that no experiment in eugenics has ever been shown to result in measurable improvements in human health. In fact, in the best-known attempt

at positive eugenics, the Nazi "Lebensborn" program, there was a higher-than-normal level of birth defects in resulting offspring.

**eukaryote** An organism that consists of one or more cells with a nucleus and other well-developed compartments. People are eukaryotes. Eukaryotes include all organisms except bacteria, viruses, and blue-green algae, which are prokaryotes. See also *prokaryote*.

**euphenics** Literally meaning "normal appearing," euphenics aims to improve the outcome of a genetic disease by altering the environment. For example, people with phenylketonuria (PKU) can avoid the expression of their disease by staying on a low-phenylalanine diet, avoiding major souces of phenylalanine such as diet soft drinks sweetened with aspartame.

**euphoria** Elevated mood. Euphoria is a desirable and natural occurence when it results from happy or exciting events. An excessive degree of euphoria that is not linked to events is characteristic of hypomania or mania, abnormal mood states associated with bipolar disorders. See also *bipolar disorders*.

**euploid** The normal number of chromosomes for a species. In humans, the euploid number of chromosomes is 46; with the notable exception of the unfertilized egg and sperm, in which it is 23.

**European typhus** See *typhus, epidemic*.

**Eustachian tube** The tube that runs from the middle ear to the pharynx. The function of the Eustachian tube is to protect, aerate, and drain the middle ear and mastoid. Occlusion of the Eustachian tube leads to the development of middle-ear inflammation (otitis media). The pharynx is subdivided into three parts: the upper part, called the nasopharynx; the middle part, called the oropharynx; and the lower part, called the hypopharynx. The Eustachian tube opens into the nasopharynx. The Eustachian tube measures only 17 to 18 mm, and is horizontal at birth. As it grows to double that length, it grows to be positioned at an incline of 45 degrees in adulthood. For this reason the nasopharyngeal opening in an adult is significantly below the tympanic opening, found in the middle ear near the eardrum. The shorter length and the horizontality of the Eustachian tube in infancy protects the middle ear poorly, makes for poor drainage of fluid from the middle ear, and predisposes infants and young children to middle-ear infection. The greater length and particularly the slope of the tube as it grows serve more effectively to protect, aerate, and drain the middle ear. The Eustachian tube in the adult is opened by two muscles, the tensor palati and the levator palati, but the anatomy of children permits only the tensor palati to work. This is a particular problem for children born with cleft palate, who have poor function of that muscle: They usually suffer from Eustachian-tube and middle-ear problems until the levator palati begins to function. The Eustachian tube serves to adjust the pressure of the air within the middle ear to that of ambient air. It is harder to get air into the middle ear than get it out, which is why we have more trouble with our ears when a plane is descending than when it takes off. The Eustachian tube is also called the otopharyngeal tube (because it connects the ear to the pharynx); the auditory tube; or, in Latin, the tuba acustica, tuba auditiva, or tuba auditoria.

**euthanasia** While the old dictionary definition for this term is "dying well," today euthanasia more commonly refers to hastening the death of a terminally ill patient. See also *active euthanasia, assisted suicide, eugenics.*

**euthyroid** The state of having normal thyroid gland function.

**evacuation supplies kit** See *disaster supplies.*

**evening primrose oil** A natural source of essential fatty acids (EFOs). Evening primrose oil contains a higher level of arachnoidic acid than some other EFO sources, so people with seizure disorders may wish to avoid its use.

**event, adverse** In pharmacology, an adverse event is any unexpected or dangerous reaction to a drug.

**evolution** The continuing process of change.

**evolution, biologic** See *biologic evolution.* See also *cultural evolution.*

**evolution, cultural** See *cultural evolution.*

**evolutionarily conserved gene** A gene that has remained essentially unchanged throughout evolution. Conservation of a gene indicates that it is unique and essential: There is not an extra copy of that gene with which evolution can tinker, and changes in the gene are likely to be lethal.

**evolutionarily conserved sequence** A base sequence in a DNA molecule (or an amino acid sequence in a protein) that has remained essentially unchanged throughout evolution.

**Ewing sarcoma** See *sarcoma, Ewing.*

**exaggerated startle disease** See *hyperexplexia.*

**exanthem** A rash.

**exanthem subitum** A sudden rash. See *measles.*

**excess iron** Iron overload can damage the heart, liver, gonads, and other organs. Iron overload is a particular risk for people with certain genetic conditions, such as hemochromatosis, and for people receiving repeated blood transfusions. According to the National Academy of Sciences, the recommended dietary allowance of iron is 15 mg for women and 10 mg per day for men. Iron supplements meant for adults (such as for pregnant women) are a major cause of poisoning in children. Care should be taken to keep iron supplements safely away from children.

**exclamation point hair** Exclamation point hair is a key diagnostic finding in a disorder called alopecia areata. These hairs can be found in areas of hair loss, and are short, broken-off hairs that are narrower closer to the scalp, and therefore mimic an exclamation point. See *alopecia areata.*

**exercise treadmill** A machine used to obtain a continuous EKG (electrocardiogram) recording of the heart as the patient performs increasing levels of exercise. The exercise treadmill permits the detection of abnormal heart rhythms (arrhythmias), and provides a screening test for the presence of narrowed arteries to the heart (coronary arteries). Narrowing of these arteries can limit the supply of oxygenated blood to the heart muscle during exercise.

**exercise, aerobic** Brisk exercise that promotes the circulation of oxygen through the blood. Examples of aerobic exercises including walking, running, swimming, and cycling.

**exercise-induced asthma** See *asthma, exercise-induced.*

**exercise-induced bronchospasm** See *asthma, exercise-induced.*

**exfoliate 1** To peel off scaly skin spontaneously. The skin exfoliates from the palms and soles in Kawasaki disease and Reiter syndrome. **2** To deliberately wear away the top layer of skin, as many be done gently by a facial technologist who is applying a topical skin treatment for cosmetic purposes, or more severely by a dermatologist treating acne. In the latter case, the most common exfoliating methods are sanding and chemical peels.

**exogenous** Outside.

**exogenous DNA** DNA originating outside an organism.

**exon** A region of DNA in a gene that is transcribed (read) into mature messenger RNA. An exon is the protein-coding part of a gene, as opposed to an intron.

**exonuclease** An enzyme that cleaves nucleotide bases sequentially from the free ends of a nucleic acid (DNA or RNA).

**exophthalmos**   Protruding eyeball. A common finding in hyperthyroidism and Graves disease.

**exotropia**   Divergent gaze, also called external strabismus or, pejoratively, wall-eyed.

**exposure**   In cognitive behavioral therapy (CBT), the process of exposing oneself to an event or place that causes anxiety or panic. The intention of controlled exposure is to gradually lower the level of stress and anxiety associated with the stimulus, to eventually prevent panic attacks, obsessive-compulsive behaviors, and other unwanted reactions. See also *cognitive behavior therapy*.

**exposure and response prevention**   A cognitive behavior therapy technique that uses planned exposures and exercises to reduce unwanted responses. Abbreviated as E&RP. See also *cognitive behavior therapy, exposure*.

**expression, gene**   When a gene is expressed, the information it encodes is translated into protein or RNA structures present and operating in the cell. Expressed genes include genes that are transcribed into messenger RNA (mRNA) and then translated into protein, as well as those genes that are transcribed into RNA (such transfer and ribosomal RNAs) but not translated into protein.

**expressivity**   The consistency of a genetic disease. For example, Marfan disease shows variable expressivity. Some persons with Marfan merely have long fingers and toes, while others have the full-blown disease, with dislocation of the lens and dissecting aneurysm of the aorta.

**expulsion, stage of**   The second and final stage of labor, lasting from the full dilatation of the cervix until the baby is completely out of the birth canal.

**extension**   The process of straightening or the state of being straight. Extension of the hip and knee joints is necessary to stand up from the sitting position.

**external ear**   See *ear, outer*.

**external jugular vein**   The more superficial of the two jugular veins in the neck that drain blood from the head, brain, face, and neck, and convey it toward the heart. The external jugular vein collects most of the blood from the outside of the skull and the deep parts of the face. It lies outside the sternocleidomastoid muscle, passes down the neck, and joins the subclavian vein.

**external radiation therapy**   Radiation therapy using a machine located outside the body to aim high-energy rays at a tumor.

**extracorporeal shock wave lithotripsy**   See *lithotripsy, extracorporeal shock wave*.

**extrapyramidal side effects**   Physical symptoms, including tremor, slurred speech, akathesia, dystonia, anxiety, distress, paranoia, and bradyphrenia, that are primarily associated with improper dosing of or unusual reactions to neuroleptic (antipsychotic) medications.

**extrapyramidal system**   That part of the nervous system that regulates muscle reflexes.

**extrauterine pregnancy**   See *ectopic pregnancy*.

**extremity**   The uttermost parts of the body: the hands and feet.

**exudative angina**   See *croup*.

**eye**   The organ of sight. The eye has a number of components, which include the cornea, iris, pupil, lens, retina, macula, optic nerve, and vitreous humor. The cornea is the clear front window of the eye that transmits and focuses light into the eye. The iris is the colored part of the eye; it helps regulate the amount of light that enters the eye. The pupil is the dark aperture in the iris that determines how much light is let into the eye. The lens is the transparent structure inside the eye that focuses light rays onto the retina. The retina is the nerve layer that lines the back of the eye, senses light, and creates impulses that travel through the optic nerve to the brain. The macula is a small area in the retina that contains special light-sensitive cells, and allows us to see fine details clearly. The optic nerve is the nerve that connects the eye to the brain. It carries the impulses formed by the retina to the visual cortex of the brain. The vitreous humor is a clear, jelly-like substance that fills the middle of the eye.

**eye chart test**   This test measures how well you see at various distances. The eye chart itself (see *chart, Snellen's*) is imprinted with block letters that line-by-line decrease in size, corresponding to the distance at which that line of letters is normally visible.

**eye chart, Snellen's**   See *chart, Snellen's*.

**Eye Institute, National**   See *National Institutes of Health*.

**eye-drop test**   There are many types of eye drops and many types of eye-drop tests. One of the most common eye-drop tests is pupil dilation. See *dilation, pupil*.

**eyelids, adult ptosis of the**   Drooping of the upper eyelids in adults, most commonly due to separation of the tendon of the lid-lifting (levator) muscle from the eyelid. This may occur with age, after cataract or other eye surgery, or due to an injury, eye tumor, or a complication of other diseases involving the levator muscle or its nerve supply, such as diabetes. If treatment is necessary, it is usually surgical. Sometimes a small tuck in the lifting muscle and eyelid can raise the lid sufficiently. More severe ptosis requires reattachment and strengthening of the levator muscle.

**eyelids, congenital ptosis of the**   Drooping of the upper eyelids at birth. The lids may droop only slightly, or they may cover the pupils and restrict or even block vision. Moderate or severe ptosis calls for treatment to permit normal vision development. If not corrected, amblyopia ("lazy eye") may develop, which can lead to permanently poor vision. Ptosis at birth is often caused by poor development of the levator muscle that lifts the eyelid. Children with ptosis may tip their heads back into a chin-up position to see underneath the eyelids, or raise their eyebrows in an attempt to lift up the lids. Congenital ptosis rarely improves with time. Mild or moderate ptosis usually does not require surgery early in life. Treatment is usually surgery to tighten the eyelid-lifting muscles, the levators. If the levator is very weak, the lid can be attached or suspended from under the eyebrow so that the forehead muscles can do the lifting. Even after surgery, focusing problems can develop as the eyes grow and change shape. All children with ptosis, whether they have had surgery or not, should therefore regularly visit an ophthalmologist.

**eyes, cataracts**   See *cataract*.

**eyes, flashing lights in the**   There are a number of causes of spontaneous flashing-light sensations in the eye.

A sensation of flashing lights can be caused when the vitreous humor (the clear, jelly-like substance that fills the middle of the eye) shrinks and tugs on the retina. These flashes of light can appear off and on for several weeks or months. With age, it is more common to experience flashes. They usually do not reflect a serious problem. However, if one notices the sudden appearance of light flashes or a sudden increase in flashing lights, one should see an ophthalmologist immediately to see whether the retina has been torn or whether there is another cause. Flashes of light that appear as jagged lines or "heat waves" in both eyes, often lasting 10 to 20 minutes, are different. They are usually caused by migraine, a spasm of blood vessels in the brain. Jagged lines or "heat waves" can also occur without a headache, in which case they are termed ophthalmic migraine, or migraine without headache.

**eyes, glaucoma**   See *glaucoma*.

**eyes, spots in front of the**   Also known as "floaters," spots are usually the images formed by deposits of protein drifting about in the vitreous humor, the clear, jelly-like substance that fills the middle of the eye. The appearance of permanent or recurring white or black spots in the same area of your field of vision may be an early warning sign of cataracts or other serious problems.

**Eygel**   See *erythromycin*.

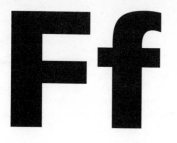

# Ff

**F**  The symbol for the coefficient of inbreeding. See *coefficient of inbreeding*.

**Fabry disease**  See *Anderson-Fabry disease*.

**face, masklike**  An expressionless face with little or no sense of animation; a face more like a mask than a normal face. A masklike face is seen in a number of disorders, including Parkinson disease and myotonic dystrophy. Also known as masklike facies.

**facelift**  A surgical procedure designed to make the face appear younger by pulling loose facial skin taut. Recovery time is usually 1 week, and the results last approximately 10 years. Additional procedures to supplement the facelift, including necklift, blepharoplasty (eyelid surgery), liposuction, autologous fat injection, removal of buccal (cheek) fat pads, forehead lift, and browlift; chemical or laser peel; and malar (cheek), submalar, or chin implants, may be necessary to achieve the desired results. Although infrequent, risks and complications of facelift surgery include bleeding; hematoma; bruising; infection; neurological dysfunction (loss of muscle function or sensation), which is usually temporary; widened or thickened scars; loss of hair around the incision site; asymmetry (unevenness between two sides); and skin necrosis (loss of skin from tissue death).

**facial canal introitus**  In anatomy, an introitus is an entrance, one that goes into a canal or hollow organ. The introitus of the facial canal is the entrance to the facial canal, a passage in the temporal bone of the skull through which the facial nerve (the seventh cranial nerve) travels.

**facial nerve**  The seventh cranial nerve, a mixed nerve that has fibers both going out and coming in (both efferent and afferent fibers). It supplies the muscles of facial expression.

**facial nerve paralysis**  Loss of voluntary movement of the muscles of one side of the face due to abnormal function of the facial nerve. Paralysis of the facial nerve causes a characteristic drooping of one side of the face, inability to wrinkle the forehead, inability to whistle, inability to close the eye, and deviation of the mouth toward the other side of the face. Paralysis of the facial nerve is called Bell palsy. The cause of facial-nerve paralysis is not known, but it is thought to be related to a virus (or to various viruses). The disease typically starts suddenly, and causes paralysis of the muscles of the side of the face on which the facial nerve is affected. Treatment is directed toward protecting the eye on the affected side from dryness during sleep. Massage of affected muscles can reduce soreness. Sometimes steroid medication, such as Prednisone, is given to reduce inflammation during the first weeks of illness. The prognosis is generally good, with about 80 percent of patients recovering within weeks to months.

**facies**  Face.

**factor VIII**  A coagulation (clotting) factor. Classic hemophilia (hemophilia A) is due to a congenital deficiency in the amount or activity of factor VIII. Factor VIII is also known as antihemophiliac factor (AHF) or antihemophiliac globulin (AHG). The gene for factor VIII (and that for classic hemophilia) is on the X chromosome, so females with the gene can be silent carriers without symptoms, while males with the gene can be hemophiliacs.

**factor, rheumatoid**  An antibody that is measurable in the blood. It is commonly used as a blood test for the diagnosis of rheumatoid arthritis. Rheumatoid factor is present in about 80 percent of adults (but a much lower proportion of children) with rheumatoid arthritis. It is also present in patients with other connective tissue diseases, such as systemic lupus erythematosus, and in some with infectious diseases, including infectious hepatitis.

**FAE**  Fetal alcohol effect.

**Fahr syndrome**  See *cerebral calcification, nonarteriosclerotic*.

**failure to thrive**  Refers to a child whose physical growth is significantly less than that of peers. There is no official consensus on what constitutes FTT. It usually refers to a child whose growth is below the 3rd or 5th percentiles for its age, or whose growth has fallen off precipitously and crossed two major growth percentiles (for example, from above the 75th percentile to below the 25th percentile). Failure to thrive in early infancy sometimes results in death, and in older infancy or childhood is an important disease marker. Causes of failure to thrive are probably many, including unrecognized food allergies leading to refusal of food, and vomiting; undiagnosed metabolic disorders; and disease. A specific type of failure to thrive is sometimes seen in abandoned or institutionalized infants who seem to "give up" and become listless and unwilling to nurse. It is assumed that this phenomenon is emotional in nature, although other factors may also be at work. Treatment of failure to thrive requires discovering and treating its underlying causes. In the interim, IV feeding is necessary in some cases, while in others supplemental high-calorie feedings can help.

**failure, heart**  See *congestive heart failure*.

**fainting**  Partial or complete loss of consciousness, with interruption of awareness of oneself and one's surroundings. When the loss of consciousness is temporary and there is spontaneous recovery, it is referred to as syncope or, in nonmedical quarters, fainting. Syncope accounts for one in every 30 visits to an emergency room. See *syncope*.

**falciparum malaria**  The most dangerous type of malaria.

**FALDH deficiency**  See *Sjogren-Larsson syndrome*.

**Fallopian tubes**  The two tubes, one on each side, that transport the egg from the ovary to the uterus. The Fallopian tubes have small hair-like projections called cilia on the cells of the lining. These tubal cilia are essential to the movement of the egg through the tube into the uterus. If the tubal cilia are damaged by infection, the egg may not get pushed along normally, but may stay in the tube. Infection can also cause partial or complete blockage of the tube with scar tissue, physically preventing the egg from getting to the uterus. Infection, endometriosis, tumors, scar tissue in the pelvis (pelvic adhesions), and any other process that damages the Fallopian tube or narrows its diameter increases the chance of an ectopic pregnancy: a pregnancy developing in the Fallopian tube or another abnormal location outside the uterus.

**false negative**  A result that appears negative but fails to reveal a situation. For example, if a particular test designed to detect cancer returns a negative result but the person actually does have cancer, that would be a false negative.

**false positive**  A result that is erroneously positive when a situation is normal. For example, if a particular test designed to detect cancer returns a positive result but the person does not have cancer, that would be a false positive.

**false rib**  One of the last five pairs of ribs. A rib is said to be false if it does not attach to the sternum (the breastbone). The upper three false ribs connect to the costal cartilages of the ribs just above them. The last two false ribs, however, usually have no ventral attachment to anchor them in front, and so are called floating, fluctuating, or vertebral ribs.

**familial**  A condition that is more common in certain families than in the general population.

**familial adenomatous polyposis**  A genetic disease characterized by the presence of numerous precancerous polyps in the colon and rectum. Also called familial polyposis. Abbreviated as FAP.

**familial breast cancer**  See *breast cancer, familial*. See also *breast cancer susceptibility genes, BRCA1, BRCA2*.

**familial cancer**  Cancer or a predisposition (tendency) to it that runs in families.

**familial hypercholesterolemia**  This is the most common inherited type of hyperlipidemia (high lipid levels in the blood). It is recognizable in childhood. Familial hypercholesterolemia is due to genetic defects in the receptor (target) for low-density lipoprotein (LDL). Familial hypercholesterolemia predisposes a person to premature arteriosclerosis, including coronary artery disease, and can lead to heart attacks at an unusually young age. Persons with familial hypercholesterolemia can reduce their risk by adhering to a very low cholesterol diet under a doctor's supervision, and may also need to take medications that reduce their cholesterol level.

**familial Mediterranean fever**  An inherited disorder of unknown cause featuring short recurring bouts of fever, together with pain in the joints, chest, or abdomen. Between attacks, the patient seems healthy, which makes FMF difficult to diagnose. The gene for FMF is an autosomal recessive gene on chromosome 16. FMF is found in persons of Mediterranean ethnic background.

**familial mental retardation 1**  See *FMR1*. See also *Fragile X syndrome*.

**familial mental retardation protein**  See *FMRP*. See also *Fragile X syndrome*.

**familial neurovisceral lipidosis**  See *Landing disease*.

**familial polyposis**  See *familial adenomatous polyposis*.

**family planning**  See *birth control*. See also *contraceptive, natural family planning*.

**FAO deficiency**  See *Sjogren-Larsson syndrome*.

**FAP**  Familial adenomatous polyposis.

**Farber disease**  A polyneuropathic disorder characterized by nodules under the skin, mental retardation, slow motor development, cherry-red spots on the eyes, and respiratory problems. It is an autosomal recessive disorder. Respiratory tract insufficiency usually causes death before the age of 20. Also known as lipogranulomatosis. See also *glycosphingolipidoses*.

**farsightedness** An error of refraction in the human eye, which causes light rays to focus behind the retina instead of on it. A person who is farsighted has normal vision at a distance, but has trouble focusing on nearby objects. It can be corrected with refractive lenses, either glasses or contact lenses, and in some cases by surgery. Also known as hyperopia.

**fart** A commonly used term for passing gas. Excess gas in the intestinal tract is medically termed flatulence. What constitutes excess gas is difficult to define, since symptom-free individuals have recorded approximately 14 passages of gas per 24 hours.

**FAS** Fetal alcohol syndrome.

**fascia** A lining tissue under the skin that covers a surface of underlying tissues. Fascia also encloses muscles.

**fasciitis** Inflammation of the fascia.

**fasciitis, eosinophilic** See *eosinophilic fasciitis*.

**fasciitis, plantar** Inflammation of the plantar fascia (fasciitis), the bowstring-like tissue stretching from the heel underneath the sole. Plantar fasciitis is often due to a bony spur that projects from the underside of the heel and makes walking painful. Spurs under the sole typically cause localized tenderness and pain, which is made worse by stepping down on the heel. Plantar fasciitis and heel spurs may occur alone, or may be related to underlying diseases that cause arthritis, such as Reiter disease, ankylosing spondylitis, and diffuse idiopathic skeletal hyperostosis. Treatment is designed to decrease the inflammation and avoid reinjury. Icing reduces pain and inflammation. Anti-inflammatory agents, such as ibuprofen or injections of cortisone, can help. Infrequently, surgery is done on chronically inflamed spurs. A donut-shaped shoe insert can take pressure off the plantar spur and lessen the plantar fasciitis.

**fasting blood glucose** A method for learning how much glucose (sugar) is in a blood sample taken after an overnight fast. The fasting blood glucose test is commonly used in the detection of diabetes mellitus. A blood sample is taken in a lab, doctor's office, or hospital. The test is done in the morning before the person has eaten. The normal range for blood glucose is from 70 to 110 mg/dl, depending on the type of blood being tested. If the level is over 140 mg/dl, it usually means the person has diabetes, although newborns and some pregnant women may have a higher glucose level without diabetes.

**fat** **1** With proteins and carbohydrates, one of the three nutrients used as energy sources by the body. The energy produced by fats is nine calories per gram. Proteins and carbohydrates each provide four calories per gram. **2** Total fat; the sum of saturated, monounsaturated, and polyunsaturated fats. Intake of monounsaturated and polyunsaturated fats can help to reduce blood cholesterol when substituted for saturated fats in the diet. **3** A slang term for obese or adipose. **4** In chemistry, compounds formed from chemicals called fatty acids. These fats compose a greasy, solid material found in animal tissues and in some plants. Fats are the major component of flabby material of our bodies, commonly known as blubber.

**fatty alcohol: NAD+ oxidoreductase deficiency** See *Sjogren-Larsson syndrome*.

**fatty aldehyde dehydrogenase deficiency** See *Sjogren-Larsson syndrome*.

**fatty liver of pregnancy, acute** See *acute fatty liver of pregnancy*.

**fauces** The throat.

**fava bean** The broad bean, to which many people react adversely. Fava beans look like large, tan lima beans. They are popular in Mediterranean and Middle Eastern cuisines, are eaten raw when very young, can be cooked in soups and many other dishes, or may be made into fava brittle as candy. Fava beans are the main commercial source of the drug L-dopa. See also *favism*.

**favism** A condition characterized by hemolytic anemia (breakup of red blood cells) after eating fava beans or being exposed to the pollen of the fava plant. This dangerous reaction occurs exclusively in people with a deficiency of the enzyme glucose-6-phosphate dehydrogenase (G6PD), an X-linked genetic trait. However, not all G6PD-deficient families appear at risk for favism, indicating the additional need for a single autosomal (not X-linked) gene to create the susceptibility to favism. The active hemolytic principle in fava beans is likely dopa-quinone. Differences in susceptibility to favism may be related to differences in the enzymatic system that converts L-dopa to dopa-quinone.

**FDA** The Food and Drug Administration.

**febrile** Feverish.

**febrile seizure** See *seizure, febrile*.

**fecal occult blood test** A test to check for hidden blood in the stool.

**feces** The proper medical term for the excrement discharged from the intestines.

**fecund** Fruitful. Just as a writer is prolific, a woman may be fecund, able to reproduce plentifully.

**fecundity** The ability to have children, usually many of them, with ease.

**feedback** Many biologic processes are controlled by feedback, just as the temperature in a home (from a furnace or air conditioner) can be regulated by a thermostat. This principle is the basis for the practice of biofeedback. See also *biofeedback*.

**feeding, breast** See *breastfeeding*.

**feet** As a measure of length, the plural of foot. See also *foot*.

**female** An individual of the sex that bears young or that produces ova or eggs. However, female can be defined by physical appearance, by chromosome constitution or by gender identification. See *female chromosome complement*.

**female chromosome complement** The large majority of females have a 46, XX chromosome complement: 46 chromosomes, including two X chromosomes. A minority of females have other chromosome constitutions, such as 45, X (45 chromosomes with only one X chromosome) or 47, XXX (47 chromosomes with three X chromosomes).

**female genital mutilation** See *circumcision, female*.

**female gonad** See *ovary*.

**female internal genitalia** The internal genital structures of the female include the ovaries, the Fallopian tubes, the uterus, and the vagina.

**female organs of reproduction** The ovaries, which produce eggs (ova) and female hormones; the Fallopian tubes, which transport the egg from the ovaries to the uterus; the uterus, which receives the egg for fertilization and provides a growth environment for the developing embryo and fetus; the cervix, the lower, narrow part of the uterus that opens into the vagina; and the vagina, the muscular canal extending from the cervix to the outside of the body that enables sperm to enter the female reproductive tract.

**female pelvis** The female pelvis is usually more delicate, wider, and not as high as the male pelvis. The angle of the female pubic arch is wide and round. The female sacrum is wider than the male's, and the iliac bone is flatter. The pelvic basin of the female is more spacious and less funnel-shaped. From a purely anatomic viewpoint, the female pelvis is better suited to accommodate the fetus during pregnancy and permit the baby to be born.

**female urethral meatus** See *female urethral opening*.

**female urethral opening** The urethra is the transport tube leading from the bladder to discharge urine outside the body. In females, the urethra is shorter than in the male. The meatus (opening) of the female urethra is above the vaginal opening.

**femoral** Having to do with the femur.

**femoral vein** The large vein in the groin that passes with the femoral artery under the inguinal ligament to enter the abdomen, at which point it becomes the external iliac vein. The femoral vein is a continuation of the popliteal vein, and carries blood back to the heart from the lower extremities.

**femur** The single bone in the thigh, that part of the leg that extends from the hip to the knee. The femur is the largest bone in the human body, and is familiarly known as the thigh bone.

**fenestration** Literally, the making of a window: Fenestration refers to the creation of a new opening.

**ferritin** A blood protein that serves as an indicator of the amount of iron stored in the body.

**ferrocalcinosis, cerebrovascular** See *cerebral calcification, nonarteriosclerotic*.

**fertile** Able to conceive and bear offspring.

**fertility** The ability to have children.

**fertilization** The process of combining the male gamete, or sperm, with the female gamete, or ovum. The product of this combination is a cell called a zygote.

**fetal alcohol effect** A diagnosis of possible FAE is considered when a child has some signs of fetal alcohol syndrome but does not meet all of the necessary criteria for FAS, and there is a history of alcohol exposure before birth. Although FAE is considered a "softer" diagnosis than FAS, it can still have severe and life-long consequences for the child, including mental retardation and facial difference. Frequent ear infections and hearing loss are also present in nearly half of all children with FAE.

**fetal alcohol syndrome** The syndrome of damage to the child before birth as a result of the mother drinking alcohol during pregnancy. FAS always involves brain damage, impaired growth, and head and face abnormalities. Most children with FAS also have frequent ear infections and some degree of hearing loss. FAS is one of the leading causes of mental retardation in the US. Other than special education and surgery to correct major physical defects, there is no treatment for FAS. No amount of alcohol has been proven safe during pregnancy. Women who are or may become pregnant are advised to avoid alcohol.

To establish the diagnosis of FAS, the following signs must be present: small size and weight before and after birth (pre- and postnatal growth retardation); brain involvement, with evidence for delay in development, intellectual impairment, or neurologic abnormalities; and specific appearance of the head and face. At least two of the following groups of signs must be present: small head size (microcephaly); small eyes (microphthalmia) and/or short eye openings (palpebral fissures); underdevelopment of the upper lip, indistinct groove between the lip and nose (the philtrum), and flattened cheekbones.

**fetal circulation**   The blood circulation in the fetus before birth. Before birth, the blood from the heart that is headed for the lungs in the aptly named pulmonary artery is shunted away from the lungs and returned to the aorta. This arterial shunting occurs through a short vessel called the ductus arteriosus. When the shunt is open, it is said to be patent. The ductus arteriosus usually tourniquets itself off at or shortly after birth. After closure of the ductus, blood is permitted from that time on to course freely to the lungs. Sometimes, however, the patent ductus arteriosus (PDA) persists, and simply will not close by itself. Surgery is then done to tie off the ductus. PDA ligation is a closed-heart operation. Historically, it was one of the earliest surgical procedures performed in children with cardiovascular disease.

**fetal distress**   Compromise of the fetus during the antepartum period (before labor) or intrapartum period (during the birth process). Fetal distress can be detected due to abnormal slowing of labor, the presence of meconium (dark green fecal material from the fetus) or other abnormal substances in the amniotic fluid, or via fetal monitoring with an electronic device.

**fetal dystocia**   Difficult labor and delivery caused by the presence of an especially large fetus compared to the mother's anatomy, or a fetus whose shape or position causes difficulty.

**fetal mortality rate**   The ratio of fetal deaths divided by the sum of all births in that year. In the United States, the fetal mortality rate has plummeted from 19.2 per 1,000 births in 1950 to 9.2 per 1,000 births in 1980. However, the fetal mortality rate is higher in certain ethnic groups and among mothers with health problems during pregnancy, especially if the mother does not receive adequate personal and prenatal health care. The fetal mortality rate is considered a good measure of the quality of health care in a country or a medical facility.

**fetal movement**   Movement of the fetus in the womb. The first fetal movements felt by the mother usually occur between 18 and 22 weeks of pregnancy. Also known as quickening.

**fetoprotein, alpha-**   See *alpha-fetoprotein*.

**fetoscope**   There are two types of fetoscopes: One is a fiberoptic scope for looking directly at the fetus within the uterus; the other is a stethoscope designed for listening to the fetal heart beat.

**fetoscopy**   A technique for looking directly at the fetus within the uterus using a fetoscope.

**fetus**   The unborn offspring from the end of the eighth week after conception, when the major structures have formed, until birth. Up until the eighth week, the developing offspring is called an embryo.

**fever**   Technically, any body temperature above the normal oral measurement of 98.6 degrees F (37 degrees C) or the normal rectal temperature of 99 degrees F. However, fever is not considered medically significant until the temperature is above 100.4° F (38° C). Fever is part of the body's own disease-fighting arsenal: Rising body temperatures apparently are capable of killing off many disease-producing organisms. For that reason, low fevers should normally go untreated, although you may need to see your doctor to be sure if the fever is accompanied by any other troubling symptoms. As fevers range to 104 degrees F and above, however, there can be unwanted consequences, particularly for children. These can include delirium and convulsions. A fever of this sort demands immediate home treatment and then medical attention. Home treatment possibilities include the use of aspirin or, in children, non-aspirin pain-killers such as acetaminophen, cool baths, or sponging to reduce the fever while seeking medical help. Fever may occur with almost any type of infection or illness. The temperature is measured with a thermometer. Also called pyrexia.

**fever blisters**   Common with a wide range of infectious diseases but particularly with herpes simplex 1 virus infection, fever blisters are sores around the mouth. They will heal rapidly if kept clean and dry. Topical ointments are available to ease the pain of long-lasting fever blisters. Also called cold sores or canker sores.

**fever therapy**   Using abnormal elevations in body temperature as a tool to treat disease. This was done in the past by deliberately raising the patient's temperature to cause fever. Fever therapy is rarely, if ever, used nowadays. Sometimes, however, a patient with a very high fever from an infection upon recovery from the infection enters into a seemingly impossible remission from an unrelated disease or is even cured of it.

**fever with renal syndrome, hemorrhagic**   See *hemorrhagic fever with renal syndrome*.

**fever, breakbone**   See *dengue fever*.

**fever, cat scratch** See *cat scratch fever*.

**fever, dandy** See *dengue fever*.

**fever, dengue** See *dengue fever*.

**fever, dengue hemorrhagic** See *dengue hemorrhagic fever*.

**fever, Ebola virus** See *Ebola virus*. See also *hemorrhagic fever with renal syndrome*.

**fever, epidemic hemorrhagic** See *hemorrhagic fever with renal syndrome*.

**fever, five-day** See *trench fever*. See also *Bartonella quintana*.

**fever, hemorrhagic** See *hemorrhagic fever with renal syndrome*.

**fever, intermittent** A type of fever that rises and falls, often becoming worst at night and being accompanied by drenching sweats.

**fever, Lassa** An acute viral infection found in the tropics, especially in West Africa. It is caused by a single-stranded RNA virus from the Arenaviridae family, and is animal-borne (zoonotic). Lassa fever is a grave health concern because it can cause a very potentially fatal illness, is highly contagious, and can rapidly spread. The number of Lassa virus infections per year in West Africa has been roughly estimated at 100,000 to 300,000, with at least 5,000 deaths yearly. The Lassa virus has been found in a rodent known as the "multimammate rat" of the genus Mastomys. People can become infected by eating this infected rat or by eating food contaminated by rat excretions. Person-to-person transmission also occurs by direct contact, contamination of skin breaks with infected blood, and aerosol spreads (virus particles moving through the air). The first symptoms typically occur one to three weeks after the patient comes into contact with the virus, and can include increasingly high fever, sore throat, cough, eye inflammation (conjunctivitis), facial swelling, retrosternal pain (behind the breastbone), back pain, abdominal pain, vomiting, diarrhea, and general weakness lasting for several days. Neurological symptoms have also been described, including hearing loss, tremors, and encephalitis (brain inflammation). The most common complication of Lassa fever is deafness. Because the symptoms are so varied and nonspecific, clinical diagnosis is often difficult. If a person has traveled to West Africa and has a severe fever within three weeks after returning, the illness should be reported to a doctor. The key agent for treatment is Ribavirin, an antiviral drug, which is most effective when given early in the course of the disease. Patients are also given supportive care with fluid balance, oxygen as needed, treatment of any other complicating infections, etc. Medical isolation procedures should be followed, due to the highly contagious nature of Lassa fever. These procedures are termed VHF isolation precautions or barrier nursing methods, and include protective clothing such as masks, gloves, gowns, and goggles; infection control measures such as complete equipment sterilization; and isolating infected patients from contact with unprotected persons until the disease has run its course. Patients may excrete the virus weeks after recovery. Their bodily fluids should therefore be monitored for the virus before they leave the hospital.

**fever, Mediterranean** See *familial Mediterranean fever*.

**fever, Meuse** See *trench fever*. See also *Bartonella quintana*.

**fever, Philippine hemorrhagic** See *dengue hemorrhagic fever*.

**fever, Q** See *Q fever*.

**fever, quintan** See *trench fever*. See also *Bartonella quintana*.

**fever, remittent** A type of fever that gradually decreases in intensity over time.

**fever, Rocky Mountain spotted** See *Rocky Mountain spotted fever*.

**fever, shinbone** See *trench fever*. See also *Bartonella quintana*.

**fever, Southeast Asian hemorrhagic** See *dengue hemorrhagic fever*.

**fever, splenic** See *anthrax*.

**fever, spotted** See *Rocky Mountain spotted fever*.

**fever, Thai hemorrhagic** See *dengue hemorrhagic fever*.

**fever, tick** See *Rocky Mountain spotted fever*.

**fever, trench** See *trench fever*. See also *Bartonella quintana*.

**fever, undulant** See *Brucellosis*.

**fever, Wolhynia** See *trench fever*. See also *Bartonella quintana*.

**Fexofenadine** A nonsedating antihistamine drug (brand name: Allegra) prescribed to treat allergies.

**FGFR2** Fibroblast growth factor receptor 2.

**FGM** Female genital mutilation. See *circumcision, female*.

**fiber** The parts of fruits and vegetables that cannot be digested. This fiber is of vital importance to digestion, helping the body move food through the digestive tract, reducing serum cholesterol, and contributing to disease protection. Also called bulk or roughage.

**fiber and bowel disorders** High fiber diets help delay the progression of diverticulosis and, at least, reduce the bouts of diverticulitis. In many cases, it helps reduce the symptoms of irritable bowel syndrome (IBS, also called spastic colitis, mucus colitis, and nervous colon syndrome).

**fiber and cancer** It is generally accepted that a diet high in fiber is protective, or at least reduces the incidence, of colon polyps and colon cancer.

**fiber and cholesterol** Soluble fiber substances are effective in helping reduce the level of blood cholesterol. This is especially true with oat bran, fruits, psyllium, and legumes. Diets high in soluble fiber may lower cholesterol and low-density lipoproteins (the "bad" lipoproteins) by 8 to 15 percent.

**fiber and constipation** Insoluble fiber retains water in the colon, resulting in a softer and larger stool. It is used effectively in treating constipation resulting from poor dietary habits. Bran is particularly rich in insoluble fiber.

**fiber and diabetes** Soluble fibers found in oat bran, apples, citrus fruits, pears, peas/beans, psyllium, and other foods slow down the digestion of carbohydrates (sugars), which results in better glucose metabolism. Some patients with adult-onset diabetes may be successfully treated with a high-fiber diet alone, and those on insulin can often reduce their insulin requirements by adhering to a high-fiber diet.

**fiber, soluble and insoluble** Fiber is classified as soluble or insoluble. Soluble fiber can be digested within the gastrointestinal tract, while insoluble fiber cannot. Soluble fiber is found in oat bran, apples, citrus, pears, peas/beans, psyllium, and other foods. Insoluble fiber is found in wheat bran, cabbage, peas and beans, and other foods. Both are important diet components for optimal health.

**fibrates** Cholesterol-lowering drugs that are primarily effective in lowering triglycerides and, to a lesser extent, in increasing HDL-cholesterol levels. Gemfibrozil (brand name: Lopid), the fibrate most widely used in the US, can be very effective for patients with high triglyceride levels,

but is not very effective for lowering the LDL-cholesterol. As a result, it is used less often than other drugs in patients with heart disease for whom LDL-cholesterol lowering is the main goal of treatment. Gemfibrozil therapy by itself is not recommended by the Food and Drug Administration for patients with heart disease. Fibrates are usually given in two daily doses, 30 minutes before the morning and evening meals. The reductions in triglycerides generally are in the range of 20 to 50 percent, with increases in HDL-cholesterol of 10 to 15 percent. Fibrates are generally well tolerated by most patients. Gastrointestinal complaints are the most common side effect, and fibrates appear to increase the likelihood of developing cholesterol gallstones. Fibrates can increase the effect of medications that thin the blood, and this should be monitored closely by your physician.

**fibril** The diminutive of fiber. A small fiber, a fine thread.

**fibrillation** In matters of the heart (cardiology), incoordinate twitching of muscle fibers.

**fibrillation, atrial** An abnormal and irregular heart rhythm whereby electrical signals are generated chaotically throughout the upper chambers (atria) of the heart. Although many persons with atrial fibrillation have no symptoms, the most common symptom is palpitations: an uncomfortable awareness of the rapid and irregular heartbeat. Atrial fibrillation can cause blood clots that travel from the heart to the brain, resulting in stroke. Treatment of atrial fibrillation involves controlling the risk factors, medications to slow the heart rate and/or convert the heart to normal rhythm, and preventing complications of blood clotting.

**fibrillation, auricular** Essentially the same as atrial fibrillation.

**fibrillation, ventricular** An abnormal irregular heart rhythm whereby there are very rapid uncoordinated fluttering contractions of the lower chambers (ventricles) of the heart. Ventricular fibrillation disrupts the synchrony between the heartbeat and the pulse beat. Ventricular fibrillation is commonly associated with heart attacks or scarring of the heart muscle from previous heart attack. Ventricular fibrillation is life threatening.

**fibrin** The protein formed during normal blood clotting that is the essence of the clot.

**fibrinogen** The protein from which fibrin is formed/generated in normal blood clotting

**fibroblast growth factor receptor 2** A gene on chromosome 10. Mutations to FGFR2 cause the best-known type of acrocephalosyndactyly, Apert syndrome.

Different mutations in FGFR2 are responsible for two other genetic diseases, namely, Pfeiffer syndrome (another type of acrocephalosyndactyly) and Crouzon syndrome (purely a craniofacial disorder with no hand or foot problems). All are inherited as dominant traits. See also *acrocephalosyndactyly, Apert syndrome, Crouzon syndrome, Pfeiffer syndrome*.

**fibroid** A benign uterine tumor, medically known as a leiomyoma (plural: leiomyomata) of the uterus. Although fibroids are not cancerous, they are sometimes removed if they cause discomfort or as a preventative measure if uterine cancer runs in the patient's family. In most cases fibroids exist without the patients' knowledge, and with no harmful consequences.

**fibroma** A mass of interlacing fibrous cells that have a spindle shape.

**fibroma, cemento-ossifying** A lesion that continues to grow, sometimes to very large size, unless treated. It has a hard, fibrous consistency. Most frequently seen in the jaw or mouth area, sometimes in connection with fracture or injury. Treatment is by surgery. Abbreviated COF.

**fibroma, collagenous** See *fibroma, desmoplastic*.

**fibroma, desmoplastic** A rare type of primary bone tumor with the structure of a fibroma.

**fibroma, nonossifying** A growing lesion with a fibroma structure. Treatment is by surgery.

**fibroma, ossifying** See *fibroma, cemento-ossifying*.

**fibromatosis** See *fibroma*.

**fibromyalgia** A syndrome characterized by chronic pain, stiffness, and tenderness of muscles, tendons, and joints, without detectable inflammation. Fibromyalgia does not cause body damage or deformity. However, undue fatigue plagues 90 percent of patients with fibromyalgia. Sleep disorder is also common in patients with fibromyalgia. Fibromyalgia can be associated with other rheumatic conditions, and irritable bowel syndrome (IBS) can occur with fibromyalgia. There is no definitive medical test for the diagnosis of fibromyalgia, so diagnosis is made by eliminating other possible causes of these symptoms. Treatment is most effective when it incorporates combinations of education, stress reduction, exercise, and medication. Also known as fibrositis.

**fibrosarcoma** A form of bone cancer that occurs mainly in middle-aged and elderly people. It usually starts in the pelvis.

**fibrosis, radiation** Scarring of the lungs from radiation. Radiation fibrosis is a sequel of radiation pneumonitis (inflammation of the lungs due to radiation), as from radiation therapy. Radiation pneumonitis typically occurs after radiation treatments for cancer within the chest or breast, and usually manifests itself two weeks to six months after completion of radiation therapy. Symptoms include shortness of breath upon activity, cough, and fever. Radiation pneumonitis frequently is discovered as an incidental finding on chest X-ray in patients who have no symptoms. Radiation fibrosis typically occurs a year after the completion of radiation treatments. Whereas radiation pneumonitis is often reversible with medications that reduce inflammation, such as cortisone drugs (prednisone and others), radiation fibrosis is usually irreversible and permanent.

**fibrositis** See *fibromyalgia*.

**fibrous dysplasia, monostotic** Excessive growth of hard, fibrous tissue that replaces normal bone tissue in a single bone. It is sometimes associated with certain endocrine disorders. Symptoms include pain and fracturing of the bones.

**fibrous dysplasia, polyostotic** Excessive growth of hard, fibrous tissue that replaces normal bone tissue in more than one bone. It is sometimes associated with certain endocrine disorders. Symptoms include pain and fracturing of the bones.

**fibula** The smaller of the two bones in the lower leg.

**fièvre boutonneuse** See *typhus, African tick*.

**fifth cranial nerve** See *trigeminal nerve*.

**fifth disease** Caused by a virus known as parvovirus B 19, the symptoms of fifth disease include low-grade fever, fatigue, a "slapped cheeks" rash, and a rash over the whole body. While the illness is not serious in children, 80 percent of adults have joint aches and pains (arthritis), which may become long-term with stiffness in the morning, redness and swelling of the same joints on both sides of the body (a "symmetrical" arthritis), most commonly involving the knees, fingers, and wrists. Pregnant women (who have not previously had the illness) should avoid contact with patients who have fifth disease, as the fifth disease virus can infect the fetus prior to birth. While no birth defects have been reported as a result of fifth disease, it can cause the death of the unborn fetus. The risk of fetal death is 5 to 10 percent if the mother becomes infected. The name "fifth disease" derives from the pre-vaccination era, when it was frequently the fifth disease that a child would develop. Also known as Erythema infectiosum.

**film**   Slang shortening of X-ray film, an X-ray, a radiograph.

**film, AP**   An X-ray picture in which the beams pass from front to back (anteroposterior), as opposed to a PA (posteroanterior) film, in which the rays pass through the body from back to front.

**film, lateral**   An X-ray picture taken from the side.

**film, PA**   An X-ray picture in which the beams pass from back to front (posteroanterior), as opposed to an AP (anteroposterior) film, in which the rays pass through the body from front to back.

**filoviridae**   See *filovirus*.

**filovirus**   One of a family of viruses (the family filoviridae) that cause hemorrhagic fever. Filoviruses have single-stranded RNA as their genetic material. Ebola virus and the Marburg virus are both filoviruses.

**finasteride**   A medication (brand names: Proscar, Propecia) prescribed to treat male-pattern baldness and benign prostatic hyperplasia (BPH).

**fine needle aspiration**   The use of a thin needle to withdraw tissue from the body.

**fingernail**   A fingernail is produced by living skin cells in the finger. It consists of several parts, including the nail plate (the visible part of the nail), the nail bed (the skin beneath the nail plate), the cuticle (the tissue that overlaps the plate and rims the base of the nail), the nail folds (the skin folds that frame and support the nail on three sides), the lunula (the whitish half-moon at the base of the nail), and the matrix (the hidden part of the nail unit under the cuticle). Fingernails grow from the matrix. They are composed largely of keratin, a hardened protein that is also found in skin and hair. As new cells grow in the matrix, the older cells are pushed out and compacted, taking on the familiar flattened, hardened form of the fingernail. The average growth rate for nails is 0.1 mm each day (or one centimeter in 100 days). The exact rate of nail growth depends on numerous factors, including the age and sex of the individual, and the time of year. Fingernails generally grow faster in young people, in males, and in the summer. Fingernails grow faster than toenails. The fingernails on the right hand of a right-handed person grow faster than those on their left hand, and vice versa. See also *nail, nail care*.

**fingers, six**   See *hexadactyly*. See also *polydactyly*.

**fire ants**   Originally from South America, fire ants are red or yellowish ants of small-to-medium size with a severe sting that burns like fire. They normally feed on small insects but they may also eat seeds and seedling plants, damage grain and vegetable crops, invade kitchens, and attack newly hatched poultry and the young of ground-nesting wild birds. Fire ants can kill newborn domestic and wild animals. Each colony is composed of a queen, winged males and females and three kinds of workers. A nest averages about 25,000 workers, but far larger populations are common. Semipermanent nests are large mounds of excavated soil with openings for ventilation. Since nests may number 50 or more in a heavily infested field, cultivating becomes difficult or impossible. Fire ants belong to the genus Solenopsis, and are also called thief ants. The severe sting of this ant burns like fire, and can trigger an allergic reaction. Avoidance and prompt treatment are essential.

**fire supplies kit**   See *disaster supplies*.

**fire, St. Anthony's**   An intensely painful burning sensation in the limbs and extremities caused by ergot, the consequence of a fungus (Claviceps purpurea) that contaminates rye and wheat. See also *ergot*.

**first cranial nerve**   See *olfactory nerve*.

**first do no harm**   Slogan used in medicine, often in the Latin wording "primum non nocere." This fundamental medical precept derives from Hippocrates.

**first stage of labor**   The part of labor when the cervix dilates fully to approximately 10 centimeters in diameter. The first stage of labor is also called the stage of dilatation.

**FISH**   Fluorescent in situ hybridization.

**fish bowl granuloma**   See *granuloma, fish bowl*.

**Fisher's exact test**   A statistical test of independence much used in medical research. It tests the independence of rows and columns in a 2 X 2 contingency table (a table with two horizontal rows crossing two vertical columns, creating four places for data) based on the exact sampling distribution of the observed frequencies. Hence it is an "exact" test.

**fish-odor syndrome**   An inborn error of metabolism associated with an offensive body odor, similar to the smell of rotting fish, due to the excessive excretion of trimethylaminuria (TMA) in urine, sweat, and breath. Persons with this syndrome may experience tachycardia (fast heart rate) and severe hypertension (high blood pressure) after eating cheese (which contains tyramine, as does red wine and some other foods) and after using nasal sprays containing epinephrine. This syndrome is caused by a mutation in the gene for an enzyme, flavin-containing monooxygenase-3 (FMO3), which is encoded by a gene on chromosome No. 1. The FMO3 enzyme normally metabolizes tyramine. The syndrome is associated with various psychosocial reactions, including social isolation, clinical depression, and attempted suicide.

**fistula** An abnormal passageway. For example, with an anal fistula the hallmark is an opening in the skin near the anus: This opening may lead to a tunnel into the rectal canal, or to a passage that ends in a blind pouch.

**five-day fever** See *trench fever*.

**flail chest** A condition that occurs when enough ribs are broken (usually from a crush injury) to compromise the rigidity of the chest wall. On inspiration, the chest wall moves inward instead of outward, and does the opposite on expiration.

**flat feet** Absence of an arch in the sole of the foot, causing the foot to lie flat when the person is standing. All babies have flat feet, because their arches are not yet built up (and their feet tend to be plump). This condition may persist into adulthood, or an arch may form as the child grows. Flat feet can also be acquired, as in jobs that require a great deal of walking and carrying heavy objects. People with flat feet sometimes experience clumsiness and fatigue from prolonged walking or running. Wearing shoes with built-in arch supports can help. People with weakness in the ankle as well as flat feet may find that their feet turn in or roll toward the middle, damaging shoes and causing discomfort. Shoes with both built-in arch supports and rigid counters (side supports) are helpful. Exercises may also be useful in reducing discomfort.

**flatulence** The passing of gas from the intestinal tract. See also *flatus*.

**flatus** Gas in the intestinal tract, or passed through the anus. The intestinal gases are hydrogen, nitrogen, carbon dioxide, and methane, all of which are odorless. The occasional unpleasant smell of flatus is the result of trace gases, such as indole, skatole and, most commonly, hydrogen sulfide.

**flavin-containing monooxygenase-3** See *fish-odor syndrome*.

**flaviviridae** A family of viruses that cause hemorrhagic fever and are transmitted by mosquitoes and ticks. Flaviviruses have single-stranded RNA as their genetic material. The virus of yellow fever, for example, is a flavivirus.

**flavivirus** A virus from the family flaviviridae. See also *flaviviridae*.

**flavoproteins** See *enzymes, yellow*.

**flexion** The process of bending, or the state of being bent. Flexion of the fingers results in a clenched fist.

**Flexner Report** "Medical Education in the United States and Canada," quite possibly the most important written document in the history of American and Canadian medical education. The 1910 report is named for its author, professional educator Abraham Flexner. Flexner researched and wrote his report for the Carnegie Foundation. At the time of the Report, many medical schools were proprietary schools operated more for profit than for education. In their stead, Flexner proposed medical schools in the German tradition of strong biomedical sciences, together with hands-on clinical training. The Flexner Report caused many medical schools to close down, and most of the remaining schools were reformed to conform to the Flexnerian model.

**floating rib** See *false rib*.

**flood supplies kit** See *disaster supplies*.

**floppy baby syndrome** A general medical reference to an abnormal condition of newborns and infants manifested by inadequate tone of the muscles. It can be due to a multitude of different neurologic and muscle problems. See also *hypotonia*.

**flow cytometry** Analysis of biological material by detection of the light-absorbing or fluorescing properties of cells, or of subcellular fractions such as chromosomes, as they pass in a narrow stream through a laser beam. Flow cytometry can be used with automated sorting devices to sort successive droplets of the stream into different fractions, depending on the fluorescence emitted by each droplet.

**flow karyotyping** Use of flow cytometry to analyze and/or separate chromosomes on the basis of their DNA content.

**flu** Short for influenza. See *influenza*.

**flu shot** See *influenza vaccine*.

**flu vaccine** See *influenza vaccine*.

**flu, stomach** So-called "stomach flu" actually has nothing to do with the influenza (flu) virus. This term is sometimes used to describe gastrointestinal illnesses caused by other microorganisms.

**fluctuating rib** See *false rib*.

**fluid, cerebrospinal** See *cerebrospinal fluid*.

**fluorescent in situ hybridization** An important molecular cytogenetic method for identifying chromosomes and parts of chromosomes, and for deciphering chromosome rearrangements. Fluorescent means emitting light that comes from a reaction within the emitter. Abbreviated as FISH.

**fluorescent microscope** A microscope equipped to examine material that fluoresces under ultraviolet (UV) light.

**fluoroscopy** An X-ray procedure that makes it possible to see internal organs in motion. Fluoroscopy uses X-rays to produce real-time video images. After the X-rays pass through the patient, instead of using film, they are captured by a device called an image intensifier and converted into light. The light is then captured by a TV camera and displayed on a video monitor.

**fluorouracil** An anticancer drug. Its chemical name is 5-fluorouracil, commonly called 5-FU.

**flush** **1** A redness of the skin, typically over the cheeks or neck. A flush is usually temporary and brought on by excitement, exercise, fever, or embarrassment. Flushing is an involuntary (uncontrollable) response of the nervous system, leading to widening of the capillaries of the involved skin. Also referred to as a blush (or, as a verb, to blush). Flushing may also be caused by medications or other substances that cause widening of the capillaries, such as niacin. **2** To wash out a wound or body area.

**fluvastin** A cholesterol-lowering drug (brand name: Lescol) prescribed to prevent medical problems associated with high cholesterol levels, such as atherosclerosis and heart disease. It is also used to treat inherited lipid disorders and similar disorders caused by liver or kidney disease.

**FMF** See *familial Mediterranean fever*.

**FMO3** Flavin-containing monooxygenase-3. See *fish-odor syndrome*.

**FMR1** The gene responsible for the production of a protein called FMRP. Lack of FMRP is one of the results of Fragile X syndrome, an inheritable genetic disorder. See also *Fragile X syndrome*.

**FMRP** Familial mental retardation protein. See also *Fragile X syndrome*.

**focused H and P** In medical slang, H and P stand for the history (H) and physical (P), namely the medical history and the physical examination of the patient. A focused H and P specifies that the doctor focuses upon the patient's present problem, rather than doing a complete clinical exam. For example, if a patient is complaining of an earache, the doctor concentrates on the ear.

**Fogarty International Center** See *National Institutes of Health*.

**folate** See *folic acid*.

**Foley catheter** See *catheter, Foley*.

**folic acid** A B vitamin that is an important factor in nucleic acid synthesis. A deficiency of folic acid causes megaloblastic anemia. Lack of folic acid during pregnancy can lead to neural tube birth defects, particularly spina bifida.

**follicle-stimulating hormone** A hormone produced by the pituitary gland that controls estrogen production by the ovaries. Abbreviated as FSH. See also *gonadotropin*.

**follicles** Shafts in the scalp through which hair grows.

**follicular cyst of the ovary** See *cyst of the ovary, follicular*.

**Fondation Jean Dausset** The Centre d'Etudes du Polymorphisme Humain (CEPH), an internationally renowned research laboratory created in Paris in 1984 by Professor Jean Dausset to provide the scientific community with resources for human genome mapping.

**Fong disease** An hereditary condition characterized by abnormally formed (dysplastic) or absent nails, and by absent or underdeveloped (hypoplastic) kneecaps. Other features of the syndrome include iliac horns; abnormality of the elbows, interfering with full range of motion (pronation and supination); and kidney disease resembling glomerulonephritis, which is often mild but can be progressive and lead to renal failure. Fong disease is inherited as a dominant gene, so the disease can be transmitted by an affected parent. Its gene locus is linked genetically to the ABO blood group locus, and is now known to be in chromosome region 9q34. Also called nail-patella syndrome and Turner-Kieser syndrome.

**fontanel** A "soft spot" of the skull of a newborn infant, where the cartilage has not yet hardened into bone between the skull bones. There are normally two fontanels, both in the midline of the skull. The anterior fontanel is well in front of the posterior fontanel. The posterior fontanel closes first, at latest by the age of eight weeks in a full-term baby. The anterior fontanel closes at around 18 months of age on average, but it can close normally as early as nine months. If fontanels close too early or too late, that may be a sign of a problem. Also known as the fontanelle.

**food** Any substance eaten to provide nutritional support for the body.

**Food and Drug Administration** An agency within the US Public Health Service, which is a part of the Department of Health and Human Services. The FDA provides a number of health-related services, including inspecting food and food-processing facilities to ensure wholesomeness and safety; scrutinizing feed and drugs for pets and farm animals; ensuring that cosmetics will not cause harm; monitoring the health of nation's blood supply; ensuring that medicines, medical devices, and biologicals (such as insulin and vaccines) are safe and effective; and testing radiation-emitting products such as microwave ovens to protect the public. It also oversees health and safety labeling of these products. All new prescription and over-the-counter drugs are subject to FDA approval. The FDA must determine that a new drug produces the benefits it's supposed to without causing side effects that would outweigh those benefits. It does so by looking at the results of clinical trials done outside the FDA. When serious adverse effects from a medication are reported, the FDA has the power to force the manufacturer to make changes in the drug, change its safety labeling or marketing practices, or remove the medication from the market.

**food poisoning** Disease caused by food-borne infectious organisms, such as the Clostridium botulinum bacteria that produces deadly botulism toxin. Food poisoning is a major public health threat, causing thousands of people to become seriously ill each year, and killing many. Symptoms may include stomach upset, nausea, vomiting, weakness, and more, depending on the organism involved. Improper food storage and preparation raise the risk of food poisoning. Food poisoning is most dangerous to children, the elderly, and people with impaired immune systems. See also *botulism*, *E. coli*, *Salmonellosis*.

**food, functional** Foods that are potentially healthful, including any modified food or ingredient that may provide a health benefit beyond the traditional nutrients it contains. Functional foods include such items as cereals, breads, beverages that are fortified with vitamins, some herbs, and nutraceuticals.

**food, "super"** Foods with alleged healing or health-promoting capabilities. The healing power of foods is a popular concept. Medicinal or nutritionally high-powered foods have been part and parcel of the natural products industry for a long time and, through emerging scientific research and particularly through growing public interest, they have reached the mainstream. Not all items advertised as "super" foods or healing foods have been proven to promote health, however, and some may be contraindicated for people with certain health conditions. Before making drastic changes to your diet, always consult with your physician or a professional nutritionist.

**foot** **1** The extremity at the end of the leg, with which the person stands and walks. The foot is a particularly complex structure, made up of dozens of bones that work together with muscles and tendons to execute precise movements. The bones of the foot include the 10 metatarsals and the 28 phalanges (toe bones). **2** In length, 12 inches or a third of a yard. The foot was originally the length of a man's foot, and served as a measurement of land. Abbreviated as ft.

**foot drop brace** See *ankle-foot orthosis*.

**foot fungus** See *athlete's foot*.

**foot, athlete's** See *athlete's foot*.

**footling presentation** See *delivery, footling*.

**foramen** A natural opening. Although a foramen is usually through bone, it can be an opening through other types of tissue, as with the foramen ovale.

**foramen magnum** The large hole at the base of the skull, which allows passage of the spinal cord.

**foramen of Magendie** An opening from the fourth ventricle in the brain to the central canal of the upper end of the spinal cord.

**foramen ovale** An oval opening between the two upper chambers of the heart (the atria) that is a normal feature of the fetal and newborn circulation. The foramen ovale normally closes by three months of age.

**foramen, interventricular** An opening between the lateral and third ventricles in the brain.

**foramina of Luschka** A pair of openings from the fourth ventricle of the brain to the central canal of the upper end of the spinal cord.

**forceps** An instrument with two blades and a handle, which is used for handling, grasping, or compressing.

**forceps, obstetrical** A forceps designed as an aid in the vaginal delivery of a baby. Today, forceps are used only when there is an intractable interruption of the normal birth process, as they can cause injury to the fetus.

**forearm** The portion of the upper limb from the elbow to the wrist. The forearm has two bones: the radius and ulna.

**foreign body airway obstruction**  Partial or complete blockage of the breathing tubes to the lungs due to the presence of a foreign body, such as food, a bead, or a toy. See *airway obstruction*.

**foreskin**  The fold of skin that covers the head (glans) of the penis. The inside of the foreskin has preputial glands, a special type of sebaceous (oil) glands that secrete an oily lubricant. This lubricant probably has protective qualities, as does the foreskin itself. However, uncircumcised men must retract the foreskin periodically to remove build-up of this lubricant, which is known as smegma. Only about 1 in every 20 boys is born with a retractable foreskin, as the tissue development of the foreskin is usually not complete at birth. The foreskin is thus not fully separable from the glans in most newborn boys. By one year of age, the foreskin can be retracted in 50 percent of boys, and by three years of age, the foreskin can be retracted in 80 percent to 90 percent of uncircumcised boys. The foreskin is often surgically removed at birth, or may instead be removed at puberty in some cultures. Also called the prepuce. See also *circumcision, male*.

**foreskin and glans, inflammation of the**  See *balanoposthitis*. See also *balanitis, posthitis*.

**foreskin, inflammation of the**  See *posthitis*. See also *balanoposthitis*.

**foreskin, tight**  See *phimosis*.

**Forestier disease**  See *diffuse idiopathic skeletal hyperostosis*.

**formula**  A prepared substitute for breast milk, which may be based on cow's milk, goat's milk, soy milk, or another food product. Formula does not contain the special immunity factors found in breast milk that help the baby to fight off infections, and it may not include all the vitamins, minerals, and enzymes found in human breast milk. For that reason, experts in infant nutrition agree that breast-feeding is best, particularly in families with a history of allergies.

**formula feeding**  Feeding an infant or toddler prepared formula instead of or in addition to breast-feeding. Formula feeding is indicated when the mother has an illness that could be passed on to the baby through breast milk or through the close physical proximity required for breast-feeding. Otherwise, experts in infant nutrition agree that breast-feeding is best.

**formulary**  In the context of managed care, a list of prescription drugs that the HMO or managed-care group is willing to cover in its prescription payment plan. If a doctor prescribes a drug that is not in the formulary, payment may be denied unless the patient applies for an exception to the formulary rules.

**fornices**  Plural form of fornix. See *fornix*.

**fornix**  In anatomy, any vaultlike or arched structure.

**fornix cerebri**  An arching fibrous band in the brain, connecting the two lobes of the cerebrum. Each of the two fornices in the brain is an arched tract of nerves.

**fornix conjunctivae**  The loose arching folds that connect the conjunctival membrane lining the inside the eyelid with the conjunctival membrane covering the eyeball.

**fornix uteri**  The anterior (front) and posterior (back) recesses into which the upper vagina is divided. These vaultlike recesses are formed by protrusion of the cervix into the vagina. The fornix uteri is also known as the fornix vaginae (the vaginal fornix).

**fornix vaginae**  See *fornix uteri*.

**fosphenytoin**  An antispasmodic drug (brand name: Cerebyx).

**founder effect**  The positive effect on gene frequency when a population (colony) has only a small number of original settlers, one or more of whom had that gene. For example, the gene for Huntington disease was introduced into the Lake Maracaibo region in Venezuela early in the 19th century. There are now over 100 persons with Huntington disease and at least 900 persons at risk for that disease in that region, the largest known aggregation of the Huntington gene in the world.

**fourth cranial nerve**  See *trochlear nerve*.

**fourth stage of labor**  The hour or two after delivery when the tone of the uterus is reestablished as the uterus contracts down again, expelling any remaining contents. These contractions are hastened by breast-feeding, which stimulates production of the hormone oxytocin.

**fourth ventricle**  One cavity in a system of four communicating cavities within the brain, which are continuous with the central canal of the spinal cord. The fourth ventricle is the most inferior (lowest) of these. It extends from the aqueduct of the midbrain to the central canal of the upper end of the spinal cord, with which it communicates by the two foramina of Luschka and the foramen of Magendie. It is filled with cerebrospinal fluid, which is formed by structures called choroid plexuses located in the walls and roofs of the ventricle.

**fraction, ejection**  See *ejection fraction*.

**fracture**   A break in the bone or cartilage. Although usually a result of trauma, a fracture can be the result of an acquired disease of bone, such as osteoporosis, or of abnormal formation of bone in a congenital disease of bone, such as osteogenesis imperfecta ("brittle bone disease"). Fractures are classified according to their character and location as, for example, greenstick fracture of the radius.

**fracture, buckle**   See *fracture, torus*.

**fracture, clay-shoveler's**   An uncommon breakage of the spine, of the vertebrae from the lower neck or upper back, as a result of stress. Clay-shoveler's fracture usually occurs in laborers who lift heavy weights rapidly with their arms extended. Examples of such activities include shoveling soil, rubble, or snow up and back over the head; using a pickax or scythe; and pulling out roots. The sheer force of the trapezius and rhomboid muscles pulling on the spine at the base of the neck actually tears off the bone of the spine. Symptoms of clay-shoveler's fracture include burning, "knife-like" pain at the level of the fractured spine between the upper shoulder blades. The pain can sharply increase with repeated activity that strains the muscles of the upper back. The broken spine and nearby muscles are exquisitely tender. Clay-shoveler's fracture is diagnosed by X-ray examination of the spine. While the intense pain gradually subsides in days to weeks, the area can intermittently develop burning pain with certain activities that involve prolonged extension of the arms, such as computer work. Most patients require no treatment other than rest and avoiding activities that stress the area of the fracture. Pain medications, physical therapy, and massage can be helpful. Occasionally surgical removal of the tip of the broken spine is performed for those with long-standing pain.

**fracture, comminuted**   A fracture in which bone is broken, splintered, or crushed into a number of pieces.

**fracture, compound**   A fracture in which the bone is sticking through the skin. Also known as an open fracture.

**fracture, compression**   A fracture caused by compression, the act of pressing together. Compression fractures of the vertebrae are especially common in the elderly.

**fracture, greenstick**   A fracture in which one side of a bone is broken while the other is bent (like a green stick).

**fracture, open**   See *fracture, compound*.

**fracture, Salter-Harris**   A traumatic fracture of the physeal and/or epiphyseal growth plate.

**fracture, spiral**   See *fracture, torsion*. See also *fracture, toddler's*.

**fracture, stress**   A fracture caused by repetitive stress, as may occur in sports, strenuous exercise, or heavy physical labor. It is especially common in the metatarsal bones of the foot, particularly in runners. Osteoporosis increases the possibility of stress fractures. Treatment is by rest, disuse, and sometimes splinting or casting to prevent reinjury during healing.

**fracture, supracondylar-intercondylar**   A fracture of bone within a moving joint, such as the knee or elbow.

**fracture, toddler's**   A torsion fracture of the tibia, without bone displacement.

**fracture, torsion**   A fracture in which a bone has been twisted apart. Also called a spiral fracture. See also *fracture, toddler's*.

**fracture, torus**   A fracture in which one side of the bone bends, but does not actually break. Torus fractures normally heal on their own within a month, with rest and disuse, although they can cause soreness and discomfort.

**fracture, transverse**   A fracture in which the break is across the bone, at a right angle to the long axis of the bone.

**fracture, Y**   A fracture with a Y-like shape that occurs at the end of a bone.

**fragile site**   A term denoting a heritable point on a chromosome where gaps and breaks tend to occur.

**fragile X chromosome**   An X chromosome with a fragile site, which is associated with a frequent form of mental retardation. It is due a trinucleotide repeat (a recurring motif of three bases) in the DNA at that spot. Not all people who inherit the fragile site have Fragile X syndrome, and it is not yet known what genetic or environmental factors cause actual breaks or deletions at this fragile site. Also known as FRAXA. See also *Fragile X syndrome*.

**Fragile X syndrome**   The most common heritable form of mental retardation, occurring in about 1 in 2,000 males and a smaller percentage of females. Characteristics of Fragile X syndrome in boys include prominent or long ears, a long face, delayed speech, large testes (*macroorchidism*), hyperactivity, tactile defensiveness, gross motor delays, and autistic-like behaviors. Much less is known about girls with Fragile X syndrome. Only about half of all females who carry the genetic mutation have symptoms themselves. Of those, half are of normal intelligence, and only one-fourth have an IQ under

70. Few Fragile X girls have autistic symptoms, although they tend to be shy and quiet. Fragile X syndrome is due to a dynamic mutation (a trinucleotide repeat) at an inherited fragile site on the X chromosome, and so is an X-linked disorder. Because the mutation is dynamic, it can change in length and hence in severity from generation to generation, from person to person, and even within a given individual. Fragile X syndrome is diagnosed with a genetic test. Also known as FRAXA (as is the fragile X chromosome itself) and Martin-Bell syndrome.

**frambesia**   See *yaws*.

**free radical**   An unstable compound whose behavior is characterized by rapid reactions. Free radicals are often blamed for such physical phenomena as cell degeneration and malfunction. Their full role in physical health is not understood.

**frenulum**   A physical structure that has a restraining function. For example, the lingual frenulum attaches the tongue to the floor of the mouth, and appears to restrain it.

**Freudian**   Adjective from the name of the founder of psychoanalysis, Sigmund Freud. Used to refer to a particular type of psychoanalysis that concentrates on finding the roots of adult behavior in childhood conflicts, or to interpretations of behavior based on Freud's precepts. Freudian psychoanalysis is no longer normally used as a diagnostic and treatment tool for mental or neurological disorders in the US, as these illnesses are now recognized to be biological in origin. It is still practiced as a method for gaining increased self-knowledge, however.

**Frey syndrome**   Sweating on one side of the forehead, face, scalp, and neck that occurs soon after ingesting food, as a result of damage to a nerve that goes to the large saliva gland in the cheek (the parotid gland). Frey syndrome is the most common cause of sweating after eating (gustatory sweating). Gustatory sweating is also a rare complication of diabetes mellitus, in which case the sweating is on both sides of the head, and the severity of the sweating may be mild or substantial. This distressing problem can be difficult to treat. Treatments used include oxybutynin chloride, propantheline bromide, and clonidine (brand name: Catapres). Recently, some success has been reported with topical applications of glycopyrrolate: the lotion is applied to the skin of the forehead and face, sparing the eyes and mouth.

**frostbite**   Damage to tissues as a result of exposure to extreme cold. The tissues become injured from blood clotting and ice-crystal formation. Severe frostbite can result in death of the tissues (gangrene).

**frozen shoulder**   Permanent severe limitation of the range of motion of the shoulder due to scarring around the shoulder joint (adhesive capsulitis). Frozen shoulder is an unwanted consequence of rotator cuff disease: damage to the rotator cuff, the set of four tendons that stabilize the shoulder joint and help move the shoulder in diverse directions.

**FSH**   Follicle-stimulating hormone.

**ft.**   Abbreviation for foot, a measure of length.

**FTT**   Failure to thrive.

**fucosidosis**   An inherited enzyme disorder characterized by lack of the enzyme fucosidase. Without this enzyme, many substances build up in the body. Fucosidosis is an autosomal recessive disorder. The gene involved in the 12 different mutations known to cause fucosidosis, FUCA1, has been mapped to chromosome 1 at the spot 1p24.

**fugue state**   An altered state of consciousness in which a person may move about purposely and even speak, but is not fully aware. A fugue state is usually a type of complex partial seizure. See also *seizure, complex partial*.

**functional food**   See *food, functional*.

**functional gene test**   A test for a specific protein which indicates not only that the corresponding gene is present, but also that it is active.

**fundus**   Latin word for the bottom. In medicine, fundus refers to the bottom or base of an organ. For example, the fundus of the eye is the retina. However, the fundus of the stomach is inexplicably the upper portion.

**fungal nail infection**   See *dermatophytic onychomycosis*.

**fungiform**   Mushroom-shaped.

**fungiform papillae**   Broad, flat structures that house taste buds in the central portion of the dorsum (back) of the tongue. These papillae were thought to resemble little mushrooms.

**fungus**   A plantlike organism that feeds on organic matter. An example of a common fungus is the yeast organism that causes thrush and diaper rash (diaper dermatitis).

**fungus, foot**   See *athlete's foot*.

**funnel chest**   "Caved-in" chest. Usually an unimportant isolated finding evident at birth, funnel chest can occasionally be part of a connective-tissue disorder such as Marfan syndrome. Also known as pectus excavatum.

**funny bone** Actually a sensation rather than a bone. When the elbow is bumped, the ulnar nerve running past the elbow is stimulated to produce a strange, almost painful, "electric" sensation.

**furosemide** A diuretic medication (brand name: Lasix) prescribed to rid the body of excess fluid. It may be recommended to treat fluid accumulation as a result of kidney trouble, fluid in the lungs, congestive heart failure, high blood pressure, and other conditions. See also *diuretic, loop.*

**furuncle** A boil.

**fusiform** Formed like a spindle: wider in the middle and tapering toward the ends. An aneurysm may be fusiform.

**fusiform aneurysm** A vascular outpouching shaped like a spindle. A fusiform widening of an artery or vein.

**fusospirillary gingivitis** See *acute membranous gingivitis.*

**fusospirillosis** See *acute membranous gingivitis.*

**fusospirochetal gingivitis** See *acute membranous gingivitis.*

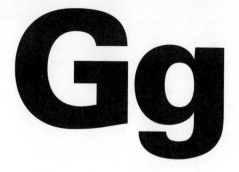

**G** Abbreviation for guanine. See *guanine*.

**G proteins** Molecules that have been described as "biological traffic lights." Located inside the cell, G proteins are able to respond to signals outside the cell—light, smell, or hormones—and translate (transduce) these signals into action within the cell.

**gait** Manner of walking. Observation of gait can provide early diagnostic clues for a number of disorders, including cerebral palsy, Parkinson disease, and Rett syndrome.

**galactose** A sugar found in milk.

**galactosemia** Inherited disorder due to defective metabolism (processing) of the sugar galactose. Newborns in the US are screened for galactosemia. The disease can be fatal, if undetected, and is treated by avoiding galactose in the diet.

**galactosylceramidosis** See *Krabbe disease*.

**gallbladder** A pear-shaped organ that stores bile. It is located below the liver.

**gallbladder absence** See *agenesis of the gallbladder*.

**gallbladder agenesis** See *agenesis of the gallbladder*.

**gallium** A rare metal with the atomic weight of 69. There are several isotopic forms of gallium that differ from it in atomic weight. One is gallium-68, which is produced by cyclotrons and emits gamma rays. The citrate form of gallium-68 is used as a radiotracer to locate sites of inflammation and tumor tissue within the body.

**gallop rhythm** Heart rhythm that resembles the gallop of a horse.

**gallstones** Gallstones are "pebbles" within the gallbladder, or in the ducts that lead from the gallbladder to the intestine. Gallstones are a frequent cause of abdominal pain, as well as of inflammation and infection of the gallbladder and the pancreas. Gallstone disease is common. About 20 percent of the world's population develop gallstones during their lives. There are two types of gallstones: cholesterol stones, composed of at least 60 percent cholesterol, which are common in the US and Western Europe; and pigment stones, which are brown or black owing to their high content of colored pigment (bilirubin), and which account for over 90 percent of gallstones in Asia.

**gallstones and ERCP** See *Endoscopic Retrograde Cholangio-Pancreatography*.

**gallstones, microscopic** See *biliary sand, biliary sludge*.

**gamete** The sperm or egg. In humans, the gametes normally have 23 chromosomes.

**gamma knife** A tool that uses highly focused radiation to perform neurosurgery without making an incision. It is used to treat many types of brain tumors as well as arteriovenous malformations in the brain. It is being used experimentally to treat Parkinson disease, chronic pain, and other disorders. See also *radiation therapy, stereotactic*.

**ganglion** 1 An aggregation of nerve cell bodies. 2 A tendon cyst, commonly near the wrist.

**gangliosidosis, GM1** See *Landing disease*.

**gangliosidosis, GM2** See *Tay-Sachs disease*, *Sandhoff disease*.

**gangrene** The state of tissue death due to loss of adequate blood supply.

**Gareis-Mason syndrome** See *MASA syndrome*. See also *adducted thumbs*.

**gargoylism** See *Hurler syndrome*.

**gas chromatography** See *chromatography, gas*.

**gas, intestinal** See *flatulence, flatus*.

**gas, laughing** See *nitrous oxide*.

**gastrectomy** Surgery to remove part or all of the stomach.

**gastric** Having to do with the stomach.

**gastric atrophy** A condition in which the stomach muscles shrink and become weak. It results in a lack of digestive juices.

**gastric cancer** See *cancer, gastric*.

**gastric emptying study** A study that evaluates the process of emptying food from the stomach. For a gastric emptying study, a patient eats a meal in which the solid food, liquid food, or both are mixed with a small amount of radioactive material. A scanner that acts like a Geiger counter is placed over the stomach to monitor the amount of radioactivity in the stomach for several hours after the test meal. In patients with abnormal emptying of the stomach, the food and radioactive material stay in the stomach longer than normal (usually for hours) before emptying into the small intestine.

**gastric stapling**   A surgical procedure that converts the upper part of the stomach into a very small pouch, forcing an obese person to eat only tiny portions yet still feel full. It is normally done only in severe cases, and in combination with diet and exercise. As the name suggests, surgical staples are used in this procedure. A similar operation is called gastric banding. Both operations have a potential for serious side effects.

**gastric ulcer**   A hole in the lining of the stomach, corroded by the acidic digestive juices secreted by the stomach cells. Ulcer formation is related to H. pylori bacteria in the stomach, anti-inflammatory medications, and the smoking of cigarettes. Ulcer pain may not correlate with the presence or severity of ulceration. Diagnosis is made with barium X-ray or with the use of a viewing tube slipped through the throat to the stomach (endoscopy).

**gastritis**   Inflammation of the stomach.

**gastroenteritis**   Inflammation of the stomach and the intestines. Can cause nausea, vomiting, and/or diarrhea. Gastroenteritis has numerous causes, including infectious organisms (viruses, bacteria, etc.), food poisoning, and stress.

**gastroenterologist**   A doctor who specializes in diagnosing and treating diseases of the digestive system.

**gastroesophageal reflux**   The return of stomach contents back up into the esophagus. This frequently causes heartburn because of irritation of the esophagus by stomach acid. Gastroesophageal reflux disease (GERD) can lead to scarring and stricture of the esophagus, which requires stretching (dilating) of the esophagus. 10 percent of patients with GERD develop Barrett esophagus, which increases the risk of cancer of the esophagus. 80 percent of patients with GERD also have a hiatal hernia.

**gastrointestinal tract**   The stomach and intestines. Abbreviated as GI tract.

**gastroparesis**   Gastroparesis is a medical condition in which the muscle of the stomach is paralyzed by a disease of the stomach muscle itself, or of the nerves controlling the muscle. As a consequence, food and secretions do not empty normally from the stomach, and there is nausea

and vomiting. Abdominal bloating and pain can result. Gastroparesis may be associated with paralysis of other parts of the gastrointestinal tract (the small intestine and colon). The most common cause of gastroparesis is diabetes mellitus. A nuclear medicine test designed to study gastric emptying is the most common means of diagnosis of gastroparesis. Gastroparesis is treated with medications to increase the contractions of the stomach's muscle, occasionally with surgery, and experimentally with electrical pacing.

**gastroscope**   A flexible, lighted instrument that is put through the mouth and esophagus to view the stomach. Tissue from the stomach can be removed through the gastroscope.

**gastrostomy**   A surgical opening into the stomach. This opening may be used for feeding, usually via a feeding tube called a gastrostomy tube. Feeding can also be done by percutaneous endoscopic gastrostomy (PEG).

**gastrostomy, percutaneous endoscopic**   A surgical procedure for placing a feeding tube without having to perform an open laparotomy operation on the abdomen. The aim of PEG is to feed those who cannot swallow. PEG may be done by a surgeon, otolaryngologist, or gastroenterologist. It is done in a hospital or outpatient surgical facility. Local anesthesia—usually lidocaine or another spray—is used to anesthetize the throat. An endoscope is passed through the mouth, throat, and esophagus to the stomach. The surgeon then makes a small incision in the skin of the abdomen, pushes an IV tube through the skin into the stomach, and then sutures (ties) it in place. The patient can usually go home the same day or the next morning. Possible complications include wound infection, and dislodging or malfunction of the tube. PEG takes less time, carries less risk, and costs less than a classic surgical gastrostomy, which requires opening the abdomen.

**Gaucher disease**   A progressive genetic disease caused by a defect in an enzyme called glucocerebrosidase, which is needed to break down the chemical glucocerebroside. The enzyme defect in persons with Gaucher disease leads to the accumulation of glucocerebroside in the spleen, liver, and lymph nodes. The most common early sign is enlargement of the spleen. Other signs include low red blood–cell counts (anemia), a decrease in blood platelets, increased pigmentation of the skin, and a yellow fatty spot on the white of the eye (a pinguecula). Severe bone involvement can lead to pain and collapse of the bone of the hips, shoulders, and spine. The Gaucher disease gene is on chromosome 1, and the disease is a recessive trait. Both parents must carry the gene and transmit it for their child to have the disease. The parents' risk of a child with the disease is one in four with each pregnancy. This type of Gaucher disease (noncerebral juvenile Gaucher disease) is most common in Ashkenazi Jews, and is the most common genetic disease among Jews in the United States. Also known as glucosylceramidosis.

**GD**   Gaucher disease.

**Gemfibrozil**   A fibrate medication (brand name: Lopid) given to reduce the level of triglyceride fats in the blood, ordinarily used in patients whose cholesterol levels have not responded to dietary changes. Gemfibrozil is associated with a number of potentially serious side effects, so patients taking this medication should be carefully monitored. See also *fibrates.*

**gene**   A gene can be defined in various ways. In classical genetics, a gene is a unit of inheritance. In molecular genetics, a gene is a sequence of chromosomal DNA required to make a functional product. Humans have 50,000 to 100,000 genes.

**gene deletion**   The total loss or absence of a gene. Gene deletion plays a role in birth defects and in the development of cancer.

**gene duplication**   An extra copy of a gene. Gene duplication is a key mechanism in evolution. Once a gene is duplicated, the identical genes can undergo changes and diverge to create two different genes.

**gene expression**   A gene speaks. When a gene is expressed, the information encoded in the gene is translated into protein or RNA structures present and operating in the cell. Expressed genes include genes that are transcribed into messenger RNA (mRNA) and then translated into protein, as well as those genes that are transcribed into RNA, such as transfer and ribosomal RNAs, but not translated into protein.

**gene family**   A group of genes related in structure, and often in function. The genes in a family are descended from an ancestral gene. For example, the hemoglobin genes belong to one gene family created by gene duplication and divergence.

**gene mapping**   The charting of the relative positions of genes on a DNA molecule or chromosome and the distance, in linkage units or physical units, between them.

**gene markers**   Detectable genetic traits or distinctive segments of DNA that serve as landmarks for a target gene. Markers are on the same chromosome as the target gene. They must be near enough to the target gene to be genetically linked to it; to be inherited, usually together with that gene, and so serve as signposts to it.

**gene product**   The RNA or protein that results from the expression of a gene. The amount of gene product is a measure of the degree of gene activity.

**gene testing**   The testing of a sample of blood (or another fluid or tissue) for evidence of a gene. The evidence can be biochemical, chromosomal, or genetic. The aim is to learn whether a gene for a disease is present or absent.

**gene therapy**   The treatment of disease by replacing, altering, or supplementing a gene that is absent or abnormal, and that is responsible for the disease. In studies of gene therapy for cancer, researchers are trying to bolster the body's natural capacity to combat cancer and make the tumor more sensitive to other kinds of therapy. Gene therapy, still in its early stages, holds great promise for the treatment of many diseases. The first gene therapy was done successfully in humans in 1990.

**gene, evolutionarily conserved**   A gene that has remained essentially unchanged throughout evolution. Conservation of a gene indicates that it is unique and essential. There is not an extra copy of that gene with which evolution can tinker. And changes in the gene are likely to be lethal.

**gene, marker**   A detectable genetic trait or segment of DNA that can be identified and tracked. A marker gene can serve as a flag for another gene, sometimes called the target gene. A marker gene must be on the same chromosome as the target gene, and near enough to it so that the two genes (the marker and the target) are genetically linked and are usually inherited together.

**gene, zygotic lethal**   A gene that is fatal for the zygote, the initial cell formed by the union of a sperm and an ovum. The zygote would normally develop into an embryo, as instructed by the genetic material within the unified cell. However, a zygotic lethal gene scotches prenatal development at its earliest point. A zygotic lethal gene is a mutated version of a normal gene essential to the survival of the zygote. The extent of the mutation can range from a change in a single base in the DNA to deletion of the entire gene.

**general paresis**   Progressive dementia and generalized paralysis due to chronic inflammation of the covering and substance of the brain (meningoencephalitis). General paresis is a part of late (tertiary) syphilis, occurring a decade or more after the initial infection.

**genes, breast cancer susceptibility**   See *breast cancer susceptibility genes.* See also *BRCA1*; *BRCA2*; *breast cancer, familial.*

**genetic** Having to do with genes, structures found in every cell of the body. Each gene contains information that directs the activities of cells and controls the way an individual develops.

**genetic code** The correspondence of the base triplets (trios composed of A, T, G, or C) in DNA with the amino acids.

**genetic counseling** Counseling services provided to individuals who may be at increased risk of having a genetic disease or of passing the disease on to their future offspring. Genetic counselors help patients assess risk and make decisions about testing, reproduction, and coping with genetic disorders.

**genetic infantile agranulocytosis** See *severe congenital neutropenia*.

**genetic screening** Testing a population to identify individuals at risk for a genetic disease or for transmitting it. For example, newborns may be screened for phenylketonuria (PKU), Jews for Tay-Sachs disease gene, and people of African descent for the sickle cell gene.

**genetic transport disease** Within the body, many molecules are able to pass across the membranes that surround cells. These molecules can accomplish this feat because of specific transport systems that include special receptors on the membrane of the cell, and special carrier proteins. The receptor recognizes the molecule and receives it on the cell membrane, and the molecule then hitches a ride through the cell membrane on the back of a carrier protein. With such remarkable specificity, it is little wonder that sometimes there are defects in transport systems. Several dozen different diseases are now known to be due to transport defects. An example of a transport disease is cystinuria, the most common defect known in the transport of an amino acid (namely, cystine), and a significant cause of kidney stones.

**genital** Pertaining to the external and internal organs of reproduction.

**genital herpes** A viral infection transmitted through intimate contact with the moist mucous linings of the genitals. This contact can involve the mouth, the vagina, or the genital skin. The herpes simplex type 2 virus enters the mucous membranes through microscopic tears. Once inside, the virus travels to nerve roots near the spinal cord and settles there permanently. When an infected person has a herpes outbreak, the virus travels down the nerve fibers to the site of the original infection; when it reaches the skin, the classic redness and blisters occur. The outbreak of herpes is closely related to the functioning of the immune system. Women who have suppressed immune systems, either through stress, disease, or medications, have more frequent and longer-lasting outbreaks. Commonly called herpes.

**genital warts** Warts confined primarily to the moist skin of the genitals or around the anus. These warts are due to viruses belonging to the family of human papillomaviruses (HPVs) which are transmitted through sexual contact. The virus can also be transmitted from mother to baby during childbirth. Most people infected with HPV have no symptoms, but these viruses increase a woman's risk for cancer of the cervix. HPV infection is the most common sexually transmitted disease in the US. It is also the leading cause of abnormal PAP smears and precancerous changes of the cervix in women. There is no cure for HPV infection, although antiviral medications can reduce outbreaks and topical preparations can speed healing. Once contracted, the virus can stay with a person for life. Also known as condyloma acuminatum, condylomata.

**genitalia** The male or female reproductive organs. The genitalia include internal structures, such as the ovaries, and external structures, such as the penis.

**genitalia, female internal** The internal genital structures of the female, including the ovaries, the Fallopian tubes, the uterus, the cervix, and the vagina.

**genitourinary** Pertaining to the genital and urinary systems.

**genome** All the genetic information, the entire genetic complement, all the DNA possessed by any organism. There is, for example, the human genome, the elephant genome, the mouse genome, the yeast genome, the genome of a bacteria, and so on. Humans (and many other higher animals) actually have two genomes—a chromosomal genome and a mitochondrial genome—that together make up their genome.

**Genome Research Institute, National Human** See *National Human Genome Research Institute*.

**genome, chromosomal** All the genetic information in the chromosomes of an organism. For humans, that is all the DNA contained in our normal complement of 46 rod-like chromosomes in virtually every cell in the body. (Mature red blood cells, for one exception, have no nucleus and, therefore, no chromosomes.) The chromosomal genome is synonymous with the nuclear genome. Together with the mitochondrial genome, it constitutes the genome of the human being.

**genome, human** All the genetic information, the entire genetic complement, all the DNA in a person. Humanity's

DNA is the treasury of human inheritance. It is this extraordinary repository of genetic information that the Human Genome Project in the US, and comparable programs in other countries that belong to HUGO (the Human Genome Organization), are designed to fully fathom. See also *Human Genome Project*.

**genome, mitochondrial**   The sum of the genetic information contained in the chromosome of the mitochondrion, a structure located in the cytoplasm outside the nucleus of the cell where the better known complement of chromosomes resides. The mitochondrial genome is composed of mitochondrial DNA (mDNA), a double-stranded circular molecule that contains a limited number of genes. During fertilization mDNA is transmitted only by the mother. Together, the mitochondrial genome and the nuclear chromosomal genome constitute the entire human genome.

**genomic library**   A collection of clones made from a set of randomly generated overlapping DNA fragments, representing the entire genome of an organism.

**genotype**   The genetic constitution (genome) of a cell, an individual, or an organism. The genotype is distinct from its expressed features, or phenotype. The genotype of a person is that person's genetic makeup. It can pertain to all genes or to a specific gene.

**genu**   The Latin word for knee, as in genu recurvatum (hyperextension of the knee), genu valgum (knock knee), and genu varum (bowleg). See *knee*.

**GERD**   GastroEsophageal Reflux Disease.

**germ cell tumor**   A type of brain tumor.

**germ cells**   The eggs and sperm: the reproductive cells. Each mature germ cell is haploid, in that it has a single set of 23 chromosomes containing half the usual amount of DNA and half the usual number of genes. Except for the eggs and sperm, each cell in the human body contains the entire human genome.

**German measles**   See *rubella*.

**German measles immunization**   See *MMR*.

**germinoma**   A type of germ-cell tumor.

**gestalt therapy**   An older psychotherapeutic concept that stresses understanding mental processes as holistic entities (*gestalt*s) rather than discrete steps. Gestalt therapy often uses group therapy techniques to help patients gain this type of insight. See also *group therapy*.

**gestation**   From conception to birth.

**gestational diabetes**   See *diabetes, gestational*.

**giant cell arteritis**   See *arteritis, cranial*.

**giant platelet syndrome**   See *Bernard-Soulier syndrome*.

**gigantism**   **1** Extreme growth in height. Gigantism is usually associated with disorders of the pituitary gland, which secretes human growth hormone (somatotrophin) during childhood, before the bones fuse. **2** Extreme growth of specific body parts. See *gigantism, focal*.

**gigantism, eunuchoid**   A form of extreme growth caused by delayed onset of puberty. Treatment is with hormones.

**gigantism, focal**   Extreme growth of specific body parts, such as one arm, the tongue, or a combination of parts, as seen in Beckwith-Wiedemann syndrome or acromegaly. This type of gigantism may occur before or after the bones fuse. If it occurs afterward, it causes disfigurement. Surgery for mass reduction can help improve function, and other treatments may be available for specific conditions.

**gigantism, pituitary**   Extreme growth in height caused by oversecretion of the growth hormone (somatotrophin) by the anterior pituitary gland. Other symptoms include thickening of the skin, enlargement of the bones, and elongation of the jaw and other areas. Pituitary gigantism may be caused by an adenoma of the pituitary, a tumor of the pituitary, or other causes. Treatment is usually possible via hormones, surgery, or both. See also *acromegaly*.

**Gilbert disease**   See *Gilbert syndrome*.

**Gilbert syndrome**   A common but harmless genetic condition in which UDP-glucuronosyltransferase, a liver enzyme essential to the disposal of bilirubin, is abnormal. This enzyme abnormality causes mild elevations of bilirubin pigment in the blood, and the elevated bilirubin pigment can sometimes cause mild yellowing (jaundice) of the eyes. People with Gilbert syndrome are otherwise entirely normal, with no other signs or symptoms. Their liver enzyme levels in blood serum are entirely normal also. The gene for Gilbert syndrome has been mapped to chromosome 2. A single dose of the Gilbert gene is sufficient to produce Gilbert syndrome, so it is an autosomal dominant trait. People who have Gilbert syndrome have a 50 percent chance of transmitting the Gilbert gene to each of their children. There is no need for treatment in Gilbert syndrome, and the prognosis is excellent. Gilbert syndrome is found frequently in people in the US and Europe. It is usually detected by accident in the course of routine blood screening. Also known as Gilbert disease.

gingiva	The gums.

gingivitis	Gum disease with inflammation of the gums. On inspection, the gums will appear red and puffy, and will usually bleed during tooth-brushing or dental examination. Treatment is by improved cleaning, with more-frequent and longer brushing and flossing, and/or the use of electronic tooth-cleaning equipment. Antiseptic mouthwashes may also be recommended. See also *acute membranous gingivitis, gum disease.*

gingivitis, acute membranous	See *acute membranous gingivitis.*

gingivitis, acute necrotizing ulcerative	See *acute membranous gingivitis.*

gingivitis, fusospirillary	See *acute membranous gingivitis.*

gingivitis, fusospirochetal	See *acute membranous gingivitis.*

gingivitis, necrotizing	See *acute membranous gingivitis.*

gingivitis, phagedenic	See *acute membranous gingivitis.*

gingivitis, ulcerative	See *acute membranous gingivitis.*

gingivitis, Vincent	See *acute membranous gingivitis.*

gland	A group of cells that secrete a substance needed by the body.

gland, mammary	One of the glands within the breast that secrete milk when prompted to do so by special hormones. Mammary glands are slightly tender to the touch, and may become more so during menstruation or pregnancy. They become enlarged when engorged with milk. See also *mastitis.*

gland, parotid	See *parotid gland.*

gland, prostate	A gland in the male reproductive system, just below the bladder. It surrounds part of the urethra, the canal that empties the bladder. The prostate gland secretes an alkaline liquid that becomes part of the semen. See also *prostate enlargement; prostatitis.*

gland, sudoriferous	See *gland, sweat.*

gland, sweat	The sweat (sudoriferous) glands are small tubular structures situated in the subcutaneous tissue within and under the skin. They discharge sweat through tiny openings in the surface of the skin. The sweat itself is a transparent, colorless, acidic fluid that contains some fatty acids and mineral matter.

gland, thyroid	The thyroid gland is located in the lower part of the neck below the Adam's apple. It is wrapped around the windpipe (the trachea). It has the shape of a butterfly, since it is formed by two wings (lobes) attached by a middle part. Thyroid hormones are essential for the function of every cell in the body. They help regulate growth and the rate of chemical reactions (metabolism) in the body. The thyroid makes and stores hormones that help regulate heart rate, blood pressure, body temperature, and the rate at which food is converted into energy. Thyroid hormones also help children grow and develop. The thyroid uses iodine, a mineral found in some foods and in iodized salt, to make several of its hormones.

glands, Meibomian	Little glands in the eyelids that make a lubricant, which they discharge through tiny openings in the edges of the lids. The lubricant is a fatty substance called sebum, and is characteristic of sebaceous glands. The Meibomian glands can become inflamed, a condition termed meibomianitis or meibomitis. Chronic inflammation leads to cysts of the Meibomian glands, or chalazions. Also known as the palpebral glands, tarsal glands, or tarsoconjunctival glands. See also *cyst, Meibomian.*

glands, palpebral	See *glands, Meibomian.*

glands, sebaceous	Skin glands that empty an oily secretion called sebum into the hair follicles near the surface of the skin. Sebum helps to keep skin moist and protected. See also *cyst, sebaceous.*

glands, tarsal	See *glands, Meibomian.*

glandular fever	See *mononucleosis.* See also *Epstein-Barr virus.*

glans	1 The glans penis, the rounded head of the penis. 2 The rounded head of the clitoris.

glans and foreskin, inflammation of the	See *balanoposthitis.*

glans penis, inflammation of the	See *balanitis.*

glaucoma	An eye condition in which the fluid pressure inside the eye rises because of slowed fluid drainage from the eye. Untreated, it may damage the optic nerve and other parts of the eye, causing vision loss or even blindness. There are several types, including open-angle glaucoma and acute angle-closure glaucoma. Glaucoma treatment may include medication, surgery, or laser surgery. Eye drops or pills alone can usually control glaucoma, although they can't cure it. Some drugs are designed to reduce pressure by slowing the flow of fluid into the eye, while others help to improve fluid drainage. These drugs may stop working over time or cause side effects, so the eye-care professional may select other drugs, change the dose, or use other means to deal with the glaucoma. Surgery to help fluid escape from the eye was once extensively used, but except for laser surgery, it is now reserved for the most difficult cases. In laser surgery for glaucoma, a laser beam of light is focused on the part of the anterior chamber where the fluid leaves the eye. This results in a series of small changes, making it easier for fluid to exit. Over time, the effect of laser surgery may wear off.

**glaucoma detection**　The common "air puff" test is a simple measure of eye pressure administered in routine eye examinations. However, this screening test alone cannot detect glaucoma. Glaucoma is found most often during an eye examination after drops have been put into the eyes to dilate (enlarge) the pupils. This allows the eye-care professional to see more of the inside of the eye, and to check for physical signs of glaucoma.

**glaucoma, acute angle-closure**　See *acute angle-closure glaucoma.*

**glaucoma, angle-closure**　See *angle-closure glaucoma.*

**glaucoma, risk factors**　High-risk groups for glaucoma include everyone with a family history of glaucoma, everyone over the age of 60, and any African-American over the age of 40. Glaucoma is five times more likely to occur in African-Americans than in whites, and about four times more likely to cause blindness. Persons of Asian or Eskimo ancestry are at particularly high risk for developing angle-closure glaucoma. Patients belonging to a high-risk group for glaucoma should have their eyes examined through dilated pupils every two years by an eye-care professional.

**glaucoma, symptoms of**　There are no symptoms in the early stages of glaucoma. Vision stays normal, and there is no pain. As the disease progresses, however, a person with glaucoma may notice that side vision is gradually failing; objects in front may still be seen clearly, but objects to the side may be missed. As the disease worsens, the field of vision narrows, and blindness may result.

**gliaden**　A protein found in wheat and some other grains, which is part of the wheat gluten. People with celiac disease, Crohn disease, and related conditions may be sensitive to gliaden in the diet.

**glial cells**　The type of connective tissue found in the central nervous system, the glial cells make physical connections and bring in nutrients that support the neurons in their work. Each part of the CNS has its own special glial cells. These cells make up 40 percent of the brain and spinal cord.

**glioblastoma multiforme**　A highly malignant type of brain tumor that derives from glial cells. Early symptoms include sleepiness, headache, and vomiting.

**glioma**　Any brain tumor that begins in the glial cells in the brain.

**globe, pale**　See *globus pallidus.*

**globus**　The sensation of having a lump in the throat when nothing really is there. Although this symptom can be all in the patient's imagination, globus can also be a symptom of disease, such as reflux laryngitis. Also known as globus hystericus.

**globus hystericus**　See *globus.*

**globus major**　The head of the epididymis, the structure just behind the testis.

**globus minor**　The tail of the epididymis, a cordlike structure just behind the testis.

**globus pallidus**　A comparatively pale-looking, spherical area in the brain. The globus pallidus is specifically part of the lentiform nucleus, which in turn is part of the striate body, a component of the basal ganglia. Also called the pale globe, the palladum, and the paleostriatum.

**glossitis**　Inflammation of the tongue.

**glossolalia**　Nonsensical sounds that mimic the rhythms and inflections of actual speech. Glossolalia may be seen in deep sleep or in trance states. It is also the scientific term for the religious phenomena known as "speaking in tongues."

**glossopharyngeal nerve**　The ninth cranial nerve, which supplies the tongue, throat, and one of the salivary glands (the parotid gland). Problems with the glossopharyngeal nerve result in trouble tasting and swallowing.

**glottis**　The middle part of the larynx, where the vocal cords are located.

**glucocerebrosidase deficiency**　An enzyme deficiency that causes type 1 Gaucher disease. See *Gaucher disease.*

**glucocorticoid**　See *corticosteroid.*

**glucosamine** A molecule derived from the sugar glucose by the addition of an amino (NH2) group. Glucosamine is a component of a number of structures, including the blood group substances and cartilage. Glucosamine is currently in use as a nutritional supplement (often in combination with chondroitin) and is touted as a remedy for arthritic symptoms. Studies of human glucosamine use are still preliminary and inconclusive, although the results of animal studies have led to its widespread use among veterinarians.

**glucose** The simple sugar that is the chief source of energy. Found in the blood, it is the main sugar the body manufactures. The body makes glucose from all three elements of food—protein, fats, and carbohydrates—but the largest amount of glucose derives from carbohydrates. Glucose serves as the major source of energy for living cells. It is carried to each cell through the bloodstream. Cells cannot use glucose without the help of insulin, however. Also known as dextrose.

**glucose tolerance test** A test of carbohydrate metabolism much used in the diagnosis of diabetes, among other disorders. Abbreviated as GTT. After the patient has fasted overnight, but before breakfast, a specific amount (100 grams) of glucose is given by mouth, and the blood levels of this sugar are measured every hour. Normally, the blood glucose should return to normal within two to two and one-half hours. The GTT depends on a number of factors, including the ability of the intestine to absorb glucose, the power of the liver to take up and store glucose, the capacity of the pancreas to produce insulin, and the amount of "active" insulin.

**glucose, fasting blood** See *fasting blood glucose*.

**glucose-6-phosphate dehydrogenase** An enzyme that assists in deanimizing amino acids. Deficiency of G6PD is the commonest disease-causing enzyme defect in humans, affecting an estimated 400 million people. The G6PD gene is on the X chromosome. Males with the enzyme deficiency develop anemia due to breakup of their red blood cells when they are exposed to oxidant drugs such as the antimalarial primaquine, the sulfonamide antibiotics or sulfones, naphthalene moth balls, or fava beans. See also *favism*.

**glucosylceramidosis** See *Gaucher disease*.

**glucuronosyltransferase, UDP-** A liver enzyme essential to the disposal of bilirubin. An abnormality of UDP-glucuronosyltransferase results in a condition called Gilbert syndrome. See also *Gilbert syndrome*.

**gluteal** Pertaining to the buttock region, which is formed by the gluteus maximus, gluteus medius, and gluteus minimus muscles.

**gluten** A protein found in wheat or related grains. Gluten can be found in a large variety of processed foods, including soups, salad dressings, and natural flavorings. Unidentified starches, hydrolyzed proteins, and binders and fillers used in medications or vitamins can be unsuspected sources of gluten. People with celiac sprue, Crohn disease, or related disorders may need to avoid gluten products. See also *gliaden*.

**gluten enteropathy** See *celiac sprue*.

**glycosaminoglycans** Negatively charged chains of polysaccharides (modified sugars) that are composed of repeating disaccharide units. Better known by the abbreviation GAGs, important glycosaminoglycans in the human body include chondroitin sulfate, dermatan sulfate, heparan sulfate, heparin, hyaluronate, and keratan sulfate. They are involved as lubricants and components of bone, cartilage, blood vessels, and certain types of cells. Also known as mucopolysaccharides.

**glycosphingolipidoses** A group of hereditary diseases involving overproduction or accumulation of fatty substances called sphingolipids in the brain and nervous system. See also *Anderson-Fabry disease; Farber disease; Gaucher disease; histiocytosis, lipid; Krabbe disease, Landing disease; leukodystrophy, metachromatic; Tay-Sachs disease; Sandhoff disease*.

**GM2-gangliosidosis, B variant** See *Tay-Sachs disease*.

**GM2-gangliosidosis, type 1** See *Tay-Sachs disease*.

**goiter** Noncancerous enlargement of the thyroid gland. A goiter can be associated with normal, elevated (hyperthyroidism), or decreased (hypothyroidism) thyroid hormone levels in the blood.

**goiter, diffuse toxic** See *Graves disease*.

**goiter, exophthalmic** See *Graves disease*.

**goiter, iodide** Just as too little iodine can cause thyroid disease, so may prolonged intake of too much iodine lead to the development of goiter and abnormally low thyroid activity (hypothyroidism). Certain foods and medications contain large amounts of iodine. Examples include seaweed; iodine-rich expectorants (such as SSKI and Lugol solution) used in the treatment of cough, asthma, chronic pulmonary disease; and amiodarone (brand name: Cardorone), an iodine-rich medication used in the control of abnormal heart rhythms.

**goiter, toxic multinodular** A condition in which the thyroid gland contains multiple lumps (nodules) that are overactive and that produce excess thyroid hormones. Also known as Parry disease or Plummer disease.

**goiter-deafness syndrome**  See *Pendred syndrome*.

**golfer's cramp**  A dystonia that affects the muscles of the hand and sometimes the forearm, and only occurs when playing golf. Similar focal dystonias have also been called typist's cramp, pianist's cramp, musician's cramp, and writer's cramp.

**gonad**  A reproductive gland that produces germ cells (gametes): an ovary or testis.

**gonad, female**  See *ovary*.

**gonad, indifferent**  In embryonic life, the gonad in males and females is initially identical. This gonad is said to be "indifferent" before it differentiates into a definitive testis or ovary. An indifferent gonad becomes a testis if the embryo has a Y chromosome, but if the embryo has no Y chromosome, the indifferent gonad becomes an ovary. Thus, an XY chromosome complement leads to testes, while an XX chromosome complement leads to ovaries. People with just one X chromosome and no Y are females with Turner syndrome, and are infertile. The absence of a Y chromosome permits the indifferent gonad to become an ovary, but both X chromosomes are needed for the ovary to function normally.

**gonad, male**  The male gonad, the testicle (or testis), is one of a pair of reproductive glands located behind the penis in a pouch of skin (the scrotum). The testicles produce and store sperm, and they are also the body's main source of male hormones. These hormones control the development of the reproductive organs and other male characteristics, such as body and facial hair, low voice, and wide shoulders.

**gonadotropin**  Hormones that are secreted by the pituitary gland, and that affect the function of the male or female gonads. See *follicle-stimulating hormone, human chorionic gonadotropin, luteinizing hormone*.

**gonadotropin, human chorionic**  See *human chorionic gonadotropin*.

**gonorrhea**  A bacterial infection transmitted by sexual contact. Gonorrhea is one of the oldest known sexually transmitted diseases, and is caused by the Neisseria gonorrhoeae bacteria. Gonorrhea cannot be transmitted via toilet seats or other inanimate objects. Men with gonorrhea may have a yellowish discharge from the penis, accompanied by itching and burning. More than half of women with gonorrhea do not have any symptoms. If symptoms occur, they may include burning or frequent urination, yellowish vaginal discharge, redness and swelling of the genitals, and a burning or itching of the vaginal area. Untreated, gonorrhea can lead to severe pelvic infections, and even sterility. Complications in later

life can include inflammation of the heart valves, arthritis, and eye infections. Gonorrhea can also cause eye infections in babies born of infected mothers. From 25 to 40 percent of women with gonorrhea are also infected with another bacterial STD, chlamydia. Treatment of gonorrhea is with antibiotics.

**goose bumps**  A temporary local change in the skin that starts with a stimulus, such as cold or fear. That stimulus causes a nerve discharge from the sympathetic nervous system, which is part of the autonomic nervous system. The nerve discharge causes contraction of the hair erector muscles (arrectores pilorum), elevating the hair follicles above the rest of the skin. These tiny elevations are what we perceive as goose bumps. Some biologists believe that goose bumps evolved as part of the fight-or-flight reaction. A similar phenomenon, bristling, makes fur-covered animals look larger and more frightening. Also called cutis anserina, gooseflesh, horripilation.

**gooseflesh**  See *goose bumps*.

**Gottron sign**  A scaly, patchy redness over the knuckles seen in patients with dermatomyositis, an inflammatory muscle disorder. See *polymyositis*.

**gout**  A condition characterized by abnormally elevated levels of uric acid in the blood, recurring attacks of joint inflammation (arthritis), deposits of hard lumps of uric acid in and around the joints, and decreased kidney function and kidney stones. Uric acid is a breakdown product of purines, which are part of many foods we eat. The tendency to develop gout and elevated blood uric–acid levels (hyperuricemia) is often inherited, and can be promoted by obesity, weight gain, alcohol intake, high blood pressure, abnormal kidney function, and drugs. The most reliable diagnostic test for gout is the identification of crystals in joints, body fluids, and tissues. See also *gouty arthritis*.

**gout, tophaceous**  A form of chronic gout characterized by the deposit of nodular masses of uric acid crystals (tophi) in different soft tissue areas of the body. Even though tophi are most commonly found as hard nodules around the fingers, at the tips of the elbows, and around the big toe, tophi nodules can appear anywhere in the body. They have been reported in unexpected areas, such as in the ears, vocal cords, or around the spinal cord.

**gouty arthritis**  An attack of joint inflammation due to deposits of uric acid crystals in the joint fluid (synovial fluid) and joint lining (synovial lining). Intense joint inflammation occurs as white blood cells engulf the uric acid crystals, causing pain, heat, and redness of the joint tissues. The term "gout" commonly is used to refer to these painful arthritis attacks, but gouty arthritis is only one manifestation of gout.

**Gower syndrome**  See *syncope, situational*.

**graft**  Healthy skin, bone, or other tissue taken from one part of the body to replace diseased or injured tissue removed from another part of the body. For example, skin grafts can be used to cover areas of skin that have been burned.

**graft-versus-host disease**  A complication of bone marrow transplants in which the donor bone marrow attacks the host's organs and tissues. Graft-versus-host disease is seen most often in cases where the blood-marrow donor is unrelated to the patient, or when the donor is related to the patient but not a perfect match. Treatment is by immunotherapy. Although this can be a life-threatening condition, it can also be beneficial for patients with leukemia. Abbreviated as GVHD.

**grand mal seizure**  See *seizure, tonic-clonic; seizure disorders*.

**granular leukocyte**  See *granulocyte*.

**granulation**  That part of the healing process in which lumpy, pink tissue containing new connective tissue and capillaries forms around the edges of a wound. Granulation of a wound is normal and desirable.

**granulocyte**  A type of white blood cell filled with microscopic granules, little sacs containing enzymes that digest microorganisms. Granulocytes are part of the innate immune system, and have somewhat nonspecific, broad-based activity. They do not respond exclusively to specific antigens, as do B-cells and T-cells. Neutrophils, eosinophils, and basophils are all types of granulocytes. They are named by the staining features of their granules in the laboratory: Neutrophils have subtle, "neutral" granules; eosinophils have prominent granules that stain readily with the acid dye eosin; and basophils have prominent granules that stain readily with basic (nonacidic) dyes. These classifications date back to a time when certain structures could be identified in cells by histochemistry, but the functions of these intracellular structures were still not known. However, these classifications are still widely used.

**granulocytopenia**  A marked decrease in the number of granulocytes, resulting in a syndrome of frequent chronic bacterial infections of the skin, lungs, throat, and so on. Granulocytopenia can be genetic and inherited, or it can be acquired as, for example, an aspect of leukemia. Granulocytopenia can more specifically involve neutropenia (shortage of neutrophils), eosinopenia (shortage of eosinophils), and/or basopenia (shortage of basophils).

The term neutropenia is sometimes used interchangeably with granulocytopenia. See also *agranulocytosis; agranulocytosis, infantile genetic; neutropenia; severe congenital neutropenia*.

**granuloma**  One of several forms of localized, nodular inflammation found in tissues. Granulomas have a typical pattern when examined under a microscope. They can be caused by a variety of biologic, chemical, and physical irritants of tissue. See also *granuloma, calcified; granuloma, fish bowl*.

**granuloma, calcified**  A granuloma containing calcium deposits. Since it usually takes some time for calcium to be deposited in a granuloma, a calcified granuloma is generally assumed to be an old granuloma.

**granuloma, fish bowl**  Localized nodular skin inflammation (small, reddish, raised areas of skin) caused by a bacterium called mycobacterium marinum. Fish bowl granuloma is typically acquired by occupational or recreational exposure to salt or fresh water; often it is the result of minor trauma during the care of aquariums. The diagnosis is suggested by the history of exposure, and confirmed by culturing tissue specimens which yield the microscopic organism, mycobacterium marinum. The infection can be treated with a variety of antibiotics, including doxycycline, minocycline, clarithromycin, rifampin, and trimethoprim-sulfamethoxazole. Also known as swimming pool granuloma.

**granuloma, swimming pool**  See *granuloma, fish bowl*.

**granulomatosis, allergic**  See *Churg-Strauss syndrome*.

**granulomatosis, Wegener**  An inflammatory disease of small arteries and veins (vasculitis) that classically involves vessels supplying the tissues of the lungs, nasal passages (sinuses), and kidneys. Symptoms include fatigue, weight loss, fevers, shortness of breath, bloody sputum, joint pains, and sinus inflammation, sometimes with nasal ulcerations and bloody nasal discharge. Wegener granulomatosis most commonly affects young or middle-aged adults. The diagnosis of Wegener granulomatosis is confirmed by finding evidence of vasculitis and abnormal cellular formations called granulomas on biopsy of tissue involved by the inflammatory process. Wegener granulomatosis is a serious disease. Without treatment, it can be fatal within months. Treatment is directed toward stopping the inflammation process by suppressing the immune system.

**granulomatous colitis**  Crohn disease of the colon. See *Crohn disease*.

**Graves disease** The most common cause of hyperthyroidism (too much thyroid hormone), Graves disease is due to generalized overactivity of an enlarged thyroid gland, or goiter. There are three components to Graves disease: hyperthyroidism, protrusion of the eyes (ophthalmopathy), and skin lesions (dermopathy). Ophthalmopathy can cause sensitivity to light and a "sandy" feeling in the eyes. With further protrusion of the eyes, double vision and vision loss may occur. The ophthalmopathy tends to worsen with smoking. Dermopathy is a rare, painless, reddish lumpy skin rash that occurs on the front of the leg. Graves disease can run in families. Factors that can trigger Graves disease include stress, smoking, radiation to the neck, medications (such as interleukin-2 and interferon-alpha), and infectious organisms such as viruses. Graves disease can be diagnosed by a typical thyroid scan (diffuse increase uptake); by finding the characteristic triad of ophthalmopathy, dermopathy, and hyperthyroidism; or by testing the blood for thyroid-stimulating immunoglobulin (TSI) and finding abnormally high levels. Treatment is with antithyroid medications, removal of thyroid tissue via surgery (subtotal thyroidectomy), or radioiodine (RAI). Also known as diffuse toxic goiter.

**gravid** Pregnant.

**gray matter** The cortex of the brain, which contains nerve cell bodies. The gray matter is so named in contrast to the white matter, the part of the brain that contains myelinated nerve fibers.

**Gray's Anatomy** A book entitled *Anatomy Descriptive and Surgical,* by Henry Gray, appeared in 1858. Little could Dr. Gray have suspected that his textbook of human anatomy would still be in print today, and perhaps the best known of all medical books. Known as "Gray's Anatomy" to generations of medical students, the book is a scientific and artistic masterpiece. Gray let the natural beauty and grace of the body's interconnected systems and structures shine forth. The illustrations are superb; the text is clear (and, some might say, dull). It is one of the great reference works of all time, used by physicians, students, artists, and anyone interested in human anatomy.

**Great Plague** The "Great Plague" that swept London in 1665 was probably not really the plague, but rather typhus. The plague was a highly contagious, infectious, virulent, devastating disease caused by the Yersinia pestis bacteria, which mainly infects rats and other rodents that serve as the prime reservoir for the bacteria. Fleas function as the prime vectors, carrying the bacteria from one species to another. The fleas bite the rodents infected with Y. pestis, and then the fleas bite people. Transmission of the plague to people can also occur from eating infected animals, such as squirrels. Once someone has the plague,

they can transmit it to another person via aerosol droplets. See also *bubonic plague, typhus*.

**great saphenous vein** The larger of the two saphenous veins, the principal veins that run up the leg near the surface. The great saphenous vein goes from the foot all the way up to the saphenous opening, an oval aperture in the broad fascia of the thigh. The vein then passes through this fibrous membrane. Also called the large saphenous vein.

**greenstick fracture** See *fracture, greenstick*.

**groin** The area where the thigh meets the hip.

**gross anatomy** See *anatomy, gross*.

**gross hematuria** See *hematuria, gross*.

**Group A strep** See *streptococcus pyogenes*.

**Group B strep** See *streptococcus, group B*.

**group therapy** 1 A type of psychiatric care in which several patients meet with one or more therapists at the same time. Patients form a support group for each other as well as receiving expert care and advice. The group therapy model is particularly appropriate for psychiatric illnesses that are support-intensive, such as anxiety disorders, but is not well-suited for treatment of some other psychiatric disorders. 2 A type of psychoanalysis in which patients analyze each other with the assistance of one or more psychotherapists, as in an "encounter group." See also *gestalt therapy*.

**growing pains** Mysterious pains in growing children, usually in the legs. These pains are similar to what the weekend gardener suffers from on Monday: an overuse problem. If children exceed their regular threshold in playing, they will be sore, just as adults are sore. Growing pains are typically somewhat diffuse, and are not associated with physical changes of the area, such as swelling or redness. The pains usually are easily relieved by massage, acetaminophen, or rest. If pain persists for over a week or there are physical changes, the child should be seen by a physician.

**gtt.** Abbreviation for drops, as of a liquid medication. See also *Appendix A, "Prescription Abbreviations."*

**guanine** One member of the base pair guanine-cytosine (G-C) in DNA.

**guarding, abdominal** See *abdominal guarding*.

**guided imagery** An alternative medicine technique in which patients use their imagination to visualize improved health, or to "attack" a disease, such as a tumor. Some studies indicate that the positive thinking can have an effect on disease outcome, so this technique is now utilized as complementary medicine in some oncology centers and other medical facilities.

**Guillain-Barre syndrome** A disorder characterized by progressive symmetrical paralysis and loss of reflexes, usually beginning in the legs. In most cases the patient has a complete or nearly complete recovery. The paralysis characteristically involves more than one limb, most commonly the legs, is progressive, and usually ascending. There is areflexia (loss of reflexes) or hyporeflexia (diminution of reflexes) in the legs and arms. Guillain-Barre syndrome is not associated with fever. Usually occurring after a respiratory infection, it is apparently caused by a misdirected immune response that results in the direct destruction of the myelin sheath surrounding the peripheral nerves, or of the axon of the nerve itself. The syndrome sometimes follows other triggering events, including vaccinations. Among the vaccines reportedly associated with Guillain-Barre syndrome are the 1976–1977 swine flu vaccine, oral poliovirus vaccine, and tetanus toxoid. Aside from vaccinations, infection with the bacteria Campylobacter jejuni, and viral infections can trigger Guillain-Barre syndrome. Other conditions that may mimic Guillain-Barre need to be ruled out before diagnosis is made. Treatment is by plasmapheresis or intravenous gamma globulin (IVIG). See also *demyelination, Landry ascending paralysis.*

**gum disease** Inflammation of the soft tissue (gingiva) and abnormal loss of bone that surrounds the teeth and holds them in place. Gum disease is caused by toxins secreted by bacteria in the hard substance called plaque that accumulates over time along the gum line. Plaque is a mixture of food, saliva, and bacteria. Early symptoms of gum disease include gum bleeding without pain. Pain is a symptom of more advanced gum disease, as the loss of bone around the teeth leads to the formation of gum pockets. Bacteria in these pockets cause gum infection, swelling, pain, and further bone destruction. Advanced gum disease can cause loss of otherwise healthy teeth. See also *acute membranous gingivitis, gingivitis.*

**gustatory sweating** See *sweating, gustatory.*

**Guthrie test** Blood test for phenylketonuria (PKU). See *phenylketonuria.*

**gutta percha** A natural material derived from tree sap that can be formed to various shapes under heat. As it does not cause allergic reactions, it is often used to pack the empty spaces left when a root canal is performed.

**GVHD** Graft-versus-host disease.

**gyn** Short for gynecology and gynecologist.

**gynecoid** Like a woman, womanly, female.

**gynecoid obesity** Overweight with fat distribution generally characteristic of a woman, with the largest accumulation around the hips, and so on.

**gynecoid pelvis** A pelvis that is generally characteristic of a woman in its bone structure, and therefore its shape. The gynecoid pelvis is more delicate, wider, and not as high as the male pelvis. The angle of the female pubic arch is wide and round. The female sacrum is wider than the male's, and the iliac bone is flatter. The pelvic basin of the female is more spacious and less funnel-shaped. From a purely anatomic viewpoint, the female pelvis is better suited to accommodate the fetus during pregnancy and to permit the baby to be born.

**gynecologic oncologist** A doctor who specializes in treating cancers of the female reproductive organs.

**gynecologist** A doctor who specializes in treating diseases of the female reproductive organs, and providing well-woman health care that focuses primarily on the reproductive organs. In some health plans and HMOs, women may choose to see a gynecologist as their primary care physician, in which case he or she will also provide routine medical care or referrals.

**gynecology** The branch of medicine particularly concerned with the health of the female organs of reproduction.

**gynecomastia** Excessive development of the male breasts. Temporary enlargement of the breasts is not unusual or abnormal in boys during adolescence or during recovery from malnutrition. Gynecomastia may be abnormal as, for example, in Klinefelter syndrome.

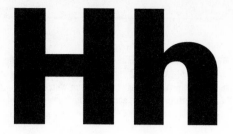

**H and H**   Popular shorthand for hemoglobin and hematocrit, two very common and important blood tests. Sometimes written as H&H.

**H and P**   Medical shorthand for history and physical: the initial clinical evaluation and examination of the patient.

**H. flu**   See *Haemophilus influenzae type B*.

**H. flu immunization**   See *Haemophilus influenzae type B immunization*.

**H. heilmannii**   Helicobacter heilmannii.

**Haemophilus influenzae type B**   Abbreviated as HIB, a bacteria capable of causing a range of diseases, including ear infections, soft tissue infection (cellulitis), upper respiratory infections, and pneumonia; as well as such serious, invasive infections as meningitis with potential brain damage, and epiglottitis with airway obstruction. More than 90 percent of all HIB infections occur in children 5 years of age or younger—the peak attack rate is at 6 to 12 months of age. See also *Haemophilus influenzae type B immunization*.

**Haemophilus influenzae type B immunization**   An immunization designed to prevent diseases caused by Haemophilus influenzae type B (HIB). In the US, the HIB vaccine is usually given at two, four, and six months of age, with a final booster at 12 to 15 months of age. The HIB vaccine rarely causes severe reactions, and it has almost eradicated HIB-related diseases in children. Before the vaccine, some 20,000 cases of HIB invasive disease in preschool children were reported every year in the US, compared to fewer than 300 cases after the advent of the vaccine. The HIB vaccine joins (conjugates) sugars from the HIB bacteria with a protein from another bacteria. The protein stimulates the baby's immature immune cells to produce antibodies to the HIB sugars, protecting the child from HIB infection.

**hair follicle**   See *follicles*.

**hair, exclamation point**   See *exclamation point hair*. See also *alopecia areata*.

**hair, lanugal**   See *lanugo*.

**hairball**   A wad of swallowed hair. Hairballs sometimes cause blockage of the digestive system, especially at the exit of the stomach. Interestingly, in some Asian cultures hairballs are felt to have medicinal properties. Also called a trichobezoar.

**hairy cell leukemia**   See *leukemia, hairy cell*.

**hallux**   The big toe.

**hallux valgus**   The big toe (hallux) is bent outward (valgus) so that it overlaps the second toe. Hallux valgus may be accompanied by a bunion (localized painful swelling), and is frequently associated with inflammation. It can be related to inflammation of the nearby bursa (bursitis) or degenerative joint disease (osteoarthritis).

**hallux varus**   An inward bending (varus) of the joint of the big toe.

**hammer toe**   A flexed (curly) toe, but with no abnormal rotation of the toe. May require surgical correction.

**hamstrings**   The prominent tendons at the back of the knee. They are the sidewalls of the hollow behind the knee (the popliteal space). Both hamstrings connect to muscles that flex the knee. A pulled hamstring is a common athletic injury.

**hand-foot-and-mouth disease**   A viral syndrome with a rash on the hands and feet and in the mouth. The internal rash (enanthem) consists of blisters and little ulcers. These may involve not only the lining of the mouth, but also the gums, palate, and tongue. The external rash on the body (exanthem) typically affects the hands, feet, and sometimes the buttocks. There may also be sore throat, irritability, decreased appetite, and fever. Hand-foot-and-mouth disease is caused by various viruses, including several types of coxsackievirus: most often Coxsackievirus A16, but also Coxsackieviruses A5, A9, A10, B1 and B3, or enterovirus 71. The incubation period is short, on the order of four to six days. The disease is most frequent in summer and fall. The rate of clinical expression in hand-foot-and-mouth disease is high, with the enanthem-exanthem pattern evident in nearly 100 percent of preschoolers, nearly 40 percent of school-age children, and about 10 percent of adults. The illness is characteristically mild and self-limited, and is usually over and done within a week when due to Coxsackievirus A16. In outbreaks due to enterovirus 71, the illness may be more severe, with such complications as viral meningitis, encephalitis, and paralytic disease. Also called hand-foot-and-mouth syndrome; or hand, foot, and mouth disease or syndrome.

**hand-foot-and-mouth syndrome**   See *hand-foot-and-mouth disease*.

**Hand-Schuller-Christian disease**   See *histiocytosis, histiocytosis X*.

**Hansen disease**  See *leprosy*.

**hantavirus**  A group of viruses that cause hemorrhagic fever and pneumonia. The hantaviruses include the hantaan virus that causes Korean (and Manchurian) hemorrhagic fever. Hantaviruses are transmitted to humans by direct or indirect contact with the saliva and excreta of rodents, such as deer mice, field mice, and ground voles.

**hantavirus pulmonary syndrome**  A severe lung condition caused by hantavirus infection. In 1993, this disease struck the Four Corners area (where the states of Arizona, New Mexico, Nevada, and Utah meet) with devastating, frequently fatal consequences. As the name indicates, it is due to a hantavirus. The HPS outbreak in Four Corners followed two years of more rain, more foliage, and more deer mice than usual. Abbreviated as HPS.

**haploid**  A set of chromosomes with only one member of each chromosome pair. The sperm and egg are haploid and, in humans, have 23 chromosomes.

**hard measles**  See *measles*.

**hard palate**  The first section of the bony part of the roof of the mouth, located in front of the soft palate.

**Hardy-Weinberg law**  A basic concept in population genetics, the Hardy-Weinberg law relates the gene frequency to the genotype frequency. It can be used, for example, to determine allele frequency and heterozygote frequency when the incidence of a genetic disorder is known.

**Hashimoto disease**  A progressive disease of the thyroid gland characterized by the presence of antibodies in the bloodstream that are directed against the thyroid, and by infiltration of the thyroid gland by lymphoctes (white blood cells activated by the immune system). Hashimoto disease predominantly affects women, and can be inherited. Also known as autoimmune thyroiditis, Hashimoto thyroiditis.

**HAV**  Hepatitis A virus.

**Havrix**  A vaccine made of killed hepatitis A virus, intended to stimulate the body's immune system to produce antibodies against the hepatitis A virus.

**hay fever**  A seasonal allergy to airborne particles, characterized by runny, itchy nose and eyes; sneezing, itchy throat, excess mucus, and nasal congestion. It is not caused by hay, nor does it produce a fever. See also *allergic rhinitis*.

**Hb**  Standard abbreviation for hemoglobin.

**HBIG**  Hepatitis B immune globulin, which contains antibodies to hepatitis B virus. HBIG offers prompt, but short-lived, protection against infection with the virus. It may be given in cases of accidents that carry a transmission risk, as when health-care workers get a needle stick.

**HBO**  Hyperbaric oxygen. See *hyperbaric oxygen therapy*.

**HBV**  Hepatitis B virus.

**HCFA**  The Health Care Finance Administration, the part of the US Department of Health and Human Services (HHS) responsible for administering Medicare and Medicaid. See also *Medicare, Medicaid*.

**hCG**  Human chorionic gonadotropin.

**HCM**  Hypertrophic cardiomyopathy.

**Hct**  Abbreviation for hematocrit.

**HCV**  Hepatitis C virus.

**HDL**  High-density lipoprotein.

**HDL cholesterol**  Lipoproteins, which are combinations of fats (lipids) and proteins, are the form in which lipids are transported in the blood. High-density lipoproteins (HDLs) transport cholesterol from the tissues of the body to the liver, so it can be gotten rid of in the bile. HDL cholesterol is therefore considered the "good" cholesterol: The higher the HDL cholesterol level, the lower the risk of coronary artery disease.

**HDV**  Hepatitis D virus.

**head bones**  See *bones of the head*.

**head lice**  *Pediculus humanus capitis,* parasitic insects found on the heads of people. Head lice are most commonly found on the scalp behind the ears, and near the neckline at the back of the neck. Head lice hold on to hair with hook-like claws at the end of each of their six legs. Head lice are rarely found on the body, eyelashes, or eyebrows. These insects lay their sticky, white eggs on the hair shaft close to the root, while hatched lice stay mostly on the scalp.

**head lice infestation**  The condition of being infested with head lice, also called pediculosis. Head lice infection is very common and easily acquired by coming in close contact with someone who has head lice, infested clothing, or infested belongings. Preschool and elementary-age children and their families are infested most often. Girls acquire head lice more often than boys, women more than men. African-Americans rarely have head lice.

Symptoms of head lice infestation include a tickling feeling of something moving in the hair, itching caused by an allergic reaction to the bites, irritability, and sores on the head caused by scratching. Although the lice are very small, they can be seen on the scalp when they move. The eggs (nits) are easily seen on the hair shaft. Treatment is by a combination of topical insecticidal medication and manual removal of all nits with a lice comb or the fingers. Baby oil can make this job easier. Both medication and complete nit removal are necessary to prevent reinfestation. All clothing, bedding, and furniture surfaces must also be washed or sprayed with insecticide. Note that pyrethin-based medications such as 1 percent lindane solution (brand name: Qwell) contain benzene, which can be toxic to brain tissue and has been linked to childhood leukemia. For this reason these medications are no longer generally recommended for use as a treatment for head lice.

**headache**   A pain in the head. A headache can have many causes. Causes include muscle tension, swollen blood vessels (as in a vascular, or migraine, headache), medications, allergies, sinus infection or pressure, exertion, hormonal cycles, or even inflammation of the brain or a brain tumor. Treatment depends on the type and severity of the headache, and on the age of the patient.

**headache, cervicogenic**   A headache that has its origins in the muscles, tendons, and nerves of the neck. It may be a simple tension headache, or it may result from actual damage to neck joints, ligaments, muscles, tendons, or the trigeminal nerve. Treatment for chronic cervicogenic headaches includes massage, physical therapy, analgesic medication, and in some extreme cases, injected nerve-block medication or surgery. See also *headache, tension*.

**headache, cluster**   See *cluster headache*.

**headache, febrile**   A headache associated with fever. Because this can sometimes indicate inflammation of the brain, as in encephalitis, see your doctor immediately if you experience this type of headache.

**headache, migraine**   See *migraine headache*.

**headache, muscle tension**   See *headache, tension*.

**headache, rebound**   Headaches experienced by those who have taken ergotamine or analgesic medications for migraines or other health conditions, and who have built up a tolerance for these medications. Often the headache occurs right after the medication wears off. Treatment is by using the medication less frequently, or switching to a different pain reliever. Some patients with acute ergotamide rebound headaches find relief with injected phenothiazine or long-acting steroid medication.

**headache, sinus**   A headache caused by pressure within the sinus cavities of the head, usually in connection with sinus infection. The sufferer has pain and tenderness in the sinus area, discharge from the nose, and sometimes a swollen face. Vascular headaches are often mistaken for sinus headaches. Treatment is by treating the underlying condition, which is often an allergic reaction, and by nasal vasoconstrictors and analgesic medication, such as aspirin (in adults only), acetaminophen, ibuprofen, or naproxen sodium. Analgesics containing caffeine may be stronger.

**headache, stress**   See *headache, tension*.

**headache, tension**   A headache caused by contraction of the muscles in the back of the neck, on the scalp, and sometimes in the jaw. Tension headaches are usually related to stress. Treatment is via stress reduction, massage, and analgesic medication, such as aspirin (in adults only), acetaminophen, ibuprofen, or naproxen sodium. Analgesics containing caffeine may be stronger. For chronic tension headaches, some doctors recommend tricyclic antidepressants, such as amitriptyline, which work to defuse stress and to lessen pain. Also called muscle tension headache, stress headache.

**headache, thunderclap**   A sudden and excruciatingly painful headache. Some doctors feel that in the absence of a known headache disorder, such as migraines, a thunderclap headache may sometimes signal a ruptured aneurysm in the brain. See your physician immediately if you experience this type of headache.

**headache, vascular**   A group of headaches felt to involve abnormal sensitivity of the blood vessels (arteries) in the brain to various triggers, resulting in rapid changes in the artery size due to spasm (constriction). Other arteries in the brain and scalp then open (dilate), and throbbing pain is perceived in the head. Migraine headaches are the most common type of vascular headache. See also *migraine headache*.

**health**   As officially defined by the World Health Organization, a state of complete physical, mental, and social well-being, not merely the absence of disease or infirmity.

**Health and Human Services**   See *HHS*.

**Health Care Finance Administration**   See *HCFA*.

**health care proxy**   An advance medical directive in the form of a legal document designates another person (a proxy) to make health care decisions in case you are rendered incapable of making your own wishes known. The health care proxy has, in essence, the same rights to request or refuse treatment that you would have if you were capable of making and communicating decisions.

**health outcomes research**   Research that measures the value of a particular course of therapy.

**health, child**   See *child health*. See also *pediatrics*.

**heart**   The muscle that pumps blood received from veins into arteries throughout the body. It is positioned in the chest behind the sternum (breastbone); in front of the trachea, esophagus, and aorta; and above the diaphragm muscle that separates the chest and abdominal cavities. The normal heart is about the size of a closed fist, and weighs about 10.5 ounces. It is cone-shaped, with the point of the cone pointing down to the left. Two-thirds of the heart lies in the left side of the chest, with the balance in the right chest. The heart is composed of specialized cardiac muscle, and it is four-chambered, with a right atrium and ventricle, and an anatomically separate left atrium and ventricle. The blood flows from the systemic veins into the right atrium, thence to the right ventricle, from which it is pumped to the lungs, then returned into the left atrium, thence to the left ventricle, from which it is driven into the systemic arteries. The heart is thus functionally composed of two hearts: the right heart and the left heart. The right heart consists of the right atrium, which receives deoxygenated blood from the body, and the right ventricle which pumps it to the lungs under low pressure; and the left heart, which consists of the left atrium, which receives oxygenated blood from the lung, and the left ventricle, which pumps it out to the body under high pressure.

**heart attack**   See *cardiac arrest*. See also *myocardial infarction, acute*.

**heart block**   A block in the conduction of the normal electrical impulses in the heart.

**heart conduction system**   See *cardiac conduction system*.

**heart failure**   Inability of the heart to keep up with the demands on it and, specifically, failure of the heart to pump blood with normal efficiency. When this occurs, the heart is unable to provide adequate blood flow to other organs. Heart failure may be due to failure of the right or left or both ventricles. Signs and symptoms depend on which side of the heart is failing. They can include shortness of breath (dyspnea), asthma due to the heart (cardiac asthma), pooling of blood (stasis) in the general body (systemic) circulation or in the liver's (portal) circulation, swelling (edema), blueness or duskiness (cyanosis), and enlargement (hypertrophy) of the heart. There are many causes of congestive heart failure, including coronary artery disease leading to heart attacks and

heart muscle weakness; primary heart muscle weakness from viral infections or toxins, such as prolonged alcohol exposure; heart valve disease, causing heart muscle weakness due to too much leaking of blood, or heart muscle stiffness from a blocked valve; and hypertension (high blood pressure). Rarer causes include hyperthyroidism (high thyroid hormone), vitamin deficiency, and excess amphetamine ("speed") use. The aim of therapy is to improve the pumping function of the heart. General treatment includes salt restriction, diuretics to get rid of excess fluid, digoxin to strengthen the heart, and other medications. Specific treatment of congestive heart failure needs to be directed toward the specific underlying cause of the problem.

**heart murmur**   An unusual, "whooshing" heart sound, which may be innocent, or may reflect disease or malformation. It is created by blood flow through heart valves, by blood flow through chamber narrowings, or by unusual connections seen with congenital heart disease. It is usually heard by the doctor, while he or she listens to the chest with a stethoscope.

**heart rate**   The number of heartbeats per unit of time, usually per minute. The heart rate is based on the number of contractions of the ventricles (the lower chambers of the heart). The heart rate may be too fast (tachycardia) or too slow (bradycardia). The pulse is a bulge of an artery from waves of blood that course through the blood vessels each time the heart beats. The pulse is often taken at the wrist to estimate the heart rate.

**heart septum**   The septum of the heart is the dividing wall between the right and left sides of the heart. That portion of the septum that separates the right and left atria of the heart is termed the atrial or interatrial septum, whereas the portion of the septum that lies between the right and left ventricles of the heart is called the ventricular or interventricular septum.

**heart transplant**   A painstaking operation in which a diseased or malfunctioning heart is replaced with a healthy donor heart taken from a deceased person.

**heart valves**   There are four heart valves, and all are one-way valves. Blood entering the heart first passes through the tricuspid valve, and then the pulmonary valve. After returning from the lungs, the blood passes through the mitral (bicuspid) valve, and exits via the aortic valve.

**heart ventricle**   One of the two lower chambers of the heart. The right ventricle receives blood from the right atrium and pumps it into the lungs via the pulmonary artery, while the left ventricle receives blood from the left atrium and pumps it into the circulation system via the aorta.

**heart, artificial**   A man-made heart used to replace a diseased or malfunctioning heart when a donor organ is not available.

**heart, left**   The left atrium and left ventricle.

**Heart, Lung, and Blood Institute, National**   See *National Institutes of Health*.

**heart, right**   The right atrium and right ventricle.

**heartburn**   Heartburn has nothing to do with the heart. It is an uncomfortable feeling of burning and warmth that occurs in waves, rising up behind the breastbone (sternum) and moving toward the neck. It is usually due to gastroesophageal reflux, the return of stomach acid into the esophagus.

**heart-lung machine**   A machine that does the work both of the heart and of the lungs: pumping and oxygenating blood. Blood returning to the heart is diverted through the machine before being returned to the arterial circulation. Such machines may be used during open heart surgery. Also called a pump-oxygenator.

**heat prostration**   See *hyperthermia*.

**heatstroke**   See *hyperthermia*.

**Heberden disease**   **1** Angina pectoris, chest pain that is often severe and crushing, due to an inadequate supply of oxygen to the heart muscle. See *angina*. **2** Osteoarthritis of the small joints with nodules (Heberden nodes) in and about the last joint of the finger.

**Heberden node**   A small fixed bump on the finger, at the last joint of the finger, a Heberden node is a calcified spur of the joint (articular) cartilage, and is associated with osteoarthritis.

**Hecht syndrome**   An inherited disorder transmitted as an autosomal dominant trait, in which short, tight muscles make it impossible to open the mouth fully or keep the fingers straight when the hand is flexed back. The small mouth creates feeding problems. The hands may be so tightly fisted that infants with Hecht syndrome crawl on their knuckles. Also called trismus pseudocamptodactyly syndrome.

**heel bone**   See *bone, heel*.

**heel spur**   A bony spur projecting from the back or underside of the heel that can make walking painful. Spurs at the back of the heel are associated with inflammation of the Achilles tendon (Achilles tendinitis), and cause tenderness and pain at the back of the heel, made worse by pushing off the ball of the foot. Spurs under the sole (in the plantar area) are associated with inflammation of the plantar fascia, the bowstring-like tissue stretching from the heel underneath the sole. These spurs cause localized tenderness and pain that is made worse by stepping down on the heel. Not all heel spurs cause symptoms. Some are discovered on X-rays taken for other purposes. Heel spurs and plantar fasciitis can occur alone or be related to underlying diseases that cause arthritis, such as Reiter disease, ankylosing spondylitis, or diffuse idiopathic skeletal hyperostosis. Treatment is designed to decrease inflammation and avoid reinjury. Icing reduces pain and inflammation. Anti-inflammatory agents, such as ibuprofen or injections of cortisone, can help. Heel lifts reduce stress on the Achilles tendon and relieve painful spurs at the back of the heel. Donut-shaped shoe inserts take pressure off plantar spurs. Surgery is occasionally done on chronically inflamed spurs.

**Heimlich maneuver**   An emergency procedure used in cases of airway obstruction, as when a piece of food is lodged in a person's windpipe, causing choking. To perform the Heimlich maneuver, stand behind the person who is choking and wrap your arms around his or her waist, placing one fist just below the breastbone with the thumb side toward the person's abdomen. Place your other hand over this first and use it to pull sharply into the top of the choking person's stomach. Repeat as necessary. If the Heimlich maneuver is unsuccessful, an emergency tracheostomy may be necessary to prevent suffocation. See also *airway obstruction, tracheostomy*.

**Helicobacter heilmannii**   A bacteria that infects most cats, dogs, and pigs, causing them stomach inflammation (gastritis). H. heilmannii is not usually transmitted from animals to people, but people who have been infected by H. heilmannii are known to have developed gastric ulcers. Antibiotics can cure H. heilmannii infections.

**Helicobacter pylori**   Bacteria that cause stomach inflammation (gastritis) and ulcers in the stomach. This bacteria, the most common cause of ulcers worldwide, is often referred to as H. pylori. H. pylori infection may be acquired from contaminated food and water, or through person-to-person contact. It is common in people who live in crowded conditions with poor sanitation. In the US, 30 percent of the adult population is infected. One out of six patients with H. pylori infection develops ulcers of the duodenum or the stomach. This bacteria is also believed to be associated with stomach cancer and a rare type of lymph gland tumor called gastric MALT lymphoma. Infected persons usually carry H. pylori indefinitely, unless treated with medications to eradicate the bacteria.

**HELLP syndrome**   A combination of breakage of red blood cells (hemolysis; the "H" in the acronym), elevated liver enzymes (EL), and low platelet count (LP). The

HELLP syndrome is a recognized complication of preeclampsia and eclampsia (toxemia) of pregnancy, occurring in 25 percent of these pregnancies. Common symptoms in women with the HELLP syndrome include a general sense of feeling unwell (malaise), nausea and/or vomiting, and pain in the upper abdomen. Increased fluid in the tissues (edema) is also frequent. Protein is found in the urine of most women with the HELLP syndrome. Blood pressure may be elevated. Occasionally, coma can result from seriously low blood sugar (hypoglycemia). The first order of treatment is management of blood-clotting issues. If HELLP syndrome develops at or after 34 weeks of gestation, fetal growth is restricted, the fetus' lungs are mature, or the mother's health is in jeopardy, urgent delivery is the treatment. After delivery, the mother's status is monitored closely. HELLP syndrome can be complicated by liver rupture, anemia, bleeding, and death. HELLP syndrome can also develop during the early period after delivery of a baby. Women with a history of HELLP syndrome are considered at increased risk for complications in future pregnancies.

**helper T cells**  See *T-4 cells.*

**helper/supressor ratio**  The ratio of T-helper (T-4) cells to supressor (T-8) cells in the bloodstream. Results of testing for each type are compared to gauge the progress of HIV infection (AIDS). Both types of cells are helpful to the immune response, so as levels of both decline, the prognosis worsens.

**hemangioma**  A birth irregularity in which a localized tissue mass (tumor) becomes rich in small blood vessels. The hemangioma may be visible through the skin as a birthmark, known colloquially as a "strawberry mark." Most hemangiomas that occur at birth disappear after a few months or years. See also *hemangioma, senile.*

**hemangioma, capillary**  A type of hemangioma that is composed nearly entirely of tiny capillary vessels.

**hemangioma, cavernous**  A type of hemangioma composed of blood-filled "lakes" and channels.

**hemangioma, senile**  A type of hemangioma that develops in an elderly patient rather than at birth.

**hemarthrosis**  Blood in a joint.

**hematemesis**  Bloody vomit.

**hematocrit**  The proportion, by volume, of the blood that consists of red blood cells. Abbreviated as hct, the hematocrit is expressed as a percentage. For example, an hematocrit of 25 percent means that there are 25 milliliters of red blood cells in 100 milliliters of blood: a

quarter of the blood consists of red cells. The normal ranges for hematocrit depend on the age and, after adolescence, the sex of the patient. The normal ranges are 55 to 68 percent for newborns, 47 to 65 percent at one week of age, 37 to 49 percent at one month of age, 30 to 36 percent at three months of age, 29 to 41 percent at one year of age, 36 to 40 percent at 10 years of age, 42 to 54 percent in adult males, and 38 to 46 percent in adult females. The values returned on hematocrit tests may vary slightly between laboratories.

**hematologist**  A doctor who specializes in treating diseases of the blood.

**hematoma**  A localized swelling, filled with blood. The blood is usually clotted or partially clotted, and exists within an organ or in a soft tissue space, such as muscle. A hematoma is caused by a break in the wall of a blood vessel. The break may be spontaneous, as in the case of an aneurysm, or caused by trauma. Treatment depends on the location and size of the hematoma, but usually involves draining the accumulated blood. Hematoma in or near the brain is particularly dangerous.

**hematoma, epidural**  A hematoma between the cranium (skull) and the brain's tissue-like covering, which is known as the dura. Epidural hematoma is usually caused by a full-on blow to the head, and is often associated with a skull fracture. Diagnosis is usually by CAT scan. Treatment is by trepanation: drilling through the skull to drain the excess blood.

**hematoma, extradural**  See *hematoma, epidural.*

**hematoma, intracerebral**  Bleeding and bruising within the brain. Diagnosis is usually by CAT scan. Treatment is by surgery.

**hematoma, intracranial**  A hematoma within the brain cavity (cranium, skull) or within the brain itself. See *hematoma, epidural; hematoma, intracerebral; hematoma, subdural.*

**hematoma, subcutaneous**  A bruise.

**hematoma, subdural**  Bleeding into the subdural space between the brain and its tissue-like covering, the dura. If the hematoma causes increased pressure on the brain, slurred speech, impaired gait, and dizziness may result. Subdural hematomas can be caused by minor accidents to the head, major trauma, or the spontaneous bursting of a blood vessel in the brain (aneurysm). They usually go unnoticed: When they do cause problems, the incident that caused the bleeding is often long past. Diagnosis is usually by CAT scan. Treatment is by trepanation: drilling through the skull to drain the excess blood.

**hematopoiesis**  The formation and development of blood cells.

**hematuria**  Blood in the urine. Hematuria may or may not be accompanied by pain, but it is always abnormal and should be further investigated. Painful hematuria can be caused by a number of disorders, including infections and stones in the urinary tract. Painless hematuria can also be due to many causes, including cancer. See also *hematuria, gross; microhematuria*.

**hematuria, gross**  Blood in the urine that can be seen with the naked eye. Hematuria may or may not be accompanied by pain, but it is always abnormal and should be further investigated. See also *hematuria, microhematuria*.

**hemiparesis**  Weakness on one side of the body.

**hemiplegia**  Paralysis on one side of the body.

**hemizygous**  Having only a single set of genes as, for example, on the single X chromosome in the male.

**hemochromatosis**  An inherited disorder in the way the body absorbs and stores iron. The excess iron gives the skin a bronze color, and damages the liver and other organs. Diabetes is also a part of the syndrome, due to damage to the pancreas. Treatment is usually via chelation to remove excess iron from the blood. Also known as bronze diabetes.

**hemodialysis**  See *dialysis*.

**hemoglobin**  The oxygen-carrying protein pigment in the blood, specifically in the red blood cells. Hemoglobin is abbreviated as Hb, and is usually measured as total hemoglobin expressed as the amount of hemoglobin in grams (gm) per deciliter (dl) of whole blood. The normal ranges for hemoglobin depend on the age and, beginning in adolescence, the sex of the person. The normal ranges are 17 to 22 gm/dl for newborns, 15 to 20 gm/dl at 1 week of age, 11 to 15 gm/dl at 1 month of age, 11 to 13 gm/dl in children, 14 to 18 gm/dl for adult men, 12 to 16 gm/dl for adult women, 12.4 to 14.9 gm/dl for men after middle age, and 11.7 to 13.8 gm/dl for women after middle age. Values returned on hemoglobin tests may vary slightly between laboratories, as some laboratories do not differentiate between adult and "after middle age" hemoglobin values.

**hemoglobin A**  The main type of hemoglobin found after early infancy. The A stands for Adult.

**hemoglobin F**  The main type of hemoglobin found in the fetus and newborn baby. The F stands for Fetal.

**hemoglobin S**  The most common type of abnormal hemoglobin, hemoglobin S is found in people with sickle cell trait and sickle cell anemia. It differs from hemoglobin A only by a single amino acid substitution. See *anemia, sickle cell; sickle cell trait*.

**hemoglobinuria**  Hemoglobin in the urine.

**hemolysis**  Breakdown of red blood cells.

**hemolytic anemia**  Anemia due to the destruction, rather than underproduction, of red blood cells.

**hemolytic disease of the newborn**  Abnormal breakup of red blood cells in the fetus or newborn. This is usually due to antibodies made by the mother that are directed against the baby's red cells. It is typically caused by Rh incompatibility: differences between the Rh blood group of mother and baby. Severe hemolytic disease can cause anemia and heart failure. Less-severe cases include jaundice, and can lead to brain damage if left untreated. Also known as erythroblastosis.

**hemolytic jaundice, congenital**  See *spherocytosis, hereditary*.

**hemophagocytic lymphohistiocytosis**  A rare, cancer-like disorder in which both histiocytes and lymphocytes start to proliferate and attack body tissues or organs. It can be an inherited condition, or it can occur as a result of immunosuppression (as in organ transplants) or infection. Most patients are young children. Treatment is by chemotherapy, and in some cases bone-marrow transplantation. See also *histiocytosis*.

**hemophilia**  A set of inherited disorders in which the ability of blood to clot normally is impaired.

**hemophilia A**  Classic hemophilia due to profound deficiency of factor VIII in the blood, which is necessary for normal clotting. The hemophilia A gene is on the X chromosome, so females carry the gene. Each son of a female carrier stands a 50 percent chance of receiving the gene and having hemophilia. Treatment is by blood products that introduce clotting factor and replace lost blood. However, use of contaminated blood products exposed many people with hemophilia to HIV infection in the 1980s and 1990s. Hemophilia A has affected the Russian royal house and other descendants of Queen Victoria.

**hemophilia B**  Hemophilia due to deficiency of coagulation factor IX in the blood. The hemophilia B gene is also on the X chromosome, so females carry the gene. Each son of a female carrier stands a 50 percent chance of receiving the gene and having hemophilia. Treatment is by blood products that introduce clotting factor and replace lost blood. Also called Christmas disease (so-named for the first patient studied in detail with the disease).

**hemoptysis** Spitting up blood or blood-tinged sputum from the respiratory tract.

**hemorrhage** Abnormal bleeding or an abnormal flow of blood. A hemorrhage can be internal, and therefore invisible, or external, and therefore visible on the body.

**hemorrhagic fever with renal syndrome** A set of diseases characterized by the abrupt onset of high fever and chills, headache, cold and cough; and pain in the muscles, joints, and abdomen with nausea and vomiting. These symptoms are followed by bleeding into the kidney (renal syndrome) and elsewhere. Some victims have bleeding from the eyes, mouth, nose, and/or through the pores of the skin. Viruses known to cause hemorrhagic fever with renal syndrome include the arboviruses, hantaviruses, and the Ebola virus. One thing these three types of viruses have in common is transmission from animal or insect host to humans. See also *arborvirus, Ebola virus, hantavirus.*

**hemorrhagic fever, epidemic** See *hemorrhagic fever with renal syndrome.*

**hemorrhoids** Dilated (enlarged) veins in the walls of the anus and sometimes around the rectum, usually caused by untreated constipation but occasionally associated with chronic diarrhea. Symptoms start with bleeding after defecation. If untreated, hemorrhoids can worsen, protruding from the anus. In their worst stage, they must be returned manually to the anal cavity. Fissures can develop, and may cause intense discomfort. Treatment is by changing the diet to prevent constipation and avoid further irritation, the use of topical medication, and sometimes surgery. Also known as piles.

**Henoch-Schonlein purpura** See *anaphylactoid purpura.*

**heparin** One of several glycosaminoglycans (GAGs), the heparins are anticlotting agents produced naturally by the liver and some other cells in the body. Heparin may also be purified or synthesized for use as a medication. As a drug, heparin is useful in preventing blood clots that travel from their site of origin through the blood stream to clog another vessel (thromboembolic complications); it is used also in the early treatment of blood clots in the lungs (pulmonary embolisms) and clotting-related heart conditions. Until recently, only heparin with particles of various sizes was available (unfractionated heparin, or UFH). See also *glycosaminoglycans; heparin, low-weight.*

**heparin, low-weight** A newer form of the drug heparin (brand name: Loverox, Fragmin) that has a lower molecular weight than normal heparin. Fewer blood tests are needed, and it may be superior to regular (unfractionated) heparin in cases of unstable angina and other cardiac diseases. See also *heparin.*

**hepatic** Having to do with the liver.

**hepatic ductular hypoplasia, syndromatic** See *Alagille syndrome.*

**hepatitis** Inflammation of the liver.

**hepatitis A** Inflammation of the liver caused by the hepatitis A virus (HAV), which is usually transmitted by food or drink that has been handled by an infected person whose hygiene is poor. Symptoms include nausea, fever, and jaundice (yellowing of the skin and/or eyes), although some patients have no symptoms at all. It does not lead to chronic disease. Diagnosis is by blood test. When immediate protection against hepatitis A infection is needed, immunoglobulin (gamma globulin) is used. Immunoglobulin is effective only if given within two weeks of exposure, and lasts but two to four months. Immunoglobulin can be used to protect household contacts of someone with acute viral hepatitis, and by travelers who must depart for regions with poor sanitation and high hepatitis A rates before vaccines can take effect. Travelers can receive immunoglobulin and hepatitis A vaccine simultaneously. Also called infectious hepatitis, epidemic jaundice. See also *hepatitis A immunization.*

**hepatitis A immunization** A vaccine that may be considered for individuals in high-risk settings, including frequent world travelers, sexually active individuals with multiple partners, homosexual men, IV drug users, employees of daycare centers, certain health-care workers, and sewage workers. Two hepatitis A vaccines (brand names: Havrix and Vaqta) are commercially available in the US. Both are highly effective and provide protection even after one dose. Two doses are recommended for adults, and three doses for children under 18 years of age to provide prolonged protection.

**hepatitis B** Inflammation of the liver due to the hepatitis B virus (HBV), once thought to be passed only through blood products. It is now known that hepatitis B can also be transmitted via needle sticks, body piercing and tattooing with unsterilized instruments, the dialysis process, sexual and even less intimate close contact, and childbirth. Symptoms include fatigue, jaundice, nausea, vomiting, dark urine, light stools. Diagnosis is by blood test. Treatment is via antiviral drugs and/or hepatitis B immunoglobulin (HBIG). Chronic hepatitis B may be treated with interferon. Health-care workers accidentally exposed to materials infected with hepatitis B, and individuals with known sexual contact with hepatitis B patients, are usually given both HBIG and the hepatitis B vaccine to provide both immediate and long-term protection. HBV infection can be prevented by the hepatitis B vaccine, and by avoiding activities that could lead to getting the virus.

**hepatitis B immunization**  A vaccine that protects against both hepatitis B and hepatitis D. It gives prolonged protection, but three shots over a half year are usually required. Until recently, the hepatitis B vaccine (brand names: Energix-B and Recombivax-HB) was given to all newborn infants in the US and the UK. In 1999 the program was stopped, presumably temporarily, because of questions about a preservative in the vaccine that contains trace amounts of mercury. Adults in high-risk situations, including health-care workers, dentists, intimate and household contacts of patients with chronic hepatitis B infection, male homosexuals, individuals with multiple sexual partners, dialysis patients, IV drug users, and recipients of repeated transfusions, may also want to get this vaccine.

**hepatitis C**  Inflammation of the liver due to the hepatitis C virus (HCV), which is usually spread by blood transfusion, hemodialysis, and needle sticks. HCV causes most transfusion-associated hepatitis, and the damage it does to the liver can lead to cirrhosis and cancer. Transmission of the virus by sexual contact is rare. At least half of HCV patients develop chronic hepatitis C infection. Diagnosis is by blood test. Treatment is via antiviral drugs. Chronic hepatitis C may be treated with interferon, sometimes in combination with antivirals. There is no vaccine for hepatitis C. Previously known as non-A, non-B hepatitis.

**hepatitis D**  Liver inflammation due to the hepatitis D virus (HDV), which only causes disease in patients who already have the hepatitis B virus. Transmission is via infected blood, needles, or sexual contact with an infected person. Symptoms are identical to those of hepatitis B. Chronic infection with HDV is currently treated with interferon, although this treatment is not very successful. HDV infection can be prevented by the hepatitis B vaccine, and by avoiding activities that could lead to getting the virus.

**hepatitis E**  A rare form of liver inflammation caused by infection with the hepatitis E virus (HEV). It is transmitted via food or drink handled by an infected person, or through infected water supplies in areas where fecal matter may get into the water. There is no vaccine or treatment for hepatitis E, although antiviral drugs may be tried.

**hepatitis F**  A rare form of liver inflammation caused by infection with the so-called hepatitis F virus, which may be

a mutation of hepatitis B. There is no vaccine or treatment for hepatitis F, although antiviral drugs may be tried.

**hepatitis G**  A rare form of liver inflammation caused by infection with the so-called hepatitis G virus, which may be a mutation of hepatitis B. There is no vaccine or treatment for hepatitis G, although antiviral drugs may be tried.

**hepatitis, infectious**  See *hepatitis A*. (Although all forms of hepatitis are infectious.)

**hepatitis, non-A, non-B**  The old name for hepatitis C, before the causative virus had been identified.

**hepatitis, viral**  Liver inflammation caused by viruses. Specific hepatitis viruses have been labeled A, B, C, D, E, F, and G. Some other viruses, such as the Epstein-Barr virus and cytomegalovirus, can also cause hepatitis, but the liver is not their primary target.

**hepatomegaly**  An enlarged liver.

**hepatosplenomegaly**  Enlargement of the liver and spleen.

**hepatotoxic**  Injurious to the liver. For example, acetaminophen (brand name: Tylenol) can be hepatotoxic.

**herbal remedy**  A medication prepared from plants, including most of the world's traditional remedies for disease. Most people think of herbal remedies as products sold over the counter as "supplements," such as saw palmetto extract or goldenseal ointment. However, many over-the-counter and prescription drugs, including aspirin and digoxin, are based on ingredients originally derived from plants. Lab tests have shown that some herbal remedies are indeed effective against illness. One should use these drugs as carefully as prescription medicines, taking care to avoid overdose, interactions with other medications, and misuse. See also *dietary supplement, herbalism*.

**herbalism**  The practice of making or prescribing herbal remedies for medical conditions. Practitioners of herbalism may be licensed MDs, naturopaths, or osteopaths. They may also be unlicensed. Interested consumers should seek out knowledgeable, and preferably licensed, herbalists.

**herbalist**  One versed in herbal lore and, in regard to therapy, an herb doctor. See also *herbalism*.

**hereditary angioedema**  See *angioedema, hereditary*.

**hereditary angioneurotic edema**  See *angioedema, hereditary*.

**hereditary hemorrhagic telangectasia** Abbreviated as HHT, this is a genetic disease characterized by widening (dilatation) of capillaries and small arteries (arterioles). This action produces small red spots called telangectases in the skin and mucous membranes, particularly in the nose and gastrointestinal tract. These spots are fragile, and bleed easily. Recurrent nosebleeds and chronic gastrointestinal bleeding are the usual major problems. Other organs may also have these spots and bleed. HHT is an autosomal dominant disorder, so the HHT gene is found on a nonsex (autosomal) chromosome, specifically chromosome 9q34.1. One copy of this gene is enough to cause the disease. Also known as Osler-Rendu-Weber syndrome or Rendu-Osler-Weber syndrome.

**hereditary multiple exostoses** See *osteochondromatosis*.

**hereditary mutation** A gene change that occurs in a germ cell (an egg or sperm), and is then incorporated into every cell in the developing body of the new organism. Hereditary mutations play a role in cancer as, for example, in eye tumor retinoblastoma and Wilms' tumor of the kidney. Also known as a germline mutation.

**hereditary spherocytosis** See *spherocytosis, hereditary*.

**heredity** Genetic transmission from parent to child.

**heritability** The degree to which something is inherited.

**heritable** Capable of being transmitted from parent to child.

**Hermansky-Pudlak syndrome** A genetic (inherited) disorder characterized by lack of skin and/or eye pigment (albinism), bruising and prolonged bleeding due to blood platelets that are deficient in so-called dense bodies, and fibrosis of the lungs. In HPS, there is occasionally also inflammatory bowel disease and/or impaired kidney function. The lack of pigment in the eye impairs vision and often leads to involuntary rhythmic eye movements called nystagmus. The most serious health problems in HPS are the tendency to bruise easily and bleed, and the progressive deterioration in lung function. Women with HPS may need medical intervention during their menstrual cycle or at childbirth. HPS patients are advised to avoid blood anticoagulants, including aspirin. Drugs are needed to prevent excessive bleeding during dental extractions and other surgical procedures. Inflammatory bowel disease with the onset of symptoms between 10 and 30 years of age can complicate HPS, and usually responds poorly to therapy. HPS patients have a biochemical storage disorder. They accumulate a fatty product called ceroid lipofuscin that causes inflammation. Prolonged inflammation of the lungs leads to fibrosis, which impairs their ability to expel air and to exchange carbon dioxide for oxygen. The lung problems in HPS begin with restrictive airway disease, and progress inexorably to death, usually in the fourth or fifth decade. HPS occurs in many countries, but is especially common in certain areas in the Swiss Alps and Puerto Rico. In northwestern Puerto Rico, 1 in 21 individuals carries the HPS gene, and 1 in every 1,800 is affected with HPS. Puerto Rican patients with HPS have all been found to have one specific, small region of DNA duplication involving a gene on chromosome 10, in bands 10q23.1-q23.3. Non-Puerto Ricans with HPS do not have this particular mutation. A number of different mutations in the HPS gene are now known to lead to HPS. HPS is inherited as an autosomal recessive condition, affecting males and females. Both parents are carriers of the HPS gene along with a normal gene, and the risk to each of their children is one in four to receive both of the parents' HPS genes and have the disease. Diagnosis is by examining the blood platelets under an electron microscope. There is currently no treatment for HPS, other than care aimed at easing symptoms and avoiding problems. HPS is also known as albinism with hemorrhagic diathesis and pigmented reticuloendithelial cells, and as delta-storage pool disease.

**hernia** A general term referring to a protrusion of a tissue through the wall of the cavity in which it is normally contained. Also called rupture.

**hernia, hiatus** Protrusion of the stomach up into the opening normally occupied by the esophagus in the diaphragm, the muscle that separates the chest cavity from the abdomen. This type of hernia can be congenital, or it may be acquired through strenuous physical activity. Symptoms usually start with a tingling or burning sensation, although patients may be able to see a bulge where the hernia is located. If extreme pain is present, emergency surgery may be needed. Treatment is via conventional or laproscopic (minimally invasive) surgery.

**hernia, Velpeau** A protrusion of tissue in front of the femoral blood vessels in the groin. Treatment is via surgery.

**herniated disk** A disk, situated between two vertebrae, that protrudes to press on a nerve root. A herniated disk may cause sciatica (pain in the lower back, leg, and behind the knee). If warranted, treatment may be via surgery.

**herniation** Abnormal protrusion of tissue through an opening.

**heroin** A semisynthetic drug derived from, but more potent than, morphine. In 1898, heroin was introduced commercially as a painkiller. It is still used in this capacity in Europe, but is not used medically in the US. Heroin is now better known as a drug of abuse than for its medical uses. Heroin may be injected into a vein, injected under the skin, snorted, or smoked. It is highly addictive, and overdose is an ever-present possibility due to the varying purity of street drugs. See also *heroin addiction*.

**heroin addiction**  Physical addiction to heroin, often with concurrent use of other opiates when heroin itself is not available. Treatment is by withdrawal, either gradual or sudden. Medication may be used to ease the physical effects of withdrawal, which include cramping, nausea, and intense craving. Opiate blocker drugs, such as reboxetine (brand name: ReVia), may be used to speed up the withdrawal process and help the addict maintain compliance. Counseling, 12-step groups such as Narcotics Anonymous, nutritional support, and often antidepressant medication to help reregulate the nervous system are helpful adjunct treatments. Another method of treating addiction is to prescribe methadone, a synthetic opioid liquid, as a substitute for heroin. In some European countries heroin itself is prescribed for addicts.

**herpetiform virus**  A virus with the characteristic shape and behavior of a virus in the herpes family. Not all members of the herpes virus family have been identified. Some herpatiform viruses may eventually be called herpesviruses, while others are merely similar. See *herpesvirus*.

**herpes**  **1** Infection with one of the human herpes viruses, particularly herpes simplex 1 or 2. **2** The family of herpesviruses.

**herpes simplex type 1**  A herpes virus that causes cold sores and fever blisters in and around the mouth. In rare cases, as when a patient's immune system is severely compromised, this virus can cause infection of the brain (encephalitis). Also known as human herpesvirus 1 (HHV-1). See also *fever blisters*.

**herpes simplex type 2**  A herpes virus that causes genital herpes, which is characterized by sores in the genital area. In rare cases, as when a patient's immune system is severely compromised, this virus can cause infection of the brain (encephalitis). Treatment is by topical or oral antiviral medication. Also known as human herpesvirus 2 (HHV-2). See also *genital herpes*.

**herpes zoster**  The herpes virus that causes chicken pox (varicella), herpes zoster is also known as human herpesvirus 3 (HHV-3). Herpes zoster and chicken pox are usually contracted in childhood, at which time the virus infects nerves (namely, the dorsal root ganglia). It remains latent for years, but can then be reactivated to cause shingles: blisters over the distribution of the affected nerve. Shingles is often accompanied by intense pain and itching. Also called shingles, zona, and zoster. See also *chicken pox, chicken pox immunization, shingles*.

**herpes, genital**  See *genital herpes*.

**herpesvirus**  One of a family of viruses that contain DNA and that cause infections in humans (human herpesviruses) or animals. Herpes viruses are common, and often live in the host's tissue for years or even decades without causing symptoms.

**hetero-**  Prefix meaning different. The opposite is homo-, meaning same. For example, heterogeneous and homogeneous, heterosexual and homosexual, and so on.

**heterochromatin**  A genetically inactive part of the genome, heterochromatin was so named because its chromosomal material (chromatin) stained more darkly throughout the cell cycle than most chromosomal material (euchromatin). There are two types: constitutive heterochromatin and facultative heterochromatin.

**heterochromatin, constituitive**  Heterochromatin that is fixed and irreversible. Regions of constituitive heterochromatin are located at very specific spots in the genome (on chromosomes 1, 9, and 16; on the Y chromosome; on the tiny short arms of chromosomes 13, 14, 15, 21, and 22; and near the centromeres of chromosomes). It consists of DNA that contains many tandem (not inverted) repeats of a short basic repeating unit known as satellite DNA.

**heterochromatin, facultative**  Heterochromatin that need not always be heterochromatic but has the ability to return to the normal euchromatic state. The inactive X chromosome is made up of facultative heterochromatin. When a woman transmits that X to a son, it reverts to euchromatin and become genetically active.

**heterochromia iridis**  A difference of color between the iris of one eye and the other: a person with one brown and one blue eye has heterochromia iridis.

**heterochromia iridis, sectoral**  A difference in color within an iris.

**heterokaryon**  A cell with two separate nuclei formed by the experimental fusion of two genetically different cells. For example, heterokaryons composed of nuclei from Hurler syndrome and Hunter syndrome, both diseases of mucopolysaccharide metabolism, have normal mucopolysaccharide metabolism. This proves that the two syndromes affect different proteins, and so can correct each other in the heterokaryon.

**heteromorphism** Something different in form. Chromosome heteromorphisms are normal variations in the appearance of chromosomes.

**heteroploid** A different chromosome number than the normal number of chromosomes.

**heterosexual** A person sexually attracted to persons of the opposite sex, also used to describe the act or habit of opposite-sex attraction. Colloquially known as straight.

**heterosexuality** Sexuality directed toward someone of the opposite sex.

**heterozygote** An individual with different genes at a particular spot (locus) on a pair of chromosomes. A heterozygote for cystic fibrosis (CF) has the CF gene on one chromosome 7 and the normal paired gene on the other chromosome 7.

**heterozygous** The state of being a heterozygote.

**HEV** Hepatitis E virus.

**Hex-A deficiency** Hexosaminidase A deficiency. See *Tay-Sachs disease*.

**hexadactyly** The presence of an extra digit: a sixth finger or toe. It is a very common birth defect. The sixth digit can be located in three different locations: on either side of the extremity, or somewhere in between. With the hand, for example, the extra finger can be out beyond the little finger (ulnar hexadactyly), out beyond the thumb (radial hexadactyly), or between two of the normally expected fingers (intercalary hexadactyly). Hexadactyly can be absolutely harmless and is easily remedied. For example, ulnar hexadactyly with just a rudimentary tag of a sixth digit can be very simply treated by tying it off with one suture. However, hexadactyly can also signal one of a number of congenital malformations affecting the baby. In this case, treatment may not be so simple, and the prognostic outlook may not be as good. See also *polydactyly*.

**hexoseaminidase A** An enzyme, deficiency of which causes Tay-Sachs disease. See *Tay-Sachs disease*.

**HHS** The Department of Health and Human Services of the US government, which has jurisdiction over public health, welfare, and civil rights issues, and is the highest-level government body with such jurisdiction. Agencies under HHS include the Public Health Service (PHS) and the Social Security Administration (SSA).

**HHV-1** Human herpesvirus 1. See *herpes simplex type 1*.

**HHV-2** Human herpesvirus 2. See *herpes simplex type 2*.

**HHV-3** Human herpesvirus 3. See *herpes zoster*.

**HHV-4** Human herpesvirus 4. See *Epstein-Barr virus*.

**HHV-5** Human herpesvirus 5. See *cytomegalovirus*.

**HHV-6** Human herpesvirus 6.

**HHV-7** Human herpesvirus 7.

**HHV-8** Human herpesvirus 8.

**hiatus hernia** See *hernia, hiatus*.

**HIB** Haemophilus influenzae type B.

**HIB immunization** See *Haemophilus influenzae type B immunization*.

**hibernation reaction** See *seasonal affective disorder*.

**hiccough** An extraordinary type of breathing movement involving a sudden intake of air (inspiration) due to an involuntary contraction of the diaphragm, accompanied by closure of the vocal apparatus (glottis) of the larynx. It results from a sudden contraction of the diaphragm. Closure of the glottis then halts the incoming air. The column of air strikes the closed glottis to produce the characteristic sound. Hiccoughs are often rhythmic. If self-limited, they are just a minor nuisance, but prolonged hiccups can become a major medical problem. In some patients with tic disorders, hiccoughs can be a tic. Also known as a hiccup or singultus.

**hiccup** See *hiccough*.

**hidradenitis suppurativa** An illness characterized by multiple abscesses that form under the armpits and in the groin area.

**high altitude** Altitude of 8,000 feet or more, at which altitude sickness may occur.

**high blood pressure** A repeatedly elevated blood pressure exceeding 140 over 90 mmHg. Also called hypertension, chronic high blood pressure can stealthily cause blood vessel changes in the back of the eye (retina), abnormal thickening of the heart muscle, kidney failure, and brain damage. No specific cause for high blood pressure is found in 95 percent of patients. High blood pressure is treated with salt restriction, regular aerobic exercise, and medication.

**Highly Sensitive test** See *HS test*.

**hip bursitis** Pain caused by an inflamed and/or infected fluid-filled sac that normally functions as a gliding surface to reduce friction between tissues that move within the hip. Bursitis is usually not infectious, but the bursa can become infected. Treatment of noninfectious bursitis includes rest, ice, and medications for inflammation and pain. Infectious bursitis is treated with antibiotics, aspiration, and surgery.

**hip pointer**   A bruise of the upper edge of the ilium, one of the hip bones. Also known as an iliac crest contusion.

**hippocampus**   An area buried deep in the forebrain that helps regulate emotion and memory.

**Hirschsprung disease**   An abnormal condition present at birth, which is due to absence of the normal nerves (ganglia) in the bowel wall. Nerves can be missing starting at the anus and extending up a variable distance of the bowel. This results in enlargement of the bowel above the point of missing nerve, as the nerves normally assist in the natural movement of the muscles in the lining of the bowels to move bowel contents through. Hirschsprung disease is the most common cause of lower intestinal blockage in the newborn, and later may cause chronic constipation or diarrhea. Also known as congenital aganglionic megacolon.

**hirsute**   Having an overabundance of hair.

**Hirudin**   An anticlotting agent that prevents blood clots from traveling through the blood stream to clog up a vessel (thromboembolic complications). Hirudin is the active principle in the secretion of leeches. Desirudin and lepirudin (brand name: Refludan) are genetically engineered recombinant forms of hirudin.

**His disease**   See *trench fever*. See also *Bartonella quintana*.

**histamine**   A substance that plays a major role in many allergic reactions, histamine dilates blood vessels and makes the vessel walls abnormally permeable. It is part of the body's natural reaction to non-self items, such as pollens.

**histamine cephalalgia**   See *cluster headache*.

**histiocyte**   A type of white blood cell, also called a macrophage, that is created by the bone marrow. They usually stay in place, but when histiocytes are stimulated by infection or inflammation they become active, attacking bacteria and other foreign matter in the body. See also *histiocytosis*.

**histiocytosis**   A rare but potentially deadly disorder with similarities to cancer, in which histiocytes start to multiply, and attack the person's own tissues or organs. The result can be tissue damage, pain, the development of tumor-like lumps called granulomas, fatigue, and other

symptoms. If histiocytosis affects the pituitary gland, diabetes insipidus may also develop. Treatment is by radiation and chemotherapy, although for reasons unknown, some cases go into remission without treatment.

**histiocytosis X**   Histiocytosis variants, including eosinophilic granuloma, Letterer Siwe disease, and Hand-Schuller-Christian disease. See *histiocytosis*.

**histiocytosis, Hand-Schuller-Christian**   See *histiocytosis, histiocytosis X*.

**histiocytosis, Langerhans cell**   Histiocytosis in which the active histiocytes normally occur in the skin. See *histiocytosis*.

**histiocytosis, Letterer Siwe**   See *histiocytosis, histiocytosis X*.

**histiocytosis, lipid**   A form of histiocytosis that affects lipid (fat) storage. Also known as Niemann-Pick disease, Erdheim-Chester disease.

**histiocytosis, malignant**   Histiocytosis in which the histiocytes actually become cancerous. Treatment is by radiation and chemotherapy, and in some cases bone-marrow transplantation. See also *histiocytosis*.

**histiocytosis, sinus**   A variant of histiocytosis in which the lymph nodes are the main site of histiocyte proliferation. The sinuses become filled with and distended by masses of histiocytes. See also *histiocytosis*.

**histocompatible**   Literally, tissue compatible. If a tissue donor and tissue recipient are histocompatible, a transplant will be easily accepted.

**histology**   The study of the form of structures as seen under the microscope. Also called microscopic anatomy, as opposed to gross anatomy, which involves structures that can be observed with the naked eye.

**histones**   Proteins associated with DNA in chromosomes.

**histoplasma**   A fungus found worldwide. In the US, it is so common in the Midwest and south that in parts of Kentucky and Tennessee nearly 90 percent of adults have a positive histoplasma skin test. It is carried in bird and bat droppings, and deposited in the soil. Although people can contract histoplasma from their environment, it cannot be passed from person to person.

**histoplasmosis**   Infection with histoplasma. Most patients have no symptoms. However, histoplasma can cause acute or chronic lung disease, eye problems, or histoplasmosis infection in a variety of body tissues. Histoplasmosis is an opportunistic infection that causes particular problems for people with AIDS. Symptoms include fatigue, lowered white blood-cell count, fever, and weight loss. Diagnosis is by skin or blood test. Treatment is via antifungal medications, usually for life in those with compromised immune systems.

**history**  In medicine, the patient's past and present, which hopefully contain helpful clues to ensure future health.

**history, developmental**  An account of how and when a person met developmental milestones, such as walking and talking. For adults, information on social-emotional development may be included. Used primarily in the diagnosis of developmental disorders.

**history, family**  An account of current and past family structure and of relationships within the family. May also include the family history of disease or behavioral disturbance. Useful in the diagnosis of developmental and medical disorders, and particularly helpful in cases of psychiatric or neurological illness.

**history, medical**  A complete account of all medical events and problems a person has experienced, including psychiatric illness. Especially helpful when differential diagnosis is needed.

**history, social**  An account of a patient that puts his illness or behavior in context. It may include aspects of the patient's developmental, family, and medical history, as well as relevant information on life events, social class, race, religion, and occupation. Useful for designing treatment plans, especially for psychiatric or neurological illness.

**His-Werner disease**  See *trench fever*. See also *Bartonella quintana*.

**HIV**  Human immunodeficiency virus, the initial cause of AIDS. HIV is a retrovirus, so it has an RNA genome and a reverse transcriptase enzyme. Using the reverse transcriptase, the virus uses its RNA as a template for making complementary DNA. This DNA can then integrate itself into the DNA of the host organism. This makes HIV particularly difficult to target with medications or vaccines, as it differs ever so slightly in each patient. Also known as the AIDS virus, human lymphotropic virus type III, lymphadenopathy-associated virus, and lymphadenopathy virus. See also *AIDS*.

**HIV infection, acute**  The body's initial reaction to infection by the HIV virus, this is a flu-like syndrome that occurs immediately after a person contracts human immunodeficiency virus 1. Symptoms include fever, sore throat, headache, skin rash, and swollen glands (lymphadenopathy). This syndrome precedes the development

of detectable antibodies to HIV in the blood (seroconversion). It normally takes weeks or months for antibodies to develop after HIV infection. When antibodies to HIV appear in the blood, a person will test positive in the standard ELISA test for HIV. See also *AIDS, AIDS-related complex*.

**HIV infection, primary**  During primary infection with the human immunodeficiency virus (HIV), detectable antibodies to HIV appear in the blood. This is called seroconversion. It normally takes several weeks to several months for antibodies to the virus to develop after HIV transmission. When antibodies to HIV appear in the blood, a person will test positive in the standard ELISA test for HIV. Primary HIV infection may or may not include the symptoms of acute HIV. See also *AIDS; HIV infection, acute*.

**hives**  Raised, itching areas of skin, often a sign of an allergic reaction. Treatment, if necessary, is usually by oral or topical antihistamines. Also known as urticaria, welts, or nettle rash.

**HLA**  Human leukocyte antigens, the major human histocompatibility system. HLA-typing is done before transplantation to determine the degree of tissue compatibility between donor and recipient.

**HMS**  Hereditary multiple exostoses. See *osteochondromatosis*.

**Hodgkin disease**  A malignant disease of the lymph nodes (lymphoma) that occurs most often in patients who are in their 20s or 30s. It can spread through the body, probably via the lymphatic ducts. Symptoms include enlarged lymph nodes, weight loss, night sweats, and itching. Treatment is via radiation and/or chemotherapy. Hodgkin disease is life-threatening if untreated, but has a very high cure rate. Also called Hodgkin lymphoma.

**Hodgkin lymphoma**  See *Hodgkin disease*.

**holandric inheritance**  Inheritance of genes on the Y chromosome. Since only males normally have a Y chromosome, Y-linked genes can only be transmitted from father to son.

**Holter monitor**  A type of portable heart monitor, the Holter monitor is a small electrocardiogram (EKG) device worn in a pouch around the neck or waist. It keeps a record of the heart rhythm, typically over a 24-hour period, while the patient keeps a diary recording activities and symptoms. The EKG recording is then correlated with the person's activities and symptoms. It is useful for identifying heart disturbances that are sporadic and not readily identified with the usual resting EKG.

**homeobox** A short stretch of nucleotides (DNA or RNA) with an almost identical base sequence in all genes that contain that stretch. Homeoboxes occur in many organisms, and appear to determine when particular groups of genes are expressed during development.

**homeopath** A person who practices homeopathy.

**homeopathy** Founded in the 19th century, homeopathy is based on the concept that disease can be treated with minute doses of drugs thought capable of producing in healthy people the same symptoms as those of the disease being treated. This principle is similar to the concept behind exposure therapy for allergies, but the amounts of active medication used in homeopathy are so small as to be almost undetectable. Scientific studies of homeopathy have returned mixed results. It is a mainstream medical practice in the UK, but considered "alternative medicine" in the US.

**homo-** Prefix meaning same. The opposite is hetero-, meaning different. For example, heterogeneous and homogeneous, heterosexual and homosexual, and so on.

**homocystine** An amino acid produced by the human body, usually as a byproduct of consuming meat. It is normally converted into other amino acids. An abnormal accumulation of homocystine, which can be measured in the blood, can be a marker for developing heart disease.

**homocystinuria** A genetic disease due to an enzyme deficiency that permits a buildup of the amino acid homocystine. Progressive mental retardation is common in untreated cases. The finding of vascular disease and premature arteriosclerosis in persons with homocystinuria led to the theory that homocystine may be a factor in heart disease.

**homolog** One chromosome of a pair. Also spelled homologue.

**homologies** Similarities in DNA or protein sequences between individuals or between species.

**homologous** The relationship between two chromosomes that are paired, and so are homologs of each other.

**homologous chromosomes** A pair of chromosomes containing the same gene sequences, each derived from one parent.

**homosexual** A person who is sexually attracted to persons of the same sex.

**homosexuality** Sexuality directed toward someone of the same sex.

**horizontal** Parallel to the floor, a plane passing through the standing body parallel to the floor. A person lying on a bed is considered in a horizontal position. See also *Appendix B, "Anatomic Orientation Terms."*

**hormone** Chemical substances produced in the body that control and regulate the activity of certain cells or organs. Many hormones are secreted by special glands, such as thyroid hormone (produced by the thyroid gland). Hormones are essential for every activity of daily living, including the processes of digestion, metabolism, growth, reproduction, and mood control. Many hormones, such as the neurotransmitters, are active in more than one physical process.

**hormone replacement therapy** The use of medications containing both estrogen and progestogen to reduce or stop short-term changes associated with menopause, such as hot flashes, disturbed sleep, and vaginal dryness. By taking the hormone progestogen along with estrogen, one reduces substantially the risk of endometrial cancer. Progestogen protects the uterus by keeping the endometrium from thickening, an effect that can be caused by estrogen. Abbreviated as HRT.

**hormone therapy** Treatment of disease or symptoms with synthetic or naturally derived hormones. Hormone therapy may be used to treat some forms of cancer, taking advantage of the fact that certain cancers depend on hormones to grow. It may be used also for thyroid disorders, problems associated with menopause, and illnesses associated with hormone production or use. The treatment may include giving hormones to the patient, or using medications that decrease the level of hormones in the body.

**hormone, aldosterone** See *aldosterone.*

**hormone, androgenic** Any hormone that promotes the development and maintenance of male sex characteristics. Testosterone is an androgen.

**hormone, antidiuretic** See *antidiuretic hormone.* See also *ADH secretion, inappropriate.*

**hormone, cortisol** See *cortisol.*

**hormone, erythropoietin** See *erythropoietin.*

**hormone, estrogenic** A female hormone produced by the ovaries, or an equivalent hormone synthesized in the laboratory. See also *estrogen.*

**hormone, follicle-stimulating** See *follicle-stimulating hormone.*

**hormone, glucocorticoid** See *corticosteroid.*

**hormone, human chorionic gonadotropin** See *human chorionic gonadotropin*.

**hormone, mineralocorticoid** A group of hormones, the most important being aldosterone, that regulate the balance of water and electrolytes (ions such as sodium and potassium) in the body. The mineralocorticoid hormones act specifically on the tubules of the kidney. See also *corticosteroid*.

**hormone, parathormone** See *parathormone*.

**hormone, parathyrin** See *parathormone*.

**hormone, parathyroid** See *parathormone*.

**hormone, progesterone** See *progesterone*.

**hormone, secretin** See *secretin*.

**hormone, T3** Triiodothyronine, a thyroid hormone. See *triiodothyronine*.

**hormone, T4** See *thyroxine*.

**hormone, thyroid** A chemical substance made by the thyroid gland which is located in the front of the neck. The two most important thyroid hormones are thyroxine (T4) and triiodothyronine (T3). See *thyroxine, triiodothyronine*.

**hormone, thyroid stimulating** See *thyroid stimulating hormone*.

**hormone, thyrotropin** See *thyroid stimulating hormone*.

**hormone, thyroxine** See *thyroxine*.

**hormone, triiodothyronine** See *triiodothyronine*.

**hormone, TSH** See *thyroid stimulating hormone*.

**Horner syndrome** A complex of abnormal findings, including the sinking in of one eyeball, drooping of the upper eyelid on the same side (ipsilateral ptosis), and constriction of the pupil of that eye (miosis), together with lack of sweating (anhidosis), and flushing of the affected side of the face. Horner syndrome is due to paralysis of cervical sympathetic nerves. Also called Horner-Bernard syndrome, Bernard syndrome, Bernard-Horner syndrome, and Horner ptosis.

**Horner-Bernard syndrome** See *Horner syndrome*.

**Horner ptosis** See *Horner syndrome*.

**hornet stings** Stings from hornets can trigger allergic reactions that vary greatly in severity. Avoidance and prompt treatment are essential. For those with severe reactions, injectable adrenaline should always be kept on hand. In selected cases, allergy injection therapy is highly effective.

**horripilation** See *goose bumps*.

**hospital** A place for receiving medical or surgical care, usually as an inpatient (resident). An ill American may be put "in the hospital," while his ailing British counterpart would say he is "in hospital."

**hospitalist** A hospital-based general physician. Hospitalists assume the care of hospitalized patients in the place of patients' primary care physician. In the most prevalent American model of hospitalist care, several doctors practice together as a group and work full-time caring for inpatients.

**hot flashes** A sudden wave of mild or intense body heat caused by rushes of hormones. Hot flashes result from blood vessels opening and constricting, an action triggered by hormonal changes caused by decreased levels of estrogen. They can occur at any time, and may last from a few seconds to a half-hour. They are a symptom of menopause.

**Hôtel-Dieu** A name often given to a hospital in France during the Middle Ages. Hôtel-Dieu literally means the hotel of God. In Paris, the Hôtel-Dieu is a venerable and famed hospital.

**housemaid's knee** See *patellofemoral syndrome*.

**HPS** Hantavirus pulmonary syndrome.

**HPS** Hermansky-Pudlak syndrome.

**HPV** Human papilloma virus.

**HRT** Hormone replacement therapy.

**HS** Hereditary spherocytosis. See *spherocytosis, hereditary*.

**HS test** Abbreviation for the Highly Sensitive test for detecting and measuring the level of P-24 antigen in the blood serum of people infected with the HIV virus. It is 10 times more sensitive than the Coulter test for P-24 antigen, and may be used to track the progression of AIDS. See also *P-24 antigen*.

**ht** Abbreviation for height, and also for heart.

**HUGO** Human Genome Organization, the international organization concerned with researching and mapping the human genes.

**human chorionic gonadotropin** Abbreviated as hCG, this hormone is made by chorionic cells in the fetal part of the placenta. Human chorionic gonadotropin is directed at the gonads and stimulates them. hCG becomes detectable by immunologic means within days of fertilization, and forms the foundation of most common pregnancy tests. The level of hCG in maternal serum also enters as one component in the "double" and the "triple" screens used during pregnancy to assign risks of Down syndrome and other fetal disorders. See also *gonadotropin*.

**Human Development, National Institute of Child Health and** See *National Institutes of Health*.

**human gene therapy** See *gene therapy*.

**human genome** See *genome, human*.

**Human Genome Project** An international effort aimed at identifying and sequencing (ordering) all of the bases in the human genome. American participation in this monumental undertaking has been supported by funds from the National Institutes of Health (NIH) and the Department of Energy (DOE).

**Human Genome Research Institute, National** See *National Institutes of Health*.

**human herpesvirus 1** See *herpes simplex type 1*.

**human herpesvirus 2** See *herpes simplex type 2*.

**human herpesvirus 3** See *herpes zoster*.

**human herpesvirus 4** See *Epstein-Barr virus*.

**human herpesvirus 5** See *cytomegalovirus*.

**human herpesvirus 6** A herpes virus that apparently lies dormant in many people, human herpesvirus 6 is most likely to cause problems when the immune system is compromised by disease, as in AIDS patients, or by deliberate immune suppression, as in organ transplant patients. There are two forms of HHV-6: A and B. A is rare, and acquired in adulthood. B is relatively common, usually acquired in childhood, and associated with roseola. Both A and B can reactivate at a later date, and are believed to contribute to diseases of the bone marrow and/or central nervous system in some patients, including fatal encephalitis, chronic fatigue syndrome, and possibly multiple sclerosis. Diagnosis is by rapid blood culture or other blood test. Treatment is experimental at this time, but antiviral drugs or beta interferon may be tried. Abbreviated as HHV-6. See also *measles*.

**human herpesvirus 7** Closely related to HHV-6, human herpesvirus 7 has also been linked to roseola.

Researchers believe it may also cause seizures and other central nervous system symptoms in children. Diagnosis is by rapid blood culture or other blood test. Treatment is experimental at this time, but antiviral drugs or beta interferon may be tried. Abbreviated as HHV-7. See also *measles*.

**human herpesvirus 8** A herpesvirus that may contribute to Kaposi sarcoma, an otherwise rare form of cancer that is sometimes seen in AIDS patients, and to some B-cell lymphomas. Diagnosis is by rapid blood culture or other blood test. Treatment is experimental at this time, but antiviral drugs or beta interferon may be tried. Also known as Kaposi sarcoma-associated herpesvirus, or KSHV. Abbreviated as HHV-8.

**human immunodeficiency virus** See *HIV*.

**human lymphotropic virus III** See *HIV*.

**human papilloma virus** A family of over 60 viruses responsible for causing warts. The majority of human papilloma viruses produce warts on the hands, fingers, or face. Most are innocuous, causing nothing more than cosmetic concerns. Several types of HPV are confined primarily to the moist skin of the genitals, producing genital warts and elevating the risk for cancer of the cervix. The papilloma viruses that cause wartlike growths on the genitals are sexually transmitted.

**humerus** The long bone in the upper arm, which extends from the shoulder to the elbow.

**humidifier** A machine that puts moisture in the air.

**humor** In medicine, humor refers to a fluid or semifluid substance. Thus, the aqueous humor is the fluid normally present in the front and rear chambers of the eye.

**humor, aqueous** The fluid normally present in the front and rear chambers of the eye.

**humoral** Pertaining to elements in the blood or other body fluids.

**humoralism** An ancient theory holding that health came from balance between the bodily liquids. These liquids were termed humors. Disease arose when imbalance occurred between the humors. The humors were phlegm (water), blood, gall (black bile, thought to be secreted by the kidneys and spleen), and choler (yellow bile secreted by the liver). The humoral theory was devised well before Hippocrates, and was not definitively demolished until 1858. Doctors now know that health rests on a cellular and molecular foundation, although the word "humor" lives on as a medical term for liquid or semiliquid substances in the body, and as a euphemism for mood (such as being "in good humor"). Also called humorism.

**humorism**   See *humoralism*.

**Hunter syndrome**   An inherited form of mucopolysaccharidosis that is carried by females, but can affect both males and females. All forms of Hunter syndrome are characterized by inability to break down heparan and dermatan sulfates, causing them to be deposited in the central nervous system and peripheral tissues. Signs and symptoms may include coarse, thickened facial features; short stature and sometimes dwarfism; hyperactivity and behavior problems; hydrocephalus; seizures; and differences in the skeleton, GI tract, eyes, ears, skin, and heart. Two distinct types of Hunter syndrome have been identified so far. The first causes progressive mental retardation, physical disability, and death before age 15 for most patients; the second does not cause death and may not cause mental retardation. Also known as mucopolysaccharidosis II (MPS II), iduronate 2-sulfatase (IDS) deficiency, sulfoiduronate sulfatase (SIDS) deficiency. See also *mucopolysaccharidosis*.

**Huntington chorea**   See *Huntington disease*.

**Huntington disease**   An inherited genetic disorder characterized by mental and physical deterioration, and leading to death. Although HD is usually an adult-onset disease, it can affect children as well. Mood disturbance is usually the first symptom seen, with bipolar disorder–like mood swings that may include mania, depression, extreme irritability or angry outbursts, and psychosis. Other symptoms include chorea (restless, wiggling, turning movements), muscle stiffness and slowness of movement, and difficulties with memory and other cognitive processes. The HD gene is located on chromosome 4, and is an autosomal dominant gene. Only one copy need be inherited to cause the illness. Diagnosis is by genetic testing, and family members of people with Huntington disease may also want to know whether they carry the HD gene. At this time, there is no cure for HD, although medication may be used to control symptoms of the illness, such as mood swings and chorea. See also *chorea*.

**Hurler syndrome**   An inherited error of metabolism in which there is a lack of the enzyme alpha-L-iduronidase. This enzyme normally breaks down mucopolysaccharides. Without it, there is an abnormal accumulation of mucopolysaccharides in the brain and other places, causing mental retardation, skeletal deformities, and other problems. This usually leads to death of individuals with Hurler syndrome by their early teen years. Scheie syndrome (MPS 1S) and Hurler-Scheie syndrome are variants on the same form of mucopolysaccharidosis. Recently, patients with Hurler syndrome have been treated with bone-marrow transplants, with some success. Surgery may also be necessary. Also known as

mucopolysaccharidosis Type 1 (MPS1), MPS 1H; previously known as gargoylism. See also *mucopolysaccharidosis*.

**hurricane supplies**   See *disaster supplies*.

**hybrid**   The result of a cross between genetically unlike parents.

**hybridoma**   A cell hybrid resulting from the fusion of a cancer cell and a normal lymphocyte (a type of white blood cell). The hybridoma is immortal in the laboratory and makes the same products as its parent cells forever.

**hydatid mole**   An abnormal pregnancy that eventuates in a mass of cysts resembling a bunch of grapes. The embryo dies, and future malignancy is a possibility.

**hydatidiform mole**   See *hydatid mole*.

**hydrocele**   Accumulation of fluid in the coat around the testis. Small hydroceles tend to disappear by one year of age, while larger hydroceles may persist and warrant surgery.

**hydrocephalus**   An abnormal buildup of cerebrospinal fluid (CSF) in the ventricles and/or subarachnoid space of the brain. The fluid often increases intracranial pressure (ICP), which can compress and damage the brain. This increased pressure is most commonly caused by obstruction of the flow of CSF, but may also be due to overproduction of CSF, a condition known as choroid plexus papilloma, or failure of the brain to reabsorb CSF. Hydrocephalus can arise before birth or at any time afterward. Causes include birth defects (particularly spina bifida), hemorrhage into the brain, infection, meningitis, tumor, and head injury. Most forms of hydrocephalus are the result of obstructed CSF flow in the ventricular system. Symptoms of hydrocephalus depend on the person's age. In infants, the most obvious sign is usually an abnormally large head; other symptoms may include vomiting, sleepiness, irritability, an inability to look upward, and seizures. In older children and adults there is no head enlargement from hydrocephalus, but symptoms may include headache, nausea, vomiting, and sometimes blurred vision. There may be problems with balance, delayed development in walking or talking, and poor coordination. Irritability, fatigue, seizures, and personality changes (such as an inability to concentrate or remember things) may also develop. Drowsiness and double vision are common symptoms as hydrocephalus progresses. Treatment involves insertion of a shunt to let the excess fluid exit, thereby relieving the pressure on the brain. The shunt is a flexible, plastic tube with a one-way valve. It is inserted into the ventricular system of the brain to divert the flow of CSF into another area of the body, where the CSF can drain and be absorbed into the bloodstream. The outlook with hydrocephalus depends on the cause, and on the timing of the diagnosis and treatment. Many children treated for hydrocephalus are able to lead normal lives with few, if any, limitations. In some cases, cognitive impairments in language and nonlanguage functions may occur. Problems with shunts, such as infection or malfunction, require revision of the shunt. Hydrocephalus is sometimes called "water on the brain." See also *hydrocephalus, acquired; hydrocephalus, congenital.*

**hydrocephalus ex-vacuo** Hydrocephalus that occurs when there is damage to the brain caused by stroke or injury, in which there may be an actual shrinkage of brain substance. Hydrocephalus ex-vacuo is essentially only hydrocephalus by default: the CSF pressure itself is normal. In old age or persons with Alzheimer disease, the entire brain may shrink and the CSF fills up the space created by the shrinkage. This is not due to hydrocephalus. See also *hydrocephalus; hydrocephalus, normal pressure.*

**hydrocephalus, acquired** Hydrocephalus as a result of something blocking the drainage of CSF after birth. Culprits can include a brain tumor, an arachnoid cyst, inflammation of the brain, hemorrhage, or head trauma. Bacterial meningitis is a particularly common cause, and is treated with high-dose antibiotics.

**hydrocephalus, communicating** Hydrocephalus in which the excess CSF gathers in the subarachnoid space rather than the ventricles of the brain.

**hydrocephalus, congenital** Hydrocephalus as a result of a birth defect or brain malformation. There are many possible causes for congenital hydrocephalus, including infection with viruses (cytomegalovirus, toxoplasmosis, and rubella, among others) or inheritance as an X-linked genetic trait. Some children with congenital hydrocephalus have other birth defects, including deadly and life-threatening problems.

**hydrocephalus, normal pressure** Hydrocephalus that occurs because of a gradual blockage of CSF drainage pathways in the brain. Although the ventricles enlarge, intracranial pressure remains within normal range. It can occur as a complication of brain infection or bleeding (hemorrhage). In some patients, no predisposing cause can be identified. Normal pressure hydrocephalus is characterized by memory loss (dementia), gait disorder, urinary incontinence, and a general slowing of activity. Abbreviated as NPH. See also *hydrocephalus, hydrocephalus ex-vacuo.*

**hydrocephaly** See *hydrocephalus.*

**hydronephrosis** Distention of the kidney with urine. Hydronephrosis is caused by obstruction of urine outflow (for example, by a stone blocking the ureter).

**hydrops fetalis** Gross edema (swelling), usually with anemia, of the fetus. It can be due to Rh blood group incompatibility, in which antibodies crossing the placenta from the mother destroy the red blood cells of the fetus. It can also be caused by alpha thalassemia, a lethal form of the genetic disorder thalassemia, in which alpha-chain polypeptides needed to make fetal or adult hemoglobin are not produced. See also *Rh incompatibility; thalassemia, alpha.*

**hydroxyapatite** An essential ingredient of normal bone and teeth, hydroxyapatite makes up bone mineral and the matrix of teeth and gives them their rigidity. See also *hydroxyapatite crystal disease.*

**hydroxyapatite crystal disease** Inflammation caused by hydroxyapatite crystals. Hydroxyapatite molecules can group together (crystallize) to form microscopic clumps. If these tiny crystals of hydroxyapatite are deposited by mistake in or around joints, they may cause inflammation of the joints and nearby tissues, such as tendons and ligaments. This is sometimes the cause of rotator cuff problems in the shoulder.

**hygiene** The science of preventive medicine and the preservation of health. Also commonly used as a euphemism for cleanliness and proper sanitation.

**hymen** A thin membrane which may completely or partially cover the vaginal opening before first sexual intercourse, but which usually disappears before puberty.

**hyoglossus** The muscle that permits the tongue to be held on the floor of the mouth.

**hyper-** Prefix meaning high, beyond, excessive, above normal. For example, hypercalcemia is high calcium in the blood. The opposite of hyper- is hypo-, as in hypocalcemia.

**hyperactivity** A higher than normal level of activity. An organ can be described as hyperactive if it is more active than is usual. Behavior also can be described as hyperactive. See also *attention deficit hyperactivity disorder.*

**hyperadrenocorticism** See *Cushing syndrome.*

**hyperaldosteronism** See *aldosteronism.*

**hyperbaric oxygen chamber** A pressurized chamber in which a patient receives pure oxygen, either directly or through a mask, tent, or tube. The oxygen is delivered at high pressure, more than 1.4 times normal atmospheric pressure. See also *hyperbaric oxygen therapy.*

**hyperbaric oxygen therapy**   The use of a hyperbaric oxygen chamber to treat any of a number of conditions, notably carbon monoxide poisoning, decompression sickness ("the bends"), smoke inhalation, and gas gangrene. It also helps to heal skin grafts and major burn injuries. The patient is enclosed in the chamber and receives appropriately pressurized pure oxygen for a specified length of time. Hyperbaric oxygen therapy activates white blood cells, and so it is sometimes used in cases of antibiotic-resistant or severe infection, such as for necrotizing fasciitis. Abbreviated as HBO.

**hyperbilirubinemia**   An elevated level of the pigment bilirubin in the blood. A sufficient elevation will produce jaundice. Some degree of hyperbilirubinemia is very common right after birth, especially in premature babies. Treatment is by exposure of the skin to special lights.

**hyperbilirubinemia I**   See *Gilbert syndrome*.

**hypercalcemia**   A higher-than-normal level of calcium in the blood. This can cause a number of nonspecific symptoms, including loss of appetite, nausea, thirst, fatigue, muscle weakness, restlessness, and confusion. Excessive intake of calcium may cause muscle weakness and constipation, affect the conduction of electrical impulses in the heart (heart block), lead to calcium stones (nephrocalcinosis) in the urinary tract, impair kidney function, and interfere with the absorption of iron, predisposing the person to iron deficiency. According to the National Academy of Sciences, adequate intake of calcium is 1 gram daily for both men and women. The upper limit for calcium intake is 2.5 grams daily.

**hypercholesterolemia**   High blood cholesterol. See *familial hypercholesterolemia*.

**hypercoagulability, estrogen-associated**   See *estrogen-associated hypercoagulability*.

**hypercoagulable state**   Medical term for a condition in which there is an abnormally increased tendency toward blood clotting (coagulation). There are numerous hypercoagulable states. Each has different causes, and each increases a person's chances of developing blood clots, such as those associated with thrombophlebitis (clot in the veins). These causes include medications (particularly female hormones and birth control pills), surgery (especially hip, knee, and urinary system procedures), pregnancy, phospholipid antibodies in blood (anticardiolipin antibodies, lupus anticoagulant), cancer (although most patients with a hypercoagulable state do not have cancer), elevated blood homocysteine levels, and inherited protein deficiencies, such as antithrombin III, factor V Leiden, protein S, or protein C. Treatment is by avoiding the triggering mechanism, and sometimes by blood-thinning medication. See also *estrogen-associated hypercoagulability*.

**hyperekplexia**   See *hyperexplexia*.

**hyperemesis gravidarum**   Excessive vomiting in early pregnancy. By definition, hyperemesis gravidarum leads to the loss of 5 percent or more of the woman's body weight. It affects about 1 in every 300 pregnant women, and is more common in young women, in first pregnancies, and in women carrying multiple fetuses. Hyperemesis gravidarum usually stops on its own and is of little clinical consequence. Sometimes, however, hyperemesis can keep the mother from getting necessary fluids and nutrition. Some women with hyperemesis gravidarum have high concentrations of the hormones human chorionic gonadotropin (hCG), estrogen, or thyroid hormone in their blood. A few also have clinical manifestations of hyperthyroidism (overactive thyroid state). Treatment of mild hyperemesis gravidarum is usually with dietary measures, rest, and antacids. Very severe hyperemesis gravidarum may call for intravenous fluid and nutrition.

**hyperexplexia**   A genetic disorder in which babies have an exaggerated startle reflex. Symptoms visible at birth include muscle stiffness (hypertonia), an exaggerated response to being startled, strong brain-stem reflexes (especially head-retraction reflex), and in some cases seizures. Hypertonia is evident when the limbs move, disappears during sleep, and diminishes over the first year of life. The startle reflex is sometimes accompanied by sudden stiffness (acute generalized hypertonia), which can cause the affected person to fall to the ground like a log. Additional findings include a tendency to umbilical and inguinal hernias (presumably due to increased pressure within the abdomen) and congenital dislocation of the hip. The exaggerated startle response persists throughout life. The gene responsible has been found on chromosome number 5, in bands 5q33.2-q33.3. Treatment is with medications. The neurological features can usually be controlled with clonazepam (brand name: Klonopin). In some cases, antispasmodic medications or tranquilizers have also been found useful. Also known as exaggerated startle disease, hyperekplexia, Kok disease, startle disease, and stiff baby syndrome.

**hyperglycemia**   Elevated level of the sugar glucose in the blood. Hyperglycemia is often found in diabetes mellitus. See also *diabetes mellitus*.

**hyperkalemia**   Elevated blood potassium.

**hyperlipidemia**   High lipid (fat) levels in the blood.

**hypermagnesemia**   Excess magnesium. Persons with impaired kidney function should be especially careful about their magnesium intake because they can accumulate magnesium, a dangerous (and sometimes fatal) situation. According to the National Academy of Sciences, the recommended dietary allowance of magnesium is 420 milligrams per day for men and 320 milligrams per day for women. The upper limit for magnesium supplements is 350 milligrams daily, in addition to the magnesium from food and water.

**hypermobility syndrome** A common, mostly harmless childhood condition in which joints can move beyond the normal range of motion. Symptoms can include pains in knees, fingers, hips, and elbows, and the affected joints may sprain or dislocate. Scoliosis (curvature of the spine) is more frequent. Hypermobility syndrome usually disappears by adulthood. Also called the joint hypermobility syndrome.

**hypernatremia** Elevated blood sodium.

**hyperopia** See *farsightedness*.

**hyperostosis** Overgrowth of bone. Hyperostosis is a nonspecific term that does not refer to any particular condition. Also known as exostosis.

**hyperphosphatemia** A higher-than-normal blood level of phosphate. Phosphate molecules are particularly important as part of larger molecules in cell energy cycles. Higher-than-normal levels can be caused by ingestion of phosphate-rich foods, such as dairy products, or by kidney failure.

**hyperpigmentation** Dark spots on the skin. Hyperpigmentation is primarily a cosmetic concern that can be covered with makeup, although in some cases (such as the café au lait spots associated with neurofibromatosis) it can be a sign of an underlying medical problem. If treatment of hyperpigmentation is desired, a dermatologist may be able to use dermabrasion, laser treatments, or bleaching agents to effect change.

**hyperplasia** A precancerous condition in which there is an increase in the number of normal cells lining the uterus.

**hyperplasia of the prostate, nodular** See *benign prostatic hyperplasia*.

**hyperplasia, benign prostatic** See *benign prostatic hyperplasia*.

**hyperplasia, endometrial** A condition characterized by overgrowth of the lining of the uterus.

**hypertension** High blood pressure, defined as a repeatedly elevated blood pressure exceeding 140 over

90 mmHg. Chronic hypertension can stealthily cause blood vessel changes in the back of the eye (retina), abnormal thickening of the heart muscle, kidney failure, and brain damage. No specific cause for high blood pressure is found in 95 percent of patients. Treatment is via salt restriction, regular aerobic exercise, and medication.

**hypertension, pulmonary** High blood pressure in the pulmonary arteries. Normally the pressure in the pulmonary arteries is low compared to that in the aorta. Pulmonary hypertension can irrevocably damage the lungs.

**hyperthermia** **1** Overheating of the body due to extreme weather conditions. Unrelieved hyperthermia can lead to collapse and death, particularly in the elderly. Prevention via air conditioning, ventilation, and by drinking extra water is the key for vulnerable persons. In emergency cases, injections of saline solution and rapid cooling of the body may be necessary. Also known as heatstroke or heat prostration. **2** Medical treatment for cancer, which involves heating a tumor or heating the whole body of the patient to kill cancerous cells.

**hyperthermia, malignant** A series of potentially fatal problems that can occur during surgery, malignant hyperthermia is caused by a reaction to anesthesia. The body's metabolism rises suddenly, causing a sudden jump in body temperature, and muscle rigidity. The result can be damage to tissues and organs (including the brain), or death. The propensity to malignant hyperthermia is inherited. Treatment is by administering dantrolene sodium (brand name: Dantrium), and rapidly cooling the patient.

**hyperthyroid** Excess of thyroid hormone resulting from an overactive thyroid gland, or from taking too much thyroid hormone. Symptoms can include increased heart rate, weight loss, depression, and cognitive slowing. Treatment is by medication, the use of radioactive iodine, thyroid surgery, or by reducing the dose of thyroid hormone.

**hypertonia** Increased tightness of muscle tone. Untreated hypertonia can lead to loss of function and deformity. Treatment is by physical and/or occupational therapy, and in some cases muscle-relaxant medication. Injections of botulism toxin (botox) are a recent treatment for chronic hypertonia in cerebral palsy and other disorders. Also known as spacticity.

**hypertonic solution** A solution containing more salt than is found in normal cells and blood.

**hypertrophic cardiomyopathy** See *cardiomyopathy, hypertrophic*.

**hypertrophy, benign prostatic** See *benign prostatic hyperplasia.*

**hyperuricemia** Abnormally elevated blood level of uric acid. Uric acid is a breakdown product of purines, which are part of many foods we eat. Hyperuricemia may indicate an increased risk of gout, but many patients with hyperuricemia do not develop gout, and some patients with repeated gout attacks have normal or low blood uric acid levels. People with hyperuricemia should avoid taking aspirin. Treatment is by dietary change, and for those without gout or kidney problems, medications that lower uric acid level.

**hyperventilation** Overbreathing due to anxiety. Hyperventilation causes dizziness, lightheadedness, a sense of unsteadiness, and tingling around the mouth and fingertips. Hyperventilation can be severe enough to mimic the early warning symptoms of a heart attack, and so is a common cause of emergency room visits in the US. Relief can be had by breathing in and out of a paper bag to increase the level of carbon dioxide in the blood.

**hypo-** Prefix meaning low, under, beneath, down, or below normal. For example, hyposensitivity is undersensitivity. The opposite of hypo- is hyper.

**hypocalcemia** Lower-than-normal levels of blood calcium, which makes the nervous system highly irritable, as evidenced by tetany: spasms of the hands and feet, muscle cramps, abdominal cramps, and overly active reflexes. Chronic calcium deficiency contributes to poor mineralization of bones, soft bones (osteomalacia), and osteoporosis. In children, it leads to rickets and impaired growth. Treatment is by increased dietary intake of calcium or calcium supplementation. Food sources of calcium include dairy foods, some leafy green vegetables, canned salmon, clams, oysters, calcium-fortified foods, and tofu. According to the National Academy of Sciences, adequate intake of calcium is 1 gram daily for both men and women. The upper limit for calcium intake is 2.5 grams daily.

**hypochondria** The condition of being obsessed with imaginary medical complaints. A person with hypochondria tends to misinterpret minor physical changes as symptoms of major illness. It is closely related to, and may be a subtype of, obsessive-compulsive disorder. Treatment with antidepressant medication and/or cognitive behavioral therapy is often successful. See also *obsessive-compulsive disorder.*

**hypochondroplasia** A type of short-limb dwarfism, with shortening especially of the ends of the limbs. See *dwarfism, hypochondroplastic.*

**hypoglossal nerve** The twelfth cranial nerve, which supplies the muscles of the tongue.

**hypoglossal neuropathy** Disease of the hypoglossal nerve. Paralysis of the hypoglossal nerve affects the tongue, making speech sound thick and causing the tongue to deviate toward the paralyzed side. In time, the tongue diminishes in size (atrophies).

**hypoglycemia** Low level of the sugar glucose in the blood. Symptoms include fatigue, dizziness, confusion, increased heart rate, and a cold, clammy feeling. Hypoglycemia is usually a complication of diabetes, in which the body does not produce enough insulin to fully metabolize glucose. Treatment is by careful diet, including small meals or snacks throughout the day; or by changing the dose or timing of insulin or other drugs that affect blood-sugar levels.

**hypokalemia** Low blood potassium.

**hypomagnesemia** Magnesium deficiency, which can occur due to inadequate intake or impaired intestinal absorption of magnesium. Hypomagnesemia is often associated with low calcium (hypocalcemia) and low potassium (hypokalemia). It causes increased irritability of the nervous system with tetany: spasms of the hands and feet, muscular twitching and cramps, spasm of the larynx, and so on. According to the National Academy of Sciences, the recommended dietary allowance of magnesium is 420 milligrams per day for men and 320 milligrams per day for women. The upper limit of magnesium supplements is 350 milligrams daily, in addition to magnesium from food and water.

**hyponatremia** Low blood sodium.

**hypophosphatemia** A lower-than-normal blood level of phosphate. The opposite of hyperphosphatemia.

**hypopigmentation** Lack of color in the skin or eyes. Hypopigmentation is characteristic of the various forms of albinism, and of several genetic diseases. See *albinism, Hermansky-Pudlak syndrome.*

**hypoplasia** Underdevelopment or incomplete development of a tissue or organ. For example, hypoplasia of the enamel of the teeth indicates that the enamel coating is thinner than normal, or missing in some but not all areas. Hypoplasia is less drastic than aplasia, where there is no development at all.

**hypoplasia of the thymus and parathyroids** See *DiGeorge syndrome.*

**hypoplasia, syndromatic hepatic ductular** See *Alagille syndrome.*

**hypoplastic left heart syndrome**   A form of congenital heart disease in which the whole left half of the heart—including the aorta, aortic valve, left ventricle, and mitral valve—is underdeveloped (hypoplastic). Blood returning from the lungs has to flow through an opening in the wall between the upper chambers of the heart (an atrial septal defect, or ASD). The right ventricle pumps blood into the pulmonary artery, and blood reaches the aorta through a shunt (the ductus arteriosus). The child may seem normal at birth, but will have trouble within a few days of when the ductus arteriosus closes. The infant becomes ashen, has rapid and difficult breathing, and has problems feeding. This heart defect is usually fatal within the first days or months of life without a sequence of surgeries or a heart transplant. See also *atrial septal defect, ductus arteriosus*.

**hypospadias**   A birth defect of the male urethra, which normally travels through the full length of the penis, carrying urine to an opening at the center of the tip. In hypospadias, the urethra opens on the underside of the penis or below the penis. In first-degree hypospadias, the urethral opening is below the tip, but nearby and on the glans. In second-degree hypospadias, the urethra opens closer to the body, on the underside of the shaft of the penis. In third-degree or perineal hypospadias, the urethral opening is below the penis on the skin. Males with first- or second-degree hypospadias can simply sit to urinate. If hypospadias is more significant, treatment is by surgery to repair and reconstruct the urethra.

**hypotension**   Blood pressure that is below the normal expected for an individual in a given environment. Blood pressure normally varies greatly with activity, age, medications, and underlying medical conditions. Hypotension can result from conditions of the nervous system, conditions that do not begin in the nervous system, and drugs. Neurological conditions that can lead to low blood pressure include changing position from lying to more vertical (postural hypotension), stroke, shock, lightheadedness after urinating or defecating, Parkinson disease, neuropathy, and simply fright. Nonneurological conditions that can cause low blood pressure include bleeding, infections, dehydration, heart disease, adrenal insufficiency, pregnancy, prolonged bed rest, poisoning, toxic shock syndrome, and blood transfusion reactions. Hypotensive drugs include blood pressure drugs; diuretics (water pills); heart medications, especially calcium antagonists such as nifedipine (brand name: Procardia); beta blockers such as propranolol (brand name: Inderal); antidepressants, such as amitriptylene (brand name: Elavil); and alcohol. Hypotension is the opposite of hypertension (abnormally high blood pressure). Treatment is not usually necessary, although people with mildly low blood pressure may want to be careful about

their activities. When necessary, medication is available. See also *hypotension, orthostatic*.

**hypotension, orthostatic**   A temporary lowering of blood pressure, usually related to suddenly standing up. Orthostatic hypotension may be experienced by healthy people who rise quickly from a chair, especially after a meal. It is more common in older people. The change in position causes a temporary reduction in blood flow, and therefore a shortage of oxygen to the brain. This leads to lightheadedness and, sometimes, a temporary loss of consciousness. Symptoms include dizziness, feeling as though one is about to black out, and tunnel vision. The symptoms are typically worse when standing, and improve with lying down. Tilt-table testing can be used to confirm orthostatic hypotension. Tilt-table testing involves placing the patient on a table with a foot support. The table is tilted upward, and blood pressure and pulse are measured while symptoms are recorded in various positions. No treatment is necessary for orthostatic hypotension. If someone with orthostatic hypotension faints, he or she will regain consciousness by simply sitting or lying down. The person is thereafter advised to exercise caution and slow the process of changing positions from lying to sitting to standing. This simple technique can allow the body to correct for the more vertical position by a gradual adjustment of the circulation of the legs. It can be especially important in older people. Also called postural hypotension.

**hypotension, postural**   See *hypotension, orthostatic*.

**hypothalamus**   The area of the brain that controls body temperature, hunger, and thirst.

**hypothermia**   Abnormally low body temperature. Someone who falls asleep in a snowbank may become hypothermic, and the condition can be fatal. Hypothermia is intentionally produced to slow the metabolism during some types of surgery.

**hypothyroid**   Deficiency of thyroid hormone.

**hypothyroidism, congenital**   Underactivity of the thyroid gland at birth, resulting in growth retardation, developmental delay, and other abnormal features. It is usually caused by an underdeveloped or malformed thyroid gland. The condition is detected today by newborn thyroid screening. Treatment is with thyroid hormone medication. Also known as cretinism.

**hypothyroidism, infantile**   Underactivity of the thyroid gland that starts after birth, as manifested by delays in growth and development, and by myxedema. Myxedema is a dry, waxy type of swelling, often including swollen lips and nose. Treatment is with thyroid hormone medication. Also known as Brissaud infantilism, infantile myxedema.

**hypotonia** Decreased muscle tone and strength; in a word, floppiness. Hypotonia is a common finding in cerebral palsy and other neuromuscular disorders. Untreated hypotonia can lead to hip dislocation and other problems. Treatment is via physical therapy. In some cases, braces may be needed to permit a full range of movement despite hypotonia.

**hypotonic solution** One with less salt than in normal cells and blood.

**hypovolemia** Abnormal decrease in the volume of blood plasma.

**hypovolemic shock** See *shock*.

**hypoxia** A lower-than-normal concentration of oxygen in arterial blood, as opposed to anoxia, a complete lack of blood oxygen.

**hypoxia-ischemia** Blood flow to cells and organs that is not sufficient to maintain their normal function, combined with a lower-than-normal concentration of oxygen in arterial blood.

**hypoxic-ischemic encephalopathy** Damage to cells in the central nervous system from inadequate oxygen during birth, as from having the umbilical cord wrapped around the neck (nuchal cord). Hypoxic-ischemic encephalopathy may cause death in the newborn period, or may result in developmental delay, mental retardation, or cerebral palsy. However, most infants born with a nuchal cord are completely healthy and normal.

**hysterectomy** An operation to remove the uterus, and sometimes also the cervix.

**hysterectomy, abdominal** Surgical removal of the uterus through an incision made in the abdominal wall, as opposed to a vaginal hysterectomy.

**hysterectomy, complete** See *hysterectomy, total*.

**hysterectomy, partial** Surgical removal of the uterus, but not the cervix. Also called a subtotal hysterectomy.

**hysterectomy, subtotal** See *hysterectomy, partial*.

**hysterectomy, total** Complete surgical removal of the uterus and cervix. Also called a complete hysterectomy.

**hysterectomy, vaginal** Removal of the uterus through a surgical incision within the vagina. With a vaginal hysterectomy, the scar is not outwardly visible. A vaginal hysterectomy is in contrast to an abdominal hysterectomy.

# Ii

thought to be a substance called filaggrin (FLG), which may act as the keratin matrix protein in cells of the layers of the skin known as stratum corneum. Also known as ichthyosis vulgaris.

**ichthyosis vulgaris**   See *ichthyosis simplex.*

**ichthyosis, spasticity, oligophrenia syndrome**   See *Sjogren-Larsson syndrome.*

**ichthyosis-keratitis-deafness syndrome**   See *keratitis-ichthyosis-deafness syndrome.*

**ICSI**   Intracytoplasmic sperm injection.

**icterus**   Jaundice.

**iatr-**   Prefix relating to a physician or medicine.

**iatrapistic**   A lack of faith in doctors.

**iatrogenic**   Due to the activity of a physician or therapy. For example, an iatrogenic illness is one caused by a medicine or doctor.

**iatromelia**   Ineffective or negligent medical treatment.

**iatromisia**   An intense dislike of doctors.

**IBD**   Inflammatory bowel disease. See *colitis, Crohn disease.*

**IBS**   Irritable bowel syndrome.

**ibuprofen**   A nonsteroidal anti-inflammatory drug (NSAID) commonly used to treat pain, swelling, and fever. Common brand names include Advil, Motrin, and Nuprin.

**I-cell disease**   A rare genetic disease that is similar to, but more severe than, pseudo-Hurler polydystrophy. I-cell disease is caused by an autosomal recessive mutation on one or more genes involved in lysosomal enzyme activity within the cells. When this enzyme activity does not occur properly, waste products build up within cells. Mental and motor retardation are marked, and death usually results within the first year. Diagnosis is by examining the level of lysosomal enzyme in the blood serum, or by other biochemical means. Prenatal and carrier detection is also possible. There is no known treatment for I-cell disease. Also known as mucolipidosis II. See also *mucolipidoses.*

**ichthyosis simplex**   A genetic skin disease that is inherited as an autosomal (non-sex-linked) trait. It is characterized by scaly areas of skin. The scaly skin usually first appears after three months of age. The palms and soles are often affected. Areas that tend to be spared include the armpits, the inside area at the bend of the elbow, and the skin behind the knee. Many people with this disease also have asthma, eczema, or hay fever. The gene responsible for this disease has been mapped to chromosome band 1q21. The product of this gene is

**ICU**   Intensive care unit.

**ICU psychosis**   A disorder in which patients in an intensive care unit (ICU) or a similar hospital setting may experience anxiety, become paranoid, hear voices, see things that are not there, become severely disoriented in time and place, become very agitated, or even become violent. One patient in every three who spends more than five days in an ICU experiences some form of psychotic reaction, according to current estimates. It is a form of delirium, or acute brain failure. Organic factors, including dehydration, low blood oxygen (hypoxia), heart failure, infection, and drugs can cause or contribute to delirium. Other factors that are believed to play into ICU psychosis are sensory deprivation, sensory overload, pain (particularly if poorly controlled), sleep deprivation, disruption of the normal day-night rhythm, and simply the loss of control over their lives that patients often feel in an ICU. ICU psychosis often goes away with the coming of morning or sleep. Although it may linger through the day, severe agitation usually occurs only at night. (This phenomenon, also known as sundowning, is common in nursing homes as well.) Treatment of ICU psychosis depends on the cause. Family members, familiar objects, and calm words may help. Dehydration calls for fluids. Heart failure needs treatment with digitalis. Infections must be diagnosed and treated. Sedation with antipsychotics may help. To prevent ICU psychosis, many critical care units have taken such steps as instituting visiting hours, minimizing shift changes in the nursing staff caring for a patient, and coordinating lighting with the normal day-night cycle. ICU psychosis usually goes away when the patient leaves the ICU.

**ID**   Intradermal.

**IDDM**   Insulin-dependent diabetes mellitus.

**idiocy, amaurotic familial**   See *Tay-Sachs disease.*

**idiopathic**   The cause is unknown.

**idiopathic hypertrophic subaortic stenosis**   A form of heart disease that causes narrowing of the left ventricle of the heart just below the aortic valve (subaortic steno-sis). Treatment options include drugs and surgery. See also *subaortic stenosis*.

**idiopathic sclerosing cholangitis** See *primary sclerosing cholangitis*.

**ideopathic torsion dystonia** See *dystonia, ideo-pathic torsion*.

**IgE** Immunoglobulin E.

**IHSS** Idiopathic hypertrophic subaortic stenosis.

**IL-1** Interleukin-1.

**IL-2** Interleukin-2.

**IL-3** Interleukin-3.

**IL-4** Interleukin-4.

**ileitis, Crohn** Inflammation of the ileum due to Crohn disease. See *Crohn disease*.

**ileitis, terminal** Inflammation of the end of the small intestine (the terminal ileum) due to Crohn disease. See *Crohn disease*.

**ileocolitis, Crohn** Crohn disease involving both the ileum and the large intestine. See *Crohn disease*.

**ileum** Part of the small intestine beyond the jejunum and before the large intestine (colon).

**ileus** Obstruction of the intestine due to its being para-lyzed. The paralysis does not need to be complete to cause ileus, but the intestine must be so inactive that food can-not pass through it, which leads to blockage of the intes-tine. Ileus commonly follows some types of surgery. It can also result from certain drugs, injuries, and illnesses. Irrespective of the cause, ileus causes constipation and bloating. On listening to the abdomen with a stethoscope, no bowel sounds are heard, because the bowel is inactive. Also known as paralytic ileus.

**ileus, meconium** Obstruction of the intestine due to overly thick meconium, a dark, sticky substance that is normally present in the intestine at birth. Meconium is passed in the feces after birth after trypsin and other enzymes from the pancreas have acted on it. Meconium ileus occurs when the infant has a deficiency of trypsin and other digestive enzymes from the pancreas, as in cys-tic fibrosis.

**ileus, paralytic** See *ileus*.

**iliac** Pertaining to the ilium.

**iliac horns** Horn-like malformations on the crest of both iliac bones of the pelvis, a characteristic finding in Fong disease. See *Fong disease*.

**ilium** The upper part of the pelvis, which forms the receptacle of the hip.

**illness, acute** An illness with an abrupt onset, and usually a short course.

**illness, altitude** See *altitude sickness*.

**illness, chronic** An illness that has persisted for a long period of time. It is a continuing disease process.

**IM** Intramuscular.

**Ilotycin** See *erythromycin*.

**Imdur** See *isosorbide mononitrate*.

**Imitrex** See *sumatriptin*.

**immune** Protected against infection, usually by the presence of antibodies.

**immune response** Any reaction by the immune sys-tem.

**immune system** A complex system that is responsible for distinguishing us from everything foreign to us, and for protecting us against infections and foreign sub-stances.

**immunity** The condition of being immune. Immunity can be innate—for example, humans are innately immune to canine distemper—or conferred by a previ-ous infection or immunization.

**immunization** Immunizations (vaccinations) work by stimulating the immune system of the body to fight dis-ease. The healthy immune system is able to recognize invading bacteria and viruses, and produces antibodies to destroy or disable them. Immunizations prepare the immune system to ward off a disease. To immunize against viral diseases, the virus used in the vaccine has been weakened or killed. To immunize against bacterial diseases, it is generally possible to use only a small por-tion of the dead bacteria to stimulate antibodies against the whole bacteria. The effectiveness of immunizations can be improved by periodic repeat injections, called "boosters." For information about specific immuniza-tions, see the name of the disease (for example, hepatitis B immunization).

**immunization, anthrax** See *anthrax immunization*.

**immunization, chicken pox** See *chicken pox vacci-nation*.

**immunization, children's** See *children's immunizations.*

**immunization, DPT** See *DPT immunization.*

**immunization, DT** Diphtheria and tetanus vaccine, usually reserved for individuals who have had a significant adverse reaction to a DPT (diptheria-pertussis-tetanus) shot, or who have a personal or family history of a seizure disorder, brain disease, or neurological disorder. See also *diphtheria, DPT immunization, DTaP immunization, tetanus.*

**immunization, DTaP** See *DTaP immunization.*

**immunization, flu** See *influenza vaccine.*

**immunization, German measles** See *MMR.* See also *rubella.*

**immunization, H. flu** See *Haemophilus influenzae type B immunization.*

**immunization, Haemophilus influenzae type B** See *Haemophilus influenzae type B immunization.*

**immunization, hepatitis A** See *hepatitis A immunization.* See also *hepatitis A.*

**immunization, hepatitis B** See *hepatitis B immunization.* See also *hepatitis B.*

**immunization, HIB** See *Haemophilus influenzae type B immunization.*

**immunization, infectious hepatitis** See *hepatitis A immunization.* See also *hepatitis A.*

**immunization, influenza** See *influenza vaccine.* See also *influenza.*

**immunization, measles** See *MMR.* See also *measles.*

**immunization, MMR** See *MMR.* See also *measles, mumps, rubella.*

**immunization, mumps** See *MMR.* See also *mumps.*

**immunization, pneumococcal pneumonia** See *pneumococcal pneumonia immunization.*

**immunization, polio** See *polio immunization.*

**immunization, rubella** See *MMR.* See also *rubella.*

**immunization, serum hepatitis** See *hepatitis B immunization.* See also *hepatitis B.*

**immunization, Td** See *Td immunization.* See also *tetanus, diphtheria.*

**immunization, varicella** See *chicken pox immunization.*

**immunocompetent** Able to develop an immune response. The opposite of immunodeficient.

**immunodeficiency** Inability to mount a normal immune response. Immunodeficiency can be due to a genetic disease, or acquired, as in AIDS.

**immunodeficient** Lacking immunity, and so susceptible to infection.

**immunodepression** See *immunosuppression.*

**immunogenetics** The genetics (inheritance) of the immune response. For example, immunogenetics includes the study of the Rh, ABO, and other blood groups.

**immunoglobulin E** Antibody of a specific class used to fight invading allergic substances (allergens). An allergic person frequently has elevated blood levels of IgE. IgE antibodies attack and engage the invading army of allergens. Abbreviated as IgE.

**immunologist** A physician or other degreed professional who is knowledgeable about immunology.

**immunology** The study of all aspects of the immune system, including its structure and function, disorders of the immune system, blood banking, immunization, and organ transplantation.

**immunosuppression** Lowering the immune response, for example, with radiation or medications.

**immunosuppressive agent** A medication that slows or halts immune system activity. Immunosuppressive agents may be given to prevent the body from mounting an immune response after an organ transplant, for example.

**immunotherapy** Treatment to stimulate or restore the ability of the immune system to fight infection and disease. See *biological therapy.*

**immunotherapy, allergy** Stimulation of the immune system with gradually increasing doses of the substances to which a person is allergic. The aim is to modify or stop the allergy by reducing the strength of the IgE response. This form of treatment is very effective for allergies to pollen, mites, animal dander, and especially stinging insects. Allergy immunotherapy usually takes six months to a year to become effective, and injections are usually required for three to five years.

**impact** To lodge firmly or wedge in.

**impaction, dental** See *dental impaction.*

**imperforate anus** See *anus, imperforate*.

**impetigo** A skin infection caused by the staphylococcus or, more rarely, streptococcus bacteria. The first sign of impetigo is a patch of red, itchy skin. Pustules develop on this area, soon forming crusty, yellow-brown sores that can spread to cover entire areas of the face, arms, and other body parts. Most patients are children. Treatment is by topical antibiotics.

**implant, cochlear** See *cochlear implant*.

**implantable cardiac defibrillator** See *cardiac defibrillator, implantable*.

**implantable pacemaker** See *pacemaker, internal*.

**impotence** A consistent inability to sustain an erection sufficient for sexual intercourse, inability to achieve ejaculation, or both. Impotence can be a total inability to achieve erection or ejaculation, an inconsistent ability to do so, or a tendency to sustain only brief erections. Impotence usually has a physical cause, such as disease, injury, drug side effects, or a disorder that impairs blood flow in the penis. Impotence can also have an emotional cause. Impotence is treatable in all age groups. Also known as erectile dysfunction.

**imprinting** A remarkable phenomenon that occurs in animals, and theoretically in humans, in the first hours of life. The newborn creature bonds to the type of animals it meets at birth, and begins to pattern its behavior after them. In humans, this is often called bonding, and usually refers to the relationship between the newborn and its parents.

**in** Abbreviation for inch.

**in situ** In the normal location. An in situ tumor is one that is confined to its site of origin, and that has not invaded neighboring tissue or gone elsewhere in the body. For example, squamous cell carcinoma in situ is an early stage of skin cancer.

**in situ hybridization** The use of a DNA or RNA probe to detect the complementary DNA sequence.

**in situ, carcinoma** Cancer that involves only the place in which it began, and that has not spread.

**in vitro** The opposite of in vivo (in a living organism), in vitro literally means in glass, as in a test tube. An in vitro test is one done in the lab.

**in vitro fertilization** A laboratory procedure in which sperm cells are put in a special dish with unfertilized eggs to achieve fertilization. The embryos that result can be transferred into the uterus or frozen (cryopreserved) for future use. Abbreviated as IVF.

**in vivo** In the living organism, as opposed to in vitro (in the laboratory).

**inactivated polio vaccine** See *polio immunization*.

**inappropriate ADH secretion** See *ADH secretion, inappropriate*.

**inborn errors of metabolism** See *metabolism, inborn errors of*.

**inbreeding** The mating of two closely related persons. Also called consanguinity.

**inbreeding, coefficient of** See *coefficient of inbreeding*.

**incest** Sexual activity between individuals so closely related that marriage is legally prohibited. Incest involving a child is a form of child abuse.

**inch** In length, 1/12 of a foot, or 1/36 of a yard; equivalent to 2.54 centimeters. Abbreviated as in.

**incidence** The frequency with which something, such as a disease or trait, appears in a particular population or area.

**incision** A cut. When making an incision, a surgeon is making a cut.

**incompetent cervix** See *cervix, incompetent*.

**incontinence** Inability to control excretions.

**incontinence of urine** See *enuresis; incontinence, urinary*. See also *bedwetting*.

**incontinence, fecal** Inability to hold feces in the rectum. This is due to failure of voluntary control over the anal sphincters, permitting untimely passage of feces and gas. Also called rectal incontinence. See *encopresis*.

**incontinence, urinary** Inability to hold urine in the bladder. This is due to failure of voluntary control over the urinary sphincters resulting in involuntary passage of urine (wetting). See *enuresis*. See also *bedwetting*.

**incontinent** Unable to control excretions, to hold urine in the bladder, or to keep feces in the rectum.

**incontinentia pigmenti** A genetic disease that begins soon after birth with the development of blisters on the trunk and limbs. These blisters then heal, but leave dark (hyperpigmented) streaks and marble-like whorls on the skin. Other key features of IP include dental and nail abnormalities, bald patches, and in about one-third of cases, mental retardation. IP is an X-linked dominant trait with male lethality, meaning that those male fetuses who do inherit the gene die before birth. The IP gene is in band q28 on the X chromosome. Mothers with IP have an equal chance of having a normal or IP daughter or a normal son. Also known as Bloch-Sulzberger syndrome.

**index case** A person who first draws attention to his or her family. For example, if your eye doctor discovers you have glaucoma, and subsequently other cases of glaucoma are found in your family, you are the index case. Also called the propositus (if male) or proposita (if female).

**indifferent gonad** See *gonad, indifferent*.

**induced menopause** See *menopause, chemical; menopause, induced*.

**infant** The young child, from birth to 24 months of age.

**infant mortality rate** The number of children dying at less than one year of age, divided by the number of live births that year. The infant mortality rate in the United States, which was 12.5 per 1,000 live births in 1980, fell to 9.2 per 1,000 live births in 1990.

**infantile genetic agranulocytosis** See *agranulocytosis, infantile genetic*.

**infantile hip dislocation** See *congenital hip dislocation*.

**infantile hypothyroidism** See *hypothyroidism, infantile*.

**infantile myxedema** See *hypothyroidism, infantile*.

**infantile paralysis** See *polio*.

**infantilism, Brissaud** See *hypothyroidism, infantile*.

**infarct** An area of tissue death due to a local lack of oxygen. See also *infarction*.

**infarction** The formation of an infarct, an area of tissue death due to a local lack of oxygen. See also *infarct*.

**infarction, acute myocardial** See *acute myocardial infarction*.

**infection, acute HIV** See *HIV infection, acute*.

**infection, ear** See *acute otitis media*.

**infection, group B strep** See *streptococcus, group B*.

**infection, middle ear** See *acute otitis media*.

**infection, opportunistic** An infection that grasps the opportunity to cause disease, presented when a person's immune system is weak. These opportunistic microorganisms may be dormant in the body, or may cause few problems for healthy individuals. Opportunistic infections are a particular problem for organ transplant patients and those with diseases that affect the immune system, particularly AIDS. Toxoplasmosis and cytomegalovirus are examples of opportunistic infections.

**infection, pinworm** See *pinworm infestation*. See also *enterobiasis*.

**infection, primary HIV** See *HIV infection, primary*.

**infection, rotavirus** See *rotavirus*.

**infection, urinary tract** See *urinary tract infection*.

**infection, Vincent** See *acute membranous gingivitis*.

**Infectious Diseases, National Institute of Allergy and** See *National Institutes of Health*.

**infectious hepatitis** See *hepatitis A*.

**infectious hepatitis immunization** See *hepatitis A, immunization*. See also *Havrix*.

**infectious mononucleosis** See *mononucleosis*.

**inferior** In medicine, inferior means below, downward, or toward the feet, as opposed to superior. The liver is inferior to the lungs. See also *Appendix B, "Anatomic Orientation Terms."*

**infertility** Diminished or absent ability to conceive and bear offspring. Infertility can have many causes. In most cases of possible female infertility, the problem is found to originate with the male partner's sperm motility. Some cases are due to physical problems or malformations of the female reproductive system. Others are due to genetic difficulties, such as Rh incompatibility between mother and fetus. Most types of infertility are treatable. In some cases, in vitro fertilization and other lab procedures may be used to ensure fertilization, and special medical care or medication may be required to enable the pregnancy to come to term.

**infiltrate** To penetrate. If an IV infiltrates, the IV fluid penetrates the surrounding tissue.

**infiltrating ductal carcinoma of the breast** See *breast, infiltrating ductal carcinoma of*.

**infiltrating lobular carcinoma of the breast** See *breast, infiltrating lobular carcinoma of the*.

**inflammation** A localized redness, warmth, swelling, and pain as a result of infection, irritation, or injury. Inflammation can be external or internal.

**inflammatory bowel disease** See *bowel disease, inflammatory*. See also *colitis, Crohn disease*.

**influenza** Popularly known as the flu, influenza is an illness caused by viruses that infect the respiratory tract. These viruses are divided into three types, designated A, B, and C. Symptoms include fever, appetite loss, an achy feeling throughout the body, and weakness. Most people who get the flu recover completely in one to two weeks, but some people develop serious and potentially life-threatening medical complications, such as pneumonia. Much of the illness and death caused by influenza can be prevented by annual influenza vaccinations.

**influenza vaccine** A vaccine recommended for persons at high risk for serious complications from influenza virus infection, including everyone age 65 or older; and people with chronic diseases of the heart, lung, or kidneys; diabetes; immunosuppression; or severe forms of anemia. The vaccine is also recommended for residents of nursing homes and other chronic-care facilities; children and teenagers receiving long-term aspirin therapy, who may therefore be at risk for developing Reye syndrome after an influenza virus infection; women who will be in the second or third trimester of pregnancy during the influenza season; and people in close or frequent contact with anyone at high risk, including physicians, nurses, other personnel in both hospital and outpatient-care settings, employees of nursing homes and chronic-care facilities, providers of home care to persons at high risk, and household members (including children) of persons in high-risk groups. People with an allergy to eggs should not receive influenza vaccine.

**informatics** The application of computers and statistics to the management of information. For example, in the Human Genome Project, informatics has permitted the development and use of methods to search databases quickly, analyze DNA sequence information, and predict protein sequence and structure from DNA sequence data.

**infraspinatus muscle** A muscle that assists the lifting of the arm while turning the arm outward (external rotation). The tendon of the infraspinatus muscle is one of four tendons that stabilize the shoulder joint and constitute the rotator cuff.

**inguinal** Having to do with the groin.

**inguinal canal** A passage in the lower anterior abdominal wall, which in the male allows passage of the spermatic cord and in the female contains the round ligament. Because of the weakness it creates in the abdominal wall, it is the most frequent site for a hernia.

**inguinal orchiectomy** Surgery to remove the testicle, with the incision made through the groin.

**inheritance, holandric** See *inheritance, Y-linked*.

**inheritance, mitochondrial** The inheritance of a trait encoded in the mitochondrial genome. Mitochondrial inheritance does not obey the classic rules of genetics. Persons with a mitochondrial disease may be male or female but are always related in the maternal line, and no male with the disease can transmit it to his children. The mitochondria are structures in the cell's cytoplasm, located outside the nucleus, and are responsible for energy production (metabolism). Mitochondrial disorders are therefore primarily disorders of metabolism. See also *mitochondria, mitochondrial diseases*.

**inheritance, multifactorial** A type of hereditary pattern seen when there is more than one genetic factor and, sometimes, environmental influence. Many common traits and many common diseases are multifactorial. Skin color, for example, is multifactorially determined, as is intelligence. Type 2 diabetes is multifactorial, because it is due to inherited (genetic) factors but usually requires environmental factors, such as obesity, to develop.

**inheritance, Y-linked** Inheritance of genes on the Y chromosome. Since only males normally have a Y chromosome, Y-linked genes can be transmitted only from father to son. Also called holandric inheritance.

**inherited metabolic diseases** See *metabolism, inborn errors of*.

**inhibitor, protease** See *protease inhibitor*.

**injury, cold** See *cold injury*. See also *chilblains, frostbite*, and *trench foot*.

**inner ear** See *ear, inner*. See also *ear*.

**INR** International normalized ratio.

**insect stings** Stings from large stinging insects, such as bees, hornets, yellow jackets, and wasps, which can trigger allergic reactions. These reactions vary greatly in severity. Avoidance and prompt treatment are essential. In selected cases, allergy injection therapy is highly effective.

**insemination** The deposition of semen in the female reproductive tract. Under normal circumstances, the deposit is made within the vagina or the cervix. By artificial means, such as intrauterine insemination, the deposit can be made directly into the uterus.

**insemination, artificial** See *artificial insemination*.

**insemination, heterologous** See *artificial insemination by donor*.

**insemination, homologous** See *artificial insemination by husband*.

**insemination, intrauterine**  See *artificial insemination*.

**insertion**  A chromosome abnormality due to insertion of a segment from one chromosome into another chromosome.

**insufficiency, pancreatic**  See *pancreatic insufficiency*.

**insulin**  A hormone made by the beta cells in what are called the islets of Langerhans of the pancreas, insulin controls the amount of sugar (glucose) in the blood. Insulin helps the body use glucose for energy. Cells cannot utilize glucose without insulin. If the beta cells that make insulin degenerate, preventing the body from making enough insulin on its own, type I (insulin-dependent) diabetes mellitus results. A person with this type of diabetes must inject insulin from other sources. Synthetic insulin is available for this purpose. See also *diabetes mellitus, insulin shock*.

**insulin shock**  A condition that may occur if a diabetic person takes too much insulin, does not eat on schedule, or is affected hormonally by emotional or other physical factors. In insulin shock, the level of sugar in the blood plummets, severely affecting brain cells. Hands and feet may tingle and become numb, vision can blur, the patient may sweat profusely and complain of headache, and the patient is likely to feel faint or even to pass out. Immediate treatment is imperative. A person in insulin shock needs sugar, which can be taken in the form of fruit juice, candy, a soft drink, or a prescribed glucose pill. Also known as insulin reaction. See also *diabetes mellitus*.

**insulin-dependent diabetes mellitus**  See *diabetes, insulin-dependent*. Abbreviated as IDDM.

**intelligence quotient**  See *IQ*.

**intelligence test**  A questionnaire or series of exercises designed to measure intelligence. It is generally understood that intelligence tests are less a measure of innate ability to learn as of what the person tested has already learned. There are many types of intelligence tests, and they may measure learning and/or ability in a wide variety of areas and skills. Scores may be presented as an IQ (intelligence quotient), a mental age, or on a scale.

**intelligence, nonverbal**  Innate or learned ability to understand and carry out motor tasks, such as solving physical puzzles. Also known as performance IQ.

**intelligence, verbal**  Innate or learned ability to understand and answer questions given in writing or verbally.

**intensive care unit psychosis**  See *ICU psychosis*.

**interatrial septum**  The partition separating the upper chambers (atria) of the heart.

**intercostal muscle**  Muscle tissue between two ribs.

**interferon**  A naturally occurring substance that interferes with the ability of viruses to reproduce. Interferon also boosts the immune system. There are a number of different interferons, and they fall into three main classes: alpha, beta, and gamma. All are proteins (lymphokines) normally produced by the body in response to infection. The interferons have been synthesized, using recombinant DNA technology.

**interferon therapy**  The goal of interferon therapy is to eradicate a virus from an infected person. Using interferon to eradicate the hepatitis B virus may, for example, prevent the future development of cirrhosis and cancer of the liver. This may require months and even years of interferon treatment, and may not be effective in many patients. In therapeutic doses, interferon can be hard to tolerate. Side effects include flu-like symptoms (fatigue, headache, and aches) and, less regularly, low thyroid activity, arthritis, low platelet count, and depression that can attain suicidal proportions. Some of these side effects, particularly depression, can be successfully treated with additional medication.

**interleukin**  One of several similar protein substances that may be used in biological therapy, interleukins stimulate the growth and activities of certain kinds of white blood cells that are involved in the immune response. Interleukins can be thought of as chemical messengers that give orders to the immune system.

**interleukin-1**  A protein produced by various cells, including macrophages, interleukin-1 raises body temperature, spurs the production of interferon, and stimulates growth of disease-fighting cells, among other functions. Abbreviated as IL-1.

**interleukin-2**  A protein that can improve the body's response to disease. It stimulates division of activated T-cells. Abbreviated as IL-2.

**interleukin-3**  A protein that stimulates the immune system to develop mast cells and bone-marrow cells. Abbreviated as IL-3.

**interleukin-4**  A protein that stimulates the immune system to develop mast cells, resting T-cells, and activated B-cells. Abbreviated as IL-4.

**intermittent claudication**  See *claudication, intermittent*.

**internal cardiac defibrillator**  See *cardiac defibrillator, implantable*.

**internal ear** See *ear, inner*. See also *ear*.

**internal genitalia, female** See *genitalia, female internal*.

**internal jugular vein** The deeper of the two jugular veins in the neck that drain blood from the head, brain, face, and neck, and then convey it toward the heart. The internal jugular vein collects blood from the brain, the outside of the face, and the neck. It runs down the inside of the neck outside the internal and common carotid arteries, and unites with the subclavian vein to form the innominate vein. See also *jugular veins*.

**internal medicine** A medical specialty dedicated to the diagnosis and medical treatment of adults. A physician who specializes in internal medicine is referred to as an internist. A minimum of seven years of medical school and postgraduate training are focused on learning the prevention, diagnosis, and treatment of diseases of adults. Subspecialties of internal medicine include allergy and immunology, cardiology (heart), endocrinology (hormone disorders), hematology (blood disorders), infectious diseases, gastroenterology (diseases of the gut), nephrology (kidney diseases), oncology (cancer), pulmonology (lung disorders), and rheumatology (arthritis and musculoskeletal disorders).

**internal pacemaker** See *pacemaker, internal*.

**internal radiation therapy** See *radiation therapy, internal*.

**international normalized ratio** A system established by the World Health Organization (WHO) and the International Committee on Thrombosis and Hemostasis for reporting the results of blood coagulation (clotting) tests. Under the INR system, all results are standardized. For example, a person taking the anticoagulant warfarin (brand name: Coumadin) would regularly have blood tested to measure the INR.

**internist** A physician who specializes in the diagnosis and medical treatment of adults. See also *internal medicine*.

**interphase** The interval in the cell cycle between two cell divisions, during which the individual chromosomes cannot be distinguished. Interphase was once thought to be a resting phase, but it is actually the time when DNA is replicated in the cell nucleus.

**interstitial cystitis** See *cystitis, interstitial*.

**interstitial radiation** See *radiation therapy, interstitial*.

**intervening sequence** See *intron*.

**interventional radiology** See *radiology, interventional*.

**interventricular foramen** An opening between the lateral and third ventricles in the system of four communicating cavities within the brain that are continuous with the central canal of the spinal cord.

**interventricular septum** The stout wall separating the lower chambers (the ventricles) of the heart from one another. A hole in the interventricular septum is termed a ventricular septal defect (VSD).

**intestinal gas** See *flatulence, flatus*.

**intestinal obstruction** Blockage of the intestine by infolding (intussusception), malformation, tumor, digestive problems, a foreign body, or inflammation. Symptoms can include crampy abdominal pain, lack of ability to eliminate normal feces, and eventually shock. On examining the abdomen, the doctor may feel a mass. Abdominal X-rays may suggest intestinal obstruction, but a barium enema may be needed to show the actual cause. Treatment depends on the cause of the obstruction. See also *intussusception*.

**intestinal pseudo-obstruction** Symptoms of intestinal obstruction with no sign of actual physical obstruction. This condition may be due to problems with the nerves that control intestinal muscles, or other causes. Treatment depends on the cause.

**intestine** The long, tubelike organ in the abdomen that completes the process of digestion. It consists of the small and large intestines, and extends from the stomach to the anus. See also *intestine, large; intestine, small*.

**intestine, large** The tubelike organ that completes the process of digestion, receiving material from the small intestine. It has four parts: the cecum (caecum), the appendix (vermiform appendix), the colon, and the rectum. Once the products of digestion enter the cecum through the ileocecal valve, they move rapidly past the appendix, which juts out from the intestine near the cecum. The colon absorbs any remaining water and forms the stool, which is sent to the rectum for elimination. The walls of the large intestine are muscular, and contract to move material along its length. See also *intestine; intestine, small*.

**intestine, small** The tubelike organ that receives the products of digestion from the stomach. It has three parts: the duodenum, the jejunum, and the ileum. The duodenum is rich in glands that produce digestive enzymes, and also receives bile from the liver. Digested material moves from the duodenum to the ileum through the jejunum. The ileum ends with the ileocecal valve, which prevents food passed into the large intestine from traveling back into the small intestine. The walls of the small intestine are muscular, and contract to move digested food along its length. The intestinal tube is lined with a mucus-like tissue that sends forth tiny, finger-like projections called villi. The villi increase the surface available for absorbing nutrients from digested food. See also *intestine; intestine, large*.

**intolerance, food**   Difficulty in digesting a food. Common offenders include milk products, wheat and other grains that contain gluten, and foods that tend to cause intestinal gas, such as cabbage or beans. Food intolerance is often mistaken for food allergy, but does not involve a histamine response against the food.

**intolerance, lactose**   See *lactose intolerance*.

**intra-arterial pressure**   See *arterial tension*.

**intracranial**   Inside the skull (the cranium).

**intracranial hemorrhage**   Bleeding inside the head.

**intractable**   Unstoppable. For example, intractable diarrhea or intractable pain.

**intracytoplasmic sperm injection**   A laboratory procedure in which a single sperm is injected directly into a single egg cell to achieve fertilization. The ICSI process is preferred when sperm motility is the primary bar to fertility.

**intradermal**   In the skin. An intradermal injection (ID) is given into the skin.

**intradermal test**   A type of skin test. An agent is injected into the skin to test the reaction to the agent (often a protein). Intradermal tests are much used to diagnose allergy and to test cellular immunity.

**intraductal papilloma**   A benign, wart-like growth that occurs in breast ducts.

**intraepithelial**   Within the layer of cells that forms the surface or lining of an organ.

**intrahepatic**   Within the liver.

**intramuscular**   Into the muscle. An intramuscular (IM) medication is given by needle into the muscle.

**intraocular**   In the eye. The intraocular pressure is the pressure within the eye.

**intraocular lens**   A lens made of plastic for replacing a lens clouded by cataract. Removal of the cataract and insertion of an intraocular lens (IOL) takes about an hour, and usually does not require hospitalization.

**intraocular pressure**   The pressure created by the continual renewal of fluids within the eye. The intraocular pressure is increased in glaucoma. In acute angle-closure glaucoma, the intraocular pressure rises because the canal into which the fluid in the front part of the eye normally drains is suddenly blocked. In chronic glaucoma, there is a gradual imbalance between the production and removal (resorption) of the fluid in the back part of the eye, causing the supply of fluid to exceed demand. See also *glaucoma*.

**intraocular tension**   See *intraocular pressure*.

**intraoperative**   During surgery.

**intraoperative blood salvage**   The recovery of blood lost into a body cavity during surgery or because of trauma. This blood can then be reintroduced into the patient's circulation, reducing the need for donor blood transfusion.

**intraoperative radiation therapy**   Radiation treatment given during surgery. Abbreviated as IORT. See also *radiation therapy*.

**intraperitoneal**   Within the peritoneal cavity, the area that contains the abdominal organs.

**intraperitoneal chemotherapy**   Treatment in which anticancer drugs are put directly into the abdomen through a thin tube. See also *chemotherapy*.

**intrastromal corneal ring**   A plastic ring designed to be implanted in the cornea, the transparent structure at the front of the eye, to flatten the cornea and thereby reduce the degree of nearsightedness (myopia). The ring is placed in the corneal stroma, the middle of the five layers of the cornea.

**intrathecal chemotherapy**   Treatment with drugs that are injected into the cerebrospinal fluid, which surrounds the brain and spinal cord. See also *chemotherapy*.

**intrauterine**   In the uterus.

**intrauterine device**   A contraceptive device inserted into the uterus to prevent conception or pregnancy. It can be a coil, loop, triangle, or T-shape. It can be plastic or metal. It is not yet known how intrauterine devices prevent pregnancy. Abbreviated as IUD.

**intrauterine growth retardation**   The growth of the fetus is abnormally slow. When born, the baby appears small for its actual age.

**intrauterine ultrasound**   Creating an image of the developing fetus within the uterus by means of measuring the vibrations returned when a device emits high-frequency sound waves. Ultrasound imaging during pregnancy has proved to be a very useful and effective diagnostic tool when there are concerns about fetal development or gestational age. It is believed to be a reasonably safe practice.

**intravenous** **1** Into a vein. Intravenous (IV) antibiotics are antibiotics in a solution that is administered directly into the venous circulation via a syringe or intravenous catheter (tube). **2** The solution that is administered intravenously. **3** The device used to administer an intravenous solution, such as the familiar IV drip used to slowly drip a bag of electrolyte solution into a dehydrated patient through a tiny plastic tube inserted directly into a vein.

**intravenous gamma globulin** See *intravenous immunoglobulin.*

**intravenous immunoglobulin** A sterile solution of concentrated antibodies extracted from healthy people that is given directly into a vein. It is used to treat disorders of the immune system, or to boost immune response to serious illness. Abbreviated as IVIG or IGG (for intravenous gamma globulin).

**intravenous pyelogram** An X-ray of the kidneys and urinary tract. Structures are made visible by the injection of a substance that blocks X-rays. Abbreviated as IVP.

**intravenous tension** The pressure of the blood within a vein. Also called venous pressure.

**intraventricular** In the ventricle of the heart or brain.

**introitus** An entrance that goes into a canal or hollow organ.

**introitus, facial canal** The entrance to the facial canal, a passage in the temporal bone of the skull through which the facial nerve travels.

**introitus, vaginal** The vaginal opening.

**intron** Part of a gene that is initially transcribed into the primary RNA transcript, but then removed from it when the exxon sequences on either side of it are spliced together. Also called an intervening sequence.

**intubate** To put a tube in.

**intussusception** Telescoping (prolapse) of a portion of the intestine within another immediately adjacent portion of intestine. This decreases the supply of blood to the affected part of the intestine, and frequently leads to intestinal obstruction. The pressure created by the two walls of the intestine pressing together causes inflammation and swelling, and reduces the blood flow. Death of

bowel tissue can occur, with significant bleeding, perforation, abdominal infection, and shock occurring very rapidly. Most cases of intussusception occur in children between five months and one year of age. Boys are affected three times more often than girls. The cause of intussusception is not known, although viral infections of the intestine may contribute to intussusception in infancy. In older children or adults, the presence of polyps or a tumor may trigger the intussusception. Early diagnosis is very important. Symptoms begin with sudden, loud crying in an infant, with the baby drawing the knees up to the chest while crying. This reaction is caused by abdominal cramping. The pain and crying is intermittent, but recurs frequently, and increases in intensity and duration. Fever is common. As the condition progresses, the infant becomes weak and then shows signs of shock, including pale color, lethargy, and sweating. About half of afflicted infants pass a bloody, mucousy ("currant jelly") stool. On examining the abdomen, the doctor may feel a mass. Abdominal X-rays may suggest intestinal obstruction, but a barium enema is needed to show the characteristic telescoping of the bowel. Treatment may or may not require surgery. In some cases, the intestinal obstruction can be reduced with a barium enema by a radiologist. (There is a risk of bowel perforation with this procedure, so it cannot be performed if perforation has already occurred.) If the obstruction cannot be reduced by a barium enema, surgery is needed to reduce the intussusception, relieve the obstruction, and remove any dead tissue. Intravenous feeding and fluid are continued until a normal bowel movement has passed. Although intussusception is life-threatening, the outlook is good with early treatment.

**invasive cervical cancer** Cancer that has spread from the surface of the cervix to tissue deeper in the cervix or to other parts of the body. See also *cancer, cervical.*

**inversion, chromosome** See *chromosome inversion.*

**inversion, paracentric chromosome** See *chromosome inversion, paracentric.*

**inversion, pericentric chromosome** See *chromosome inversion, pericentric.*

**invest** In medicine, this has nothing to do with the stock market: It means to envelop, cover, or embed.

**involution** A retrograde change. After treatment, a tumor may involute; with advancing age, there may be physical and emotional involution.

**iodide** The form to which iodine in the diet is reduced before being absorbed through the intestinal wall into bloodstream, and carried to the thyroid gland. See *iodine.*

**iodide goiter**   See *iodine excess*.

**iodine**   An essential element in the diet, iodine is essential for the manufacture of hormones by the thyroid gland. The thyroid uses iodine to make thyroxine (T4), which has four iodine molecules attached to its structure, and triiodothyronine (T3), which has three iodine molecules attached. Iodine is found in seafood, bread, iodized salt, and seaweed.

**iodine deficiency**   A lack of sufficient iodine in the diet, which can lead to inadequate production of thyroid hormone (hypothyroidism) and enlargement of the thyroid gland (goiter). Since the addition of iodine to table salt, iodine deficiency is rarely seen in the United States.

**iodine excess**   Prolonged intake of too much iodine also leads to swelling of the thyroid gland (goiter) and abnormally low thyroid activity (hypothyroidism). Certain foods and medications contain large amounts of iodine, including seaweed, iodine-rich expectorants like SSKI and Lugol's solution used to treat cough, asthma, and chronic pulmonary disease; and amiodarone (brand name: Cardorone), an iodine-rich medication used to control abnormal heart rhythms.

**ipecac, syrup of**   A solution containing a naturally occurring substance that can cause vomiting (emesis). Ipecac is derived from dried roots of a Brazilian bush, Uragoga ipecacuanha. Syrup of ipecac is used to treat a few types of poisoning. Always consult with your local Poison Control Center before administering syrup of ipecac, as many poisons cause additional harm if vomited.

**ipratropium**   An anticholinergic medication (brand name: Atrovent) used to treat bronchial spasms in bronchitis, emphysema, and chronic pulmonary disease.

**ipsilateral**   On the same side; the opposite of contralateral (the other or opposite side). For example, a tumor involving the right side of the brain may affect vision ipsilaterally, that is, in the right eye.

**IPV**   Inactivated polio vaccine. See *polio immunization*.

**IQ**   Abbreviation for intelligence quotient, an attempt to measure the intelligence of an individual. The IQ score is usually based on the results of a written test. To calculate the IQ, the person's mental age as determined by a test is divided by chronologic age, and the result is multiplied by 100. See also *intelligence test; intelligence, nonverbal; intelligence, verbal*.

**iridectomy**   Making a hole in the iris.

**iridology**   The practice of diagnosing disease by examining the iris of the eye. Although some diseases do affect the eye, iridology is not considered scientific medicine.

**iris**   The circular, colored curtain of the eye. Its opening forms the pupil. The iris helps regulate the amount of light that enters the eye.

**iris, speckled**   An iris that has small white or lightly colored spots slightly elevated on its surface. These spots are arranged in a ring concentric with the pupil, and are due to aggregation of normal connective tissue in the iris. They occur in normal children, but are far more frequent in Down syndrome. Also known as Brushfield spots.

**iritis**   Inflammation of the iris.

**iron**   An essential mineral, iron is necessary for the transport of oxygen via hemoglobin in red blood cells, and for oxidation by cells via cytochrome. Food sources of iron include meat, poultry, eggs, vegetables, and cereals, especially those fortified with iron. According to the National Academy of Sciences, the recommended dietary allowance of iron is 15 mg per day for women and 10 mg per day for men. See also *iron deficiency, iron excess, iron poisoning*.

**iron deficiency**   A common cause of anemia, since iron is necessary to make hemoglobin. Hemoglobin is the key molecule in red blood cells for the transport of oxygen. See also *anemia, iron deficiency*.

**iron excess**   Iron overload can damage the heart, liver, gonads, and other organs. Iron overload is a particular risk for people with certain genetic conditions, such as hemochromatosis, and people receiving repeated blood transfusions. According to the National Academy of Sciences, the recommended dietary allowances of iron are 15 mg per day for women and 10 mg per day for men.

**iron poisoning**   Iron supplements meant for adults, such as pregnant women, are a major cause of poisoning in children. Children should never be given supplements or multivitamins containing iron unless they have been prescribed by a doctor, and iron preparations for adults should be kept away from children.

**irrigate**   To wash out as, for example, irrigating a wound to clean it.

**irrigation of the colon**   The use of liquid solutions given by enema to remove material from the rectum or colon, ostensibly to eliminate toxins from the bowel. Unless ordered by a physician, this practice is rarely advisable. Irrigation of the colon carries a number of risks, including interference with the normal digestive process, and perforation. Also known as colonic irrigation, high colonics.

**irritable bowel syndrome**   A common gastrointestinal disorder in which gut contractions (motility) are abnormal. IBS is characterized by abdominal pain, bloating, mucus in stools, and irregular bowel habits with alternating diarrhea and constipation. These symptoms tend to be chronic, and wax and wane over the years. Although IBS can cause chronic and recurrent discomfort, it does not normally lead to any serious organ problems. Diagnosis usually involves excluding other illnesses. Treatment is directed toward relief of symptoms, and includes high-fiber diet; exercise; relaxation techniques; avoidance of caffeine, milk products, and sweeteners; and medications. Also called spastic colitis, mucus colitis, nervous colon syndrome.

**ischemia** Inadequate blood supply to a local area due to blockage of blood vessels leading to that area.

**ischiopubic bar** See *ischium*.

**ischiopubic synchondrosis** The central point of the ischium, which does not close until after the toddler years. See *ischium*.

**ischium** The bone that makes up the lower rear part of the pelvis. Also called the ischiopubic bar or bone.

**islets of Langerhans** Groups of specialized cells in the pancreas that make and secrete hormones, including insulin. These cells sit in groups (islets), with five types of cells in an islet: alpha cells that make glucagon, which raises the level of glucose (sugar) in the blood; beta cells that make insulin; delta cells that make somatostatin, which inhibits the release of numerous other hormones in the body; and PP cells and D1 cells, about which little is known. Degeneration of the insulin-producing beta cells is the main cause of type 1 (insulin-dependent) diabetes mellitus.

**ISMO** See *isosorbide mononitrate*.

**isochromosome** An abnormal chromosome with two identical arms due to duplication of one arm and loss of the other. Isochromosomes are found in some girls with Turner syndrome, and in tumors.

**isodisomy** A remarkable situation where both chromosomes in a pair are from one parent only. Isodisomy causes some birth defects and is suspected to play a role in cancer. Also called uniparental disomy.

**isolate** A group (for example, the Amish) in which mating is always between members of the group.

**isosorbide mononitrate** A nitrate medication (brand name: Imdur, ISMO, Monoket) used to treat chest pain associated with angina, and to prevent congestive heart failure.

**isotonic solution** A solution that has the same salt concentration as cells and blood.

**isotope** A form of a chemical element with a different atomic mass. Isotopes are used in a number of medical tests.

**itching** An uncomfortable sensation in the skin that feels as if something were crawling on the skin, and makes the person want to scratch the affected area. It is medically known as pruritis, so something that is itchy is pruritic.

**itching, anal** See *anal itching*.

**-itis** Suffix meaning inflammation. For example, colitis is inflammation of the colon.

**ITP** Idiopathic thrombocytopenic purpura.

**IUD** Intrauterine device.

**IUGR** Intrauterine growth retardation.

**IV** Intravenous.

**IVF** In vitro fertilization.

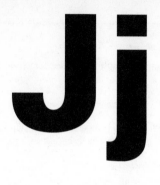

# Jj

**Jacksonian seizure** See *seizure, partial*.

**Jadassohn-Lewandowski syndrome** An inherited (genetic) condition characterized by abnormally thick, curved nails (onychogryposis); thickening of the skin (hyperkeratosis) of the palms, soles, knees and elbows; white plaques (leukoplakia) in the mouth; excess sweating (hyperhidrosis) of the hands and feet; and the presence of erupted (visible) teeth at birth (natal teeth). Jadassohn-Lewandowski syndrome is an autosomal dominant trait. The gene (named PD1) responsible is on chromosome 12, in band 12q13, and a single copy of the PD1 gene is capable of causing the disease. The basic abnormality is a mutation in a gene for keratin, a primary constituent of nails, hair, and skin. Also known as elephant nails from birth, pachyonychia congenita of the Jadassohn-Lewandowski type, pachyonychia congenita with natal teeth, type 1 pachyonychia congenita.

**jail fever** See *typhus, epidemic*.

**Jakob disease** See *Creutzfeldt-Jakob disease*.

**Jakob-Creutzfeldt disease** See *Creutzfeldt-Jakob disease*.

**JAMA** The *Journal of the American Medical Association*, one of the two leading general medical journals published in the United States. *JAMA* is published by the American Medical Association (AMA). It carries original, generally well-documented, peer-reviewed medical articles on many clinical and research topics in medicine.

**jamais vu** The illusion that the familiar does not seem familiar. See also *déjà vu*, *seizure disorders*.

**jaundice** A yellowish staining of the skin and white of the eyes (sclerae) with bilirubin, the pigment found in bile. Jaundice can be an indicator of liver or gallbladder disease, or it may result from red blood cells rupturing (hemolysis). In newborn babies it is usually, but not always, a normal condition. Also known as icterus. See also *jaundice, hemolytic; jaundice, hepatocellular; jaundice, neonatal; jaundice, obstructive; spherocytosis, hereditary*.

**jaundice, congenital hemolytic** See *spherocytosis, hereditary*.

**jaundice, hemolytic** Jaundice caused by destruction of red blood cells. This can be an inborn condition (hereditary spherocytosis) or it may be caused by a blood transfusion from a different blood group, infection in the blood, or some types of poisoning. See also *spherocytosis, hereditary*.

**jaundice, hepatocellular** Jaundice caused by liver disease, as by hepatitis. See also *hepatitis*.

**jaundice, malignant obstructive** See *jaundice, obstructive*.

**jaundice, neonatal** A certain degree of jaundice is normal in newborn babies due to the breakdown of red blood cells, which release bilirubin into the blood, and to the immaturity of the newborn's liver, which cannot effectively metabolize the bilirubin and prepare it for excretion into the urine. Normal neonatal jaundice typically appears between the second and fifth days of life, and clears with time. Frequent breastfeeding may be helpful. Diagnosis is by observation and by blood test for bilirubin level. Treatment, if warranted, is usually with timed exposure of the skin to special lights, sometimes through a device called a bilirubin blanket. Jaundice that appears during the first day of life may be due to a biliary disorder and is much more likely to require medical treatment. See also *jaundice; spherocytosis, hereditary*.

**jaundice, obstructive** Jaundice caused by obstruction of the bile ducts, as with gallstones. Additional symptoms of obstructive jaundice include dark urine, pale feces, and itching, although there is no pain. Sometimes the cause of obstructive jaundice is cancer (malignant obstructive jaundice), in which case treatment is by chemotherapy, radiation, and/or biliary drainage (surgery is rarely used).

**jaw** The movable junction of the bones below the mouth (the mandible) and the bone just above the mouth (the maxilla).

**jejunal** Having to do with the jejunum.

**jejunum** The middle part of the small intestine, located halfway between the duodenum and ileum. See also *intestine; intestine, small*.

**jet lag** Sleep disturbance and fatigue caused when the body's natural rhythms are interrupted by travel across time zones. See also *circadian clock*.

**jogger's nails** Very common, small, semicircular white spots on the nails. These spots result from injury to the base (matrix) of the nail, a structure under the visible nail where the cells that make up the visible nail are produced. The injury responsible for white spots on the nails can be due to athletic activity or poorly fitting shoes, so jogging in poorly fitting shoes causes it so often as to coin the term "jogger's nails." These spots are not a cause for concern. They eventually grow out.

**joint** The area where two bones are attached for the purpose of permitting body parts to move. A joint is usually formed of fibrous connective tissue and cartilage. Joints are grouped according to their motion: ball-and-socket joint; hinge joint; condyloid joint, which permits all forms of angular movement except axial rotation; pivot joint; gliding joint; or saddle joint. Joints can move in only four ways: Gliding, in which one bony surface glides on another without angular or rotatory movement; angular, a movement that occurs only between long bones, increasing or decreasing the angle between the bones; circumduction, which occurs in joints composed of the head of a bone and an articular cavity, with the long bone describing a series of circles and the whole forming a cone; and rotation, in which a bone moves about a central axis without moving from this axis. Also known as an articulation or arthrosis.

**joint aspiration** See *arthrocentesis*.

**joint hypermobility syndrome** See *hypermobility syndrome*.

**joint, AC** Acromioclavicular joint. See *acromioclavicular joint*.

**joint, acetabular** The hip joint. The acetabulum is the cup-shaped socket of the hip joint, and a key feature of the pelvic anatomy. The upper end of the femur (thighbone) fits right into the acetabulum, articulates with it, and thereby forms the largest ball-and-socket joint in the human body.

**joint, acromioclavicular** See *acromioclavicular joint*.

**joint, ankle** See *ankle joint*.

**joint, atlas and axis** See *atlas and axis joint*.

**joint, ball-and-socket** A joint in which the round end of a bone fits into the cavity of another bone. The hip joint is a ball-and-socket joint.

**joint, calcaneocuboid** See *calcaneocuboid joint*.

**joint, elbow** See *elbow*.

**joint, knee** See *knee*.

**joint, patellofemoral** See *patellofemoral joint*.

**joint, shoulder** See *shoulder joint*.

**joint, temporomandibular** See *temporomandibular joint*.

**joint, TM** Temporomandibular joint.

**joints of the body, principal** The principal joints of the human body include the following:

acromioclavicular

ankle (tibia-fibula and talus)

atlas and axis

atlas and occipital

calcaneocuboid

carpometacarpal

elbow (humerus, radius, and ulna)

femur and tibia

hip bone and femur

humerus and ulna

intercarpal (proximal carpal, distal carpal, and the two rows of carpal bones with each other)

intermetacarpals

intermetatarsals

interphalangeal

knee (femur, tibia, and patella)

mandible (jaw) and temporal

metacarpophalangeal

metatarsophalangeal

pubic bones

radioulnar, distal

radioulnar, middle

radioulnar, proximal

radius-ulna and carpals (wrist)

ribs, heads of

ribs, tubercles and necks of

sacrococcygeal

sacroiliac

shoulder (humerus and scapula)

symphysis

sacroiliac

scapula and humerus

sternoclavicular

sternocostal

subtalar

talus and calcaneus

talus and navicular

tarsometatarsal

tibia-fibula and talus (ankle)

tibiofibular

vertebral arches

vertebral bodies

wrist (radius-ulna and carpals)

***Journal of the American Medical Association***
See *JAMA*.

**jugular**   See *jugular veins*.

**jugular vein, external**   The more superficial of the two jugular veins in the neck. The external jugular vein collects most of the blood from the outside of the skull and the deep parts of the face. It lies outside the sternocleidomastoid muscle, passes down the neck, and joins the subclavian vein. See also *jugular veins*.

**jugular vein, internal**   The deeper of the two jugular veins in the neck. The internal jugular vein collects blood from the brain, the outside of the face, and the neck. It runs down the inside of the neck outside the internal and common carotid arteries, and unites with the subclavian vein to form the innominate vein. See also *jugular veins*.

**jugular veins**   The veins in the neck that drain blood from the head, brain, face, and neck, and then convey it toward the heart. There are an external and an internal jugular vein. The jugular veins are particularly prominent during congestive heart failure. When the patient is sitting or in a semirecumbent position, the height of the jugular veins and their pulsations provide an estimate of the central venous pressure, as well as important information about whether the heart is keeping up with the demands on it. See also *jugular vein, external; jugular vein, internal*.

**June cold**   Another term for hay fever, an allergic disorder. Also known as allergic rhinitis, summer cold.

**juvenile**   Between infantile and adult. Used in medical terms to indicate onset in childhood as, for example, in juvenile rheumatoid arthritis.

**juvenile chronic arthritis, systemic-onset**   See *arthritis, systemic-onset juvenile rheumatoid*.

**juvenile laryngeal papillomatosis**   A condition characterized by the emergence of numerous warty growths on the vocal cords in children and young adults. A baby can contract juvenile laryngeal papillomatosis by being contaminated with the human papilloma virus (HPV) during birth through the vaginal canal of a mother with genital warts. Each year, about 300 infants are thus born with the virus on their vocal cords. Treatment is usually by surgical excision. Recurrences of laryngeal papillomatosis are, unfortunately, frequent. Remission may occur after several years.

**juvenile rheumatoid arthritis**   See *arthritis, systemic-onset juvenile rheumatoid*.

**juxta-**   A prefix meaning near, nearby, close. For example, juxtaspinal is near the spinal column, and juxtavesicular is near the bladder.

**juxtaarticular**   Near a joint: a juxtaarticular fracture is a break near a joint.

**juxtaglomerular apparatus**   A collective term referring to the cells near a structure called the glomerulus in the kidney. The juxtaglomerular cells are specialised cells that stimulate the secretion of the adrenal hormone aldosterone. They play a major role in the kidney's self-regulation system.

**juxtaposition**   The act of placing two or more things side by side, or the state of being so placed. To lose a pair of juxtaposed teeth is to lose teeth that are next to one another. Also known as apposition.

**juxtapyloric**   Near the pylorus, the muscular area at the junction of the stomach and the first part of the small intestine. A juxtapyloric ulcer is located near the pylorus.

**juxtaspinal**   Near the spinal column.

**juxtavesicular**   Near the bladder.

# Kk

**k cells** See *natural killer cells*.

**kala-azar** Hindi for black fever. Kala-azar is a disease of the viscera, particularly the liver, spleen, bone marrow, and lymph nodes, due to infection by a parasite called Leishmania. Also known as visceral leishmaniasis. See also *Leishmania, leishmaniasis*.

**Kaposi sarcoma** A relatively rare type of cancer that can develop on the skin of some elderly persons or those with a weak immune system, including about 20 percent of people with AIDS. It is a vascular (angioblastic) cancer of the skin, characterized by soft, purplish plaques and papules that form tumor-like nodules. These often appear first on the feet, and then slowly spread across the skin. It is currently believed that Kaposi sarcoma is triggered by a virus. Treatment is by topical medication, cryosurgery, interferon, or radiation therapy. See also *sarcoma*.

**Kartagener syndrome** The trio of sinusitis, bronchitis, and situs inversus (lateral reversal of the position of all organs in the chest and abdomen).

**karyotype** A standard arrangement of the chromosome complement, done for chromosome analysis.

**karyotyping** Chromosome study.

**karyotyping, flow** See *flow karyotyping*. See also *flow cytometry*.

**Kawasaki disease** A syndrome that mainly affects young children, causing fever; reddening of the eyes (conjunctivitis), lips, and mucous membranes of the mouth; ulcerative gum disease (gingivitis); swollen glands in the neck (cervical lymphadenopathy); and a rash that is raised and bright red (maculoerythematous). The rash appears in a "glove-and-sock" fashion over the skin of the hands and feet. The skin then becomes hard, swollen (edematous), and peels off. Kawasaki disease affects the vascular system, and is now the main cause of acquired heart disease in children. It is most common in people of Asian descent, and is both more common and more deadly in males. Its cause is unknown; current theories include viral causes or an environmental toxin. Treatment is usually by intravenous immunoglobulin (IVIG). Also known as mucocutaneous lymph node syndrome.

**Kb** Abbreviation for kilobase.

**KB** Keratodermia blennorrhagicum.

**Keflax** See *cephalexin*.

**Kegel exercises** Exercises designed to increase muscle strength and elasticity in the female pelvis. Kegel exercises may be recommended for treatment of an incompetent cervix, vaginal looseness after pregnancy and delivery, or urinary incontinence.

**keloid** A scar that rises quite abruptly above the rest of the skin. It is irregularly shaped, tends to enlarge progressively, and may be darker in color and harder than the surrounding skin. Keloids are a response to trauma, such as a cut to the skin. In creating a normal scar, connective tissue in the skin is repaired by the formation of collagen. This occurs in the dermis, the second layer of skin. Keloids arise when extra collagen forms. Susceptibility to keloids is clearly genetic, and they are particularly common in people of African descent. If a keloid is uncomfortable or cosmetically undesirable (as in the case of a keloid scar on the face), a dermatologist may be able to reduce its prominence by using several different techniques.

**keratectomy** Removal of part of the cornea by surgical excision or by laser. See also *keratectomy, photorefractive*.

**keratectomy, photorefractive** Laser eye surgery designed to change the shape of the cornea, reducing or eliminating the need for glasses and contact lenses. The laser removes the outer layer of the cornea, and then flattens it. This is intended to correct nearsightedness (myopia) and uneven curvature of the cornea that distorts vision (astigmatism). It is an outpatient procedure done in the office with numbing eye drops. It takes about one minute to do, and about three days to heal. No eye patch need be worn afterwards. Abbreviated as PRK.

**keratin** A protein found in the upper layer of the skin, hair, and nails, and in animal horns.

**keratitis** Inflammation of the cornea.

**keratitis, rosacea** A condition affecting the eyes in about half of all people with rosacea. Symptoms include burning and grittiness of the eyes (conjunctivitis). If this is not treated, inflammation of the cornea may impair vision. See also *rosacea*.

**keratitis-ichthyosis-deafness syndrome** A very rare inherited disorder in which affected persons have gradual destruction of the cornea (keratitis), possibly leading to blindness. Localized areas of disfiguring reddish thickened skin (ichthyosis), deafness at birth, and thin or even absent scalp hair are also seen. Some patients develop carcinoma of the tongue, while others have subtle abnormalities of the nervous system. The cause of keratitis-ichthyosis-deafness (KID) syndrome is still a mystery, although it has been linked to an autosomal recessive trait.

**kerato-**  Prefix referring to the cornea, as in keratitis and keratocornea, or to nail, hair, or skin tissue, as in keratin and keratosis.

**keratoconjunctitis**  Inflammation of the eye involving both the cornea and conjunctiva.

**keratoconus**  A cone-shaped cornea with the apex of the cone being forward. Also known as conical cornea.

**keratodermia blennorrhagicum**  A skin disease that occurs in patients with Reiter syndrome. Classically, the areas of the skin involved are the palms of the hands and soles of the feet, although other body surfaces may also be affected. The inflammation of the skin can come and go. When present, it causes patches of reddish, raised pustules that can be painful and tender. These patchy areas may group together and peel periodically. Keratodermia blennorrhagicum can be treated with topical medications, including skin softeners (emollients) and medications that clear off the peeling, dry skin (keratolytic medications). Sometimes these treatments are used along with vitamin D creams, such as calcipotriene. Emotional stress and certain medications, such as propanolol (brand name: Vasotec) and hydroxychloroquine (brand name: Plaquenil) may aggravate the condition. Abbreviated as KB.

**keratoma**  An area of hardened skin, usually called a callus.

**keratoplasty**  Corneal transplant.

**keratosis**  A localized overgrowth of the upper layer of skin. Common forms of keratosis include aging and sun exposure.

**keratosis follicularis**  A rare skin disease characterized by hardening of the skin around the hair follicles, leading to baldness (alopecia). Also known as Darier disease.

**keratosis, actinic**  Overgrowth of skin due to sun exposure. The raised spots are usually red, or may match the skin but look leathery and wart-like.

**keratosis, seborrheic**  A skin disorder characterized by oily skin, and warts and skin lesions that appear to be "stuck on." The raised spots are usually yellow or brown. Treatment, if warranted, is by surgical or cryosurgical removal. Also known as seborrheic warts, verruca.

**keratosis, senile**  Thickening of the skin that is associated with old age. The raised spots are usually red, or may match the skin but look leathery and wart-like.

**keratotomy**  A surgical cut of the cornea.

**keratotomy, radial**  A surgical procedure designed to flatten the cornea, and thereby correct nearsightedness (myopia). It is called a radial keratotomy because the incisions resemble the spokes in a bicycle wheel.

**kernicterus**  Disorder due to severe jaundice in a newborn baby. High blood levels of the pigment bilirubin are deposited in the brain, resulting in damage. Although some degree of jaundice is normal between the second and fifth day of life, the level of bilirubin is monitored in newborns to determine whether treatment is needed to prevent kernicterus. When the brain is affected, it is also called bilirubin encephalopathy.

**Kernig sign**  A sign of meningitis: inflammation of the meninges covering the brain and spinal cord. The test for Kernig sign is done by having the person lie flat on the back, flex the thigh so that it is at a right angle to the trunk, and completely extend the leg at the knee joint. If the leg cannot be completely extended due to pain, this is Kernig sign.

**Keshan disease**  Condition caused by deficiency of the essential mineral selenium. Keshan disease is a potentially fatal form of cardiomyopathy (disease of the heart muscle). It was first observed in Keshan province in China, and since has been found in other areas where the selenium level in the soil is low. Treatment is by selenium supplementation.

**ketoacidosis**  Accumulation of substances called ketone bodies in the blood (ketosis), plus increased acidity of the blood (acidosis). Ketoacidosis is a potentially fatal condition that may occur when diabetes is not controlled. Symptoms include slow, deep breathing with a fruity odor to the breath; confusion; frequent urination; poor appetite; and eventually loss of consciousness. Treatment is usually in a hospital setting, and may require intravenous fluids, insulin, glucose, and dietary changes. See also *diabetes mellitus*.

**ketogenic diet**  A diet devised as a treatment for severe seizure disorders that do not respond to conventional medication. The ketogenic diet is almost entirely made up of fats and protein. All portions must be precisely weighed and timed. Because this diet can cause the buildup of ketone bodies in the blood, it is highly risky and should only be tried under close medical supervision. See also *ketone bodies, ketoacidosis, seizure disorders.*

**ketone bodies**   Acetone, acetoacetate, and B-hydroxybutyrate, three toxic, acidic chemicals that build up in the bloodstream when the body is forced to burn fat for energy instead of burning glucose. See also *ketoacidosis.*

**KID syndrome**   See *keratitis-ichthyosis-deafness syndrome.*

**Kidney Diseases, National Institute of Diabetes and Digestive and**   See *National Institutes of Health.*

**kidney scoping**         See *retrograde intrarenal surgery.*

**kidney stone**   A stone in the kidney, or a stone that originated in the kidney but has passed lower down in the urinary tract. Kidney stones are a common cause of blood in the urine and pain in the abdomen, flank, or groin. One in 20 people will have a kidney stone at some time in his or her life. The development of kidney stones is related to decreased urine volume, or to increased excretion of stone-forming components, such as calcium, oxalate, urate, cystine, xanthine, and phosphate. The stones form in the urine-collecting area (pelvis) of the kidney, and may range in size from tiny to "staghorn" stones the size of the renal pelvis itself. Factors that predispose people to kidney stones include reduction in fluid intake, increased exercise with dehydration, medications that cause high uric acid (hyperuricemia), and a history of gout. Pain from kidney stones is usually of sudden onset, very severe and intermittent, not improved by changes in position, and radiates from the back, down the flank, and into the groin. Nausea and vomiting are common. The majority of stones pass spontaneously within 48 hours. However, some stones do not. Several factors influence the ability to pass a stone, including the size of the person, prior stone passage, prostate enlargement, pregnancy, and the size of the stone. If a stone does not pass, the help of a urology specialist may be needed. Routine treatment includes relief of pain, hydration and, if there is concurrent urinary infection, antibiotics.

**kidney stones, cystine**   See *cystine kidney stones.* See also *cystinuria.*

**kidney transplant**   Replacement of a diseased, damaged, or missing kidney with a donor kidney.

**kidneys**   A pair of organs located in the right and left side of the abdomen. The kidneys remove waste products from the blood and produce urine. As blood flows through the kidneys, they filter waste products, chemicals, and unneeded water from the blood. Urine collects in the middle of each kidney, an area called the renal pelvis. It

then drains from the kidney through a long tube, the ureter, to the bladder, where it is stored until elimination. The kidneys also make substances that help control blood pressure and regulate the formation of red blood cells.

**kilobase**   A unit of length of DNA equal to 1000 nucleotide bases.

**kilocalorie**   The amount of energy required to raise the temperature of a liter of water one degree centigrade at sea level. In nutrition terms, the word calorie is commonly used instead of the more precise scientific term kilocalorie. See also *calorie.*

**Kimmelstiel-Wilson   disease**   See   *diabetic nephropathy.*

**Kimmelstiel-Wilson   syndrome**   See   *diabetic nephropathy.*

**kindred**   The extended family. The term kindred is used in preparing population studies related to disease or genetic traits.

**kinetic**   With movement, as opposed to akinetic, or without movement.

**kinetics**   The rate of change in a biochemical or other reaction, and the study of reaction rates.

**kinky hair syndrome**   See *Menkes syndrome.*

**kinship**   Relationship by marriage or, specifically, a blood tie.

**kissing bugs**   Insect carriers of the parasite called Trypanosoma cruzi, which causes Chagas disease. The bugs "kiss" people, especially babies, on the lips while they are asleep, infecting them with their parasite. See also *Chagas disease.*

**kissing disease**   Nickname for mononucleosis. See *mononucleosis.*

**kit, disaster supplies**   See *disaster supplies.*

**klebsiella**   A group of bacteria normally living in the intestinal tract. Klebsiella are frequently the cause of infections acquired in the hospital.

**Kleine-Levin syndrome**   A rare condition characterized by excessive need for sleep, food, and sexual disinhibition. Most people with Kleine-Levin syndrome are adolescent males. When awake, they may be confused, irritable, and lethargic, and some have hallucinations. The cause is unknown, although current theory holds that Kleine-Levin syndrome is caused by an inherited autosomal dominant trait that affects the hypothalamus gland. Most cases resolve over time without treatment.

**Klinefelter syndrome**   A condition in males who have XXY sex chromosomes, rather than the usual XY. Some also have additional X chromosomes, or more than one Y chromosome. Symptoms include small testes, insufficient production of testosterone, and infertility. Klinefelter boys tend to have learning and/or behavioral problems.

**Klippel-Feil syndrome**   The combination of short neck, low hairline at the nape of the neck, and limited movement of the head. It is due to a defect in the early development of the spinal column in the neck. Also known as Klippel-Feil sequence.

**Klippel-Trenaunay-Weber syndrome**   A congenital malformation syndrome characterized by three basic symptoms: enlargement of a single limb (asymmetric limb hypertrophy), abnormal nests of blood vessels that proliferate inappropriately and excessively (hemangiomata), and pigmented moles on the skin (nevi). The enlarged limb is three times more likely to be a leg than an arm, and both bone and soft tissue are enlarged. The hemangiomas range from small, innocuous capillary hemangiomas ("strawberry marks") to huge cavernous hemangiomas. The nevi are often also dark linear streaks on the skin due to too much pigment. There can be other abnormalities. Most persons with KTW syndrome do relatively well without treatment. Compression from an elastic stocking or sleeve can help. Skin ulcers and other skin problems can occur over the swollen limb, and these can also be treated. Usually treatment is conservative, unless the limb reaches gigantic proportions or secondary clotting difficulties arise due to trapping and destruction of blood platelets in a huge hemangioma. In such cases amputation may become necessary. The cause of KTW syndrome is unknown.

**Klonopin**   See *Clonazepam*.

**knee**   A joint that permits flexibility in the middle of the leg. The thigh bone (femur) meets the large shinbone (tibia) to form the main knee joint. This joint has an inner (medial) and an outer (lateral) compartment. The kneecap (patella) joins the femur to form a third joint, called the patellofemoral joint. The patella protects the front of the knee joint. The knee joint is surrounded by a joint capsule, with ligaments strapping the inside and outside of the joint (collateral ligaments) as well as crossing within the joint (cruciate ligaments). The collateral ligaments run along the sides of the knee, and limit its sideways motion. The anterior cruciate ligament (ACL) connects the tibia to the femur at the center of the knee, and functions to limit the tibia's rotation and forward motion. The posterior cruciate ligament (PCL), located just behind the ACL, limits the backward motion of the tibia. All of these ligaments provide stability and strength

to the knee joint. There is a thickened cartilage pad between the two joints formed by the femur and tibia. Called the meniscus, it acts as a smooth surface for the joint to move on. It serves to evenly load the surface during weight-bearing, and also aids in disbursing joint fluid for joint lubrication. The knee joint is surrounded by fluid-filled sacs called bursae, which serve as gliding surfaces to reduce friction of the tendons. Below the kneecap is a large tendon (patellar tendon), which attaches to the front of the tibia bone. Large blood vessels pass through the area behind the knee, which is called the popliteal space. The large muscles of the thigh move the knee. In the front of the thigh, the quadriceps muscles extend the knee joint. In the back of the thigh, the hamstring muscles flex the knee. The knee also rotates slightly under the guidance of specific muscles of the thigh. The knee is critical to normal walking, and is a weight-bearing joint. Knee pain can be caused by a number of factors, including injury, inflammation of the bursa (bursitis), strain, or problems with the sciatic nerve, which runs from the lower back to the knee. See also *bursitis, patellofemoral syndrome, sciatica.*

**knee bursitis**   Inflammation of the fluid-filled sac (bursa) within the knee. See *bursitis.*

**knee jerk**   The reflex tested by tapping just below the bent knee on the patellar tendon. Normally this causes the quadriceps muscle to contract and bring the lower leg forward. It has given rise to the saying "a knee-jerk reaction." Also known as the patellar reflex.

**knee joint**   See *knee.*

**knee, housemaid's**   See *patellofemoral syndrome.*

**knee, secretary's**   See *patellofemoral syndrome.*

**kneecap**   The patella, the small bone in the front of the knee. The patella is a little (sesamoid) bone, embedded in the tendon of insertion of the quadriceps muscle. If the patella is shattered beyond repair, it can be removed in an operation called a patellectomy.

**knock-knees**   An abnormal curve of the legs that causes the knees to touch or nearly touch while the feet are apart. The problem may arise in the bone structure itself, or in some cases it develops gradually as a result of muscle abnormalities. Knock-knees can cause movement difficulties, muscle and bone strain, and pain from overstress on the ankles. The condition can be helped via physical therapy, and in some cases corrected with surgery. Also known as genu valgum.

**knuckle**   The top of the flexed finger joint.

**Koch postulates** A set of criteria for judging whether a given bacteria is the cause of a given disease.

**Kok disease** See *hyperexplexia*.

**Koplik spots** Little spots inside the mouth that are highly characteristic of the early phase of measles (rubeola). The spots look like tiny grains of white sand, each surrounded by a red ring. They are often found on the inside of the cheek opposite the first and second upper molars. See also *measles*.

**Kostmann disease** See *severe congenital neutropenia*.

**Krabbe disease** A rare form of leukodystrophy in which the myelin sheath around nerves does not form properly, preventing proper information exchange between brain and body. Symptoms usually begin before nine months of age, and include physical rigidity, crying and extreme fussiness, seizures (particularly absence seizures), and unexplained fevers. Diagnosis is by blood test for lack or low levels of the enzyme galactosylceramide B. Also known as galactosylceramidosis, globoid-cell leukodystrophy. See also *glycosphingolipidoses*.

**Krukenberg tumor** A tumor of the ovary, caused by the spread of metastatic stomach cancer.

**KUB** Kidney, ureter, and bladder.

**KUB film** An abdominal X-ray showing the kidney, ureter, and bladder.

**kuru** A slowly progressive fatal disease of the brain due to an infectious agent that is transmitted among people in Papua New Guinea by ritual cannibalism. Kuru is an infectious form of subacute spongiform encephalopathy, and is believed to be caused by a tiny virus-like particle called a prion. It appears to be similar to bovine spongiform encephalopathy ("Mad Cow disease") and Creuztfeldt-Jakob disease. The discovery of the basis of kuru is one of the more interesting detective stories in modern medicine. Also called trembling disease.

**Kussmaul breathing** Air hunger, gasping.

**kwashiorkor** A childhood disease caused by protein deprivation. Early signs include apathy, drowsiness, and irritability. More advanced signs are poor growth, lack of stamina, loss of muscle mass, swelling, abnormal hair (sparse, thin, often streaky red or gray hair in dark-skinned children), and abnormal skin that darkens in irritated but not sun-exposed areas. Kwashiorkor disables the immune system, making the child susceptible to a host of infectious diseases. It is responsible for much illness and death among children worldwide. Also known as protein malnutrition, protein-calorie malnutrition (PCM).

**kyphoscoliosis** A combination of a humped back (kyphosis) and lateral curvature of the spine (scoliosis). It can be due to musculoskeletal disease, or to unknown causes. Treatment is by physical therapy and wearing a back brace, and in some cases by surgery. Surgery may include inserting a metal rod in the spine and restructuring some bones, and is usually followed by wearing a back cast and then a back brace for some time.

**kyphoscoliosis, ideopathic** Kyphoscoliosis that occurs during development, without a known cause.

**kyphosis** Outward curvature of the spine, causing a humped back. Treatment is by physical therapy and wearing a back brace, and in some cases by surgery. Surgery may include inserting a metal rod in the spine and restructuring some bones, and is usually followed by wearing a back cast and then a back brace for some time.

**kyphosis, fixed** Kyphosis caused by collapse of the vertebrae, usually due to musculoskeletal disease. See *kyphosis*.

**kyphosis, juvenile** See *Scheuermann disease*.

**kyphosis, mobile** Kyphosis caused by compensating for muscle weakness or structural abnormality in another area of the body. See *kyphosis*.

# Ll

**L-dopa**  See *levodopa*.

**L1 to L5**  Symbols that represent the five lumbar vertebrae, which are situated between the thoracic vertebrae and the sacral vertebrae in the spinal column.

**La Leche League**  An organization that helps and supports breast-feeding mothers with advice, ideas, and both legal and medical advocacy.

**lab results**  The reported results of a test done in a lab.

**lab test**  A test that cannot be performed in the doctor's office, usually a specialized blood draw.

**labia**  Lips, either the lips around the mouth (oral labia) or the lip-like external female genitalia (the labia majora and labia minor).

**labia majora**  The larger outside pair of labia (lips) of the vulva.

**labia minora**  The smaller (minor) inside pair of labia (lips) of the vulva.

**labia, oral**  The lips around the mouth. See *lip*.

**labia, vaginal**  The two pairs of labia (lips) at the entrance to the vagina. Together they form part of the vulva, the female external genitalia. See *labia majora, labia minora*.

**labial**  Pertaining to the lip, one of the fleshy folds that surround the opening of the mouth or the vagina.

**labial sounds**  A sound requiring the participation of one or both lips, which simply may be called a labial. All labials are consonants. Bilabial sounds, such as "p," involve both lips, whereas labiodental sounds, such as "v," involve the upper teeth and lower lip.

**labile**  Unstable.

**labile diabetes**  See *diabetes, labile*.

**labium**  A lip, the singular form of labia.

**labor**  Childbirth, the aptly named experience of delivering the baby and placenta from the uterus to the vagina to the outside world. There are two phases of labor. During the first stage (the stage of dilatation), the cervix dilates fully to a diameter of about 10 cm. In the second stage (the stage of expulsion), the fetus moves out through the cervix and vagina to be born.

**laboratory**  A place for doing tests and research procedures, and for preparing chemicals and some medications.

**labyrinth**  The maze of canals in the inner ear. The labyrinth is the portion of the ear responsible for sensing balance.

**labyrinthitis**  Inflammation of the labyrinth of the ear, which can be accompanied by vertigo.

**laceration**  Severed skin. See *cut*.

**lacrimal**  Pertaining to tears.

**lacrimal gland**  A structure located at the top of the eye socket that secretes tears. Tears flow through tiny ducts at the corner of the eye.

**lacrimation**  Shedding tears, or shedding more tears than is normal (for example, as a result of eye injury or irritation).

**lactase**  Enzyme that breaks down the milk sugar lactose.

**lactase deficiency**  Lack of an enzyme called lactase in the small intestine. Lactase is needed to digest lactose, a component of milk and some other dairy products. Lactase production normally decreases with age, more so in some persons than others. There are significant differences relative to lactase production among ethnic groups. Inadequate lactase production can cause difficulty digesting products that contain lactose, which include dairy products themselves and foods that contain dairy products as ingredients. The most common symptoms of lactase deficiency are diarrhea, bloating, and gas when dairy products are eaten. Diagnosis may be made by a trial of a lactose-free diet or by special testing. In some cases, other diseases of the intestine may need to be excluded by further medical evaluation. See also *lactose intolerance*.

**lactation**  The process of milk production. Human milk is secreted by the mammary glands, which are located within the fatty tissue of the breast. The hormone oxytocin is produced in response to the birth of a new baby, and it both stimulates uterine contractions and begins the lactation process. For the first few hours of nursing, a special fluid called colostrum is delivered; it is especially high in nutrients, fats, and antibodies to protect the newborn from infection. Thereafter, the amount of milk produced is controlled primarily by the hormone prolactin, which is produced in response to the length of time the infant nurses at the breast. See also *breast-feeding*.

**lactic acid**   A simple sugar that is the byproduct of glucose metabolism. When lactic acid accumulates rapidly in the muscle cells during or just after exercise, the result can be cramping.

**Lactobacillus**   A bacteria normally found in the mouth, intestinal tract, and vagina, Lactobacillus can also live in fermenting products, such as yogurt. Humans appear to have a symbiotic relationship with this bacteria: It's been with us so long that some types have become an important part of food digestion, although it can also contribute to cavities in the teeth if allowed to remain too long within the mouth.

**Lactobacillus acidophilus**   The bacteria found in milk and fermented milk products, particularly yogurt with "live cultures" of L. acidopholus. L. acidopholous assists with the digestive process within the intestinal tract. It can be decimated by the use of antibiotics, and many health professionals urge people to use probiotics to counter this unfortunate side effect of antibiotic use. See also *probiotics*.

**lactose intolerance**   Inability to digest lactose, a component of milk and some other dairy products. The basis for this condition is the lack of an enzyme called lactase in the small intestine. Treatment is by avoiding products that contain lactose, or by using lactase enzyme supplements before eating. See also *lactase deficiency*.

**lacuna**   A small pit, cavity, defect, or gap.

**lamella**   A thin leaf, plate, disk, or wafer.

**lamina**   A plate or layer. For example, the lamina arcus vertebrae are plates of bone within each vertebral body.

**laminaria**   A thin piece of sterile seaweed frequently used to dilate the cervix during an abortion procedure.

**lancet**   A small, pointed knife used to prick a finger for a blood test.

**Lancet**   A well-known medical journal based in England.

**Landau-Kleffner syndrome**   A seizure disorder with onset in childhood, in which the patient loses skills, such as speech, and develops behaviors characteristic of autism. See also *autism, epilepsy, seizure, seizure disorders*.

**Landing disease**   A genetic lipid storage disorder that is similar to both Hurler syndrome and Tay-Sachs disease, but affects both the brain and the viscera. Symptoms include skeletal deformities, and severe effects on the brain and organs. Death occurs by the age of two in most cases. The mutation responsible for Landing disease has been located on chromosome 3 at the spot 3p21. There is no treatment for this disease. Also known as familial neurovisceral lipidosis, GM1 gangliosidosis. See also *glycosphingolipidoses, Hurler syndrome, Tay-Sachs disease*.

**Landry ascending paralysis**   A particularly virulent form of Guillain-Barre syndrome. The disorder often begins with a flu-like illness that brings on general physical weakness, but is then characterized by rapidly progressing paralysis that starts in the legs and arms, and may move on (ascend) to affect the breathing muscles and face. As with less severe forms of Guillain-Barre, the exact cause is not yet known but is presumed to be viral and/or autoimmune. Hospitalization is usually required, and treatment is by plasmapheresis or intravenous gamma globulin (IVIG). See also *demyelination, Guillain-Barre syndrome*.

**Langerhans, islets of**   See *islets of Langerhans*.

**Lanoxicaps**   See *digoxin*.

**Lanoxin**   See *digoxin*.

**lanugo**   Downy hair on the body of the fetus and newborn baby. It is the first hair to be produced by the fetal hair follicles, usually appearing on the fetus at about five months of gestation. It is very fine, soft, and usually unpigmented. Although lanugo is normally shed before birth, around seven or eight months of gestation, it is sometimes present at birth. This is not a cause for concern: Lanugo will disappear of its own accord within a few days or weeks.

**laparoscope**   A special type of surgical instrument that can be inserted through a small incision to shine light within the abdomen. It is useful for both diagnosis and surgery, as it provides the surgeon with a good view while minimizing the amount of cutting, suturing, and abdominal exposure. Some laparoscopes can now project lighted images onto a computer screen, where they can be further enhanced.

**laparoscopy**   A type of surgery in which small incisions are made in the abdominal wall through which a laparoscope and other instruments can be placed. Laparoscopy is used particularly frequently for female sterilization in which the Fallopian tubes are tied off or cauterized, and for excising the abdominal growths that cause pain in endometriosis.

**laparotomy** An operation to open the abdomen.

**large cell carcinoma** A group of lung cancers in which the cells are large and look abnormal.

**large-cell lymphoma** See *lymphoma, large-cell.* See also *lymphoma.*

**large intestine** See *intestine, large.*

**large saphenous vein** See *saphenous vein, great.*

**laryngeal** Having to do with the larynx (voice box).

**laryngeal nerve palsy** See *laryngeal palsy.*

**laryngeal nerve, recurrent** One of the best-known branches of the vagus nerve, a long and important nerve that originates in the brain stem and runs down to the colon. After the recurrent laryngeal nerve leaves the vagus nerve, it goes down into the chest and then loops back up to supply the larynx.

**laryngeal palsy** Paralysis of the larynx (voice box) caused by damage to the recurrent laryngeal nerve or its parent nerve, the vagus nerve, which originates in the brain stem and runs down to the colon. The recurrent laryngeal nerve supplies the larynx (voice box). The larynx will be paralyzed on the side where this nerve has been damaged, unless the problem originated with damage to the vagus nerve itself. Damage to the recurrent laryngeal nerve can be the result of diseases inside the chest, such as a tumor, an aneurysm of the arch of the aorta, or an aneurysm of the left atrium of the heart.

**laryngeal papilloma** A warty growth in the larynx, usually on the vocal cords. Persistent hoarseness is a common symptom.

**laryngeal papillomatosis** The presence of numerous warty growths on the vocal cords. The disease is most common in young children. Recurrences of laryngeal papillomatosis are, unfortunately, frequent. Remission may occur after several years.

**laryngeal papillomatosis, juvenile** Papillomatosis that occurs in infancy or childhood. Laryngeal papillomatosis can be caused by human papilloma virus (HPV), which is contracted at birth via the vaginal canal of a mother with genital warts.

**laryngectomee** A person who has had his or her larynx removed. See *laryngectomy.*

**laryngectomy** Surgery to remove part or all of the larynx. The surgeon performs a tracheostomy, creating an opening called a stoma in the front of the neck. Air enters and leaves the trachea and lungs through this opening. A tracheostomy tube, also called a trach ("trake") tube, keeps the new airway open.

**laryngectomy, partial** A laryngectomy that preserves the voice. The surgeon removes only part of the voice box—just one vocal cord, part of a cord, or just the epiglottis—and the stoma is temporary. After a brief recovery period, the tracheostomy tube is removed, and the stoma closes up. The patient can then breathe and talk in the usual way. In some cases, however, the voice may be hoarse or weak.

**laryngectomy, total** A laryngectomy in which the whole voice box is removed, and the stoma is permanent. The patient breathes through the stoma, and must learn to talk in a new way.

**laryngitis, reflux** Inflammation of the larynx caused by stomach acid backing up into the esophagus. Reflux laryngitis is associated with chronic hoarseness and symptoms of esophageal irritation such as heartburn. See also *reflux.*

**laryngomalacia** A soft, floppy larynx.

**laryngoscope** A flexible, lighted tube used to examine the inside of the larynx.

**laryngoscopy** Examination of the larynx, either with a mirror (indirect laryngoscopy) or with a laryngoscope (direct laryngoscopy).

**laryngostasis** See *croup.*

**larynx** A two-inch–long, tube-shaped organ in the neck that contains the vocal cords. It is part of the respiratory system, and located between the pharynx and the trachea. Humans use the larynx when we breathe, talk, or swallow. Its outer wall of cartilage forms the area of the front of the neck referred to as the Adam's apple. The vocal cords, two bands of muscle, form a V inside the larynx. Each time a person inhales, air goes into the nose or mouth, then through the larynx, down the trachea, and into the lungs. When a person exhales, the air goes the other way. The vocal cords are relaxed during breathing, and air moves through the space between them without making any sound. The vocal cords tighten up and move closer together for speech. Air from the lungs is forced between them and makes them vibrate, producing the sound of a voice. The tongue, lips, and teeth form this sound into words. The esophagus, a tube that carries food from the mouth to the stomach, is just behind the trachea and the larynx. The openings of the esophagus and the larynx are very close together in the throat. When a person swallows, a flap called the epiglottis moves down over the larynx to keep food out of the windpipe. Also called the voice box.

**laser** A powerful beam of light used in some types of surgery to cut or destroy tissue.

**laser surgery, Yag** The use of a laser to punch a hole in the iris, relieving increased pressure within the eye. Yag laser surgery is an office procedure that may be used, for example, to treat acute angle-closure glaucoma.

**laser-assisted in situ keratomileusis** A kind of laser eye surgery designed to change the shape of the cornea to eliminate or reduce the need for glasses and contact lenses in cases of severe nearsightedness (myopia). LASIK is an outpatient procedure done with numbing eye drops. It takes about one minute to do, and only a few days to heal. No eye patch need be worn after LASIK.

**LASIK** Laser-assisted in situ keratomileusis.

**Lasix** See *furosemide*.

**Lassa fever** See *fever, Lassa*.

**lateral 1** The side of the body or body part that is farther from the middle or center (median) of the body. Typically, lateral refers to the outer side of the body part, but it is also used to refer to the side of a body part. For example, in references to the knee, lateral means the side of the knee farthest from the opposite knee. The opposite of lateral is medial. See also *Appendix B, "Anatomic Orientation Terms."* **2** In radiology, slang term for a lateral X-ray film. See *lateral X-ray*.

**lateral collateral ligament of the knee** The ligament that straps the outside of the knee joint, providing stability and strength. See also *knee*.

**lateral meniscus of the knee** A thickened crescent-shaped cartilage pad between the two joints formed by the femur (the thigh bone) and the tibia (the shinbone). It acts as a smooth surface for the joint to move on. The lateral meniscus is toward the outer side of the knee joint. It serves to evenly load the surface during weight-bearing, and also aids in disbursing joint fluid for joint lubrication. See also *knee*.

**lateral ventricle** Two in a system of four communicating cavities within the brain that are continuous with the central canal of the spinal cord. The two lateral ventricles are located in the cerebral hemispheres, one in each hemisphere. Each consists of a triangular central body and four horns. The lateral ventricles communicate with the third ventricle through an opening called the interventricular foramen. Both ventricles are filled with cerebrospinal fluid.

**lateral X-ray** An X-ray picture taken from the side of the patient.

**laughing gas** See *nitrous oxide*.

**Launois-Bensaude syndrome** See *cephalothoracic lipodystrophy*.

**lavage** Washing out. Gastric lavage, for example, is the washing out of the stomach to remove drugs or poisons.

**law, Hardy-Weinberg** See *Hardy-Weinberg law*.

**laxative** Something that loosens the bowels. Laxatives are used to combat constipation—and sometimes overused, producing diarrhea.

**lb.** Abbreviation for pound (in Latin, *libra*), a measure of weight.

**LCHAD deficiency** Deficiency of the enzyme long-chain-3-hydroxyacyl-CoA dehydrogenease, preventing normal metabolism of fatty acids. See also *acute fatty liver of pregnancy*.

**LDL** Low-density lipoprotein.

**LDL cholesterol** Lipoproteins, which are combinations of lipids (fats) and proteins, are the form in which lipids are transported in the blood. The low-density lipoproteins transport cholesterol from the liver to the tissues of the body. LDL cholesterol is therefore considered the "bad" cholesterol.

**lead poisoning** An environmental hazard capable of causing mental retardation, behavioral disturbance, and brain damage. Lead was used in household paint until 1978, and was also found in leaded gasoline, some types of batteries, water pipes, and pottery glazes. Lead paint and pipes are still found in many older homes, and lead is sometimes also found in water, food, household dust, and soil. Lead can be a workplace hazard for people in some occupations. A diet that is high in iron and calcium can help protect people against absorbing lead. Diagnosis is by blood test: A lead level over 70 is considered lead poisoning, even if the person has no apparent symptoms. Treatment is by chelation therapy, usually in the hospital. Treatment cannot repair damage to the brain done by lead poisoning, but may prevent further damage.

**left heart** See *heart, left*. See also *heart*.

**left heart hypoplasia syndrome** See *hypoplastic left heart syndrome*. See also *atrial septal defect, ductus arteriosus*.

**left ventricle** See *ventricle, left*. See also *heart*.

**leg** In popular usage, the leg extends from the top of the thigh down to the foot, but in medical terminology, the leg is only that portion of the lower extremity that runs from the knee to the ankle. The leg has two bones: the tibia and the fibula. Both are known as long bones. The larger of the two is the tibia, familiarly called the shinbone. The fibula runs alongside the tibia.

**leg, ankle, and foot bones** There are 62 lower-extremity bones. They consist of 10 hip and leg, 14 ankle, and 38 foot bones. The 10 hip and leg bones are the hip bone (innominate bone), which is a fusion of the ilium, ischium, and pubis bones; femur, tibia, fibula, and patella (kneecap) on each side. The 14 ankle bones are the talus, calcaneus, navicular, cuboid, internal cuneiform, middle cuneiform, and external cuneiform bones on each side. The 38 foot bones are the 10 metatarsals and the 28 phalanges.

**leg, lower** See *leg*.

**leg, upper** More properly called the thigh, the upper leg is the area between the knee and the hip. It has only one bone, the femur.

**Legg-Calve-Perthes disease** A hip disorder in children caused by interruption of the blood supply to the head of the femur. Also known as Legg disease and Legg-Perthes disease.

**Legg-Perthes disease** See *Legg-Calve-Perthes disease*.

**Legionella** The bacteria that causes Legionnaires disease.

**Legionnaires disease** A disease first identified at the 1976 American Legion convention and caused by bacteria found in plumbing, shower heads, and water-storage tanks. Outbreaks have also been attributed to this bacteria, now known as Legionella, thriving in condensers and evaporative cooling towers. The symptoms are much like those of pneumonia. Also known as Legionella pneumonia.

**leiomyoma** See *fibroid*.

**leiomyosarcoma** A malignant tumor that originates in smooth muscle. Smooth muscle is the major structural component of most hollow internal organs and in the walls of blood vessels. Leiomyosarcoma can occur almost anywhere in the body, but is most frequently found in the uterus and gastrointestinal tract. Complete surgical excision, if possible, is the treatment of choice.

**Leishmania** A group of parasites that cause several human diseases. See *leishmaniasis*.

**leishmaniasis** Diseases due to Leishmania parasites. Leishmaniasis can involve the organs (kala-azar), skin and mucous membranes (espundia), or skin alone. When it affects only the skin, the disorder is usually named for the place: for example, Jericho boil, Baghdad button, Delhi sore. See also *kala-azar*.

**Lennox syndrome** See *Lennox-Gastaut syndrome*.

**Lennox-Gastaut syndrome** A severe form of epilepsy that usually begins in early childhood. It is characterized by frequent seizures of multiple types, mental impairment, and a slow spike-and-wave pattern seen on an EEG. The seizures are notoriously hard to treat, and may lead to falls and injuries. These seizures can be reduced in frequency by treatment with lamotrogine, a chemically novel antiepileptic drug, or with other medication. In some cases surgery may be considered.

**lens** The transparent structure inside the eye that focuses light rays onto the retina.

**lens, intraocular** See *intraocular lens*.

**lens, objective** In a microscope, the lens nearest to the object being examined. Most light microscopes now have a turret bearing a selection of objective lenses.

**lens, ocular** In a microscope, the lens closest to the eye. Also called the eyepiece. Most light microscopes are binocular, with one ocular lens for each eye.

**Lenti-virinae** A family of retroviruses that includes the human immunodeficiency virus (HIV) 1 and 2. See also *HIV*.

**leprosy** An infectious disease of the skin, nervous system, and mucous membranes caused by the bacteria Mycobacterium leprae. It is transmitted via person-to-person contact. For thousands of years leprosy was one of the world's most feared communicable diseases, because the nerve and skin damage often led to terrible disfigurement and disability. Today leprosy can be cured, particularly if treatment is begun early. The treatment of choice is a multidrug therapy (MDT) using diaphenylsulfone (brand name: Dapsone), rifampicin (brand name: Rifadin), and clofazimine (brand name: Lamprene). Surgery can reconstruct damaged faces and limbs. Also known as Hansen disease, leprosyis.

**lesbian** A female homosexual.

**lesbianism** Female homosexuality.

**Lescol**   See *fluvastin*.

**lesion**   An area of abnormal tissue change.

**let-down reflex**   An involuntary reflex during breast-feeding that causes the milk to flow freely.

**lethal**   Deadly.

**lethal gene, zygotic**   See *gene, zygotic lethal*.

**lethargy**   Abnormal drowsiness, stupor.

**Letterer-Siwe disease**   See *histiocytosis, histiocytosis X*.

**leucemia**   A different spelling of leukemia.

**leukemia**   Cancer of the blood cells, particularly cancers characterized by uncontrolled proliferation of white blood cells in the bone marrow and sometimes also in the circulating blood. Strictly speaking, leukemia should refer only to cancer of the white blood cells (leukocytes), but in practice it can apply to malignancy of any cellular element in the blood or bone marrow, as in red cell leukemia (erythroleukemia). Treatment may be by chemotherapy, radiation therapy, biological therapy, and/or bone-marrow transplant. Some forms of leukemia are associated with viral infection.

**leukemia, accelerated phase of**   Chronic myelogenous leukemia that is progressing. The number of immature, abnormal white blood cells in the bone marrow and blood is higher than in the chronic phase, but not as high as in the blastic phase.

**leukemia, acute lymphoblastic**   See *leukemia, lymphocytic*.

**leukemia, blastic phase of**   A stage in which 30 percent or more of the cells in the bone marrow or blood are blast cells, which may form tumors.

**leukemia, chronic phase of**   A stage in which there are few blast cells in the blood or bone marrow, and few if any symptoms.

**leukemia, granulocytic**   See *leukemia, myelogenous*.

**leukemia, hairy cell**   A rare type of chronic leukemia in which the abnormal white blood cells appear to be covered with tiny hairs. The cancer most frequently affects lymphocytes. Early symptoms include fatigue, flu-like symptoms, and sometimes an enlarged spleen. Treatment includes chemotherapy, biological therapy, and surgery to remove the enlarged spleen. In some cases, bone-marrow transplantation may be tried.

**leukemia, lymphocytic**   A form of leukemia that has a sudden onset, lymphocytic leukemia starts in the bone marrow but often spreads to the lymphatic and nervous system. With aggressive treatment, which may include chemotherapy, radiation, bone-marrow transplant, and/or biological therapy, there is a high cure rate, especially for children. Also known as acute lymphoblastic leukemia (ALL).

**leukemia, myelogenous**   A condition in which the bone marrow makes too many white blood cells. Early symptoms include fatigue and night sweats. Treatment may be by radiation, chemotherapy, biological therapy, or bone-marrow transplant. Also known as chronic myelogenous leukemia (CML), and chronic granulocytic leukemia.

**leukemia, myeloid**   A condition in which cancerous cells are found in both the bone marrow and the blood. Early symptoms include fatigue and aching bones. Treatment may be by radiation, chemotherapy, biological therapy, or bone-marrow transplant. Abbreviated as AML; also known as acute nonlymphocytic leukemia (ANLL).

**leukemia, nonlymphocytic**   See *leukemia, myeloid*.

**leukemia, refractory**   Leukemia in which the high level of white blood cells is not decreasing in response to treatment.

**leukemia, smoldering**   One of a group of disorders characterized by abnormal development of one or more of the cell lines normally found in the bone marrow. Patients can develop a variety of symptoms related to anemia, low or high white cell count, infections, and bleeding problems. This condition may progress and become acute leukemia. The seven well-recognized myelodysplastic syndromes include refractory anemia (RA), refractory anemia with ringed sideroblasts (RARS), refractory anemia with excess blasts (RAEB), refractory anemia with excess blasts in transformation (RAEB-T), chronic myelomonocytic leukemia (CMML), chronic myelomonocytic leukemia in transformation (CMML-T), and unclassified myelodysplastic syndrome. Also known as myelodysplastic syndrome, preleukemia.

**leukemoid reaction**   A benign condition in which the high number of white blood cells found in a blood test resembles the numbers seen in leukemia. For example, infectious mononucleosis can return blood-test results with a leukemoid reaction.

**leuko-**   Prefix meaning white.

**leukocyte**   See *leukocytes*. See also *blood cell*.

**leukocyte count**   A white blood cell (WBC) count. See also *leukocytes*.

**leukocyte, granular** See *granulocyte*. See also *leukocytes*.

**leukocyte, polymorphonuclear** A type of white blood cell with a nucleus that is so deeply lobated or divided that the cell appears to have multiple nuclei. Informally called a poly. See also *blood cell*, *leukocytes*.

**leukocytes** Blood cells that help the body fight infections and other diseases. Also known as white blood cells (WBCs). See also *blood cell*.

**leukocytosis** Increase in the number of white blood cells.

**leukodystrophy** Disorder of the white matter of the brain. The white matter mainly consists of nerve fibers rather than nerve cells themselves, and is concerned with conduction of nerve impulses.

**leukodystrophy, globoid-cell** See *Krabbe disease*.

**leukodystrophy, metachromatic** A rare genetic disorder caused by lack of the enzyme arylsulfatase A. Without this enzyme, compounds accumulate in the brain that strip the myelin coating from nerves. Also known as sulfatidosis.

**leukopenia** Shortage of white blood cells.

**leukoplakia** A white spot or patch in the mouth.

**levo-** Prefix meaning on the left side. For example, a molecule that shows levorotation is turning or twisting to the left. The opposition of levo- is dextro-.

**levocardia** Reversal of all the abdominal and thoracic organs (situs inversus) except the heart, which is still in its usual location on the left. Levocardia virtually always results in congenital heart disease.

**levodopa** A drug (brand name: Dopar, Larodopa) used to treat Parkinson disease, Parkinsonian symptoms in other disorders, restless legs syndrome, and herpes zoster. It converts to the neurotransmitter dopamine in the brain.

**Levothroid** See *levothyroxine sodium*.

**levothyroxine sodium** A synthetic thyroid hormone used as a thyroid hormone replacement drug (brand names include Eltroxin, Levothroid, Levoxine, Levoxyl, Synthroid) to treat an underactive thyroid gland (hypothyroidism). Because not all brands of levothyroxine sodium are equivalent, it is important not to switch between brand names or even between generic formulations.

**Levoxine** See *levothyroxine sodium*.

**Levoxyl** See *levothyroxine sodium*.

**LH** Luteinizing hormone.

**LHRH** Luteinizing hormone-releasing hormone.

**LHRH agonists** Compounds that are similar to luteinizing hormone-releasing hormone (LHRH) in structure, and are able to act like LHRH.

**libido** In psychoanalysis, psychic energy or drive, especially the sexual instinct.

**library** In genetics, an unordered collection of cloned DNA from a particular organism. The relationships between these clones can be established by physical mapping. For example, you can have an E. coli library or a human DNA library. See also *genomic library*.

**Library of Medicine, National** See *National Institutes of Health*.

**library, genomic** See *genomic library*.

**lice, head** See *head lice*. See also *head lice infestation*.

**Li-Fraumeni syndrome** A syndrome characterized by inherited susceptibility to a wide spectrum of cancers, including breast cancer, soft tissue sarcomas, brain tumors, a bone tumor called osteosarcoma, leukemia, and a tumor of the adrenal gland (adrenocortical carcinoma). Li-Fraumeni syndrome is due to a mutation in a gene that normally serves to curb cancer: the p53 tumor-suppressor gene, and studying it has been of considerable importance to understanding the genetics and molecular biology of cancer.

**ligament** A tough band of connective tissue that connects various structures, such as two bones.

**ligament, anterior cruciate** The cross-shaped ligament that crosses in front of the knee joint, within the joint capsule. See also *knee*.

**ligament, lateral collateral knee** The ligament that straps the outside of the knee joint. See also *knee*.

**ligament, medial collateral knee** The ligament that straps the inner side of the knee joint. See also *knee*.

**ligament, posterior cruciate** The cross-shaped ligament within the knee joint that crosses behind the anterior cruciate ligament. See also *knee*.

**ligate** To tie, as in ligating (tying off) an artery.

**ligature** Material used to tie something in surgery. Ligatures are used to tie off blood vessels. Ligatures may be made of silk, gut, wire, or other materials.

**lightening** See *engagement*.

**lightheadedness** Feeling as if one is about to faint. Lightheadedness is medically distinct from dizziness, unsteadiness, and vertigo. See also *dizziness, unsteadiness, vertigo*.

**lights, flashing** A sensation created when the clear, jelly-like substance that fills the middle of the eye (vitreous humor) shrinks and tugs on the retina. These flashes of light can appear off and on for several weeks or months. With age, it is more common to experience flashes. They usually do not reflect a serious problem. However, if flashing lights suddenly appear or increase, an ophthalmologist should be consulted immediately to see whether the retina has been torn. Flashes of light that appear as jagged lines or "heat waves" in both eyes, often lasting 10 to 20 minutes, are different. They are usually caused by migraine, a spasm of blood vessels in the brain.

**limb** The arm or leg.

**lingual** Having to do with the tongue.

**linkage** Tendency for genes to be inherited together because of their location near one another on the same chromosome.

**linkage analysis** Study aimed at establishing linkage between genes. Today, linkage analysis serves as a way of gene-hunting and genetic testing.

**linkage map** A map of the genes on a chromosome, based on linkage analysis. A linkage map does not show the physical distances between genes, but rather their relative positions as determined by how often two gene loci are inherited together. The closer two genes are, the more often they will be inherited together. Linkage distance is measured in centimorgans (cM).

**lip** One of the two fleshy folds that surround the opening of the mouth. The upper lip is separated from the nose by the philtrum, the area that lies between the base of the nose and the pigmented edge (called the vermillion border or the carmine margin) of the upper lip. The upper and lower lips meet at the corners (angles) of the mouth, which are called the oral commissures. The oral commissure normally lies in a vertical line below the pupil. Small blind pits are sometimes seen at the corners of the mouth; they are known as angular lip pits, and are considered normal minor variants. The lips may be abnormally thin or thick. For example, children with fetal alcohol syndrome typically have a thin upper lip and flat philtrum. If the upper lip is overgrown, the corners of the mouth appear to be downturned.

**lip, cleft** A fissure in the upper lip due to failure of the lip to fuse before birth. Normally, lip fusion occurs by 35 days of uterine age. Cleft lip can be on one side only (unilateral) or on both sides (bilateral). Cleft lip often occurs in association with cleft palate. It can be easily repaired with surgery.

**lipectomy, suction-assisted** See *liposuction*.

**lipid** Fatty substance.

**lipid profile** Pattern of lipids in the blood. A lipid profile usually includes the total cholesterol, high-density lipoprotein (HDL) cholesterol, triglycerides, and the calculated low-density lipoprotein (LDL) cholesterol.

**lipid storage diseases** A series of disorders due to inborn errors in lipid metabolism. Lipid storage diseases result in the abnormal accumulation of lipids in the wrong places. Examples include Gaucher, Fabry, and Niemann-Pick diseases, and metachromatic leukodystrophy.

**lipodystrophy syndrome** A disturbance of lipid (fat) metabolism that involves the partial or total absence of fat, and often abnormal deposition and distribution of fat in the body. There are a number of different lipodystrophy syndromes. Some of them are present at birth (congenital), while others are acquired later. Some are genetic (inherited), others are not. One lipodystrophy syndrome is associated with the protease inhibitor drugs used to treat AIDS. The face, arms, and legs become thin due to loss of subcutaneous fat. The skin becomes dry, the lips crack, and weight drops. How the protease inhibitors induce this lipodystrophy syndrome is unknown. See also *cephalothoracic lipodystrophy, protease inhibitor.*

**lipodystrophy, cephalothoracic** See *cephalothoracic lipodystrophy.*

**lipoma** A benign fatty tumor.

**lipomatosis, multiple symmetric** See *cephalothoracic lipodystrophy.*

**lipoprotein** A combination of lipid and protein. Lipids travel in the blood as part of a lipoprotein.

**liposarcoma** A rare type of tumor that arises from fat cells in deep, soft tissue, such as inside the thigh. Most frequently seen in older adults, liposarcomas may be described as cell differentiated, myxoid, round cell, or pleomorphic, depending on the appearance of cells in the tumor. See also *sarcoma*.

**liposuction**  The most common cosmetic operation in the US, liposuction involves the surgical suctioning of fat deposits from specific parts of the body, the most common being the abdomen, buttocks, hips, thighs and knees, chin, upper arms, back, and calves. A hollow instrument called a cannula is inserted under the skin to break up the fat. A high-pressure vacuum is then applied to the cannula to suck out the fat. See also *liposuction, tumescent; liposuction, ultrasonic-assisted*.

**liposuction, tumescent**  A form of liposuction in which several quarts of a solution are pumped below the skin in the area from which fat is to be suctioned. The saline (salt water) solution used includes the local anesthetic lidocaine to numb the area, and the vessel-constrictor epinephrine (adrenaline) to help minimize bleeding. The fat is suctioned out through small suction tubes called microcannulas. Tumescent liposuction is now the most-used form of liposuction. Tumescent liposuction can be fatal. It has been suggested that death occurs because of the toxicity of lidocaine, or drug interactions related to lidocaine. See also *liposuction*.

**liposuction, ultrasonic-assisted**  A form of liposuction in which the cannula is energized with ultrasonic energy, causing the fat to melt away on contact. This technique has an advantage in areas of scar tissue, such as the male breast, the back, and areas where liposuction has been performed before. Its disadvantages include the need for longer incisions in the skin, a potential for skin or internal burns, greater cost, and a longer time needed to complete the procedure. See also *liposuction*.

**lips**  The lips of the mouth or the two pairs of lips at the entrance to the vagina. See *lip, labia majora, labia minora*.

**Listeria**  A group of parasitic bacteria that can infect both animals and humans. See also *Listeriosis*.

**Listeriosis**  Infection with one of the Listeria bacteria, which are capable of causing miscarriage, stillbirth, and premature birth. Listeria bacteria can cause meningoencephalitis (inflammation of the brain). Listeriosis is most dangerous to young children, frail or elderly people, and persons with weakened immune systems.

**litho-**  Prefix meaning stone. A lithotomy is an operation to remove a stone. Lithotripsy involves crushing a stone. The stone may be in the gallbladder or in the urinary tract.

**lithotomy**  Surgical removal of a stone.

**lithotripsy**  Procedure to break a stone into small particles that can be passed in the urine. Lithotripsy results

are generally good with kidney stones that are less than 5/8 inch in diameter.

**lithotripsy, extracorporeal shock wave**  A technique for shattering a kidney stone or gallstone with a shock wave produced outside the body. The stone breaks up after 800 to 2,000 shocks. Anesthesia may be necessary to control the pain, depending on the size and density of the stone, and on the energy of the shock wave needed to break it up. The urologist may opt to place a catheter (stent) in the ureter from below to facilitate passage of the shattered fragments. Abbreviated as ESWL.

**lithotripsy, percutaneous nephro-**  A technique for removing large and/or dense stones and staghorn stones. An access port is created by puncturing the kidney through the skin, and then enlarged to about 3/8 inch in diameter. There is no surgical incision. The procedure is done under anesthesia and real-time live X-ray control (fluoroscopy). Because X-rays are involved, an interventional radiologist may perform this part of the procedure. An endourologist then inserts instruments into the kidney via this port to break up the stone and remove most of the debris from the stone. Abbreviated as PNL.

**lithotriptor**  A machine used to shatter kidney stones and gallstones by physical or other means, such as with a shock wave. It is operated by a urologist.

**lithium**  A naturally occurring salt that, in purified form, is used to treat bipolar disorders, acute mania, and a variety of other disorders.

**lithium toxicity**  The therapeutic level of lithium—the amount needed to treat bipolar disorders—is perilously close to the level that can cause toxicity. Symptoms of lithium toxicity include diarrhea, vomiting, blurred vision, loss of coordination, and loss of motor control. Treatment is to immediately reduce or discontinue lithium use under medical supervision.

**livedo reticularis**  A mottled purplish discoloration of the skin. Livedo reticularis can be a normal condition that is simply more obvious when a person is exposed to the cold. It can also be an indicator of impaired circulation. Livedo reticularis has been reported in association with autoimmune diseases, such as systemic lupus erythematosus; abnormal antibodies referred to as phospholipid antibodies; and a syndrome featuring phospholipid antibodies with multiple brain strokes.

**liver**  An organ in the upper abdomen that aids in digestion, and also removes waste products and worn-out cells from the blood.

**liver of pregnancy, acute fatty**  See *acute fatty liver of pregnancy*.

**livid** Black-and-blue, as from bruising.

**living will** An advance medical directive that specifies what types of medical treatment are desired. A living will can be very specific or very general. The most common statement in a living will requests that if the patient suffers an incurable, irreversible illness, disease, or condition and the attending physician determines that the condition is terminal, life-sustaining measures that would serve only to prolong dying be withheld or discontinued. More specific living wills may include information regarding an individual's desire for services such as pain relief, antibiotics, hydration, feeding, and the use of ventilators, blood products, or cardiopulmonary resuscitation.

**LLL** 1 Left lower lobe (of the lung). 2 La Leche League. 3 The Lawrence Livermore National Laboratory, a federal research facility that focuses on health and biomedicine, science and math education, the environment, energy, and national security.

**LLQ** Left lower quadrant (quarter). The LLQ of the abdomen contains the descending portion of the colon.

**lobar** Having to do with a lobe. For example, lobar pneumonia.

**lobe** 1 A subdivision of an organ that is divided by fissures, connective tissue, or other natural boundaries. 2 A rounded projecting portion, such as the lobe of the ear.

**lobectomy** An operation to remove an entire lobe of the lung.

**Lobstein disease** See *osteogenesis imperfecta type I*.

**lobular carcinoma of the breast, infiltrating** See *breast, infiltrating lobular carcinoma of the*.

**lobule** A little lobe.

**local therapy** Therapy that affects only a tumor and the area close to it.

**local treatment** Treatment that affects the tumor and the area close to it.

**lochia** The fluid that weeps from the vagina for a week or so after delivery of a baby. At first the lochia is primarily blood, followed by a more mucousy fluid containing dried blood, and finally a clear-to-yellow discharge.

**lockjaw** Inability to move the jaw and neck normally as a result of tetanus infection. See *tetanus*.

**locomotion** Movement from one place to another, and the ability to get from one place to the next. See also *locomotive system*.

**locomotive system** The bones, the joints, and the muscles that contract and relax to move the joints and bones.

**locus** In genetics, the place a gene occupies on a chromosome. The plural is loci.

**locus minoris resistentiae** Latin for "a place of less resistance." A locus minoris resistentiae offers little resistance to microorganisms. For example, a damaged heart valve acts as a locus minoris resistentiae, a place where any bacteria in the bloodstream tend to settle.

**Lodine** See *etodolac*.

**loin** The portion of the lower back from just below the ribs to the pelvis.

**long arm of a chromosome** See *chromosome*.

**long QT syndrome** A genetic (inherited) condition that predisposes individuals to irregular heartbeats, fainting spells, and sudden death. The irregular heartbeats are typically brought on by stress or vigorous activity. It is often symptomless and undiagnosed, but long QT syndrome is well known as a cause of sudden cardiac death in young, apparently healthy people, most notably competitive athletes. QT refers to an interval seen in an electrocardiogram (EKG) test of heart function. Abbreviated as LQTS.

**long-chain-3-hydroxyacyl-CoA dehydrogenease deficiency** See *LCHAD deficiency*. See also *acute fatty liver of pregnancy*.

**longevity** Lifespan. Increased longevity means a longer life.

**longitudinal** Along the length of something; running lengthwise or, by extension, over the course of time.

**longitudinal section** A section that is cut along the long axis of a structure. The opposite is a cross-section.

**longitudinal study** A study done over the passage of time. For example, a longitudinal study of children with Down syndrome might involve the study of 100 children with this condition from birth to 10 years of age. The opposite of a cross-sectional (synchronic) study. Also called a diachronic study.

**Lorabid** See *loracarbef*.

**loracarbef** A cephalosporin antibiotic (brand name: Lorabid) used to treat bacterial infections. See also *cephalosporin antibiotic*.

**lorazepam**  A benzodiazepine tranquilizer (brand name: Ativan) used to treat anxiety, chronic insomnia, panic attacks, and sometimes irritable bowel syndrome, among other disorders. See also *benzodiazepine tranquilizer*.

**lordosis**  Inward curvature of the spine. The spine is not supposed to be absolutely straight, so some degree of curvature is normal. When the curve exceeds the usual range, it may be due to musculoskeletal disease or simple poor posture. Treatment is usually by physical therapy, although in severe cases surgery, casting, and/or bracing may be required. Also known as swayback.

**Lotrisone**  A topical medication with two active ingredients: betamethasone dipropionate, a steroid; and clotrimazole, an antifungal. It is used to treat serious skin problems caused by fungal organisms, such as severe athlete's foot or yeast rashes.

**Lou Gehrig's disease**  See *amyotrophic lateral sclerosis*.

**louse-borne typhus**  See *typhus, epidemic*.

**low blood pressure**  See *hypotension*.

**low placenta**  See *placenta previa*.

**lower GI series**  A series of diagnostic X-rays of the colon and rectum, taken after the patient is given a barium enema. See also *barium enema*.

**lower leg**  See *leg*.

**lower segment Cesarean section**  A Cesarean section in which the surgical incision is made in the lower segment of the uterus. Abbreviated as LSCS.

**low-set ear**  See *ear, low-set*.

**LP**  Lumbar puncture.

**LSCS**  Lower segment Cesarean section.

**lubricant**  An oily or slippery substance. A vaginal lubricant may be helpful for women who feel pain during intercourse because of vaginal dryness.

**lues**  See *syphilis*.

**LUL**  Left upper lobe (of the lung).

**lumbar puncture**  A procedure in which cerebrospinal fluid is removed from the spinal canal for diagnostic testing or treatment. The patient usually lies sideways for the procedure, although LPs in infants are often done upright. After local anesthesia is injected into the small of the back

(the lumbar area), a needle is inserted between two vertebrae and into the spinal canal. The needle is usually placed between the third and fourth lumbar vertebrae. Spinal fluid pressure can then be measured, and cerebrospinal fluid removed for testing. LP is particularly helpful in the diagnosis of inflammatory diseases of the central nervous system, especially meningitis and other infections. It can also provide clues to the diagnosis of stroke, spinal cord tumor, and cancer in the central nervous system. An LP can also be done for therapeutic purposes, as a way of administering antibiotics, cancer drugs, or anesthetic agents into the spinal canal. Spinal fluid is sometimes removed by LP to decrease spinal fluid pressure in patients with conditions such as normal-pressure hydrocephalus or benign intracranial hypertension. Normal values for spinal fluid examination are as follows: 15–45 mg/dl protein, 50–75 mg/dl glucose, cell count of 0 to 5 mononuclear cells, and an initial pressure of 70 to 180 mm. These normal values can be altered by injury or disease of the brain, spinal cord, or adjacent tissues. LP risks include headache, brain herniation, bleeding, and infection. These complications are uncommon, with the exception of headache, which can appear up to a day after LP. Headaches occur less frequently when the patient remains lying flat for 1 to 3 hours after the procedure. The benefits of LP depend on the exact situation, but an LP can provide lifesaving information. Also known as a spinal tap, spinal puncture, thecal puncture, rachiocentesis.

**lumbar vertebrae**  There are five lumbar vertebrae situated between the thoracic vertebrae and the sacral vertebrae in the spinal column. They are represented by the symbols L1 through L5.

**lumpectomy**  The surgical removal of a small tumor, which may be benign or cancerous. In common use, lumpectomy refers especially to removal of a lump from the breast. Lumpectomy, often with chemotherapy or radiation therapy, can be an alternative to mastectomy in cases of nonmetastatic breast cancer.

**lung transplant**  Surgery to replace a diseased or damaged lung with a healthy lung from an organ donor. Lung transplant is sometimes done in tandem with heart transplant.

**Lung, and Blood Institute, National Heart**  See *National Institutes of Health*.

**lung, collapsed**  Failure of full expansion of a once fully expanded lung. A lung may collapse due to injury (particularly puncture or gunshot wounds) or as a result of lung damage caused by disease. Also known as atelectasis.

**lungs**  A pair of three-lobed breathing organs located within the right and left sides of the chest. The lungs remove carbon dioxide from the blood and bring oxygen into the blood. Air comes into the lungs via the trachea, traveling evenly into the left and right lungs by means of the left and right bronchi. Each bronchus branches off into several smaller bronchioles, which end in many structures called alveolar sacs. It is in the tiny alveoli within these sacs that oxygen is traded for carbon dioxide in blood delivered back to the heart by the pulmonary veins. Lung function is controlled by several muscles, including the diaphragm muscle beneath the lungs, and the intercostal muscles that surround the lungs.

**lupus** A chronic inflammatory disease caused by an autoimmune condition. Patients with lupus have unusual antibodies in their blood that are targeted against their own body tissues. Lupus can cause disease of the skin, heart, lungs, kidneys, joints, and nervous system. The first symptom is a red (or dark), scaly rash on the nose and cheeks, often called a butterfly rash because of its distinctive shape. As inflammation continues, scar tissue may form, including keloid scarring in patients prone to keloid formation. The cause of lupus is unknown, although heredity, viruses, ultraviolet light, and drugs may all play a role. Lupus is more common in women than in men, and although it occurs in all ethnic groups, it is more common in people of African descent. Diagnosis is by observation of symptoms, and by testing the blood for signs of autoimmune activity. Early treatment is essential, because if it spreads beyond the skin, lupus can be painful, disabling, and fatal. Treatment is by a rheumatologist, and has two objectives: treating the difficult symptoms of the disease and treating the underlying autoimmune activity. It may include steroids and other anti-inflammatory agents, antidepressants and/or mood stabilizers, intravenous immunoglobulin, and in cases in which lupus involves the internal organs, chemotherapy. See also *lupus, discoid; lupus erythematosis, systemic*.

**lupus erythematosis, systemic** When internal organs are involved, the condition is called systemic lupus erythematosus (SLE). Eleven criteria have been established for the diagnosis of SLE. They include the presence of a malar ("butterfly") rash and/or other discoid skin rash; skin rash in reaction to sunlight exposure; ulceration of the mucus lining of the mouth, nose, or throat; two or more swollen, tender joints of the extremities (arthritis); inflammation of the lining tissue around the heart or lungs (pericarditis/pleuritis), usually associated with chest pain with breathing; abnormal amounts of protein or cellular elements in the urine, caused by kidney abnormalities; brain irritation manifested by seizures, severe mood swings, and/or psychosis; low counts of white or red blood cells, or platelets; and abnormal results on immune-system tests, including anti-DNA or anti-Sm (Smith) antibodies, falsely positive blood test for syphilis,

anticardiolipin antibodies, lupus anticoagulant, or a positive LE prep test; and positive results for antinuclear antibodies (ANA) on a blood test. SLE is also often characterized by fatigue. Psychiatric symptoms closely resemble those of a bipolar disorder, which sometimes leads to misdiagnosis. SLE is eight times more common in women than men. The causes of SLE are unknown, but heredity, infectious disease, ultraviolet light, and drugs may all play a role. Treatment is directed toward decreasing inflammation and moderating the level of autoimmune activity, and can range from anti-inflammatory medication to chemotherapy. Persons with SLE can help prevent flareups of disease by avoiding sun exposure and by not abruptly discontinuing medications. Medication can help treat specific symptoms as well, including reducing skin rash, irritation, and scarring; reducing joint inflammation; and treating psychiatric symptoms. See also *lupus*.

**lupus, discoid** A chronic inflammatory condition limited to the skin, caused by an autoimmune disease. Up to 10 percent of persons with discoid lupus eventually develop systemic lupus erythematosus (SLE). Discoid lupus can be caused by infection with the bacteria that causes tuberculosis, and in some cases is a reaction to tuberculosis skin testing. Heredity, viruses, ultraviolet light, and drugs may also be involved. Skin symptoms associated with discoid lupus include a malar (over the cheeks of the face) or "butterfly" rash; a discoid skin rash, characterized by patchy redness that can cause scarring; and photosensitivity, or skin rash in reaction to exposure to sunlight. Diagnosis of discoid lupus may be by a combination of medical history and antinuclear antibody (ANA) testing. Treatment is directed toward decreasing inflammation and/or the level of autoimmune activity. Avoiding sun exposure, antimalarial medications (hydroxychloroquine and others), local cortisone injections, Dapsone, and immune suppression medications are among the possibilities. Also known as lupus verrucosus, lupus vulgaris. See also *lupus; lupus erythematosis, systemic*.

**LUQ** Left upper quadrant (quarter). The LUQ of the abdomen contains the spleen.

**Luschka, foramina of** See *foramina of Luschka*.

**luteinizing hormone** A hormone released by the pituitary gland in response to luteinizing hormone-releasing hormone. Abbreviated as LH, it controls the length and sequence of the female menstrual cycle, including ovulation, preparation of the uterus for implantation of a fertilized egg, and ovarian production of both estrogen and progesterone. In males, it stimulates the testes to produce androgen. Also known as interstitial-cell-stimulating hormone (ICSH).

**luteinizing hormone-releasing hormone** A hormone that controls the production of luteinizing hormone in men and women. Abbreviated as LHRH. See also *luteinizing hormone.*

**luxation** Complete dislocation of a joint. A partial dislocation is a subluxation.

**Lyme disease** An inflammatory disease caused by the bacteria Borrelia burgdorferi, which is transmitted to humans by the deer tick. The first sign of Lyme disease is a red, circular, expanding rash, usually radiating from the tick bite, followed by flu-like symptoms and joint pains. Once the bacteria has entered the bloodstream, it can infect and inflame many different types of tissues, eventually causing many diverse symptoms. Early treatment with antibiotics is the best strategy for preventing major problems due to Lyme disease. You can prevent Lyme disease by avoiding areas where ticks are common, wearing protective clothing and lotion, and immediately removing any ticks that do find you. A vaccine for Lyme disease is available.

**lymph** The almost colorless fluid that travels through the lymphatic system, carrying cells that help fight infection and disease.

**lymph gland** See *lymph node.*

**lymph node** One of many small, bean-shaped organs located throughout the lymphatic system. The lymph nodes store special cells that can trap cancer cells or bacteria that are traveling through the body through the lymph. Also known as lymph glands.

**lymph node, sentinel** The first lymph node to receive lymphatic drainage from a tumor. The sentinel node for a given tumor is found by injecting a tracer substance around the tumor. This substance will travel through the lymphatic system to the first draining node, which is the sentinel node. The tracer substance may be a blue dye that can be tracked visually, or a radioactive colloid that can be followed radiologically. Biopsy of the sentinel lymph node can reveal whether cancer has spread through the lymphatic system. If the sentinel node contains tumor cells, removal of more nodes in the area may be warranted. Sentinel-lymph–node biopsy has become a standard technique for determining the nodal stage of disease in some patients with malignant melanoma.

**lymphadenitis, EBV positive** Disease of the lymph nodes caused by infection with the Epstein-Barr virus, and resembling mononucleosis. EBV-positive lymphadenitis appears in about 1 percent of all transplant patients. Treatment is by reducing the dose of immunosuppressive drugs, if any; antiviral medication; biological therapy; or

interferon. In transplant patients, lymphadenitis may be mistaken for rejection of the new organ. See also *Epstein-Barr virus, mononucleosis, lymphoproliferative disorders.*

**lymphadenitis, regional** See *cat scratch fever.*

**lymphadenopathy** Disease of the lymph nodes.

**lymphadenopathy virus** The human immunodeficiency virus (HIV). See also *HIV, AIDS.*

**lymphadenopathy-associated virus** The human immunodeficiency virus (HIV). See also *HIV, AIDS.*

**lymphangiogram** X-ray of the lymphatic system. A dye is injected to outline the lymphatic vessels and organs.

**lymphangioma** A structure consisting of a collection of blood vessels and lymph vessels that are overgrown and clumped together. Depending on its nature, a lymphangioma may grow slowly or quickly. Lymphangiomas can cause problems because of their location. For example, a lymphangioma around the larynx might cause a breathing problem.

**lymphatic system** The tissues and organs, including the bone marrow, spleen, thymus, and lymph nodes, that produce and store cells that fight infection and disease. The channels that carry lymph are also part of this system.

**lymphatics** Small, thin channels similar to blood vessels that collect and carry tissue fluid from the body. This fluid ultimately drains back into the bloodstream.

**lymphedema** A condition in which excess fluid collects in tissue and causes swelling. It may occur in the arm or leg after lymph vessels or lymph nodes in the underarm or groin are removed.

**lymphocytes** White blood cells that fight infection and disease.

**lymphocytic** Referring to lymphocytes, a type of white blood cell.

**lymphocytopenia** Having an abnormally low number of lymphocytes.

**lymphocytosis** Too many lymphocytes, a finding that may be a marker for infection or disease.

**lymphoid** Referring to lymphocytes, a type of white blood cell. Also refers to tissue in which lymphocytes develop.

**lymphoid tissue** The part of the body's immune system that helps protect it from bacteria.

**lymphoma** Tumor of the lymphoid tissue. Diagnosis is by biopsy. Treatment may be chemotherapy, radiation, surgery, or medication, depending on the age of the patient and type of tumor.

**lymphoma, AIDS-related** Lymphoid tumors that appear in people with AIDS, presumably due to immune-system impairment. Treatment is like that of other lymphomas, but must take impaired natural immunity into account.

**lymphoma, Hodgkin** See *Hodgkin disease*.

**lymphoma, large-cell** Cancer of the lymphatic tissue, characterized by unusually large cells. See also *lymphoma*.

**lymphoma, lymphoblastic** A rapidly moving, aggressive form of lymphoma most often seen in children or young adults. Treatment may be chemotherapy, radiation, surgery, medication, and/or bone-marrow transplant. Precautionary treatment of the central nervous system is usually included because of lymphoblastic lymphoma's ability to spread rapidly to the CNS.

**lymphoma, non-Hodgkin** Malignant tumors that arise in the lymphatic system. Several subtypes of cancer are classified as non-Hodgkin lymphoma. All originate in and spread via the lymphatic system. Symptoms depend on the location of the tumor, but can include swollen, but not painful, lymph nodes; gastric distress; skin problems; night sweats; unexplained weight loss; itching; and fever. Diagnosis is by biopsy of a swollen lymph node, although an X-ray, sonogram, CAT scan, or MRI may also be helpful. Treatment may be chemotherapy, radiation, bone-marrow transplantation, stem-cell rescue, medication, and recently, monoclonal antibodies, depending on the age of the patient and type of tumor. Follow-up examinations are important after lymphoma treatment. Most relapses occur in the first two years after therapy. Abbreviated as NHL.

**lymphoproliferative disorders** Malignant diseases of the lymphoid cells and of cells from the reticuloendothelial system. These disorders occur most often in people with compromised immune systems, such as patients with AIDS and recent transplant patients; they are often associated with Epstein-Barr virus infection. Treatment is by antiviral drugs, interferon, biological therapy, and by reducing the dose of immunosuppressive drugs used, if any. In transplant patients, lymphoproliferative disorders may be mistaken for rejection of the new organ. See also *Epstein-Barr virus; lymphadenitis, EBV positive*.

**lymphoreticulosis, benign** See *cat scratch fever*.

**Lyon hypothesis** See *Lyonization*.

**Lyonization** The inactivation of an X chromosome. One of the two X chromosomes in every cell in a female is randomly inactivated early in embryonic development.

**lysis** Destruction. For example, hemolysis is the destruction of red blood cells with the release of hemoglobin.

**-lytic** Suffix having to do with lysis. For example, hemolytic anemia.

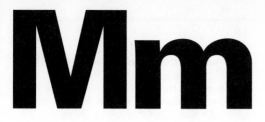

**M proteins**  Antibodies or parts of antibodies found in unusually large amounts in the blood or urine of multiple myeloma patients.

**MAC**  **1** Mycobacterium avium complex. **2** Membrane attack complex.

**Macewen operation**  A surgical operation for inguinal hernia designed by Sir William Macewen.

**Macewen sign**  A sign that helps physicians detect hydrocephalus and brain abscess. Percussion (tapping) on the skull at a particular spot near the junction of the frontal, temporal, and parietal bones yields an unusually resonant sound in the presence of hydrocephalus or a brain abscess.

**machine, heart-lung**  See *heart-lung machine*.

**macro-**  Prefix meaning large or long. Examples of terms involving macro- include macrobiotic, macrocephaly, and macrosomia. The opposite of macro- is micro-.

**macroangiopathy**  Disease of the blood vessels in which fat and blood clots build up in the large blood vessels, stick to the vessel walls, and block the flow of blood. Types of macroangiopathy include coronary artery disease (macroangiopathy in the heart), cerebrovascular disease (macroangiopathy in the brain), and peripheral vascular disease (macroangiopathy affecting, for example, vessels in the legs).

**macrobiota**  The living organisms of a region that are large enough to be seen with the naked eye.

**macrobiotic**  Refering to the macrobiota, a region's living organisms that are large enough to be seen with the naked eye.

**macrobiotic diet**  A diet that claims to lengthen life. The macrobiotic diet concept borrows from Ayurvedic principles of food combining and relies mainly on brown rice and vegetables. It is not recommended for pregnant women or children, and may not provide sufficient protein and nutrients for others.

**macrocephaly**  An abnormally large head.

**macrocytic**  Enlarged red blood cells. Folic acid deficiency is one cause of macrocytic anemia.

**macrogenitosomia**  Condition in which the external sex organs are prematurely or abnormally enlarged. In males, it is caused by an excess of the hormone androgen during fetal development. In females, the clitoris may be enlarged enough to resemble a small penis. Macrogenitosomia is associated with hormonal disorders, which may also create changes in the internal sex organs.

**macroglossia**  An abnormally large tongue. Macroglossia is sometimes said to be associated with Down syndrome, but in that disorder the tongue is actually large only in relation to a smaller-than-normal mouth cavity.

**macrognathia**  An abnormally large jaw. This condition is associated with pituitary gigantism, tumors, and other disorders. Macrognathia can often be corrected with surgery. Also called prognathic mandible.

**macrolide antibiotic**  One of a family of antibiotics produced by anaerobic bacteria. The macrolide antibiotics include erythromycin and troleandomycin. See also *clarithromycin, erythromycin.*

**macrophage**  A type of white blood cell that ingests foreign material. Macrophages are key players in the immune response to foreign invaders of the body, such as infectious microorganisms. They are normally found in the liver, spleen, and connective tissues of the body.

**macrophagic myofasciitis**  A muscle disease named for the findings seen in tissue from muscle biopsies, namely an abnormal infiltrate of macrophages surrounding muscle tissue. Muscle pain is the most frequent symptom. This can be localized to the limbs, or more diffuse. Other symptoms include joint pain, muscle weakness, fatigue, fever, and muscle tenderness. The disorder is associated with an altered immune system in some, but not all, patients. A significant number of patients had taken chloroquine or hydroxychloroquine for malaria; these drugs are known to inhibit the secretion from macrophages of a cell messenger molecule called interleukin. The cause of macrophagic myofasciitis has not been identified. A unique material that accumulates within the affected macrophages has been seen on electron microscopy, but this material has yet to be characterized. Most patients have responded within a few days or weeks to treatment with antibiotics and/or steroids.

**macroscopic**  Large enough to be seen with the naked eye, as opposed to microscopic. A big tumor may well be macroscopic, while a tiny tumor is microscopic.

**macrosomia**  Overly large body. A child with macrosomia has significant overgrowth.

**macula** A small spot. A macula on the skin is a small flat spot, whereas a macula in the eye is the light-sensitive layer of tissue at the back of the eye.

**macular vision** The macula is a special area in the center of the retina. As a person reads, light is focused onto the macula. There, millions of cells change the light into nerve signals that tell the brain what we are seeing. This is called macular or central vision. Thanks to macular vision, we are able to read, drive, and perform other activities that require fine, sharp, straight-ahead vision.

**macule** A circumscribed change in the color of skin that is neither raised nor depressed. Macules are completely flat, and can only be appreciated by visual inspection.

**Madelung disease** See *cephalothoracic lipodystrophy*.

**Magendie, foramen of** See *foramen of Magendie*.

**Magnesia** Named after a town in present-day Turkey where an ore containing magnesium carbonate was mined. Milk of Magnesia, the laxative, is magnesium hydroxide.

**magnesium** A mineral involved in many processes in the body, including nerve signaling, the building of healthy bones, and normal muscle contraction. Magnesium is contained in all unprocessed foods. High concentrations of magnesium are found in nuts, unmilled grains, and legumes, such as peas and beans. According to the National Academy of Sciences, the recommended dietary allowance of magnesium is 420 mg per day for men and 320 mg per day for women. The upper limit for magnesium as a supplement is 350 mg daily, in addition to magnesium from food and water. See also *magnesium deficiency, magnesium excess*.

**magnesium deficiency** Inadequate intake or impaired intestinal absorption of magnesium. Low magnesium (hypomagnesemia) is often associated with low calcium (hypocalcemia) and low potassium (hypokalemia). Deficiency of magnesium causes increased irritability of the nervous system with tetany, a condition characterized by spasms of the hands and feet, muscular twitching and cramps, spasm of the larynx, and other muscle symptoms. See also *magnesium*.

**magnesium excess** Too much magnesium in the body. Persons with impaired kidney function should be especially careful about their magnesium intake because they can accumulate dangerous levels of magnesium. See also *magnesium*.

**magnetic resonance imaging** A procedure that uses a magnet linked to a computer to create pictures of areas inside the body. The patient slides into a tube-like chamber, which may be open or closed. The procedure takes less than an hour. There is no pain involved, but there can be a great deal of clattering noise as the magnet moves around the walls of the tube, and many patients in a closed MRI feel claustrophobic. In some cases sedation may be used, or the noise and the mental discomfort can be reduced by listening to music through headphones. Abbreviated as MRI.

**Maimonides' Daily Prayer of a Physician** See *Daily Prayer of a Physician*.

**maintenance therapy** Chemotherapy given to leukemia patients in remission to prevent a relapse.

**major** A major may be an officer in the military but, in a larger sense, the word denotes anything that is more than something else. For example, the teres major muscle is larger than the teres minor muscle. In anatomy, wherever there is a major, a minor cannot be far behind.

**major histocompatabilty complex** A cluster of genes on chromosome 6 that are concerned with antigen production, and are critical to transplantation. The MHC includes the human leukocyte antigen (HLA) genes.

**malabsorption** Poor intestinal absorption of nutrients.

**malacia** Softening. Osteomalacia is thus softening of bone, usually due to deficiency of calcium and vitamin D.

**malady** From the French *maladie,* meaning illness.

**malaise** A vague feeling of discomfort, one that cannot be pinned down but is often sensed as "just not right."

**malar** Referring to the cheek.

**malar rash** See *butterfly rash*. See also *lupus*.

**malaria** An infectious disease that affects many millions of people, malaria is caused by protozoan parasites from the Plasmodium family. These parasites can be transmitted by the sting of the Anopheles mosquito or by a contaminated needle or transfusion. Treatment is with oral or intravenous medication, particularly chloroquine, mefloquine (brand name: Larium), or atovaquone/proguanil (brand name: Malarone). Persons carrying the sickle cell gene have some protection against malaria. Persons with a gene for hemoglobin C (another abnormal hemoglobin like sickle hemoglobin), thalassemia trait, or deficiency of the enzyme glucose-6-phosphate dehydrogenase (G6PD) are thought also to have partial protection against malaria. Among the many names for malaria are ague, jungle fever, marsh or swamp fever, and paludism.

**malaria, falciparum** The most dangerous type of malaria, this variant is caused by a parasite that is highly resistant to most antimalarial drugs. Complications can include coma, jaundice, renal failure, hypoglycemia, acidosis, severe anemia, high parasite count, and hyperpyrexia. Treatment is in a hospital setting, using intravenous medication.

**malaria, urgent** A fast-acting variant of malaria that emerged in Southeast Asia in the late 1990s. For most patients, death occurs within 24 hours of the emergence of malarial symptoms unless there is medical intervention. Treatment is in a hospital setting, using intravenous medication.

**male** Of the sex that produces sperm cells rather than eggs. However, male can also be defined by physical appearance, by chromosome constitution, or by gender identification.

**male breast cancer** See *breast cancer, male*. See also *breast cancer*.

**male chromosome complement** The large majority of males have a 46,XY chromosome complement: 46 chromosomes, including an X and a Y chromosome. A minority of males have other chromosome constitutions, such as 47,XXY (47 chromosomes, including two X chromosomes and a Y chromosome) or 47,XYY (47 chromosomes, including an X and two Y chromosomes).

**male gonad** The testicles, a pair of organs located behind the penis in a pouch of skin called the scrotum. The testicles produce and store sperm, and are also the body's main source of male hormones. These hormones control the development of the reproductive organs and other male characteristics, such as body and facial hair, low voice, and wide shoulders.

**male pelvis** The male pelvis is more robust, narrower, and taller than the female pelvis. The angle of the male pubic arch and the sacrum are narrower as well.

**malignancy** A tumor that is malignant, usually meaning cancerous.

**malignant** Resistant to treatment or severe, as in malignant hypertension. In reference to an abnormal growth, it implies a tendency to spread to other organs or areas of the body (metastasize), and implies the presence of cancer.

**malignant giant cell tumor** A type of bone tumor that is spreading to other bones or tissues. About half occur in the knee, with most of the rest in the long bones, such as the femur. Diagnosis is by examining a sample of the affected area. Treatment is by excising the affected area, usually followed by chemotherapy or radiation.

**malignant melanoma** See *melanoma*.

**malleability, brain** See *brain plasticity*.

**malleolus** Bony prominence on either side of the ankle.

**malleus** Tiny bone shaped like a minute mallet. The malleus is found in the middle ear.

**malrotated ear** See *ear, slanted*.

**malrotation of the intestine** Failure of the intestine to rotate normally during embryonic development.

**mammary gland** One of the two half-moon–shaped glands on either side of the adult female chest, which with fatty tissue and the nipple make up the breast. Within each mammary gland is a network of sacs that produce milk during lactation and send it to the nipple via a system of ducts. Undeveloped mammary glands are present in female children and in males). See also *breast, lactation*.

**mammogram** An X-ray of the breast, which is taken with a device that compresses and flattens the breast. A mammogram can help a health professional decide whether a lump in the breast is a gland, a harmless cyst, or a tumor. It can cause pressure, discomfort, and some soreness for a little while after the procedure. If the X-ray raises suspicions about cancer, a biopsy is usually the next step. Most doctors recommend regular mammograms for older female patients and for those with a family history of breast cancer.

**managed care** Any system that manages health-care delivery to control costs. Typically, managed-care systems rely on a primary care physician who acts as a gatekeeper for other services, such as specialized medical care, surgery, or physical therapy.

**mandible** The bone of the lower jaw. The joint where the mandible meets the upper jaw at the temporal bone is called the temporomandibular joint.

**maneuver, Heimlich** See *Heimlich maneuver*.

**maneuver, Valsalva** See *Valsalva maneuver*.

**mania** An abnormally elevated mood state characterized by such symptoms as inappropriate elation, increased irritability, severe insomnia, grandiose notions, increased speed and/or volume of speech, disconnected and racing thoughts, increased sexual desire, markedly increased energy and activity level, poor judgment, and inappropriate social behavior. A mild form of mania that does not require hospitalization is called hypomania. Mania that also features symptoms of depression ("agitated depression") is called mixed mania. See *bipolar disorders*. See also *mixed mania*.

**manic** In a state of mania. See *mania*.

**manic-depression** See *bipolar disorders*.

**manic-depressive disease** See *bipolar disorders*.

**manicheel tree** A dangerous tropical tree whose sap is highly poisonous and corrosive. The sap comes out when a leaf is crushed, a branch broken, or the fruit of the tree eaten. The manicheel is hazardous to stand under for shelter from the heat of the tropical sun or, worse, the rain. The leaves of the manicheel are small, round and green but bisected by a yellow vein. The fruit of the manicheel looks like a small green apple. In the event of contact with manicheel sap, one should seek immediate medical attention.

**MAO** Monoamine oxydase, an enzyme active in the nervous system. Although all of MAO's effects are not known, it does act against the neurotransmitter epinephrine.

**MAO inhibitor** One of a family of medications (brand names include: Aurorex, Nardil, Parnate) that act to limit the activity of monoamine oxydase in the nervous system. MAOIs are prescribed to treat depression, anxiety, migraine, and selected other conditions in patients who are not responsive to other medications. They interact with many over-the-counter medications and some foods, so patients taking MAOIs must be educated about what to avoid, and must follow a restricted diet.

**MAOI** Monoamine oxidase inhibitor.

**map, contig** A map depicting the relative order of a linked library of small overlapping clones, representing a complete chromosome segment.

**map, linkage** A map of the genes on a chromosome, based on linkage analysis. A linkage map does not show the physical distances between genes but rather their relative positions, as determined by how often two gene loci are inherited together. The closer two genes are, the more often they will be inherited together. Linkage distance is measured in centimorgans (cM).

**map, physical** A map of the locations of identifiable landmarks on chromosomes. Physical distance is measured in base pairs. The physical map differs from the genetic map, which is based purely on genetic linkage data. In the human genome, the lowest-resolution physical map is the banding patterns of the 24 different chromosomes. The highest-resolution physical map is the complete nucleotide sequence of all chromosomes, a future goal.

**map-dot-fingerprint type corneal dystrophy** See *Cogan corneal dystrophy*.

**maple syrup urine disease** Hereditary disease due to deficiency of an enzyme involved in amino acid metabolism, characterized by urine that smells like maple syrup. Abbreviated as MSUD.

**mapping** Charting the location of genes on chromosomes.

**mapping, gene** Charting the positions of genes on chromosomes and learning the distance, in linkage units or physical units, between genes.

**marasmus** Wasting away, as occurs with children who have kwashiorkor. Also called cachexia, it is usually a result of protein and calorie deficiency.

**Marburg disease** A severe form of hemorrhagic fever that can occur in people who work with African green monkeys. Marburg disease is caused by a filovirus. Ebola virus is also a filovirus.

**Marburg virus** The filovirus that causes Marburg disease.

**Marfan syndrome** Inherited disorder characterized by long fingers and toes, dislocation of the lens, and aortic-wall weakness and aneurysm. Parents with Marfan syndrome have a 50 percent chance of passing it on to each child. There is not yet a genetic test for Marfan syndrome, so diagnosis is complex. It usually includes several steps: generally, a detailed medical and family history, visual examination, measurement and comparison of height to limb length, eye examination, X-rays of the spine and sometimes other areas, and electrocardiogram and echocardiogram of the heart. There is no treatment specifically for Marfan syndrome, but specific problems associated with it (such as scoliosis and eye problems) may be treated individually.

**marker** An identifiable heritable spot on a chromosome. A marker can be an expressed region of DNA (a gene) or a segment of DNA with no known coding function. All that matters is that the marker can be monitored.

**marker chromosome** An abnormal chromosome that is distinctive in appearance, but not fully identified. A marker chromosome is not a marker of a specific disease; it is simply a chromosome that can be distinguished under the microscope from all the normal human chromosomes. For example, the Fragile X chromosome was once called the marker X, until it was found to cause a specific cluster of abnormalities.

**marker gene** A detectable genetic trait or segment of DNA that can be identified and tracked. A marker gene can serve as a flag for another gene, sometimes called the target gene. A marker gene must be on the same chromosome as the target gene, and near enough to it so that the marker gene and the target gene are genetically linked and usually inherited together.

**marker, blood** A sign of a disease or condition that can be isolated from a blood sample. For example, the monoclonal antibody D8/17 is a diagnostic sign of pediatric autoimmune disorders associated with strep.

**marker, tumor** Substances that can be detected in higher-than-normal amounts in the blood, urine, or body tissues of some patients with certain types of cancer. A tumor marker may be made by a tumor itself or by the body in response to the tumor. Testing for tumor markers alone is not a valid way to detect and diagnose cancer, as most tumor markers can be elevated in patients who don't have a tumor; no tumor marker is entirely specific to a particular type of cancer; and not every cancer patient has an elevated tumor-marker level, especially in the early stages of cancer, when tumor-marker levels are usually still normal. Although tumor markers are typically imperfect as screening tests to detect hidden cancers, once a particular tumor has been found with a marker, the marker may be a means of monitoring the success or failure of treatment. The tumor-marker level may also reflect the stage of the disease and how quickly the cancer is likely to progress, helping to determine the prognosis (outlook). Examples of tumor markers include alpha-fetoprotein (AFP), carcinoembryonic antigen (CEA), human chorionic gonadotropin (HCG), lactate dehydrogenase (LDH), and neuron-specific enolase (NSE).

**Maroteaux-Lamy syndrome** A form of mucopolysaccharidosis with onset before age three, Maroteaux-Lamy syndrome is characterized by an inability to metabolize dermatin sulfate. This leads to abnormal accumulation of dermatin sulfate, mostly in the peripheral tissues. The result is mild to severe changes in muscle, bone, skin, and other tissues, particularly the heart. Diagnosis is by examining leukocytes and cultured skin fibroblasts, or 24-hour urine collection to search for high levels of dermatin sulfate. There is no current treatment for Maroteaux-Lamy syndrome, but individual symptoms and problems may respond to physical therapy, medication, or surgery. Due to heart damage, death usually occurs before age 40. Also known as mucopolysaccharidosis Type VI. See also *mucopolysaccharidosis*.

**marriage, cousin** See *consanguinity*.

**marrow** See *bone marrow*.

**marsh fever** See *malaria*.

**MASA syndrome** MASA stands for mental retardation, aphasia, shuffling gait, and adducted thumbs. Features of the syndrome include mental retardation and aphasia (lack of speech); adducted (clasped) thumbs, absent extensor pollicis longus and/or brevis muscles to the thumb, shuffling gait, and leg spasticity; small body size; and lumbar lordosis (swayback). MASA is inherited as an X-linked trait, and so affects mainly boys. Alternative names for MASA include clasped thumbs and mental retardation, congenital clasped thumbs with mental retardation, adducted thumbs with mental retardation, and the Gareis-Mason syndrome. See also *adducted thumbs*.

**masklike face** An expressionless face with little or no sense of animation; a face more like a mask than a real face. A masklike face is seen in a number of disorders, including Parkinson disease and myotonic dystrophy. Also called masklike facies.

**masochism** Pleasure from one's own pain. Masochism is considered a sexual disorder, or paraphilia. Named after the 19th-century Austrian writer Leopold von Sacher-Masoch.

**MASS syndrome** MASS stands for mitral valve, aorta, skeleton, skin, and MASS syndrome is a heritable disorder of connective tissue characterized by involvement of all those structures. One basis for MASS syndrome is a mutation in the fibrillin gene.

**massage** The therapeutic practice of manipulating the muscles and limbs to ease tension and reduce pain. Massage can be a part of physical therapy, or practiced on its own. It can be highly effective for reducing the symptoms of arthritis, back pain, carpal tunnel syndrome, and other disorders of the muscles and/or nervous system.

**massage therapist** A person who practices therapeutic massage. In many US states, massage therapists can be licensed after completing a specified training program. Licensed therapists may practice independently or in a medical setting.

**masseter** The muscle that raises the lower jaw.

**mast cell** A connective tissue cell whose normal function is unknown, the mast cell is frequently injured during allergic reactions. It then releases strong chemicals, including histamine, into the tissues and blood. These chemicals are very irritating, and cause itching, swelling, and fluid leaking from cells. They can also cause muscle spasm, leading to lung- and throat-tightening (as is found in asthma), and loss of voice.

**mastectomy** A general term for removal of the breast, usually to remove cancerous tissue. The operation can be done in a hospital or in an outpatient clinic, depending on how extensive it needs to be. It takes from two to three hours, with three to five weeks for full recovery. Drainage shunts are left in the surgical incision for a few days after the operation; these are removed in three to five days if the area is healing normally. After the mastectomy, reconstructive surgery may be performed to restore a more normal appearance. Many patients choose to avoid reconstructive surgery, and instead wear special undergarments. In cases of nonmetastatic breast cancer, a lumpectomy, radiation, chemotherapy, or a combination of these treatments may prove a viable alternative to mastectomy. If a lumpectomy is chosen, the surgeon may remove some lymph-node tissue from under the arms to make sure cancer has not spread.

**mastectomy, double** Removal of both breasts.

**mastectomy, modified radical** Removal of the breast tissue and the axillary lymph nodes, which are under the arms.

**mastectomy, preventative** Removal of one or both breasts without the current presence of cancer. This surgery is sometimes chosen as a preventative measure by women who have a strong family history of breast cancer.

**mastectomy, prophylactic** See *mastectomy, preventative*.

**mastectomy, radical** Removal of all breast tissue, from just under the collarbone to the abdomen, including the chest wall muscles. The axillary lymph nodes are also removed. This operation is rarely used anymore, having first been replaced by the modified radical mastectomy and then by even less-invasive alternatives. Also known as a Halstead mastectomy.

**mastectomy, simple** Removal of one or both breasts, but not the lymph nodes.

**mastectomy, subcutaneous** Removal of breast tissue, using a minimal incision. This type of mastectomy may be used to remove small areas of suspicious or cancerous tissue, but can also be a cosmetic surgery procedure. For example, subcutaneous mastectomy can reduce the volume of enlarged male breasts or be part of a female-to-male sex-change procedure.

**masticate** To chew.

**mastitis** Inflammation of one or more mammary glands within the breast, usually in a lactating woman. It can be felt as a hard, sore spot within the breast. Mastitis can be caused by an infection in the breast or by a plugged milk duct. Treatment is by rest, applying warm compresses to the affected area, and for those who are lactating, nursing or expressing milk frequently. If mastitis recurs during nursing, contact a lactation expert through your obstetrician, midwife, or the La Leche League.

**mastoid** The rounded protrusion of bone just behind the ear, which was once thought to look like a breast.

**mastoiditis** Inflammation of the mastoid, often secondary to ear infection.

**maternal mortality rate** The number of maternal deaths related to childbearing, divided by the number of live births (or by the number of live births and fetal deaths) in that year. The maternal mortality rate in the US in 1993 and 1994 was 0.1 per 1,000 live births, or 1 mother dying per 10,000 live births.

**maternal serum alpha-fetoprotein (MSAFP)** The presence of AFP, a plasma protein normally produced by the fetus, in the mother's blood. MSAFP serves as the basis for some valuable tests. AFP is manufactured principally in the fetus's liver, but is also found in the fetal gastrointestinal tract and in the yolk sac, a structure temporarily present during embryonic development. The level of AFP is typically high in the fetus's blood, goes down in the baby's blood after birth, and by one year of age is virtually undetectable. During pregnancy, AFP crosses the placenta from the fetal circulation and appears in the mother's blood. The level of AFP in the mother's blood (the maternal serum AFP) provides a screening test for a number of disorders, including open neural tube defects, such as anencephaly and spina bifida, in which case MSAFP tends to be high; Down syndrome, in which case MSAFP tends to be low; and other chromosome abnormalities.

**matter, gray** See *gray matter*.

**matter, white** See *white matter*.

**maxilla** The major bone of the upper jaw.

**MCAT** Medical College Admissions Test.

**McBurney point** The most tender area of the abdomen of patients in the early stage of appendicitis.

**measles** An acute and highly contagious viral disease characterized by fever, runny nose, cough, red eyes, and a spreading skin rash. Measles, also known as rubeola, is a potentially disastrous disease. It can be complicated by ear infections, pneumonia, encephalitis (which can cause convulsions, mental retardation, and even death), the sudden onset of low blood platelet levels with severe bleeding (acute thrombocytopenic purpura), or a chronic brain disease that occurs months to years after an attack of measles (subacute sclerosing panencephalitis). During pregnancy, exposure to the measles virus may trigger miscarriage or premature delivery. Treatment includes rest, calamine lotion or other anti-itching preparations to soothe the skin, nonaspirin pain relievers for fever, and in some cases antibiotics. Measles can often be prevented through vaccination. Also known as hard measles, seven-day measles, eight-day measles, nine-day measles, ten-day measles, morbilli. See also *measles* *encephalitis; measles immunization; measles syndrome, atypical; MMR.*

**measles encephalitis** Inflammation of the brain due to infection with the measles virus. Measles encephalitis occurs in perhaps 1 in 1,000 cases of measles, starting up to three weeks after onset of the rash and presenting with high fever, convulsions, and coma. It usually runs a blessedly short course, with full recovery within a week, but it may eventuate in central nervous system impairment or death.

**measles immunization** A vaccine for measles only. Single-virus vaccines may be safer for children with known or suspected brain disorders or a compromised immune system, and are generally given after one year of age. For other children, the measles vaccine is usually administered with vaccines for mumps and rubella. See *MMR.*

**measles syndrome, atypical** An altered expression of measles, atypical measles syndrome begins suddenly with high fever, headache, cough, and abdominal pain. The rash may appear one to two days later, often beginning on the limbs. Swelling (edema) of the hands and feet may occur. Pneumonia is common, and may persist for three months or more. Atypical measles syndrome occurs in persons who were incompletely immunized against measles. This may happen in persons given the old killed-virus measles vaccine, which does not provide complete immunity and is no longer available, or attenuated (weakened) live measles vaccine that was inactivated due to improper storage. It can be confused with other entities, including Rocky Mountain spotted fever, meningococcal infection, various types of pneumonia, appendicitis, and juvenile rheumatoid arthritis. Abbreviated as AMS.

**measly tapeworm** See *Taenia solium.*

**meatus** An opening or passageway.

**meatus, female urethral** The meatus (opening) of the female urethra, the transport tube leading from the bladder to discharge urine outside the body, is above the vaginal opening.

**Meckel diverticulum** See *diverticulum, Meckel.*

**meconium** Dark, sticky material normally present in the intestine at birth, and passed in the feces after birth after trypsin and other enzymes from the pancreas have acted on it. The passage of meconium before birth can be a sign of fetal distress.

**meconium ileus** Obstruction of the intestine (ileus) due to overly thick meconium. Meconium ileus results from a deficiency of trypsin and other digestive enzymes from the pancreas, as in cystic fibrosis.

**MEDEVAC** See *MEDVAC.*

**medial** The side of the body or body part that is nearer to the middle or center (median) of the body. For example, when referring to the knee, medial would mean the side of the knee that is closest to the other knee. The opposite of medial is lateral. See also *Appendix B, "Anatomic Orientation Terms."*

**medial collateral ligament of the knee** The ligament that straps the inner side of the knee joint, providing stability and strength. See also *knee.*

**medial meniscus of the knee** A thickened, crescent-shaped cartilage pad between the two joints formed by the femur (the thigh bone) and the tibia (the shinbone). The medial meniscus is toward the inner side of the knee joint. The meniscus acts as a smooth surface for the joint to move on, serves to evenly load the surface during weight-bearing, and also adds in disbursing joint fluid for joint lubrication. See also *knee.*

**median** The middle, like the median strip in a highway.

**mediastinoscopy** A procedure in which the doctor inserts a tube into the chest to view the organs in the mediastinum. The tube is inserted through an incision above the breastbone. Also called a mediastinotomy.

**mediastinotomy** See *mediastinoscopy.*

**mediastinum** The area between the lungs. The organs in this area include the heart and its large veins and arteries, the trachea, the esophagus, the bronchi, and lymph nodes.

**Medicaid** Programs of public assistance to persons whose income is insufficient to pay for health care, regardless of age. Medicaid is administered on a state level, with the federal government providing matching funds to state Medicaid programs. Services and options can vary from state to state. Disabled persons who receive Social Security Income (SSI) are automatically eligible for Medicaid. To apply for Medicaid, contact your local Social Security, public health, or disability services office.

**Medical College Admissions Test** A test required of all applicants to medical school in the US and Canada, the MCAT assesses applicants' science knowledge, reasoning, and communication and writing skills. It is given under the aegis of the Association of American Medical Colleges.

**medical directives, advance** See *advance directives.*

**Medical Research Council** In the UK and some Commonwealth countries, the Medical Research Council (MRC) is the counterpart of the National Institutes of

Health (NIH) in the US. It plays an important role in funding extramural biomedical research.

**medical symbol** See *Aesculapius*.

**Medicare** The US government's national health insurance program for people aged 65 and older who receive Social Security or railroad retirement benefits, and people with certain disabilities. Medicare Part A covers inpatient hospital stays, whereas Medicare Part B covers physician and outpatient services. Currently, Medicare does not cover the cost of prescription drugs. Former federal employees and noncitizens usually cannot receive Medicare.

**medication, ACE-inhibitor** See *ACE inhibitors*.

**medication, anticoagulant** See *anticoagulent agents*.

**medication, antiplatelet** See *antiplatelet agents*.

**medication, antiviral** See *antiviral agent*.

**medication, beta-blocker** See *beta blockers*.

**medication, clot-dissolving** See *clot-dissolving medications*.

**medication, vasodilator** See *vasodilators*. See also *ACE inhibitors*.

**medicine, transfusion** See *transfusion medicine*.

**Medigap** An insurance policy in the US that supplements Medicare benefits, presumably filling the gaps in health-care coverage. Many Medigap policies are mainly intended to cover the cost of prescription drugs. Some actually duplicate Medicare coverage, however, and may be unnecessary.

**Mediterranean anemia** See *thalassemia major*.

**Mediterranean fever** See *familial Mediterranean fever*.

**MEDLARS** Medical Literature Analysis and Retrieval System, a computer system of the US National Library of Medicine (NLM) that allows rapid access to NLM's store of biomedical information. Today, through the Internet and World Wide Web, MEDLARS search services are available around the world without charge.

**MEDLINE** The best known database of the US National Library of Medicine (NLM), MEDLINE lets anyone with computer access query the NLM's store of journal references on specific topics. It currently contains nine million references, going back to the mid-1960s. Other databases

provide information on cataloging and serials, toxicological and environmental health data, AIDS, and other specialized areas. Through the World Wide Web, some 350,000 MEDLINE searches a day are done by health professionals, scientists, librarians, and the general public. A new Web service, called MEDLINEplus, links users to sources of consumer health information. MEDLINE and MEDLINEplus are part of the MEDLARS system. See also *MEDLARS*.

**medroxyprogesterone acetate** See *Depo-Provera*.

**medulla** The innermost part. The spinal medulla, for example, is that part of the spinal cord that is lodged within the vertebral canal.

**medulla oblongata** The base of the brain, which is formed by the enlarged top of the spinal cord. This part of the brain directly controls breathing, blood flow, and other essential functions.

**medulloblastoma** A type of virulent brain tumor that occurs most frequently in children. Medulloblastomas originate in residual embryonic nerve cells that begin to proliferate. Treatment is by radiation, but is rarely successful.

**MEDVAC** Acronym for medical evacuation. MEDVAC typically refers to a team that is organized with the skills necessary for proper medical evacuation in emergency situations. Also known as MEDEVAC.

**mega-** Prefix meaning abnormally large. Megalocephaly is too large a head; megacardia is an enlarged heart.

**megacolon** An abnormally enlarged colon.

**megakaryocyte** A giant cell in the bone marrow that is the ancestor of blood platelets.

**megavitamin therapy** The use of massive doses of vitamins to treat disease. Because overuse of vitamins can itself cause disease, this approach is controversial with most doctors. See also *Appendix C, "Vitamins"; orthomolecular medicine; vitamin therapy*.

**Meibomian cyst** See *cyst, Meibomian*.

**Meibomian glands** See *glands, Meibomian*.

**meibomianitis** Inflammation of the little glands in the tarsus of the eyelids. Chronic inflammation leads to cysts of the Meibomian glands, which are also called chalazions. Also known as meibomitis.

**meibomitis** See *meibomianitis*.

**meiosis** What chromosomes do during germ-cell formation to halve the chromosome number from 46 to 23. In meiosis, the 46 chromosomes in the cell divide to make two new cells with 23 chromosomes each. Before meiosis is completed, however, chromosomes pair with their corresponding chromosomes and exchange bits of genetic material. In women, X chromosomes pair; in men, the X and Y chromosomes pair. After the exchange, the chromosomes separate, and meiosis continues.

**meiotic** Pertaining to meiosis.

**meiotic nondisjunction** Failure of two members of a chromosome pair to separate during meiosis, causing both to go to a single daughter cell. This mechanism is responsible for the extra chromosome 21 in trisomy 21 (Down syndrome) and for extra and missing chromosomes that cause other birth defects and many miscarriages.

**melan-** Prefix meaning dark or black. For example, melancholia is a dark and gloomy mood, and melanin is a dark pigment.

**melancholia** Old term for depression.

**melanin** The pigment that gives human skin, hair, and eyes their color. Dark-skinned people have more melanin in their skin than light-skinned people have. Melanin is produced by cells called melanocytes. It provides some protection again skin damage from the sun, and the melanocytes increase their production of melanin in response to sun exposure. Freckles, which occur in people of all races, are small, concentrated areas of increased melanin production.

**melanocytes** Cells in the skin that produce and contain the pigment called melanin.

**melanoma** Tumors of the melanocytes, the cells that produce pigment in the skin. Melanomas can be benign or cancerous; when malignant, they are the most common type of skin cancer. They are most common in people with fair skin, but can occur in all races. Most melanomas present as a dark, mole-like spot that spreads and, unlike a mole, has an irregular border. Tendency toward melanoma may be inherited, and risk increases with overexposure to the sun and sunburn. Fair-skinned people and people with a family history of melanoma should always use a high-SPF sunscreen when outdoors. Everyone who has concerns about an unusual mole-like spot should see a doctor: detected early, melanoma is almost always treatable, but undetected melanoma can spread and become fatal.

**melanoma, amelanic** A colorless melanoma, detectable only on close examination of the skin.

**melanoma, benign** A tumor of the melanocytes that is not cancerous.

**melanoma, benign juvenile** A noncancerous, raised, pink or red scaly area on a child's skin, usually on the cheek.

**melanoma, choroidal malignant** A tumor of melanocytes in the choroid membrane that surrounds the eye.

**melanoma, nodular** A raised, distinct, bluish-black tumor that may be encircled by particularly pale skin. Nodular melanoma is seen most often in middle-aged or older adults.

**melanoma, superficial spreading** The most common type of melanoma, a raised, irregular, colored area that starts as a mole-like shape but spreads across the skin.

**MELAS syndrome** An acronym for mitochondrial encephalopathy, lactic acidosis, and stroke-like episodes, MELAS is a rare form of dementia caused by mutations in the genetic material (DNA) in the mitochondria. Most of our DNA is in the chromosomes in the cell nucleus, but another important cell structure that carries DNA is the mitochondrion. Much of the DNA in the mitochondrion is used to manufacture proteins that help to produce energy. As a result of the disturbed function of their cells' mitochondria, patients with MELAS develop brain dysfunction (encephalopathy) with seizures and headaches, as well as muscle disease with a buildup of lactic acid in the blood (lactic acidosis), temporary local paralysis (stroke-like episodes), and abnormal thinking (dementia). MELAS is diagnosed by muscle biopsy showing characteristic ragged red fibers. Brain biopsy shows stroke-like changes. MELAS can affect people at different times of life, but most patients show symptoms before age 20. Patients are managed according to which areas of the body are affected at a particular time. There is no known treatment for MELAS, which is progressive and fatal.

**melatonin** A hormone produced by the pineal gland, melatonin is intimately involved in regulating the sleeping and waking cycles, among other processes. Melatonin supplements are sometimes used by people who have chronic insomnia. Always see your doctor before taking melatonin, as it is not recommended for all patients with sleep problems.

**melena** Stools or vomit stained black by blood pigment or dark blood products.

**melioidosis** An infectious illness that is most frequent in Southeast Asia and Northern Australia, melioidosis is caused by the Pseudomonas pseudomallei bacteria. This bacteria is found in soil, rice paddies, and stagnant waters. Humans catch the disease by inhalation of contaminated dust, or when soil contaminated by the bacteria comes in contact with abraded (scraped) skin. Melioidosis most commonly involves the lungs, where the infection can form a cavity of pus (abscess). The bacteria can also spread from the skin through the bloodstream to affect the brain, eyes, heart, liver, kidneys, and joints. The common symptoms of melioidosis are not specific. They include headaches, fever, chills, cough, chest pain, and loss of appetite. Melioidosis can also cause encephalitis (brain inflammation) with seizures. Diagnosis is by a microscopic evaluation of a sputum (spit) sample in the laboratory. A blood test may detect early acute cases of melioidosis. Treatment involves antibiotics, and depends on the location of the disease. For mild illness, antibiotics such as chloramphenicol, doxycycline, sulfisoxazole, or trimethoprim-sulfamethoxazole are used. For more severe illness, a combination of chloramphenicol, doxycycline, and cotrimoxazole is recommended. Very severe illness, as with persistent blood infection, indicates use of intravenous antibiotics, including chloramphenicol. If sputum cultures remain positive for six months, surgical removal of the lung abscess with lobectomy is considered. Antibiotic treatments may be necessary for from 3 to 12 months. Melioidosis can remain latent (in hiding) for years and emerge when a person's resistance to disease is low. Also known as Whitmore disease.

**membrane**  A very thin layer of tissue that covers a surface.

**membrane attack complex**  An abnormal activation of the complement (protein) portion of the blood, forming a cascade reaction that brings blood proteins together, binds them to the cell wall, and then inserts them through the cell membrane. MAC formation allows water, ions, and other small molecules to move freely into and out of a cell, and quickly results in cell death. Abbreviated as MAC.

**membranous gingivitis, acute**  See *acute membranous gingivitis.*

**memory**  The ability to recover information about past events or knowledge, and/or the process of doing so. Often divided into short-term (also known as working or recent memory) and long-term memory: The first recovers memories of recent events, whereas the latter is concerned with the more distant past. Some medical disorders, such as Alzheimer disease, damage the cognitive systems that control memory. Usually, long-term memory is retained while short-term memory is lost; conversely, memories may become jumbled, leading to mistakes in recognizing people or places that should be

familiar. See also *memory, anterograde; memory, long-term; memory, short-term.*

**memory B cells**  Secondary immune-system components that have an affinity for a particular antigen. Like other B cells, memory B cells originate from lymphocytes that develop and are activated in the bone marrow. They become antigen-specific when stimulated by interleukin-4 (IL-4).

**memory span**  The number of items, usually words or numbers, that a person can retain and recall. Memory span is a test of working memory (short-term memory). In a typical test of memory span, an examiner reads a list of random numbers aloud at about the rate of one number per second. At the end of a sequence, the person being tested is asked to recall the items in order. The average span for normal adults is seven.

**memory, anterograde**  Loss of short-term memory with retention of memories from the distant past.

**memory, long-term**  A system for permanently storing, managing, and retrieving information for later use. Items of information stored as long-term memory may be available for a lifetime.

**memory, recent**  See *memory, short-term.*

**memory, short-term**  A system for temporarily storing and managing information required to carry out complex cognitive tasks such as learning, reasoning, and comprehension. Short-term memory is involved in the selection, initiation, and termination of information-processing functions, such as encoding, storing, and retrieving data. One test of short-term memory is memory span: the number of items, usually words or numbers, that a person can retain and recall. Also known as recent or working memory. See also *memory, memory span.*

**memory, working**  See *memory, short-term.*

**menarche**  The time in a girl's life that menstruation first begins. During the menarche period, menstruation may be irregular and unpredictable. Mood, weight, activity level, and growth rate may fluctuate with the hormone levels as well. Synonymous with female puberty.

**Mendelian**  Referring to the Austrian monk, Gregor Mendel (1822–84), who formulated the foundation of classical genetics.

**Ménière disease**  A condition characterized by recurrent vertigo accompanied by ringing in the ears (tinnitus) and deafness. Symptoms include vertigo, dizziness, nausea, vomiting, loss of hearing in the affected ear, and abnormal eye movements. Ménière disease is due to dysfunction of the semicircular canals (endolymphatic sac) in the inner ear. Treatment usually includes medications, such as anticholinergic drugs or antihistamines, to relieve the vertigo. Diuretics have been also used to lower the pressure in the endolymphatic sac. Also known as recurrent aural vertigo. See also *vertigo*.

**meninges**　The three membranes that cover the brain and spinal cord (singular: meninx). The outside meninx is called the dura mater, and is the most resilient of the three. The center layer is the pia mater, and the thin innermost layer is the arachnoid. Inflammation of the meninges (meningitis) can occur due to bacterial infection. See also *meningitis*.

**meningioma**　A type of brain tumor that starts within the meninges. These slow-growing tumors are sometimes associated with earlier head trauma.

**meningitis**　Inflammation of the meninges, usually due to a bacterial infection but sometimes from viral, protozoan, or other causes (in some cases the cause cannot be determined). Onset is usually rapid (acute), and if untreated, the disease can be fatal within a very short period of time. Early symptoms are nonspecific and flu-like. They are followed by more serious symptoms, which may include rash, stiff neck, confusion, vomiting, loss of appetite, fever, headache, and coma. Diagnosis is by observation of symptoms, and confirmed by lumbar puncture to examine the cerebrospinal fluid. Treatment depends on the cause of the inflammation. Meningitis can cause permanent damage to the brain and nervous system, and is sometimes the cause of deafness.

**meningitis, aseptic**　See *meningitis, viral.*

**meningitis, bacterial**　Inflammation of the meninges due to a bacterial infection, often with the streptococcus B bacteria. Treatment is by very strong antibiotics, and almost always takes place in a hospital setting because of the potentially fatal nature of the disease. Dehydration is a common side effect in bacterial meningitis, so intravenous fluids and/or oral electrolyte solutions may also be given.

**meningitis, cryptococcal**　Inflammation of the meninges due to infection with the fungal organism cryptococcus neoformans, which is found mainly in dirt and bird droppings. Most people have been exposed to this organism at some time, but normally it causes no problems. Often associated with AIDS, cryptococcal meningitis is considered an opportunistic infection: a disease that emerges most often when the immune system is compromised in some way. Diagnosis is by observation of symptoms, lumbar puncture, and cryptococcal titre. Treatment

takes place in the hospital, and usually consists of intravenous doses of the antibiotic amphotericin B. Once the infection is under control, patients usually remain on a maintainance dose of fluconazole (Diflucan) to prevent reinfection.

**meningitis, infectuous**　Meningitis caused by bacterial, viral, or protozoan infection. Most of the agents known to cause meningitis are infectuous, but very few people exposed to them will get meningitis. Those at greatest risk include people with AIDS, infants, transplant patients, and others whose immune systems may be compromised. For this reason, infectuous meningitis patients are almost always isolated until the risk of spreading the illness to others has passed.

**meningitis, Kernig's sign of**　This sign of meningitis is tested by having the person lie flat on the back, flexing the thigh so that it is at a right angle to the trunk, and completely extending the leg at the knee joint. If the leg cannot be completely extended because of pain, this is Kernig's sign.

**meningitis, meningococcal**　Inflammation of the meninges due to infection with the meningococcus bacteria. Bleeding beneath the skin is a special symptom associated with this type of infection, which is most common in crowded settings. This is a particularly dangerous form of meningitis, as it is highly contagious by any type of intimate contact—however, most people exposed to the bacteria will not become ill. Prompt medical attention is essential, as is avoiding the spread of infection to others. Treatment is with antibiotics, usually in a hospital setting. Prevention is by improved hygiene and vaccination.

**meningitis, neoplastic**　Inflammation of the meninges that occurs due to the spread of solid tumors to the brain or spinal cord. Treatment is with medication, usually methotrexate (brand name: Rheumatrex), and usually takes place in a hospital.

**meningitis, viral**　Inflammation of the meninges caused by a virus—usually one of the enteroviruses, such as mumps or Coxsackie virus. These viruses are shed in the feces, sputum (spit), and nasal discharges. Viral meningitis is contagious, and occurs most frequently in children. It can be a complication of infection with common childhood diseases, including chicken pox. Most patients with viral meningitis recover completely. Treatment, if warranted, is by antiviral drugs. Viral meningitis can often be prevented by improved hygiene. Also known as aseptic meningitis, infectuous meningitis.

**meningocele**　Protrusion, through a bone defect in the vertebral column, of the membranes that cover the spine and part of the spinal cord. This birth defect is due to failure of the bottom end of the neural tube to close during embryonic life. This structure gives rise to the brain and spinal cord. The risk of all neural-tube birth defects can be decreased by adequate folic acid intake during pregnancy. See also *spina bifida*.

**meningomyelocele**   Protrusion of the membranes that cover the spine and some of the spinal cord itself, due to spina bifida, a defect in the bony encasement of the vertebral column. See also *spina bifida*.

**meniscus, lateral knee**   The thickened, crescent-shaped cartilage pad between the two joints formed by the femur (the thigh bone) and the tibia (the shinbone). The meniscus acts as a smooth surface for the joint to move on. The lateral meniscus is toward the outer side of the knee joint. See also *knee*.

**meniscus, medial knee**   The thickened, crescent-shaped cartilage pad between the two joints formed by the femur (the thigh bone) and the tibia (the shinbone). The meniscus acts as a smooth surface for the joint to move on. The medial meniscus is toward the inner side of the knee joint. See also *knee*.

**Menkes syndrome**   Genetic disorder characterized by fragile, twisted hair and progressive deterioration of the brain. Menkes syndrome is due to an error in copper transport, resulting in copper deficiency. Females are carriers, and their sons with the gene have the disease. If the disorder is recognized early, injections of copper may stop further damage. Also known as kinky hair syndrome.

**menometrorrhagia**   Excessive uterine bleeding, both at the usual time of menstrual periods and at other irregular intervals. This can be a sign of cancer, endometriosis, or fibroid tumors in the uterus, which are usually benign. Women who have abnormal menstrual bleeding should always consult their physician to rule out these conditions. Anemia may also result. Treatment depends on the cause: If there does not appear to be a dangerous cause, such as cancer, then hormone supplementation or the therapeutic use of birth control pills to better control the menstrual cycle may be recommended.

**menopause**   The time, usually in middle age, when menstrual periods end. When there has been no menstruation for 12 consecutive months, and no other biological or physiological cause can be identified, the childbearing years have probably ended and menopause has begun. Natural menopause occurs when the ovaries begin decreasing their production of the sex hormones estrogen and progesterone. The timing of menopause varies. In the western world, the average age is now 51, but menopause can occur from the 30s onward. Factors influencing the time of menopause include heredity and cigarette smoking. Smokers and former smokers reach menopause an

average of two years before women who have never smoked. There is no relation between the time of a woman's first period and her age at menopause, nor is the age of menopause influenced by a woman's race, height, number of children, or use of oral contraceptives. Changes associated with menopause include night sweats, mood swings, vaginal dryness, fluctuations in sexual desire (libido), forgetfulness, trouble sleeping, and fatigue (probably from the loss of sleep). Problems that have not been proved due to the menopause include headache, dizziness, palpitations of the heart, and depression. Estrogen replacement therapy (ERT) is sometimes used to treat symptoms associated with menopause. ERT reduces or stops short-term changes such as hot flashes, disturbed sleep, and vaginal dryness. ERT can prevent osteoporosis, a consequence of lowered estrogen levels, and reduces the risk of heart disease by up to 50 percent. Vaginal ERT products help with vaginal dryness, more severe vaginal changes, and bladder effects only. The use of ERT by itself is associated with an increase in the risk of endometrial cancer (cancer of the lining of the uterus). However, by taking the hormone progestogen along with estrogen, the risk of endometrial cancer is reduced substantially. Progestogen protects the uterus by keeping the endometrium from thickening, an effect caused by estrogen. The combination therapy of estrogen plus progestogen is called hormone replacement therapy (HRT). See also *menopause transition; menopause, induced*.

**menopause transition**   Changes in female hormone production that begin about six years before the natural menopause; also called perimenopause. The levels of hormones produced by the aging ovaries fluctuate, leading to irregularity in the length of the menstrual period, the time between periods, and the level of flow, and hot flashes, a sudden warm feeling with blushing. Other changes associated with the perimenopause include night sweats, mood swings, vaginal dryness, fluctuations in sexual desire (libido), forgetfulness, trouble sleeping, and fatigue (probably from loss of sleep). Estrogen replacement therapy (ERT) or hormone replacement therapy (HRT) may be recommended if the symptoms accompanying perimenopause are difficult. See also *menopause*.

**menopause, chemical**   Menopause induced by chemotherapy or other chemicals or medications. See *menopause, induced*.

**menopause, induced**   Menopause caused by surgical removal of the ovaries, or grave damage to the ovaries by radiation, chemotherapy, or medication. Because of the abrupt cutoff of ovarian hormones, induced menopause causes the sudden onset of hot flashes and other menopause-related symptoms, such as vaginal dryness and a decline in sex drive. Induced menopause before age 40 carries with it a greater risk for heart disease and osteoporosis, since more years are spent beyond the protective cover of estrogen. Estrogen replacement therapy (ERT) may be used to treat symptoms associated with induced menopause, as may hormone replacement therapy (HRT). See also *menopause*.

**menopause, natural** Menopause that occurs when the ovaries naturally decrease their production of the sex hormones estrogen and progesterone. See *menopause*.

**menopause, radiation** See *menopause, induced*.

**menopause, surgical** See *menopause, induced*.

**menorrhagia** Excessive uterine bleeding or menstruation that lasts longer than usual.

**menstrual cramps** Cramping in the lower abdomen, usually in the first or second day of the menstrual cycle. These cramps are caused by contractions of the uterus as it expels its unneeded contents, and also by the passage of clotted blood through the cervix. Ibuprofin or other pain relievers can reduce the severity of cramps; some women report that exercise is also helpful. Severe menstrual cramps, particularly if paired with excessive bleeding or passage of large blood clots, can occasionally be a sign of endometriosis or other disorders of the female reproductive tract. Also known as dysmenorrhea.

**menstrual cycle** The monthly cycle of changes in the ovaries and the lining of the uterus (endometrium), starting with the preparation of an egg for fertilization. When the follicle of the prepared egg in the ovary breaks, it is released for fertilization, and ovulation occurs. Unless pregnancy occurs, the cycle ends with the shedding of part of the endometrium, which is menstruation. Although it is actually the end of the physical cycle, the first day of menstrual bleeding is designated as "day 1" of the menstrual cycle in medical parlance.

**menstrual irregularity** The normal menstrual cycle is about four weeks long, and often follows the phases of the moon. Its length varies from three to seven days, but is usually consistent. However, girls and teenagers who menstruate are usually irregular. This is not a cause for concern unless regular menstruation has been established and is then lost. Some adult women also have irregular cycles. This can be a benign condition, but it can also be due to problems in the uterus or ovaries, including cancer. Adults with menstrual irregularity should see their physician to rule out disease or other problems. In some cases, medication can be used to regulate a chronically irregular cycle.

**menstrual spotting** The presence of apparent menstrual blood during the wrong parts of the menstrual cycle. Some women have a tendency to bleed around

ovulation, which occurs at about the fourteenth day after the first day of menstrual bleeding. In others, spotting can be a sign of internal problems, including fibroid tumors of the uterus. Although spotting is usually benign, its onset is always a reason to see a doctor who can rule out problems.

**menstrual synchronization** A phenomenon that occurs when two or more menstruating women live together, in which the menstrual cycles of the women gradually become synchronized. The mechanism and reason for this effect is unknown, although current research lays it to the effects of female pheromones on other women's ovulation cycles.

**menstruation** The blood that is discharged from the uterus each month if pregnancy does not occur. Also called menorrhea. The time during which menstruation occurs is referred to as the menses. See also *menstrual cycle*.

**menstruation, anovular** Menstruation that occurs without ovulation. Usually the egg that remains in the ovary simply disintegrates, but in some circumstances it is fertilized and a life-threatening ovarian pregnancy results.

**menstruation, cessation of** Menstruation ends naturally in middle age with the onset of the menopause. It can also end suddenly as a result of induced menopause. Cessation of menstruation in nonmenopausal women may be due to pregnancy, illness, disorders of the hypothalamus or pituitary gland, medication, stress, overexercise, or malnutrition, among other causes. In particular, it can be a symptom of anorexia, signalling potentially dangerous changes in the body's hormonal system. Cessation of menstruation in women who have established a regular menstrual cycle, or in girls or teens who show other signs of anorexia, is always a cause for medical concern. Also known as amenorrhea.

**menstruation, retrograde** The flow of menstrual blood from the uterus into the Fallopian tubes, and potentially into the abdomen. This condition can lead to endometriosis.

**mental child injury** See *child abuse, emotional*.

**mental illness** Any disease that affects the central nervous system, causing disturbances of thought or behavior. Mental illnesses can be caused by genetic, metabolic, structural, viral, bacterial, or environmental causes. The term mental illness is also used to describe emotional disturbances caused by traumatic or distressing events, or by poor adjustment to normal life stresses. Treatment depends on the root cause of the illness, and may include medication, surgery (as in the case of brain tumors or some types of epilepsy), and various forms of therapy to help patients rebuild life skills. See also *neurobiological disorders*.

**mental retardation** The condition of having an IQ measured as below 70 to 75, and significant delays or lacks in at least two areas of adaptive skills. Mental retardation is present from childhood. Between 2 and 3 percent of the general population meet these criteria. Causes of mental retardation include fetal alcohol syndrome and fetal alcohol effect; similar brain damage caused by the use of prescription or illegal drugs during pregnancy; brain injury and disease; and genetic disorders, such as Down syndrome and Fragile X syndrome. Most people with mental retardation are mildly affected. These individuals have an IQ over 50, and are usually able to work, care for themselves, and live independently. About 13 percent require more intensive help as adults. Treatment of mental retardation depends on the underlying cause. In some cases, such as phenylketonuria and congenital hypothyroidism, special diets or medical treatments can help. In all cases, special education starting as early in infancy as possible can help people with mental retardation maximize their abilities.

**mephenytoin** An antispasmodic medication (brand name: Mesantoin). See *phenytoin*.

**Mesantoin** See *mephenytoin*. See also *phenytoin*.

**mesentery** A fold of tissue that attaches organs to the body wall. The word mesentery usually refers to the small bowel mesentery, which anchors the small intestines to the back of the abdominal wall. Blood vessels, nerves, and lymphatics branch through the mesentery to supply the intestine. Other mesenteries exist to support the sigmoid colon, appendix, transverse colon, and portions of the ascending and descending colon.

**messenger RNA** A type of RNA that acts as an intermediary between DNA and protein. The DNA of the gene is transcribed into mRNA, which then is translated into the sequence of amino acids that make up a protein.

**metabolic disorders, inherited** See *metabolism, inborn errors of*.

**metabolic rate, basal** A measure of the rate of metabolism. For example, someone with an overly active thyroid will have an elevated basal metabolic rate.

**metabolism** The whole range of biochemical processes that occur within a living organism. Metabolism consists of anabolism (the buildup of substances) and catabolism (the breakdown of substances). The term is commonly used to refer specifically to the breakdown of food and its transformation into energy.

**metabolism, inborn errors of** Genetic disorders of biochemistry, such as albinism, cystinuria, phenylketonuria (PKU), and some forms of gout, sun sensitivity, and thyroid disease. There are hundreds of known inborn errors of metabolism, and there are surely many more yet to be discovered. Advances in the diagnosis and treatment of inborn errors of metabolism have improved the outlook for many of these conditions so that early diagnosis, if possible in infancy, can be helpful. Many inborn errors of metabolism cause infants to have symptoms such as sluggishness (lethargy), poor feeding, apnea (stopping breathing) or tachypnea (fast breathing), and recurrent vomiting. Any infant with these findings, particularly a full-term infant, should be seen immediately by a doctor. Laboratory testing for metabolic disorders is done in children who are possible candidates for inborn errors of metabolism. Testing might include specific blood tests for known conditions, or general tests that indicate a metabolic problem. General indicators include hypoglycemia (low blood sugar), the predominant finding in a number of inborn errors of metabolism, and jaundice (yellowing) or other evidence of liver disease, a sign of another important group of inborn errors of metabolism. Specific patterns of birth defects characterize yet another group of inherited metabolic disorders. The great number, complexity, and varied features of the inborn errors of metabolism would fill a large book if each were considered in any detail. Although most of these disorders are individually rare, together they represent a major source of human disease and suffering.

**metacarpals** Five cylindrical bones that extend from the wrist to the fingers.

**metacentric chromosome** A chromosome with arms of equal length.

**metaphase chromosomes** Chromosomes in the stage of their cell life in which they are most condensed, and easiest to see separately. Because metaphase chromosomes are therefore easier to study than others, they are often chosen for karyotyping and chromosome analysis.

**metastasis** **1** The spread of cancerous cells from one part of the body to another. The cells may be carried by the lymphatic system or in the blood. Cells that have metastasized are still like those in the original (primary) tumor. For example, if the cancer begins in the stomach and spreads to the pancreas, the cancer cells in the pancreas will still be stomach cancer cells. **2** The tumor that is spreading via metastasis. (Plural: metastases.)

**metastasize** What cancer cells do when they spread from one part of the body to another. See also *metastasis*.

**metatarsals**   Five cylindrical bones that extend from the heel to the toes.

**methadone**   A synthetic opiate. The most common medical use for methadone is as a legal substitute for heroin in some treatment programs for drug addiction. It is administered to participating addicts daily at a drug clinic in the form of a green, tasteless liquid.

**methemoglobin**   Hemoglobin in a form incapable of carrying oxygen.

**methimazole**   An antithyroid medication (brand name: Tapazol) prescribed to treat hyperthyroidism. Also known as thiamazole.

**methotrexate**   An anti-inflammatory drug (brand name: Rheumatrex) used to treat rheumatoid arthritis, severe psoriasis, Reiter disease, severe asthma, and in high doses as a part of cancer chemotherapy programs. It is an effective but potentially dangerous medication. People taking methotrexate must have their lung, liver, and kidney function monitored regularly, and need frequent blood testing done as well. Methotrexate interacts dangerously, and potentially fatally, with many other medications, including prescription and over-the-counter nonsteroidal anti-inflammatory drugs (NSAIDs), even aspirin and ibuprofin. Folic acid supplements counteract methotrexate. It should be taken on an empty stomach.

**metorrhagia**   Uterine bleeding at irregular intervals.

**Meuse fever**   See *trench fever*. See also *Bartonella quintana*.

**MHC**   Major histocompatability complex.

**MI**   Myocardial infarction.

**micro-**   Prefix meaning small. For example, microcephaly means a small head. The opposite of micro- is macro-.

**microangiopathy**   Disease of the very small blood vessels (capillaries), in which the capillary walls become so thick and weak that they bleed, leak protein, and slow the flow of blood. For example, diabetics may develop microangiopathy in many areas, including the eye.

**microbe**   A minute organism. Microbes include bacteria, fungi, and protozoan parasites, and are best seen with a microscope.

**microcephaly**   An abnormally small head. Microcephaly is often associated with developmental delay and mental retardation. Not all causes of microcephaly are known, but it is believed to involve a chromosome defect, or an injury to the embryo or fetus caused by infection, radiation, medication, or other factors.

**microcystic corneal dystrophy**   See *Cogan corneal dystrophy*.

**microdeletion**   Loss of a tiny piece from a chromosome; this piece is too small to be seen through a microscope. Microdeletions require high-resolution chromosome banding, molecular chromosome analysis (with FISH), or DNA analysis for detection. Disorders caused by microdeletions include Angelman, DiGeorge, Prader-Willi, and Williams syndromes.

**microhematuria**   Blood in the urine that is visible only under a microscope. There is so little blood that it cannot be seen without magnification. Microhematuria is in contrast to gross hematuria, in which the blood is so plentiful that it is visible to the naked eye. Hematuria in any amount is abnormal and should be further investigated. It may or may not be accompanied by pain. See also *hematuria*.

**microorchidism**   Underdevelopment of the genitalia. Microorchidism is associated with Prader-Willi syndrome and some other genetic disorders.

**micropenis**   An abnormally small penis. In medical practice, the dimension of the penis that is measured is the length. The measurement is taken along the upper surface of the shaft of the penis to the tip, using a measuring tape or preferably a ruler. The ruler is pressed firmly into the soft tissue over the pubic bone (the symphysis pubis) since, in obese boys and men, a seemingly small penis may be partly engulfed by the fat pad at its base and actually be quite normal in length. Normal standards are available for penile length. True micropenis may reflect failure of normal hormonal stimulation or failure of normal development (a birth defect). See also *microorchidism*.

**microphallus**   See *micropenis*. See also *microorchidism*.

**microscope**   An optical instrument that augments the power of the eye to see small objects. Most optical microscopes today are compound microscopes.

**microscope, compound**   A microscope that consists of two microscopes in series, the first serving as the ocular lens (close to the eye), and the second serving as the objective lens (close to the object to be viewed).

**microscope, electron**   A microscope in which an electron beam replaces light to form the image. Electron microscopy (EM) has its pluses (greater magnification and resolution than optical microscopes) and minuses (you are not really "seeing" objects, but rather their electron densities, so artifacts may abound).

**microscope, fluorescent** A microscope equipped to examine material that fluoresces under ultraviolet (UV) light.

**microscope, simple** A microscope that has a single converging lens.

**microscopic** So small it cannot be seen without the aid of a microscope, as opposed to macroscopic, which is large enough to be seen with naked eye.

**microscopic anatomy** See *anatomy, microscopic*.

**microscopic gallstones** See *biliary sludge*.

**microsomia** Too small a body. A child with microsomia has significant undergrowth.

**micturate** To urinate.

**micturition** Urination; the act of urinating.

**micturition syncope** The temporary loss of consciousness upon urinating. See also *syncope, vasovagal reaction*.

**midbrain aqueduct** See *aqueduct of Sylvius*.

**middle ear** See *ear, middle*. See also *ear*.

**middle ear infection, acute** See *ear infection*.

**midwife** A trained person who assists women during childbirth. Many midwives also provide prenatal care for pregnant women, birth education for women and their partners, and care for mothers and newborn babies after the birth. A midwife may be a man or a woman. Depending on local law, midwives may deliver babies in the mother's home, in a special birthing center or clinic, or in a hospital. Most midwives specialize in normal, uncomplicated deliveries, referring women with health problems that could require hospitalization during birth to a hospital-based obstetrician. Others work with physicians as part of a team. Legal qualifications required to practice midwifery differ between the US states and various countries. See also *midwife, certified; midwife, certified nurse; midwife, certified professional; midwife, direct-entry; midwife, traditional*.

**midwife assistant** A person who assists a midwife with prenatal care, childbirth education, delivery, and postnatal care. Also known as a doula or labor assistant.

**midwife, certified** A midwife who has been certified by her state or national agency for credentialing midwives.

**midwife, certified nurse** A person with an AS, BS, or Master's degree in nursing who has also completed specialized training in midwifery. In the US, certified nurse midwives (CNMs) must earn certification from the American College of Nurse Midwives.

**midwife, certified professional** A midwife who has completed a degree in midwifery at a credentialed educational institution. Abbreviated as CPM.

**midwife, direct-entry** A midwife who has entered the profession as an apprentice to a practicing midwife rather than by attending a formal school program.

**midwife, empirical** See *midwife, direct-entry*.

**midwife, lay** See *midwife, direct-entry*.

**midwife, traditional** A direct-entry midwife practicing within the confines of traditional folk medicine. Traditional midwives are now very rare in the US, but preside over the majority of births in many other countries. Most have no formal medical training, but instead learned as an apprentice or through direct experience.

**migraine** Usually, periodic attacks of headaches on one or both sides of the head. These may be accompanied by nausea, vomiting, increased sensitivity of the eyes to light (photophobia), increased sensitivity to sound (phonophobia), dizziness, blurred vision, cognitive disturbances, and other symptoms. Some migraines do not include headache, and migraines may or may not be preceded by an aura. See also *migraine, abdominal; migraine aura; migraine headache; migraine, ocular*.

**migraine aura** Sensory phenomena that may occur before a migraine. Visual auras may include flashing lights, geometric patterns, or distorted vision. Some people may have aural auras that involve hearing sounds (usually buzzing), olfactory auras that involve smelling odors not actually present, or tactile auras that present as a premonitory physical sensation. Auras are caused by unusual activity in the brain. The auras experienced by migraine sufferers are similar to those associated with epilepsy.

**migraine headache** The most common type of vascular headache, migraine headaches are thought to be caused by abnormal sensitivity of arteries in the brain to various triggers, which result in arterial spasms. Other arteries in the brain and scalp then open, and throbbing pain is perceived in the head. The tendency to migraine is inherited, and appears to involve serotonin. This brain chemical (neurotransmitter) is involved in the transmission of nerve impulses that trigger the release of substances in the blood vessels. These nerve impulses cause the flashing lights and other sensory phenomena, known as an aura, that may accompany a migraine. Not all severe headaches are migraines and not all migraines are severe. Factors known to make migraines worse in some patients include stress, food sensitivities, menstruation, and the onset of menopause. Most patients feel better if they lie down and avoid bright lights. Preventive measures can include taking preventative medication (usually an antispasmodic) and avoiding any known migraine triggers. Medication is also available that can ease the pain of a current migraine. See also *headache; headache, vascular.*

**migraine, abdominal** An attack of abdominal pain that may be preceded by a migraine aura and accompanied by nausea, vomiting, and cognitive disturbance.

**migraine, classic** Migraine with aura. Accounts for no more than 20 percent of migraines. See *migraine.*

**migraine, common** Migraine without aura. The most frequent type, accounting for about 80 to 85 percent of migraines. See *migraine.*

**migraine, ocular** Migraine involving the eyes, with or without headache. Ocular migraines usually affect only one eye at a time. Image distortion generally begins in the center of the image and then moves to one side. Images "gray out" or look wavy, and sight may be temporarily lost. See also *migraine, ophthalmic.*

**migraine, ophthalmic** Migraine involving the eyes but without headache. Flashes of light may appear as jagged lines or "heat waves" in one or both eyes, and often last 10 to 20 minutes.

**migrainous neuralgia** See *cluster headache.*

**miliary aneurysm** A tiny aneurysm. Miliary aneurysms tend to affect minute arteries in the brain or in the retina of the eye.

**miliary tuberculosis** The presence of numerous sites of tuberculosis infection, each of which is minute, due to dissemination of infected material through the bloodstream in a process somewhat like the metastatis of a malignancy.

**milzbrand** See *anthrax.*

**mineralocorticoids** A group of hormones that regulate the balance of water and electrolytes (ions such as sodium and potassium) in the body. The mineralocorticoid hormones act on the tubules of the kidney.

The most important mineralocorticoid hormone is aldosterone.

**minor** Something that is less than something else. For example, the teres minor muscle is smaller than the teres major muscle. Minor also enters into the idea of a *locus minoris resistentiae*, Latin for a place of less resistance. A locus minoris resistentiae offers little resistance to microorganisms. A damaged heart valve acts as a locus minoris resistentiae, a place where any bacteria in the bloodstream tend to settle.

**minor salivary gland** A small gland that produces saliva. The mouth and palate contain numerous minor salivary glands.

**minoxidil** A medication (brand name: Loniten, Rogaine) originally developed to treat high blood pressure, minoxidil is now also prescribed in lotion form to promote hair growth. Side effects of the oral form can include increased heart rate, edema, and nausea. Side effects of the lotion are usually restricted to itching or irritation of the scalp.

**miosis** Contraction of the pupil. The opposite of mydriasis.

**miscarriage** Inadvertent loss of a pregnancy before the fetus is viable. A considerable proportion of pregnancies end in miscarriage. Also called spontaneous abortion.

**miscarriages, multiple** When couples have more than one miscarriage, there is about a 5 percent chance that one member of the couple is carrying a chromosome translocation responsible for the miscarriages. Other causes of multiple miscarriage include Rh incompatibility, teratogen exposure that continues over time, and physical problems in the mother that make it difficult to carry a fetus to term.

**missense mutation** A genetic change that results in the substitution of one amino acid in protein for another. A missense mutation is responsible for sickle hemoglobin, the molecular basis of sickle cell trait and sickle cell anemia.

**mite-borne typhus** See *typhus, scrub.*

**mitochondria** Structures located in the cell's cytoplasm outside the nucleus. The mitochondria are responsible for energy production. They consist of two sets of membranes: a smooth, continuous outer coat, and an inner membrane arranged in tubules or in folds that form plate-like double membranes (cristae). The mitochondria are the principal energy source of the cell, thanks to the cytochrome enzymes of terminal electron transport and the enzymes of the citric acid cycle, fatty acid oxidation, and oxidative phosphorylation. They not only convert nutrients into energy, but also perform many other specialized tasks. Each mitochondrion has a chromosome that is made of DNA but is otherwise quite different from the better-known chromosomes in the nucleus. The mitochondrial chromosome is much smaller than other chromosomes. It is round, whereas the chromosomes in the nucleus are shaped like rods. There are many copies of the mitochondrial chromosome in every cell, whereas there is normally only one set of chromosomes in the nucleus. All mitochondrial chromosomes are inherited from the mother.

**mitochondrial**   Referring to mitochondria.

**mitochondrial diseases**   Mutations in the mitochondrial chromosome are responsible for a number of disorders. These include the eye disease Leber hereditary optic atrophy; myoclonus epilepsy with ragged red fibers (MERRF); and mitochondrial encephalopathy, lactic acidosis, and stroke-like episodes (MELAS).

**mitochondrial DNA**   The DNA of the mitochondria. There are 2 to 10 copies of the mtDNA genome in each mitochondrion. The mtDNA molecule is double-stranded and circular. It is very small compared to the chromosomes in the nucleus, and so contains only a limited number of genes. It is specialized in the information it carries, and encodes a number of the subunits in the mitochondrial respiratory-chain complex that the cell needs to respire. It also contains genes for some ribosomal RNAs and transfer RNAs. Mutations in mtDNA can cause disease. These mutations often impair the function of oxidative-phosphorylation enzymes in the respiratory chain. This is especially manifest in tissues with a high energy expenditure, such as those of the brain and muscle. All mtDNA comes from the oocyte at fertilization. Therefore, inherited mtDNA mutations are transmitted from the mother to all offspring, male and female alike. The higher the level of mutant mtDNA in the mother's blood, the higher the frequency of clinically affected offspring, and the more severely the children tend to be affected. Each cell in the body contains different mtDNA populations. Due to the presence of multiple mitochondria in cells, each cell contains several mtDNA copies. This produces tissue variation, so a mutation in mtDNA versus normal mtDNA can vary widely among tissues in an individual. Accordingly, the percentage of mutant mtDNA must be above a certain threshold to produce clinical disease. The threshold varies from tissue to tissue, because the percent of mutant mDNAs needed to cause cell dysfunction varies according to the oxidative requirements of the tissue. Abbreviated as mtDNA.

**mitochondrial encephalopathy, MELAS**   See *MELAS syndrome*.

**mitochondrial genome**   All of the DNA in the mitochondrial chromosome.

**mitochondrial inheritance**   See *inheritance, mitochondrial*.

**mitochondrial myopathy**   A form of muscle disease that leads to progressive muscle weakness. More than 25 types of enzyme abnormalities have been defined that fall into this category. They result in a disease of cell metabolism, and are defined by a biopsy of muscle tissue that shows ragged red fibers under microscopic examination.

**mitochondrion**   Singular of mitochondria.

**mitosis**   Ordinary division of a body cell to form two daughter cells, each with the same chromosome complement as the parent cell.

**mitotic**   Pertaining to mitosis.

**mitotic nondisjunction**   Failure of the two members of a chromosome pair to separate during mitosis, causing both to go to one daughter cell while none go to the other daughter cell.

**mitral insufficiency**   Malfunction of the mitral valve. Mitral insufficiency allows the backflow of blood (regurgitation) from the left ventricle into the left atrium.

**mitral prolapse**   See *mitral valve prolapse*.

**mitral regurgitation**   Backflow of blood from the left ventricle to the left atrium due to mitral valve insufficiency.

**mitral valve**   One of the four valves of the heart, the mitral valve is situated between the left atrium and the left ventricle. It permits blood to flow from the left atrium into the left ventricle. The mitral valve has two flaps (cusps). Also known as the bicuspid valve.

**mitral valve prolapse**   Drooping down or abnormal bulging of the mitral valve's cusps during the contraction of the heart.

**mittelschmerz**   Pain between the menstrual periods.

**mixed mania**   A state of mind characterized by symptoms of both mania and depression, mixed mania is seen in bipolar disorders. It is more common in bipolar children and women than in men. A person experiencing mixed mania may feel agitated, angry, irritable, and depressed all at once. Because it combines a high activity level with depression, mixed mania poses a particular danger of suicide or self-injury. Treatment is by mood-stabilizing medication, sometimes accompanied by antidepressant or neuroleptic medication. Also known as agitated depression. See also *bipolar disorders, depression, mania.*

**ML I**   See *sialidosis.*

**ML II**   See *I-cell disease.*

**ML III**   See *pseudo-Hurler polydystrophy.*

**ML IV**   A rare genetic storage disorder seen primarily in children of Ashkenazi Jewish descent. Most patients have some degree of mental retardation and motor delays, and develop clouded eyes that may appear to be crossed. Diagnosis is by observation, and can be confirmed by culturing cells. There is currently no treatment for ML IV, but speech, occupational, and physical therapy are useful as supportive measures.

**MM**   Meningomyelocele.

**MMR**   Measles, mumps, rubella vaccine.

**modifiers, biological response**   See *biological response modifiers.*

**Mohs surgery**   A special type of surgery for skin cancer. Its purpose is to remove all of the cancerous tissue while taking as little healthy tissue as possible. It is especially helpful when the doctor is not sure of the shape and depth of the tumor. In addition, this method is used to remove large tumors, those in hard-to-treat places, and cancers that have recurred. The patient is given a local anesthetic, and the cancer is shaved off, one thin layer at a time. Each layer is checked under a microscope until the entire tumor has been removed. The degree of scarring depends on the location and size of the treated area. This method should be used only by doctors who are specially trained in Mohs surgery. Also known as Mohs technique.

**molar**   **1** One of the large teeth at the back of the mouth. The molars are well adapted to grinding. **2** Relating to or associated with a mass within the uterus formed by degeneration of partly developed products of conception.

**mold**   A large group of fungi that can proliferate on food or in moist areas. Household mold is a common trigger for allergies.

**mole**   **1** A pigmented spot on the skin. Also known as a nevus. **2** A mass within the uterus formed by partly developed products of conception.

**molecule**   The smallest unit of a substance that can exist alone and retain the character of that substance.

**molecules, recombinant DNA**   A combination of DNA molecules of different origin that are joined by using recombinant DNA technology.

**mongolism**   See *Down syndrome.*

**monilia**   A yeast-like fungus, now known as Candida.

**monitor, Holter**   See *Holter monitor.*

**mono**   Abbreviation for infectious mononucleosis. See *mononucleosis.*

**monoarticular**   Involving just one joint, as opposed to polyarticular, affecting many joints.

**monochromat**   A person with one of the many forms of colorblindness. See also *colorblindness.*

**monochromatism**   **1** Total inability to perceive color due to the lack of or damage to the cones of the eye that perceive color, or the inability of the nerves to translate information received from the cones. A person with true monochromatism perceives only black, white, and shades of gray. Complete monochromatism is usually an inherited condition. **2** One of the many types of colorblindness that affects perception of certain colors only. See *colorblindness.*

**monoclonal**   Derived from a single cell and cells identical to that cell.

**monoclonal antibodies**   Identical antibodies that are made in large amounts in the laboratory. Doctors are studying ways of using monoclonal antibodies to treat leukemia.

**monocyte**   A white blood cell that has a single nucleus and can take in (ingest) foreign material.

**mononeuritis**   Inflammation of a single nerve. The many causes of mononeuritis include diabetes mellitus, carpal tunnel syndrome, rheumatoid arthritis, and Lyme disease. The treatment of mononeuritis depends on the underlying cause. See also *mononeuritis multiplex.*

**mononeuritis multiplex**   Inflammation of two or more nerves, typically in unrelated parts of the body. Mononeuritis multiplex causes a loss of function in the muscle tissue that is innervated by the affected nerves. For example, sudden loss of the ability to lift the foot up normally while walking (foot drop) can be caused by mononeuritis multiplex, when it is accompanied by loss of nerve function elsewhere in the body. There are many causes of mononeuritis multiplex, including diabetes mellitus; infections, such as AIDS, Lyme disease, and leprosy; sarcoidosis; and connective tissue diseases, such as rheumatoid arthritis, systemic lupus erythematosus, vasculitis, Churg-Strauss syndrome, cryoglobulinemia, and Sjogren syndrome. The treatment of mononeuritis multiplex depends on the underlying cause.

**mononucleosis**   Chronic infection with the Epstein-Barr virus (EBV, human herpesvirus 4, HHV-4) in which there is an increase of white blood cells that have a single nucleus (monocytes). The infection can be spread by saliva. Its incubation period is four to eight weeks. Symptoms include fever, fatigue, sore throat, and swollen lymph glands. Mononucleosis can cause liver inflammation (hepatitis) and spleen enlargement; vigorous contact sports should be avoided to prevent spleen rupture. It is less severe in young children. Most people exposed to EBV do not develop mononucleosis; most adults carry an antibody against EBV in their blood, which means they have been infected with EBV at some time. Treatment includes rest, pain medication, and in some cases antiviral medication. Also known as mono, the kissing disease. See also *Epstein-Barr virus*.

**monosomy**   Missing one chromosome from a pair. For example, if a female has one X chromosome (X monosomy) rather than two, Turner syndrome is the result.

**monozygous twins**   Identical twins. They are called monozygous because they originate from a single fertilized egg (zygote).

**morbidity**   Illness, disease.

**morbilli**   See *measles*.

**morgue**   A place where bodies of the dead are kept before autopsy, funeral, or burial.

**morning sickness**   The common phenomenon of nausea between the sixth and twelfth weeks of pregnancy. Symptoms include nausea and vomiting. Morning sickness is believed to be caused by hormonal changes and metabolic changes involving carbohydrate digestion. Suggested treatment includes eating crackers or other high-carbohydrate foods first thing in the morning (even before getting out of bed); eating small, frequent meals; drinking extra fluids between meals; and avoiding fatty foods. If morning sickness is extreme enough to lead to weight loss during pregnancy, the condition is termed hyperemesis gravidarum, and requires immediate medical treatment. See also *hyperemesis gravidarum*.

**morning-after pill**   See *contraceptive, emergency*.

**morphology**   Literally, the study of form (structure). It is also the form itself.

**Morquio syndrome**   A form of mucopolysaccharidosis characterized by an inability to break down keratin sulfate, leading to abnormal accumulation of keratin sulfate in muscle and skeletal tissues. This can lead to abnormalities of the skeleton, muscles, skin, teeth, and muscular organs. Diagnosis is by examining leukocytes and cultured skin fibroblasts, or by checking urine for high levels of keratin sulfate. There is currently no treatment for Morquio syndrome, but physical therapy, medication, and sometimes surgery can reduce discomfort and enhance the patient's ability to move. The disorder is inherited in an autosomal recessive manner. Also known as mucopolysaccharidosis IV (MPS IV). See also *mucopolysaccharidosis*.

**mortality rate, fetal**   See *fetal mortality rate*.

**mortality rate, infant**   See *infant mortality rate*.

**mortality rate, maternal**   See *maternal mortality rate*.

**mortality rate, neonatal**   See *neonatal mortality rate*.

**mosaic**   An individual or tissue containing two or more types of genetically different cells. All females are mosaics because of X-chromosome inactivation (lyonization). Mosaic patterns can affect the way genetic disorders are expressed. For example, about 5 percent of people with Down syndrome have a mosaic variant, where only some cells have an extra chromosome 21. These individuals have fewer clinical symptoms, are more likely to have a normal IQ, and are less likely to have heart and other problems that can be associated with Down syndrome.

**motility study, antro-duodenal**   A study for detecting and recording the contractions of the muscles of the stomach and the first part of the small intestine (the duodenum). It is performed to diagnose problems in the way the muscles of the stomach and small intestine are working. An antro-duodenal motility study requires the passage of a tube through the nose, throat, esophagus, and stomach until the tip of the tube lies in the small intestine. The tube senses when the muscles of the stomach and small intestine contract and squeeze the tube tightly. The contractions are recorded for analysis by a computer.

**motion, range of**   See *range of motion*.

**motor**   Something that produces or refers to motion. For example, a motor neuron is a nerve cell that conveys an impulse to a muscle for contraction, which then moves a joint.

**mountain sickness**   See *altitude sickness*. See also *acclimatization to altitude, acute mountain sickness*.

**mouth, trench**   See *acute membranous gingivitis*.

**movement, fetal**   See *fetal movement*.

**MPH**   Master of Public Health.

**MPS**   **1** Mucopolysaccharidosis. **2** Myofascial pain syndrome.

**MPS1**   Mucopolysaccharidosis Type I. See *Hurler syndrome*.

**MPS2**   Mucopolysaccharidosis Type II. See *Hunter syndrome*.

**MPS3**   Mucopolysaccharidosis Type III. See *Sanfilippo syndrome*.

**MPS4**   Mucopolysaccharidosis Type IV. See *Morquios syndrome*.

**MRC**   **1** Medical Reserve Corps. **2** In the UK and some Commonwealth countries, the Medical Research Council.

**MRI**   Magnetic resonance imaging.

**mRNA**   Messenger RNA.

**MS**   Multiple sclerosis.

**MSAFP**   Maternal serum alpha-fetoprotein.

**mtDNA**   Mitochondrial DNA.

**mucocutaneous lymph node syndrome**   See *Kawasaki disease*.

**mucolipidosis**   Mucopolysaccharidosis-like inherited storage disorders. At least four have been definitively identified so far: neuramidase deficiency/sialidosis (ML I), I-cell disease (ML II), pseudo-Hurler polydystrophy (ML III), and ML IV. Abbreviated as ML. See also *mucopolysaccharidosis*.

**mucopolysaccharidosis**   One of several inherited metabolic disorders affecting carbohydrate use by the body. Substances derived from carbohydrates, called mucopolysacchardes or glycosaminoglycans (GAGs), accumulate in body tissues because the body lacks specific enzymes needed to metabolize or digest them. This accumulation damages and distorts tissues, stunts growth, limits muscle and joint movement, and may cause mental retardation. MPS is believed to occur in about 1 in every 25,000 births. It usually becomes obvious in early childhood, and leads to death before middle age. There are currently no treatments available for any form of MPS, although enzyme replacement therapies are being researched and bone-marrow transplants have been tried on patients with MPS I (Hurler syndrome) with some limited success. Abbreviated as MPS. See also *Hunter syndrome, Hurler syndrome, Maroteaux-Lamy syndrome, Morquio syndrome, Sanfilippo syndrome*.

**mucopolysaccharidosis Type I**   Hurler syndrome or Scheie syndrome. See *Hurler syndrome*.

**mucopolysaccharidosis Type II**   See *Hunter syndrome*.

**mucopolysaccharidosis Type III**   See *Sanfilippo syndrome*.

**mucopolysaccharidosis Type IV**   See *Morquio syndrome*.

**mucopolysaccharidosis Type V**   A designation no longer used to describe a form of MPS.

**mucopolysaccharidosis Type VI**   See *Maroteaux-Lamy syndrome*.

**mucopolysaccharidosis Type VII**   A designation no longer used to describe a form of MPS.

**mucopolysaccharidosis Type VIII**   See *Sly syndrome*.

**mucopolysaccharidosis Type IX**   See *Di Ferrante syndrome*.

**mucosa**   Having to do with a mucous membrane. For example, the oral mucosa.

**mucoviscidosis**   See *cystic fibrosis*.

**mucus**   A thick fluid produced by the lining of some organs of the body.

**multifactorial**   Referring to multiple factors in heredity or disease. Traits and conditions caused by more than one gene occuring together are multifactorial. Diseases caused by more than one factor interacting (for example, heredity and diet in diabetes) are multifactorial.

**multifactorial inheritance**   An hereditary pattern seen when more than one genetic factor is involved and, sometimes, the addition of environmental influence to multiple genetic differences. Many common traits and many common diseases are multifactorial. Skin color, for example, is multifactorially determined, as is intelligence.

**multi-infarct dementia**   Dementia brought on by a series of strokes.

**multipara**   A woman who has had two or more pregnancies resulting in potentially viable offspring. A para III has had three such pregnancies; a para VI or more is also known as a grand multipara.

**multiparous 1** Having two or more offspring at one birth. **2** Related to a multipara. See also *uniparous*.

**multiple myeloma** A malignancy of plasma cells (a form of lymphocyte) that typically involves multiple sites within the bone marrow and secretes all or part of a monoclonal antibody. Also called plasma cell myeloma.

**multiple personality disorder** See *dissociative disorder*.

**multiple sclerosis** A disease characterized by loss of myelin (demyelinization). Myelin, the coating of nerve fibers, is composed of lipids (fats) and protein. It serves as insulation, and permits efficient nerve fiber conduction. In MS, demyelinization usually affects white matter in the brain, but sometimes extends into the gray matter. When myelin is damaged, nerve fiber conduction is faulty or absent, and nerve cell death may occur. Impaired bodily functions or altered sensations associated with those demyelinated nerve fibers give rise to the symptoms of MS, which range from numbness to paralysis and blindness. People with MS experience "attacks" of symptoms that may last days, months, or longer. For many patients, the disease is progressive and leads to disablement, although some cases enter long, perhaps even permanent, remission. The cause of MS is unknown, although viral activity is suspected. Most patients are diagnosed between the ages of 20 and 40. Until recently, treatment had focused on preventing attacks. Steroids, interferon, and medications to treat specific symptoms (such as fatigue, depression, and vertigo) are standard, along with lifestyle changes to avoid stress and other triggers. New treatment options are under development, most of which involve immune system modulation or support. Some patients also use antiviral medications.

**multiple symmetric lipomatosis** See *cephalothoracic lipodystrophy*.

**mumps** An acute viral illness caused by the paramyxovirus, mumps usually presents with inflammation of the salivary glands, particularly the parotid glands. A child with mumps often looks like a chipmunk with a full mouth due to the swelling of the salivary glands near the ears. Mumps can also cause inflammation of other tissues, most frequently the covering and substance of the central nervous system (meningoencephalitis), next to the pancreas (pancreatitis) and, especially after adolescence, the ovaries (oophoritis) or the testes (orchitis). The mature testes are particularly susceptible to damage from mumps, which can lead to infertility. Mumps spreads easily through airborne particles of human saliva. Treatment is with rest and nonaspirin pain relievers to ease pain in swollen areas. Rarely, mumps can cause a form of meningitis, in which case hospitalization may be necessary. Prevention is by vaccine. See also *meningitis, MMR*.

**mumps immunization** A vaccination for mumps, which may be given individually or with the measles and rubella vaccines in the MMR immunization. See also *MMR*.

**mumps in pregnancy** Mumps vaccination is not recommended during or shortly before pregnancy because it is a live attenuated vaccine, and so carries a risk of causing mumps infection. When contracted in pregnancy, mumps can cause early miscarriage or birth defects. The most common birth defect associated with mumps is congenital deafness.

**Munchhausen by proxy** A form of Munchhausen syndrome in which a parent feigns illness in a child. In some cases the parent is simply overanxious or poorly informed. In others, a misdirected desire for attention or psychiatric illness is the cause. In a very few cases, the parent actually causes the child's illness, as by injecting toxic substances. See also *Munchhausen syndrome*.

**Munchhausen syndrome** Recurrent feigning of catastrophic illnesses. Some patients with Munchhausen syndrome actually cause their own illness, as by secretly drinking or injecting substances. Munchhausen syndrome may be caused by a misdirected desire for attention, although in some cases it arises in actual psychiatric illness. It is named for the fictitious Baron Munchhausen, who told tall tales. See also *body dysmorphic disorder, hypochondria, Munchhausen by proxy*.

**murine typhus** See *typhus, murine*.

**murmur, heart** See *heart murmur*.

**muscle** The tissue of the body that functions primarily as a source of power. There are three types of muscle in the body. Muscle that is responsible for moving extremities and external areas of the body is called skeletal muscle, heart muscle is called cardiac muscle, and muscle in the walls of arteries and the bowel is called smooth muscle. See also *cardiac muscle, skeletal muscle, smooth muscle*.

**muscle, abductor** Any muscle that pushes away from the midline of the body. For example, the abductor muscles of the arms allow them to be raised from one's sides. Abductor muscles are opposed by adductor muscles. To keep these similar-sounding terms straight, medical students learn to speak of "A B ductors" versus "A D ductors."

**muscle, adductor** Any muscle that pulls inward toward the midline of the body. For example, the adductor muscles of the leg serve to pull the legs together.

Adductor muscles are opposed by abductor muscles. To keep these similar-sounding terms straight, medical students learn to speak of "A B ductors" versus "A D ductors."

**muscle, central core disease of**   See *central core disease of muscle*.

**muscle, infraspinatus**   A muscle that assists the lifting of the arm while turning the arm outward (external rotation). The tendon of the infraspinatus muscle is one of four tendons that stabilize the shoulder joint and constitute the rotator cuff.

**muscle, papillary**   Small muscles within the heart that anchor the heart valves. The anchor ropes are the chordae tendineae, thread-like bands of fibrous tissue that attach on one end to the edges of the tricuspid and mitral valves of the heart, and on the other end to the papillary muscles.

**muscle, piriformis**   A muscle that begins at the front surface of the sacrum (the V-shaped bone between the buttocks at the base of the spine) and passes through the greater sciatic notch to attach to the top of the thigh bone (femur) at its bony prominence (the greater trochanter). The gluteus maximus muscle covers the piriformis muscle in the buttocks.

**muscle, subscapularis**   A muscle that moves the arm by turning it inward (internal rotation). The tendon of the subscapularis muscle is one of four tendons that stabilize the shoulder joint and constitute the rotator cuff.

**muscle, supraspinatus**   A muscle responsible for elevating the arm and moving it away from the body. The tendon of the supraspinatus muscle is one of four tendons that stabilize the shoulder joint and constitute the rotator cuff.

**muscle, teres minor**   A muscle that assists in the lifting of the arm during outward turning (external rotation) of the arm. The tendon of the teres minor muscle is one of four tendons that stabilize the shoulder joint and constitute the rotator cuff.

**muscles, abdominal**   A large group of muscles in the front of the abdomen that assist in breathing movements, support the muscles of the spine during lifting, and keep abdominal organs in place. Colloquially known as the abs.

**muscular**   Having to do with the muscles. Also, endowed with above-average muscle development. "Muscular system" refers to all the muscles of the body, collectively.

**muscular atrophy, post-polio**   Late muscle-wasting that occurs as part of the post-polio syndrome (PPS).

**muscular dystrophy**   One of several conditions that affect the muscles and nerves, causing muscle weakness and movement difficulties. All are caused by a genetic defect, and in some cases the gene has been identified. Many treatments are available to overcome specific problems associated with these conditions. Physical therapy, occupational therapy, assistive technology, and in some cases surgery can all help patients improve and retain physical abilities. There is no cure yet for any form of muscular dystrophy, but experimental gene therapy is currently being investigated. Abbreviated as MD.

**muscular dystrophy, Becker**   A form of muscular dystrophy that is similar to Duchenne MD, except that patients do produce some dystrophin. Progression is slower, and symptoms may appear as late as the mid-twenties. See also *muscular dystrophy, Duchenne*.

**muscular dystrophy, congenital**   A form of muscular dystrophy that is present at birth. Various types of congenital MD have been identified, each caused by a different genetic error. Congenital MD can affect males or females. Diagnosis is initially by observation of general muscle weakness (hypotonia). See also *muscular dystrophy, myotonic*.

**muscular dystrophy, distal**   One of several rare genetic muscle diseases characterized by wasting of those muscles farthest from the midline, such as the hands and feet. Distal MD begins in adulthood, and can affect males or females.

**muscular dystrophy, Duchenne**   A form of muscular dystrophy that affects males only, with symptoms appearing between the ages of two and six. The disease is caused by a genetic error that prevents the body from producing dystrophin, a protein that normally occurs in muscle tissues. Duchenne MD begins in the pelvis and upper limbs, and is characterized by clumsiness, frequent falling, an unusual gait, and general weakness. Some patients have mild mental retardation. As the disease progresses, a wheelchair may be necessary. Most patients with Duchenne MD die in their early twenties because of muscle-based breathing and heart problems.

**muscular dystrophy, Emory-Dreifuss**   A rare form of muscular dystrophy that begins in childhood or the teen years. It is a slowly progressing disorder that begins in the upper arms or upper legs. Contractures of the limbs are common in Emory-Dreifuss MD, as are serious heart problems. It is caused by a defect on the X chromosome. Although only males have the muscle problems associated with Emory-Dreifuss MD, females may have the heart problems. Accordingly, female relatives of males with this disorder should have regular heart checkups.

**muscular dystrophy, facioscapulohumeral**  A form of muscular dystrophy that begins in the muscles of the face or shoulders. Onset is in the teen years or early adulthood. Severity can range from mild to disabling, although most people with FSH retain the ability to walk, especially if they receive adequate physical therapy. However, some do experience significant problems with eating and speaking. Abbreviated as FSH.

**muscular dystrophy, limb-girdle**  A form of muscular dystrophy that begins in the patient's teens or twenties, starting with progressive weakness in the hips or shoulders. A wheelchair is usually necessary within 20 years. Limb-girdle MD can be caused by any of several genetic defects, and can affect both males and females.

**muscular dystrophy, myotonic**  A slowly progressing form of muscular dystrophy that is characterized by muscle spasms after movements. It can be congenital, or may begin any time from early childhood to adulthood. It usually becomes evident first in the face, hands, or feet. It has systemic effects, causing problems in the heart, GI tract, eyes, and hormones. Some patients have mental retardation and may be very passive. The disease is caused by an error on chromosome 19, and occurs in both males and females.

**muscular dystrophy, oculopharyngeal**  A form of muscular dystrophy that begins in the muscles of the eyes and throat. It usually appears between the ages of 40 and 60, and progresses slowly. It is caused by an error on chromosome 14, and occurs in both males and females.

**Musculoskeletal and Skin Diseases, National Institute of Arthritis and**  See *National Institutes of Health*.

**mutagen**  Something capable of causing a gene-change. Among the known mutagens are radiation, certain chemicals, and some viruses.

**mutant**  An individual with a mutant (changed) gene.

**mutation**  A change in a gene. Mutations can be caused by many factors, including random chance and environmental insult. See also *missense mutation, point mutation*.

**mute**  **1** A person who does not speak, either because of an inability to speak or an unwillingness to speak. The term is specifically applied to a person who, due to profound congenital or early deafness, is unable to use articulate language and so is deaf-mute. **2** The condition of not speaking. See also *apraxia of speech, autism, elective mutism, selective mutism*. **3** In speech, a letter that is silent, or an element of speech formed by a position of the mouth that stops the passage of the breath, such as the letters p, b, d, k, and t.

**mutism**  The inability or unwillingness to speak. See also *apraxia of speech, autism, elective mutism, selective mutism*.

**mutism, akinetic**  A state in which a person is unable to speak (mute) or move (akinetic). Akinetic mutism is often due to damage to the frontal lobes of the brain.

**myalgia**  Pain in the muscles or within muscle tissue.

**myalgia, epidemic**  See *Bornholm disease*.

**myasthenia gravis**  An autoimmune neuromuscular disorder characterized by fatigue and exhaustion of muscles. It is caused by a mistaken immune response to the body's own nicotinic acetylcholine receptors, which are found in junctions between muscles and the nervous system. The body produces antibodies that attack these receptors, preventing signals from reaching the muscles. There is currently no cure for myasthenia gravis, but today only about 10 percent of patients with MG die. A number of treatments are available that help, including steroids and other immunosuppressive medications and cholinergic medications.

**mycobacterium avium complex**  A serious opportunistic infection caused by two similar bacteria, Mycobacterium avium and Mycobacterium intercellulare, which are found in the soil and in dust particles. In persons with suppressed immune systems, such as people with AIDS, mycobacterium avium complex can spread through the bloodstream to infect lymph nodes, bone marrow, liver, spleen, spinal fluid, the lungs, and the intestinal tract. Typical symptoms of MAC include night sweats, weight loss, fever, fatigue, diarrhea, and enlarged spleen. MAC is usually found in people with CD4 counts below 100. Clarithromycin, azithromycin, ethambutal, rifampin, clofazimine, and rifabutin are some of the antibiotics commonly used in MAC prevention and treatment.

**mycoplasma**  A large group of bacteria, with more than 70 types identified. Mycoplasma are very simple one-celled organisms without an outer membrane. They penetrate and infect individual cells. Mycoplasma hominis and mycoplasma pneumoniae are among the dozen mycoplasmas that occur in humans.

**mycoplasma hominis**  A common inhabitant of the vagina that can cause infections of the female and male genital tracts. Treatment is by antibiotics, including tetracycline and erythromycin.

**mycoplasma pneumoniae**  A mycoplasma that can infect the upper respiratory tract and the lungs. It is a major cause of respiratory infection in children of school age and young adults. It is also a common cause of pneumonia in persons with HIV. Treatment is by antibiotics, including tetracycline and erythromycin.

**mycosis fungoides**  A type of non-Hodgkin lymphoma that first appears on the skin. Also called cutaneous T-cell lymphoma.

**mydriasis**  Dilation of the pupils induced by eye drops. The opposite of miosis.

**myelin**  The fatty substance that covers and protects nerves. Myelin is a layered tissue surrounding the axons, or nerve fibers. This sheath around the nerve fibers acts like a conduit in an electrical system, ensuring that messages sent by nerve fibers are not lost en route.

**myelitis**  Inflammation of the spinal cord.

**myelodysplastic syndrome**  See *leukemia, smoldering*.

**myeloencephalitis**  See *encephalomyelitis*.

**myelofibrosis**  Spontaneous scarring (fibrosis) of the bone marrow. Myelofibrosis can be associated with a variety of diseases, primarily myeloproliferative (preleukemic) disorders. Also known as agnogenic myeloid metaplasia.

**myelofibrosis, acute**  A distinct disorder characterized by acute inadequate blood-cell production (pancytopenia) and marrow fibrosis, but no enlargement of the spleen or liver.

**myelogenous**  See *myeloid*.

**myelogram**  An X-ray of the spinal cord and the bones of the spine.

**myeloid**  Referring to myelocytes, a type of white blood cells. Also called myelogenous.

**myeloma**  A tumor of cells that are normally found in the bone marrow.

**myeloproliferative disorders**  Malignant diseases of certain bone-marrow cells, including those that give rise to the red blood cells, the granulocytes, and the blood platelets. The myeloproliferative disorders include myelophthisic anemia, erythroblastic leukemia, leukemoid reaction, myelofibrosis, myeloid metaplasia, polycythemia vera, and thrombocytosis.

**myocardial infarction, acute**  A heart attack. In a myocardial infarction, the heart muscle (myocardium) experiences sudden deprivation of circulating blood, which results in death (necrosis) of myocardial tissue and other changes. The interruption of blood is usually caused by arteriosclerosis with narrowing of the coronary arteries, the culminating event being a thrombosis (clot).

**myocarditis**  Inflammation of the heart muscle.

**myocardium**  The heart muscle.

**myoclonic twitch**  A rapid, involuntary muscle contraction, particularly near the eye. Myoclonic tics resemble, and may be mistaken for, tics. Like tics, they tend to occur more often when the person is under stress; unlike tics, they are not preceded by any sensation and they cannot be delayed.

**myoclonus**  Shock-like contraction of muscle. See also *myoclonic twitch*.

**myofascial pain syndrome**  A condition characterized by chronic pain in the muscle tissues, similar to fibromyalgia. MPS is sometimes the aftermath of injury. Pain medication, anti-inflammatory medication, and therapies aimed at relaxing the muscle tissues (such as massage, chiropractic, and some forms of acupuncture) have been reported as beneficial. Abbreviated as MPS. See also *fibromyalgia*.

**myoglobin**  The pigment in muscle that carries oxygen.

**myoma**  A tumor of muscle. Can refer specifically to a benign tumor of uterine muscle, also called a leiomyoma or a fibroid.

**myometrium**  The muscular outer layer of the uterus.

**myopathy**  Any and all disease of muscle.

**myopathy, mitochondrial**  See *MELAS syndrome*.

**myopia**  Nearsightedness. Myopia can be caused by either a longer-than-normal eyeball, or a condition that prevents light rays from focusing on the retina. Most forms of myopia can be managed with corrective lenses. Surgery is available to permanently correct some forms of myopia, although long-term effectiveness and safety have not been determined.

**myotonic dystrophy**  Inherited disease characterized by irritability and prolonged contraction of muscles (myotonia), mask-like face, premature balding, cataracts, and cardiac disease. It is due to a trinucleotide repeat (a stuttering sequence of three bases) in the DNA.

**myringotomy**  A tiny surgical incision in the eardrum. Any fluid behind the eardrum can then drain, and usually thickened secretions can be removed. A small plastic ear tube is often inserted into the eardrum to keep the middle ear aerated for a prolonged period of time. These ventilating tubes usually remain in place for six months to several years. Eventually, they move out of the eardrum (extrude) and fall into the ear canal.

**myxedema, infantile**  See *hypothyroidism, infantile.*

# Nn

**Na** The chemical symbol for sodium. Sodium chloride (table salt) is NaCl.

**nail** 1 A metal nail used to hold two or more pieces of bone together, for example, after a fracture. 2 The horny plate on the end of the finger (fingernail) or toe (toenail). Each nail has a body, lateral nail folds on its sides, a lunula (the little moon-shaped feature at the base), and a proximal skin fold at its base. See also *fingernail, nail care, toenail*.

**nail care** Many nail problems are due to poor nail care. Recommendations for maintaining nail health include keeping nails clean and dry to keep bacteria and other infectious organisms from collecting under the nails, cutting nails straight across with only slight rounding at the tip, using a fine-textured file to keep nails shaped and free of snags, and avoiding nail-biting. Soak toenails that are thick and difficult to cut in warm salt water (one tsp. salt to one pint of water) for 5 to 10 minutes, and apply a 10 percent urea cream (available at the drugstore without a prescription) before trimming. Do not "dig out" ingrown toenails, especially if they are sore. Instead, seek treatment from a doctor. Nail changes, swelling, and pain can signal a serious problem. Report any nail irregularities to a doctor.

**nail fungus** See *dermatophytic onychomycosis*.

**nail-patella syndrome** See *Fong disease*.

**nails, jogger's** See *nails, white spots on the*.

**nails, ringworm of the** See *dermatophytic onychomycosis*.

**nails, white spots on the** Small, semicircular white spots on the nails are caused by injury to the base (matrix) of the nail, where the nail cells and nail are produced. The injury responsible for white spots on the nails can be due to athletic activity and poorly fitting shoes. For example, jogging in poorly fitting shoes causes this condition so often that it is known as "jogger's nails." These spots are not a cause for concern. They eventually grow out.

**named reporting** In public health, the reporting of infected persons by name to public health departments. This is standard practice for the surveillance of many infectious diseases, such as syphilis, gonorrhea, and tuberculosis, that pose a public health threat. The opposite of named reporting is anonymous testing and reporting, in which the individuals involved remain nameless.

**nares** The nostrils.

**NARP** Acronym for neuropathy, ataxia, and retinitis pigmentosa. A mitochondrial disease, caused by a mutation in mitochondrial DNA, NARP features weakness of the muscles near the trunk of the body, ataxia (wobbliness), retinal disease, seizures, and developmental delay. See also *ataxia, mitochondria, mitochondrial diseases*.

**nasal** Having to do with the nose.

**nasal decongestants** Drugs that shrink the swollen membranes in the nose, making it easier for the patient to breath. Decongestants can be taken orally or by nasal spray. Decongestant nasal spray should not be used for more than five days without the doctor's consent, and then usually only when accompanied by a nasal steroid. When decongestant nasal sprays are used for a long time and then discontinued, symptoms often worsen (a rebound effect) because the tissues become dependent on the medication.

**nasal passages** The walls of the nasal passages are coated with respiratory mucous membranes, which contain innumerable tiny hair-like cells. These act to move waves of mucus toward the throat. Dust, bacteria, and other particles inhaled from the air are trapped by the mucus in the nose, carried back, swallowed, and dropped into the gastric juices to nullify any potential harm they might do. The organs of smell are made up of patches of tissue called olfactory membranes. These are about the size of a postage stamp, and are located in a pair of clefts just under the bridge of the nose. Most air breathed in normally flows through the nose, but only a small part reaches the olfactory clefts to get a response to an odor. When a person sniffs to detect a smell, air moves faster through the nose, increasing the flow to the olfactory clefts and carrying more odor to these sensory organs.

**nasal septum** The dividing wall that runs down the middle of the nose, so that the nose normally has two sides, each of which ends in a nostril.

**nasal septum, deviated** A condition in which the dividing wall between the two nasal passages has been eroded away, causing communication between the passages. A deviated septum can be caused by a number of things, including repeated inhalation of cocaine and other harmful drugs. It can usually be repaired with surgery.

**naso-** Prefix referring to the nose. For example, nasogastric refers to the passage from the nose to the stomach.

**nasogastric** A term referring to the passage from the nose to the stomach.

**nasogastric tube** A tube that is passed through the nose, and down through the nasopharynx and esophagus into the stomach. It is a flexible tube made of rubber or plastic, and has bidirectional potential. It can be used to remove the contents of the stomach, including air, to decompress the stomach; or to remove small solid objects and fluid, such as poison, from the stomach. A nasogastric tube can also be used to put substances into the stomach, and so may be used to place nutrients directly into the stomach when a patient cannot eat by mouth.

**nasopharynx** The area of the upper throat behind the nose.

**national board exams** The United States Medical Licensing Examination (USMLE), an exam sponsored by the Federation of State Medical Boards (FSMB) of the United States and the National Board of Medical Examiners (NBME). It has replaced the examinations previously used to fulfill examination requirements for medical licensure: the Federation Licensing Examination (FLEX) and the certifying examinations of the NBME, Parts I, II, and III. The USMLE provides a common evaluation system for all applicants for medical licensure. Results of the USMLE are reported to medical licensing authorities in the US for use in granting licenses to practice medicine.

**National Institutes of Health** An important US agency devoted to medical research. Administered by the Department of Health and Human Services (HHS), the NIH consists of 24 separate Institutes and Centers. NIH's program activities are represented by these Institutes and Centers. They are as follows:

- **Center for Information Technology** As NIH's computing technology arm, CIT seeks to develop, promote, and spread the use of high-tech tools in biomedical science.

- **Center for Scientific Review** CSR provides staff and procedural support to the director of NIH for running the grant approval process. It handles scientific review of most NIH grant applications, proposals, fellowships, and projects. Formerly known as the Division of Research Grants.

- **Fogarty International Center** The FIC serves as NIH's coordinating body for international medical research and cooperation. It supports research partnerships between US biomedical scientists and their counterparts around the world.

- **National Cancer Institute** The NCI's mission is to lead a national effort against cancer. The NCI conducts basic and clinical biomedical research, trains practitioners, and conducts and supports programs to prevent, detect, diagnose, treat, and control cancer. It also provides practitioners, patients, and the public with information about cancer detection and treatment.

- **National Center for Research Resources** The NCRR conducts biomedical research, and shares its resources and findings with others in the fields of biomedical technology, clinical research, comparative medicine, and research infrastructure.

- **National Eye Institute** NEI conducts and supports research, training, and other programs related to eye diseases, visual disorders, mechanisms of visual function, preservation of sight, blindness, and the health problems and special needs of the visually impaired.

- **National Heart, Lung, and Blood Institute** The NHLBI leads a national research program covering diseases of the heart, blood vessels, lungs, and blood. It also supports basic clinical, population-based, and health-education research in the area of transfusion medicine.

- **National Human Genome Research Institute** NHGRI supports NIH's role in the Human Genome Project, a worldwide research effort designed to analyze the structure of human DNA and determine the location of the estimated 100,000 human genes. NHGRI also develops and implements technology for understanding, diagnosing, and treating genetic diseases.

- **National Institute of Allergy and Infectious Diseases** NIAID's specialty is research and research training into infectious, immune-system, and allergic diseases.

- **National Institute of Arthritis and Musculoskeletal and Skin Diseases** NIAMS specializes in research into the normal structure and function of bones, muscles, and skin, as well as diseases that affect these tissues.

- **National Institute of Child Health and Human Development** NICHD supports and conducts research on fertility, pregnancy, child growth and development, and medical rehabilitation for children affected by disease or disability.

- **National Institute of Dental Research** The NIDR leads a national research program aimed at understanding, treating, and preventing dental and craniofacial diseases.

- **National Institute of Diabetes and Digestive and Kidney Diseases**  This part of NIH conducts national programs in diabetes, endocrinology, and metabolic diseases; digestive diseases and nutrition; and kidney, urologic, and hematologic diseases. The NIDDK conducts studies on its own through the auspices of NIH, and also funds research and outreach efforts nationwide.

- **National Institute of Environmental Health Sciences**  NIEHS conducts research into interactions between environmental exposure, genetic susceptibility, and age that can cause disease or disability.

- **National Institute of General Medical Sciences**  NIGMS supports basic biomedical research that is not targeted to specific diseases or disorders. Among its most significant research results has been the development of recombinant DNA technology, forming the basis for the biotechnology industry.

- **National Institute of Mental Health**  NIMH leads a national program of research into the causes, treatment, and prevention of mental illness. It conducts basic research on the brain and behavior, as well as clinical, epidemiological, and services research.

- **National Institute of Neurological Disorders and Stroke**  NINDS supports and conducts research and research training on the normal structure and function of the nervous system, and on the causes, prevention, diagnosis, and treatment of neurological disorders.

- **National Institute of Nursing Research**  NINR supports research into clinical patient care. These research projects are aimed at understanding and mitigating the effects of acute and chronic illness and disability, promoting healthy behaviors, preventing the onset or worsening of disease, and improving the clinical environment.

- **National Institute on Aging**  NIA leads a national program of research on the biomedical, social, and behavioral aspects of the aging process; the prevention of age-related diseases and disabilities; and health promotion for older Americans.

- **National Institute on Alcohol Abuse and Alcoholism**  NIAAA conducts research into improving the treatment and prevention of alcoholism and alcohol-related problems.

- **National Institute on Deafness and Other Communication Disorders**  NIDCD conducts and supports biomedical research and research training on normal mechanisms as well as diseases and disorders of hearing, balance, smell, taste, voice, speech, and language.

- **National Institute on Drug Abuse**  NIDA conducts and supports research on the causes, prevention, and treatment of drug abuse and addiction.

- **National Library of Medicine**  The world's largest medical library, the NLM collects, organizes, and makes available biomedical science information to investigators, educators, and practitioners. It also carries out programs to strengthen medical library services in the United States. Its electronic databases, including MEDLINE, are used extensively throughout the world.

- **Warren Grant Magnuson Clinical Center**  As the clinical research facility of NIH, this center provides the patient care, services, and facilities to support human subjects research by the NIH. Also known as the National Institutes of Health Clinical Center (NIHCC).

**natural family planning**  Birth control without the use of contraceptive medications or barrier methods. There are several natural family planning methods. If applied exactly, their efficiency comes close to that of barrier methods, but not to that of birth control pills, Depo-Provera, Norplant, or the IUD. The most common method is the use of basal temperature to detect ovulation, accompanied by abstention from intercourse during and after ovulation. Also known as the basal temperature method, the rhythm method. See also *birth control.*

**natural killer cells**  Immune-system components that recognize and bind to cancer cells and other cells involved in disease processes. When they recognize a tumor cell or other target, natural killer cells surround it and release molecules that kill it by breaching the cell wall. Also known as K cells, large granular lymphocytes.

**natural menopause**  See *menopause.*

**naturopath**  A person who practices naturopathy. A naturopathic doctor (ND) has been trained to care for well and ailing patients, using naturopathic methods. In some US states, NDs must complete a program equivalent to the training received by MDs, and are therefore licensed to practice medicine. In other states, the term ND is neither defined nor regulated.

**naturopathy**  A system of therapy based on preventative care, and on the use of heat, water, light, air, and massage as primary therapies for disease. Some naturopaths use no medications, either pharmaceutical or herbal. Some recommend herbal remedies only. A few who are licensed to prescribe may recommend pharmaceuticals in those cases where they feel their use is warranted.

**nausea**  Stomach queasiness, the urge to vomit. It can be brought on by many causes, including systemic illnesses such as influenza, medications, pain, and inner ear disease.

**navel** The umbilicus; the former attachment site of the umbilical cord, usually found in approximately the center of the abdomen. The appearance of the navel depends on how the cord was cut and also on the condition of the underlying muscle. If the muscles are firm and the cut was close enough to the belly, the navel will go inward. If the muscles are weak and/or the cut was too far from the belly, the navel will protrude outward. Also called the belly button.

**NCI** National Cancer Institute.

**NCRR** National Center for Research Resources.

**nebulization, heated** Administration of medication via fine spray that has been heated to increase its water content.

**nebulizer** A device for administering a medication by spraying a fine mist into the nose. Also known as an atomizer.

**neck dissection** Surgery to remove lymph nodes and other tissues in the neck.

**neck, chronic stiff** See *torticollis*.

**necropsy** An examination of a dead body; an autopsy.

**necrosis** Death of cells or tissues. Necrosis can be due, for example, to lack of blood flow (ischemia).

**necrosis, coagulation** Tissue death due to clots in the bloodstream, which block the flow of blood to the affected area.

**necrosis, gangrenous** Tissue death due to the combined effects of blood-flow stoppage and bacterial infection.

**necrotic** Synonymous with dead. Necrotic tissue is dead tissue.

**necrotizing fasciitis** Severe bacterial infection of the fascia, the tissues that line and separate muscles, causing extensive tissue death. Necrotizing fasciitis can be caused by several different types of bacteria, particularly virulent strains of streptococcus and staphylococcus, or by several different bacterial infections occurring at once. Treatment is with high-dose antibiotics, life support, and debridement (removal) of affected tissues. Known colloquially as "flesh-eating bacteria."

**necrotizing gingivitis** See *acute membranous gingivitis*.

**needle biopsy** See *biopsy, needle*.

**needle biopsy, stereotactic** See *biopsy, stereotactic needle*.

**Nef gene** Short for negative factor gene, a gene whose absence or weakness diminishes the strength of a disease. The term was coined in respect to HIV and AIDS to describe an as-yet-unknown genetic mechanism that diminishes the strength of AIDS in some patients. Also written as NEF, NeF, or nef gene; sometimes shortened to nef.

**negative, false** A medical test result that appears to be negative, but fails to reveal a situation. An example is a biopsy for cancer that returns a negative result even though the person has cancer.

**neglect, child** See *child neglect*.

**NEI** National Eye Institute.

**Neisseria** Group of bacteria that includes the cause of gonorrhea.

**nematodes** Parasitic roundworms.

**neo-** Prefix meaning new. For example, a neonate is a newborn baby, and a neoplasm is a new growth: a tumor.

**neonatal** Pertaining to the newborn period, the first four weeks after birth.

**neonatal jaundice** See *jaundice, neonatal*.

**neonatal mortality rate** The number of children under 28 days of age who die, divided by the number of live births that year. The neonatal mortality rate in the US, which was 8.4 per 1,000 live births in 1980, declined to 5.8 per 1,000 live births in 1990.

**neonatal sepsis** A serious bacterial infection of the blood in an infant less than 4 weeks of age. Babies with sepsis may be listless, overly sleepy, floppy, weak, and very pale.

**neonate** A newborn baby.

**neonatologist** A specialist in the care of the newborn.

**neonatology** The art and science of medical care for the newborn.

**neoplasia** Abnormal new growth of cells.

**neoplasm** A tumor.

**nephrectomy** Surgery to remove the kidney.

**nephrectomy, partial**   Removal of a kidney tumor, but not the entire kidney.

**nephrectomy, radical**   Surgery to remove the kidney, the adrenal gland, nearby lymph nodes, and other surrounding tissue.

**nephrectomy, simple**   Surgery to remove the affected kidney only.

**nephritis**   Inflammation of the kidney, which causes impaired kidney function. Nephritis can be due to a variety of causes, including kidney disease, allergies, and infection. Treatment depends on the cause.

**nephritis, acute**   Sudden kidney inflammation. Diagnosis is by finding protein or urine in the blood.

**nephritis, infective tubulointerstitial**   Inflammation of the kidney due to infection. Symptoms include nausea, pain in the kidney area, fever, and chills. Early diagnosis is essential to save the kidneys. Treatment is by antibiotics or antiviral medications.

**nephritis, interstitial**   Nephritis due to disorders of the connective tissue within the kidney, severe allergic reactions, exposure to toxic substances, transplant rejection, urinary blockage, or other factors. Symptoms include fever, pain in the kidney area, blood or protein in the urine, and eventually kidney failure. Treatment depends on the cause.

**nephritis, lipomatous**   A disorder in which the nephrons of the kidney are gradually replaced with fatty tissues, preventing proper filtration of wastes and eventually resulting in kidney failure. Treatment is by dialysis.

**nephro-**   Having to do with the kidney.

**nephrolith**   A kidney stone.

**nephrolithiasis**   The process of forming a stone in the kidney or lower down in the urinary tract. Also known as urolithiasis. See also *kidney stone*.

**nephrolithotripsy, percutaneous**   See *percutaneous nephrolithotripsy*.

**nephrologist**   A medical practitioner whose specialty is nephrology.

**nephrology**   The art and science of the care of the kidneys.

**nephrons**   A key unit of the kidney, the nephrons are tiny funnel-like structures that filter wastes as they enter and progress through the kidney.

**nephropathy**   Any kidney disease.

**nephropathy, diabetic**   See *diabetic nephropathy*.

**nephrosclerosis**   Hardening (sclerosis) of the kidney, usually due to hardening of the blood vessels within it (atherosclerosis).

**nephrosis**   Noninflammatory, nonneoplastic disease of the kidney. Nephrosis can be caused by kidney disease, or it may be a complication of another disorder, particularly diabetes. Diagnosis is by urine testing for the presence of protein, blood testing for lower-than-normal levels of protein, and observation of edema. Treatment is usually with adrenal hormones. Also known as nephrotic syndrome.

**nephrotic syndrome**   See *nephrosis*.

**nephrotomogram**   A series of special X-rays of the kidneys. The X-rays are taken from different angles to show the kidneys clearly, without the shadows of the organs around them.

**nerve**   A bundle of fibers that uses electrical and chemical signals to transmit sensory and motor information from one body part to another. The fibrous portions of a nerve are covered by a sheath called myelin and/or a membrane called neurilemma. See also *nervous system*.

**nerve compression**   "Pinching" a nerve by putting too much pressure on it. For example, a woman's sciatic nerve may be painfully compressed by the weight and position of the fetus during the latter part of pregnancy.

**nerve growth factor**   A naturally occurring substance that enhances the growth and survival of cholinergic nerves.

**nerve palsy, laryngeal**   See *laryngeal palsy*.

**nerve pathways, visual**   See *optic nerve pathways*.

**nerve, abducent**   See *abducent nerve*.

**nerve, accessory**   See *accessory nerve*.

**nerve, afferent**   See *afferent nerve*.

**nerve, efferent**   See *efferent nerve*.

**nerve, eighth cranial**   See *vestibulocochlear nerve*.

**nerve, eleventh cranial**   See *accessory nerve*.

**nerve, facial**   See *facial nerve*.

**nerve, fifth cranial**   See *trigeminal nerve*.

**nerve, first cranial**  See *olfactory nerve*.

**nerve, fourth cranial**  See *trochlear nerve*.

**nerve, glossopharyngeal**  See *glossopharyngeal nerve*.

**nerve, hypoglossal**  See *hypoglossal nerve*.

**nerve, ninth cranial**  See *glossopharyngeal nerve*.

**nerve, oculomotor**  See *oculomotor nerve*.

**nerve, olfactory**  See *olfactory nerve*.

**nerve, optic**  See *optic nerve*.

**nerve, pinched**  Compression of a nerve, as between two vertebrae or within a joint, causing discomfort, pain, or impairment of sensation. Treatment is by physical therapy, and sometimes by surgery. See also *nerve compression*.

**nerve, recurrent laryngeal**  See *recurrent laryngeal nerve*. See also *vagus nerve*.

**nerve, sciatic**  See *sciatic nerve*.

**nerve, second cranial**  See *optic nerve*.

**nerve, seventh cranial**  See *facial nerve*.

**nerve, sixth cranial**  See *abducent nerve*.

**nerve, tenth cranial**  See *vagus nerve*.

**nerve, third cranial**  See *oculomotor nerve*.

**nerve, trigeminal**  See *trigeminal nerve*.

**nerve, trochlear**  See *trochlear nerve*.

**nerve, twelfth cranial**  See *hypoglossal nerve*.

**nerve, vagus**  See *vagus nerve*.

**nerve, vestibulocochlear**  See *vestibulocochlear nerve*.

**nerves, cranial**  See *cranial nerves*.

**nervous colon syndrome**  See *irritable bowel syndrome*.

**nervous system**  The collection of body tissues that record and distribute information via electrical and chemical signals. It includes the central nervous system (the brain and spinal cord) and the peripheral nervous system.

**nervous system, autonomic**  See *autonomic nervous system*. See also *sympathetic nervous system*, *parasympathetic nervous system*.

**nervous system, central**  See *central nervous system*.

**nervous system, parasympathetic**  See *parasympathetic nervous system*.

**nervous system, peripheral**  See *peripheral nervous system*.

**nervous system, sympathetic**  See *sympathetic nervous system*.

**neural**  Having to do with nerve cells.

**neural tube defect**  A birth defect caused by abnormal development during embryonic life of the neural tube, the structure that gives rise to the central nervous system. Neural tube defects include anencephaly (absence of the cranial vault, and absence of most or all of the cerebral hemispheres of the brain) and spina bifida. The risk of NTDs can be decreased if the mother's diet includes adequate folic acid during pregnancy.

**neuralgia**  Pain along the course of a nerve.

**neuralgia, ciliary**  See *cluster headache*.

**neuralgia, facial**  Severe pain, usually occurring in bursts, that emanates along the path of the trigeminal nerve. The trigeminal nerve is the chief sensory nerve of the face.

**neuralgia, migrainous**  See *cluster headache*.

**neuralgia, postherpetic**  The most common complication of shingles, postherpetic neuralgia occurs when the pain associated with shingles persists beyond one month, even after the rash is gone. The pain can be severe and debilitating, and occurs primarily in persons over the age of 50. There is some evidence that treating shingles with steroids and antiviral agents can reduce the duration and occurrence of postherpetic neuralgia. However, the decrease is minimal. The pain of postherpetic neuralgia can be reduced by a number of medications. Tricyclic antidepressant medications, such as amitriptyline (brand name: Elavil), as well as antiseizure medications such as gabapentin (brand name: Neurontin) or carbamazepine (brand name: Tegretol), have been used. Capsaicin cream, a derivative of hot chili peppers, can be applied on the area after all the blisters have healed, to reduce pain. Acupuncture and electric nerve stimulation through the skin can be helpful for some patients.

**neuralgia, spenopalatine**  See *cluster headache*.

**neuralgia, vidian**  See *cluster headache*.

**neuritis**  Inflammation of nerves.

**neurobiological disorders**  A preferred name for illnesses of the brain and nervous system that are known to be caused by genetic, metabolic, or other biological factors. Many illnesses categorized as psychiatric disorders are now known to be neurobiological in nature, including autism, bipolar disorders, obsessive-compulsive disorders, schizophrenia, and Tourette syndrome.

**neuroblastoma**  Childhood tumor of adrenal or related tissue in the nervous system.

**neurofibromatosis**  Hereditary disorder characterized by café au lait (light brown) spots on the skin, and a tendency to develop large tumors on the nerves, skin, and internal organs. Neurofibromatosis may include deformation of the bones and muscles as well. It is sometimes associated with neural tube defects or epilepsy. There are two major types of neurofibromatosis, known as NF-1 and NF-2. There are currently no treatments for either form of NF, but surgery is sometimes used to remove the tumors. Also known as von Recklinghausen disease.

**neurogenic**  Starting with or having to do with the nerves or the nervous system.

**neurological**  Having to do with the nerves or the nervous system.

**neurologist**  A doctor who specializes in the diagnosis and treatment of disorders of the nervous system.

**neuroma**  A tumor that arises in nerve cells.

**neuroma, optic**  A benign tumor of the optic nerve.

**neuron**  A nerve cell that receives and sends electrical signals over long distances within the body. A neuron receives electrical input signals from sensory cells (called sensory neurons) and from other neurons. The neuron sends electrical output signals to muscle neurons (called motoneurons or motor neurons) and to other neurons. A neuron that simply signals another neuron is called an interneuron.

**neuron-specific enolase**  A substance that has been detected in patients with certain tumors, namely neuroblastoma, small-cell lung cancer, medullary thyroid cancer, carcinoid tumors, pancreatic endocrine tumors, and melanoma. Measurement of NSE levels in patients with neuroblastoma or small-cell lung cancer can provide information about the extent of the disease and the patient's prognosis, as well as about the patient's response to treatment.

**neuropathy**  Any and all disease or malfunction of the nerves.

**neuropathy, accessory**  See *accessory neuropathy*.

**neuropathy, ataxia, and retinitis pigmentosa**  See *NARP*.

**neuropathy, hypoglossal**  See *hypoglossal neuropathy*.

**neuropsychologist**  A psychologist who has completed special training in the neurobiological causes of brain disorders, and who specializes in diagnosing and treating these illnesses by using a predominantly medical (as opposed to psychoanalytical) approach.

**neurosurgeon**  A doctor who specializes in surgery on the brain and other parts of the nervous system.

**neurosyphilis**  Neurological complications in the third (tertiary) and final phase of syphilis, which involve the central nervous system and can include psychosis, pain, and loss of physical control over a variety of bodily functions.

**neurosyphilis, tabes**  The slowly progressive degeneration of the spinal cord that occurs in the tertiary phase of syphilis, a decade or more after a person contracts the infection. Among its features are sharp, lightning-like pain; wobbliness (ataxia); deterioration of the optic nerve, leading to blindness; urinary incontinence; loss of the sense of position; and degeneration of the joints. Also known as tabes dorsalis.

**neurotoxic**  Poisonous to nerves or nerve tissue.

**neurotoxin**  A substance that causes damage to nerves or nerve tissue. For example, lead is a neurotoxin.

**neutropenia**  A marked decrease in the number of neutrophils, a type of white blood cell. Neutropenia is a sign of impaired immune-system response. See also *agranulocytosis; agranulocytosis, infantile genetic; granulocytopenia; severe congenital neutropenia*.

**neutropenia, severe congenital**  See *severe congenital neutropenia*.

**neutrophil**  A type of white blood cell. A neutrophil is a granulocyte that is filled with microscopic granules, little sacs containing enzymes that digest microorganisms.

**neutrophilia**  Too many neutrophils.

**nevus**  A pigmented spot on the skin, such as a mole. The plural of nevus is nevi.

**nevus araneus**  See *spider veins*.

**newborn screening**  Tests of newborns to detect those at increased risk for disorders such as phenylketonuria (PKU) and hypothyroidism.

**NG tube**  See *nasogastric tube*.

**NHGRI**  National Human Genome Research Institute.

**NHL**  Non-Hodgkin lymphoma. See *lymphoma, non-Hodgkin*.

**NHLBI**  National Heart, Lung, and Blood Institute.

**NIA**  National Institute on Aging.

**NIAAA**  National Institute on Alcohol Abuse and Alcoholism.

**niacin**  Nicotinic acid, one of the water-soluble B vitamins. See also *Appendix C, "Vitamins."*

**niacin deficiency**  A lack of niacin, which in its most extreme form is known as pellagra. Signs of less severe niacin deficiency may include rough, dry skin; skin rashes; and mild depression. See *pellagra*.

**niacin for high cholesterol**  When given in doses well above the RDA, niacin lowers the total cholesterol, LDL-cholesterol, and triglyceride levels, while raising the HDL-cholesterol level. It reduces LDL-cholesterol levels by 10 to 20 percent, reduces triglycerides by 20 to 50 percent, and raises HDL-cholesterol by 15 to 35 percent. Patients are usually started on low daily doses and gradually increased to an average daily dose of 1.5 to 3 grams per day. Most experts recommend starting with the immediate-release form; patients should discuss with their doctors which type is best for them. All patients taking niacin acid to lower their serum cholesterol should be closely monitored by their doctor to avoid complications. A common and troublesome side effect of nicotinic acid is flushing or hot flashes, which result from the widening of blood vessels. Most patients develop a tolerance to flushing, and in some patients, it can be decreased by taking the drug during or after meals or by the use of aspirin or other similar medications prescribed by a doctor. The effect of high blood pressure medicines may also be increased for people on niacin. If a patient is taking high blood pressure medication, it is important to set up a blood pressure–monitoring system while he or she is getting used to the new niacin regimen. A variety of gastrointestinal symptoms, including nausea, indigestion, gas, vomiting, diarrhea, and the activation of peptic ulcers have been seen with the use of niacin. Three other major adverse effects include liver problems, gout, and high blood sugar. Risk of these complications increases as the dose of nicotinic acid is increased. Doctors will probably not recommend niacin for patients with diabetes, because of the effect on blood sugar.

**NIAID**  National Institute of Allergy and Infectious Diseases.

**NIAMS**  National Institute of Arthritis and Musculoskeletal and Skin Diseases.

**NICHD**  National Institute of Child Health and Development.

**nicotinic acid**  See *niacin*.

**NIDA**  National Institute on Drug Abuse.

**NIDCD**  National Institute on Deafness and Other Communication Disorders.

**NIDDK**  National Institute of Diabetes and Digestive and Kidney Diseases.

**NIDR**  National Institute of Dental Research.

**NIEHS**  National Institute of Environmental Health Sciences.

**Niemann-Pick disease**  See *histiocytosis, lipid*.

**night blindness**  See *nyctanopia*.

**night sweats**  Severe hot flashes that occur at night and result in a drenching sweat. Night sweats can have many different causes, including medications, infections, and cancers.

**NIGMS**  National Institute of General Medical Sciences.

**NIH**  The National Institutes of Health.

**NIMH**  National Institute of Mental Health.

**NINDS**  National Institute of Neurological Disorders and Stroke.

**nine-day measles**  See *measles*.

**NINR**  National Institute of Nursing Research.

**ninth cranial nerve**  See *glossopharyngeal nerve*.

**Nipah virus**  A virus that infects pigs and people, in whom it causes a sometimes fatal form of viral encephalitis. It is similar to Hendra virus. Symptoms include high fever and aches, coma, and sometimes death. It is still not known how Nipah virus is transmitted. It may be carried from pigs to humans by mosquitoes.

**nipple**  The pigmented projection on the surface of the breast. Ducts that conduct milk from the mammary glands to the surface of the breast exit through the nipple. The surrounding flat area of pigmentation is the areola.

**nipple absence**  See *athelia*.

**nipple, supernumerary** An extra nipple. Supernumerary nipples are usually smaller than normal and vestigial (nonfunctional, without accompanying mammary glands). They tend to occur along a roughly curved line extending from near the armpit, through the center of the normal breast, and down to the lower abdomen. This distribution is very similar to the location of nipples on mammals that have multiple nipples along the underbelly.

**nits** Lice eggs. They are hard to see, and are often confused with dandruff or hair-spray droplets. Nits firmly attach to the hair shaft with a glue-like substance. They are oval, and range in color from yellow to white. Nits take about a week to hatch. All nits must be removed to prevent reinfestation with lice. They can be removed with a special comb or with the fingers. Topical preparations are available that loosen the "glue" that binds them to the hair, making removal easier. See also *head lice, head lice infestation*.

**nitrogenous base** A molecule that contains nitrogen and has the chemical properties of a base. The nitrogenous bases in DNA are adenine (A), guanine (G), thymine (T), and cytosine (C). The nitrogenous bases in RNA are the same, with one exception: adenine (A), guanine (G), uracil (U), and cytosine (C).

**nitrosoureas** A group of anticancer drugs that can cross the blood-brain barrier. Carmustine and lomustine are nitrosoureas.

**nitrous oxide** A gas that can cause general anesthesia, it should be administered with other anesthetic agents. It is not used alone today because the concentration of nitrous oxide needed to produce anesthesia is close to the concentration that seriously lowers the blood oxygen level, creating a hazardous hypoxic state. Also known as nitrous or "laughing gas."

**NK** Natural killer cells.

**NLM** National Library of Medicine.

**NMR** Nuclear Magnetic Resonance.

**nocturia** Excessive urinating at night.

**nocturnal amblyopia** See *nyctanopia*.

**nocturnal enuresis** Bedwetting. See *enuresis*.

**node** Literally a knot, a node is a collection of tissue. For example, a lymph node is a collection of lymphoid tissue. See also *nodule*.

**node, atrioventricular** See *atrioventricular node*.

**node, AV** See *atrioventricular node*.

**node, Heberden** See *Heberden node*.

**node, SA** See *sinoatrial node*.

**node, sentinel lymph** See *lymph node, sentinel*.

**node, sinoatrial** See *sinoatrial node*.

**node, sinus** See *sinoatrial node*.

**nodes, Osler** See *Osler nodes*.

**nodular** Bumpy.

**nodular hyperplasia of the prostate** See *benign prostatic hyperplasia*.

**nodule** A small collection of tissue.

**nondisjunction** Failure of paired chromosomes to separate during cell division, so that both chromosomes go to one daughter cell and none to the other. Nondisjunction causes errors in chromosome number, such as trisomy 21 (Down syndrome) and monsomy X (Turner syndrome).

**non-Hodgkin lymphoma** See *lymphoma, non-Hodgkin*.

**nonmelanoma skin cancer** Skin cancer that does not involve melanocytes. Basal cell cancer and squamous cell cancer are nonmelanoma skin cancers.

**nonossifying fibroma** See *fibroma, nonossifying*.

**Nonoxynol-9** A potent spermicide (sperm-killing solution) that may also provide some protection against the HIV virus.

**non-rapid eye movement sleep** See *NREM sleep*.

**nonseminoma** A type of testicular cancer that arises in specialized sex cells called germ cells. Nonseminomas include embryonal carcinoma, teratoma, choriocarcinoma, and yolk sac tumor.

**non-small–cell lung cancer** A general classification for squamous cell carcinoma, adenocarcinoma, and large cell carcinoma.

**nonsteroidal anti-inflammatory drug** See *NSAID*.

**Noonan syndrome** A condition characterized by a series of birth defects, including short stature after birth (postnatal growth retardation), webbing of the neck (pterygium colli), caved-in chestbone (pectus excavatum), narrowing of the artery from the heart to the lungs (pulmonic stenosis) and, in boys, testes that do not descend normally into the scrotum (cryptorchidism). Abbreviated as NS. Although NS was once called Turner-like syndrome, it is a distinctive entity that affects both sexes and carries an elevated risk of developmental and language delay, learning disability, hearing loss, and mild mental retardation. NS is inherited as a dominant condition, and an NS gene has been mapped to chromosome 12.

**normal pressure hydrocephalus** See *hydrocephalus, normal pressure*.

**normal range** Characteristic of 95 percent of values from a normal population, meaning that 5 percent of normal results will fall outside the normal range along with any truly abnormal results. The normal range for a particular test result, condition, symptom, or behavior may differ, based on the patient's age, size, sex, race, or culture.

**Norplant** A contraceptive device consisting of six matchstick-sized rods that can be implemented in a woman's upper arms. The rods release hormones that prevent conception for five years. It is the most effective reversible form of contraception. See also *birth control, contraception*.

**North Asian tick-borne rickettsiosis** See *rickettsiosis, North Asian tick-borne*.

**Northern blot** A technique in molecular biology, used mainly to separate and identify pieces of RNA. It is called a Northern blot because it is similar to another technique known as a Southern blot.

**nortriptyline** A tricyclic antidepressant medication (brand name: Avenytl, Pamelor), nortriptyline is used to treat depression, chronic pain, bulimia and other eating disorders, sleep apnea, and a number of other conditions. It may be given in combination with other medications for some disorders. Nortriptyline is potentiated by, interacts with, or strengthens medicines, so always consult your doctor before taking it with any other drug. It can have serious side effects, including liver problems, sedation, seizures, and mood swing in people with bipolar disorders.

**Norvir** See *ritonavir*.

**nose job** Slang for plastic surgery on the nose, known medically as a rhinoplasty. See *rhinoplasty*.

**nose, runny** Rhinorrhea is the medical term for this common problem. The nose makes extra mucus whenever something that is in the nose, such as pollen or dust, needs to be removed. Mucus formation is also part of the histamine reaction to allergies, and of the body's defenses during respiratory infections. Although many over-the-counter medications are available to treat a runny nose, it's usually best to allow the mucus to perform its function until the underlying condition is resolved.

**nosebleed** Bleeding from the blood vessels of the nose. The nose is rich in blood vessels, and is situated in a vulnerable position on the face. As a result, any trauma to the face can cause bleeding, which may be profuse. Nosebleeds can occur spontaneously when the nasal membranes dry out, crust, and crack, as is common in dry climates or during winter months when the air is dry and warm from household heaters. People are more susceptible to nosebleeds if they are taking medications that prevent normal blood clotting, such as coumadin, warfarin, aspirin, or any anti-inflammatory medication. Other predisposing factors include infection, trauma, allergic and nonallergic rhinitis, hypertension, alcohol abuse, and inherited bleeding problems. Also known as epistaxis.

**nosebleed, treatment of** To stop a nosebleed, you should pinch all the soft parts of the nose together between your thumb and index finger, and press firmly toward the face, compressing the pinched parts of the nose against the bones of the face. Hold the nose for at least five minutes, and repeat as necessary until the nose has stopped bleeding. Sit quietly, keeping the head higher than the level of the heart; that is, sit up or lie with the head elevated. Do not lie flat or put your head between your legs. Apply ice (crushed in a plastic bag or washcloth) to nose and cheeks.

**nosocomial** Hospital-acquired: A nosocomial infection is one caught in a hospital. Since antibiotics have come into common usage, bacteria that are resistant to them have also become common, especially in hospitals. As a result, there are now many nosocomial infections.

**nostrum** 1 Formerly, a medicine of secret composition recommended by the person who concocted it, but with no scientific proof of its effectiveness. A patent medicine was a nostrum. 2 Specifically, a worthless remedy. 3 In common use, any questionable remedy or scheme for improving matters, a pet plan for accomplishing things, or a panacea.

**NPH** Normal pressure hydrocephalus.

**NREM sleep** Non-rapid eye movement sleep: dreamless sleep. During NREM sleep, the brain waves seen on an electroencephalogram (EEG) are typically slow and of high voltage, the breathing and heart rate are slow and regular, the blood pressure is low, and the sleeper is relatively still. NREM sleep is divided into four stages of increasing depth, eventually leading to REM sleep. About 80 percent of sleep is NREM sleep. See also *REM sleep, sleep*.

**NS**   Noonan syndrome.

**NSAID**   Nonsteroidal anti-inflammatory drug. NSAID medications are commonly prescribed or purchased over the counter for the inflammation associated with conditions such as arthritis, tendinitis, and bursitis. Examples of NSAIDs include aspirin, indomethacin (brand name: Indocin), ibuprofen (brand name: Motrin), naproxen (brand name: Naprosyn), piroxicam (brand name: Feldene), and nabumetone (brand name: Relafen). The major side effects of NSAIDs are gastrointestinal problems. Some 10 to 50 percent of patients are unable to tolerate NSAID treatment because of these side effects, which include abdominal pain, diarrhea, bloating, heartburn, and upset stomach. Approximately 15 percent of patients on long-term NSAID treatment develop ulceration of the stomach and duodenum. Even though many of these patients with ulcers do not have symptoms, they are at risk of developing serious complications, such as bleeding or perforation of the stomach. The risk of serious complications is higher in elderly patients, in those with rheumatoid arthritis, in patients taking blood-thinning medications or Prednisone (cortisone medication), and in patients with heart disease or a history of bleeding ulcers. However, the NSAIDS have a much lower side-effect profile than that of steroidal anti-inflammatory drugs, such as Prednisone.

**NSE**   Neuron-specific enolase.

**NTD**   Neural tube defect.

**nucleic acid**   DNA or RNA.

**nucleosome**   Structure responsible in part for the compactness of a chromosome. Each nucleosome consists of a sequence of DNA wrapped around a core of histone, which is a type of protein.

**nucleotide**   A subunit of DNA or RNA. A nucleotide consists of a nitrogenous base (A, G, T, or C in DNA; A, G, U, or C in RNA), a phosphate molecule, and a sugar molecule (deoxyribose in DNA, and ribose in RNA). Thousands of nucleotides are linked to form a DNA or RNA molecule.

**nucleus**   1 In cell biology, the structure that houses the chromosomes. 2 In neuroanatomy, a group of nerve cells.

**null mutation**   Change in a gene that leads to nothing: for example, a change that does not result in a nonfunctioning enzyme or in physical malformation.

**nullipara**   A woman who has not given birth to a viable child.

**nurse**   1 A person trained, licensed, or skilled in nursing. 2 To feed an infant at the breast.

**nurse assistant**   A person who has completed a brief health-care training program, and who provides support services for RNs and LPNs. Also known as an orderly or, when certified by a state agency, a certified nurse aide (CNA).

**nurse practitioner**   A registered nurse (RN) who has completed an advanced training program in a medical specialty, such as pediatric care. An NP may be a primary, direct health-care provider, and can prescribe medications. Some NPs work in research rather than in direct patient care.

**nurse, licensed practical**   A nurse who has completed a one- or two-year training program in health care and has earned a state license. LPNs provide direct patient care for people with chronic illness, in nursing homes, hospitals, and home settings. They assist RNs in caring for acutely ill patients.

**nurse, registered**   A nurse who has completed a two- to four-year degree program in nursing. Registered nurses provide direct patient care for acutely or chronically ill patients. RNs may further specialize in a particular area. For example, psychiatric nurses are RNs with special training in working with mentally ill patients, and trauma nurses work with doctors and surgeons to help patients in the emergency room of a hospital. Some RNs also work in health research. Abbreviated as RN.

**nursing**   1 A profession concerned with the provision of services essential to the maintenance and restoration of health. Nurses attend to the needs of sick people. Some nurses are licensed to directly diagnose and treat disease, and others work in medical research. 2 Feeding an infant at the breast.

**nursing home**   A residential facility for people with chronic illness or disability, particularly older people who have mobility and eating problems. Also known as a convalescent home, long-term–care facility.

**nutraceutical**   A food or part of a food that allegedly provides medicinal or health benefits, including the prevention and treatment of disease. A nutraceutical may be a naturally nutrient-rich or medicinally active food, such as garlic or soybeans, or it may be a specific component of a food, such as the omega-3 fish oil that can be derived from salmon and other cold-water fish.

**nutrition** 1 The science or practice of taking in and utilizing foods. 2 A nourishing substance, such as nutritional solutions delivered to hospitalized patients via an IV or IG tube.

**nutritionist** 1 In a hospital or nursing home, a person who plans and/or formulates special meals for patients. The term can also be a euphemism for a cook who works in a medical facility but who does not have extensive training in special nutritional needs. 2 In clinical practice, a specialist in nutrition. Nutritionists can help patients with special needs, allergies, health problems, or a desire for increased energy or weight change devise healthy diets. Some nutritionists in private practice are well-trained, degreed, and licensed. Depending on state law, however, a person using the title may not be trained or licensed at all.

**nyctalopia** See *nyctanopia*.

**nyctanopia** Impaired vision in dim light and in the dark, due to impaired function of the rods in the retina. Night blindness is a classic finding from deficiency of vitamin A. Also known as day sight, nocturnal amblyopia, nyctalopia.

**nyctophobia** Pathological fear of the dark.

**nymph** A stage in the life cycle of certain arthropods, such as ticks and lice. The nymph stage comes between a nit and an adult louse. A nymph louse looks like an adult, but is smaller. Nymphs mature into adults about seven days after hatching. To live, the nymph must feed on blood.

**nystagmus** Rapid, rhythmic, repetitious, and involuntary eye movements. Nystagmus can be horizontal, vertical, or rotary.

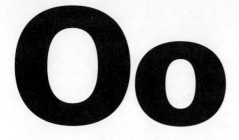

**oat-cell lung cancer**  A type of lung cancer in which the cancerous cells look like oats. Also called small-cell lung cancer.

**Oath of Maimonides**  See *Daily Prayer of a Physician*.

**OB**  Abbreviation for obstetrician or for obstetrics.

**obesity**  Overweight. People are considered to be obese if they are more than 20 percent over their ideal weight. That ideal weight must take into account the person's height, age, sex, and build. Obesity is often multifactorial, based on both genetic and behavioral factors. Accordingly, treatment of obesity usually requires more than just dietary changes. Exercise, counseling and support, and sometimes medication can supplement diet to help patients conquer weight problems. Extreme diets, on the other hand, can actually contribute to increased obesity. Overweight is a significant contributor to health problems. See *obesity-related diseases*.

**obesity, endogenous**  Overweight caused by malfunction of the hormonal or metabolic system.

**obesity, exogenous**  Overweight caused by consuming more food than the person's activity level warrants, leading to increased fat storage.

**obesity, gynecoid**  Fat distribution in a pattern generally characteristic of that of a woman, with the largest amount around the hips and thighs.

**obesity, male**  Fat distribution in a pattern generally characteristic of that of a man, as with a prominent paunch.

**obesity-related diseases**  Obesity increases the risk of developing a number of diseases, and can be a diagnostic marker for others. Diseases related to obesity include type 2 (adult-onset) diabetes; high blood pressure (hypertension); stroke (cerebrovascular accident); heart attack (myocardial infarction); heart failure (congestive heart failure); certain forms of cancer, such as prostate and colon cancer; gallstones and gall bladder disease (cholecystitis); gout and gouty arthritis; osteoarthritis (degenerative arthritis) of the knees, hips, and the lower back; sleep apnea; and Pickwickian syndrome, which is characterized by obesity, red face, underventilation, and drowsiness.

**OB/GYN**  Abbreviation for obstetrician-gynecologist.

**objective lens**  See *lens, objective*.

**observer variation**  Failure by the observer to measure accurately, resulting in error. Observer variation may be due to the observer's missing a measurement, making an incorrect measurement, or misinterpreting data. Interobserver variation is the amount of variation between the results obtained by two or more observers examining the same material. Intraobserver variation is the amount of variation one observer experiences when observing the same material more than once.

**obsessive-compulsive disorder**  A psychiatric disorder characterized by obsessive thoughts and compulsive actions, often concerned with cleaning, checking, counting, or hoarding. OCD appears to be rooted in malfunction or insult to the basal ganglia, a structure within the brain that controls automatic activities, and is believed to have genetic origins. Symptoms wax and wane, and in some patients emerge in response to, or are made worse by, an unusual immune response to streptococcus infection. Diagnosis is by interview and, with children, by observation. Treatment is by cognitive behavioral therapy and/or medication. Abbreviated as OCD. See also *PANDAS*.

**obsessive-compulsive personality disorder**  A pathologically rigid, controlling personality type.

**obstetrical forceps**  An instrument with two blades and a handle, designed to aid in the vaginal delivery of a baby.

**obstetrician**  A physician who specializes in obstetrics.

**obstetrician/gynecologist**  An obstetrician who also specializes in treating diseases of the female reproductive organs. Some OB/GYNs also provide general health care for women.

**obstetrics**  The art and science of managing pregnancy, labor, and the pueperium, the time after delivery.

**obstruction, airway**  See *airway obstruction*.

**obstructive sleep apnea**  See *sleep apnea, obstructive*.

**obtunded**  Mentally dulled. Head trauma may obtund a person.

**occipital bone**  The bone forming the rear and rear bottom of the skull.

**occiput** The back of the head.

**occular** See *ocular*.

**occult** Hidden. For example, occult blood in the stool is hidden from the eye, but can be detected by chemical tests.

**occupational therapist** A person trained and licensed to design and deliver occupational therapy services. Abbreviated OT. See also *occupational therapy*.

**occupational therapy** Therapy designed to help patients gain or relearn skills needed for activities of daily living, including self-care, handwriting and other school-related skills, and work-related skills. In occupational therapy, patients may do exercises, manipulate items that help develop normal hand motion, or learn to use assistive devices, among other activities. Abbreviated OT.

**OCD** **1** Obsessive-compulsive disorder. **2** Osteochondritis dissecans.

**OCP** Oral contraceptive pill.

**OCPD** Obsessive-compulsive personality disorder.

**ocular** Having to do with the eye.

**ocular lens** See *lens, ocular*.

**oculomotor nerve** The third cranial nerve. The oculomotor nerve is responsible for the nerve supply to muscles about the eye, including the upper eyelid muscle, which raises the eyelid; the extraocular muscle, which moves the eye inward; and the pupillary muscle, which constricts the pupil. Paralysis of the oculomotor nerve results in a drooping eyelid (ptosis), deviation of the eyeball outward (and therefore double vision), and a dilated (wide-open) pupil.

**OD** **1** Osteochondritis dissecans. **2** Overdose.

**oesophagus** Alternate spelling for esophagus.

**off-label use** In the US, the regulations of the Food and Drug Administration (FDA) permit physicians to prescribe approved medications for conditions other than those indicated on the official medication label. This practice is known as off-label use.

**ointment** A preparation that is applied onto the skin. An ointment has an oil base, whereas a cream is water-soluble.

**olecranon** Of or pertaining to the bony tip of the elbow. The olecranon is the near end of the ulna, the bone in the forearm, that forms the pointed portion of the elbow. The triceps muscle tendon of the back of the arm attaches to the olecranon. Disease can affect the olecranon. For example, inflammation of the tiny fluid-filled sac (bursa) at the tip of the elbow can occur, and is referred to as olecranon bursitis. A firm nodule can form at the tip of the elbow; it is referred to as an olecranon nodule and can be found in gout or rheumatoid arthritis. Also known as the olecranon process of the ulna.

**olfaction** The sense of smell.

**olfactory apparatus** The whole system needed to have a sense of smell, including the nose and affiliated nerves.

**olfactory nerve** The nerve that carries impulses for the sense of smell from the nose to the brain. It is the first cranial nerve.

**olgosaccharidoses** A group of inherited metabolic disorders that are similar to the mucopolysaccharidoses. These conditions include aspartylglycosaminuria (AGU), fucosidosis, mannosidosis, and multiple sulfatase deficiency.

**oligo-** Prefix meaning just a few, or scanty. For example, oligodactyly means having fewer than 10 fingers.

**oligodactyly** Fewer than the normal number of fingers or toes. Oligodactyly is the opposite of polydactyly, which means too many fingers or toes.

**oligodendrocyte** A type of cell in the central nervous system. The oligodendrocytes surround and insulate the long fibers (the axons) through which the nerves send their electrical messages.

**oligodendroglioma** A type of brain tumor that is derived from oligodendrocytes.

**oligohydramnios** The presence of less amniotic fluid than is usual.

**oligomenorrhea** Less menstrual blood flow than usual.

**oligonucleotide** A short DNA molecule composed of relatively few nucleotide bases.

**oligospermia** Fewer sperm than usual. Azospermia, by contrast, means absolutely no sperm at all.

**oliguria** Less urination than normal.

**Ollier disease** An inherited condition in which multiple growths (enchondromas) on the bones cause deformity and shortening. Surgery can help to correct limb-length inequality if it occurs. Also known as multiple enchondromatosis.

**omentum**   A sheet of fat that is covered by peritoneum. The greater omentum is attached to the bottom edge of the stomach, and hangs down in front of the intestines. Its other edge is attached to the transverse colon. The lesser omentum is attached to the top edge of the stomach, and extends to the undersurface of the liver.

**Ommaya reservoir**   A device implanted under the scalp, an Ommaya reservoir is used to deliver anticancer drugs to the fluid surrounding the brain and spinal cord.

**omphalocele**   A birth defect in which the intestine protrudes outside the abdomen at the umbilicus. It is due to the intestine's failure to return to the abdomen after the tenth week of fetal development. It can be repaired with surgery, in some cases before birth.

**OMS**   Organisation Mondiale de la Santé: The World Health Organization (WHO).

**oncogene**   A gene that plays a normal role in cell growth and, when altered, may contribute to the growth of a tumor.

**oncologist**   A doctor who specializes in treating cancer.

**onycho-**   Prefix having to do with the nails. For example, onychodystrophy is abnormal growth and development of nails.

**onychodystrophy**   Malformation of the nails.

**onychomycosis**   Fungal infection of the nails. See *dermatophytic onychomycosis.*

**onychomycosis, dermatophytic**   See *dermatophytic onychomycosis.*

**onychomycosis, proximal white subungual**   The rarest form of fungus infection of the finger- or toenail. The infection begins in the nail fold, the portion of the nail opposite the tip of the finger. Proximal white subungual onychomycosis is typically associated with HIV infection (AIDS), although it can follow injury to the nail. The most common fungus implicated is Trichophyton rubrum. Other causes include T. megninii, T. tonsiurans, T. mentagrophytes, T. schoenleinii, and Epidermophyton floccosum. Diagnosis is by observation of infection in the portion of the nailbed closest to the hand, and can be confirmed by seeing the fungus in a scraping of the tissue placed under a microscope. Proximal white subungual onychomycosis is treated by antifungal medications taken by mouth. Examples include itraconzole (brand name: Sporanox) and terbinafine (brand name: Lamisil).

**onychoosteodysplasia**   See *Fong disease.*

**oo-**   Prefix meaning egg or egg-related.

**oocyte**   A female germ cell in the works: a developing egg cell.

**oogonium**   An ancestral cell that gives rise to oocytes.

**oomphalomesenteric duct**   See *yolk stalk.*

**oophorectomy**   The removal of one or both ovaries by surgery.

**oophoritis**   Inflammation of the ovary or egg sac.

**open charting**   The practice of making medical charts available to the patient.

**open fracture**   See *fracture, compound.*

**open reading frame**   In genetics, an open reading frame in DNA has no termination codon (no signal to stop reading the nucleotide sequence), and so may be translated into protein.

**open wound**   An injury that is exposed because of broken skin. An open wound is at high risk for infection.

**opening, vaginal**   The opening to the muscular canal extending from the cervix to the outside of the body.

**operating room**   A facility equipped for performing surgery. Abbreviated as OR.

**operation, Blalock-Taussig**   See *Blalock-Taussig operation.*

**operation, Macewan**   See *Macewen operation.*

**ophthalmia**   Inflammation of the eye.

**ophthalmic**   Pertaining to the eye. An ophthalmic ointment is designed for the eye.

**ophthalmic artery**   The artery that supplies blood to the eye and adjacent structures of the face. It arises from the internal carotid artery, which courses up from deep within the front of the neck. See also *artery.*

**ophthalmic migraine**   See *migraine, ophthalmic.*

**ophthalmic veins**   The paired veins that drain the orbital (eye) cavity. The superior ophthalmic vein arises at the inner angle of the orbit, and follows the course of the ophthalmic artery into the cavernous sinus, a large channel of venous blood. The inferior ophthalmic vein arises from a venous network at the forepart of orbit, and divides into two branches, one of which also ends in the cavernous sinus. See also *vein.*

**ophthalmologist**   An eye doctor: a physician (MD) who practices ophthalmology.

**ophthalmology**   The art and science of eye medicine.

**ophthalmopathy**   Eye disease.

**ophthalmoscope**   A lighted instrument used to examine the inside of the eye, including the retina and the optic nerve.

**opiate**   A medication or illegal drug that is derived from the opium poppy, or that mimics the effect of an opiate (a synthetic opiate). Opiate drugs are narcotic sedatives that depress activity of the central nervous system, reduce pain, and induce sleep. Side effects may include oversedation, nausea, and constipation. Long-term use of opiates can produce addiction, and overuse can cause overdose, and potentially death.

**opportunistic condition**   A condition that occurs especially or exclusively in persons with a weak immune system due, for example, to AIDS, cancer, or immunosuppressive drugs, such as corticosteroids or chemotherapy. An opportunistic condition may be an infection, such as toxoplasmosis or cytomegalovirus (CMV), or a tumor, such as Kaposi sarcoma in AIDS. See also *opportunistic infection, opportunistic microorganism.*

**opportunistic infection**   An infection that occurs because of a weakened immune system. Opportunistic infections are a particular danger for people with AIDS. The HIV virus itself does not cause death, but the opportunistic infections that occur because of the virus's effect on the immune system can do so. See also *opportunistic condition, opportunistic microorganism.*

**opportunistic microorganism**   A bacteria, virus, or fungus that takes advantage of certain opportunities to cause disease. Those opportunities are called opportunistic conditions. These microorganisms are often ones that can lie dormant in body tissues for many years, such as the human herpesviruses, or that are extremely common but usually cause no symptoms of illness. When the immune system cannot raise an adequate response, these microorganisms are activated, begin to multiply, and soon overwhelm the body's weakened defenses. See also *opportunistic condition, opportunistic infection.*

**optic**   Having to do with vision.

**optic nerve**   The second cranial nerve, which connects the eye to the brain. The optic nerve carries the impulses formed by the retina, the nerve layer that lines the back of the eye, senses light, and creates impulses. These impulses are dispatched through the optic nerve to the brain, which interprets them as images. Using an ophthalmoscope, one can easily see the head of the optic nerve. It is the only visible extension of the brain, and is a part of the central nervous system rather than a peripheral nerve.

**optic nerve pathways**   The left and right branches of the optic nerves join behind the eyes, just in front of the pituitary gland, to form a cross-shaped structure called the optic chiasma. Within the optic chiasma, some of the nerve fibers cross. The fibers from the nasal (inside) half of each retina cross over, but those from the temporal (outside) half do not. Specifically, the fibers from the nasal half of the left eye and the temporal half of the right eye form the right optic tract; and the fibers from the nasal half of the right eye and the temporal half of the left form the left optic tract. The nerve fibers then continue along in the optic tracts. Just before they reach the thalamus of the brain, a few of the nerve fibers leave to enter nerve nuclei that function in visual reflexes. Most of the nerve fibers enter the thalamus, forming a junction (synapse) in the back of the thalamus. From there the visual impulses enter nerve pathways called the optic radiations, which lead to the visual (sight) cortex of the occipital (back) lobes of the brain.

**optic neuroma**   A benign tumor of the optic nerve.

**optician**   A specialist in fitting eyeglasses and making lenses to correct vision problems. An optometrist performs eye examinations and writes prescriptions for corrective lenses; an optician fills that prescription.

**optometrist**   A practitioner who provides primary eye and vision care, performs eye examinations to detect vision problems, and prescribes corrective lenses to correct those problems. Some optometrists also make and fit eyeglasses, but many leave that job to an optician. An optometrist is a Doctor of Optometry (OD), not an MD. When an optometrist detects eye disease, the patient may be referred instead to an ophthalmologist, an MD who specializes in diseases of the eye.

**OR**   Operating room. Sometimes written O.R.

**oral**   Having to do with the mouth; given by mouth, as in an oral solution.

**oral cancer**   Cancer within the mouth.

**oral contraceptive**   A birth control pill taken by mouth. Most oral contraceptives include both estrogen and progestogen. When given in certain amounts and at certain times in the menstrual cycle, these hormones prevent the ovary from releasing an egg for fertilization. Colloquially known as the Pill. See also *birth control, contraceptive.*

**oral rehydration solution**   A specially designed liquid containing water, glucose, and electrolytes. ORS is given to treat dehydration.

**oral rehydration therapy** The administration of special fluids by mouth. ORT is used to treat dehydration. See also *oral rehydration solution*.

**oral surgeon** A dentist with special training in surgery to correct problems of the mouth and jaw.

**oral-motor** Relating to the muscles of the mouth and/or to movements of the mouth.

**oral-motor apraxia of speech** See *apraxia of speech*.

**orbit** In medicine, the bony cavity in which the eyeball sits.

**orbital ridge** The bony ridge beneath the eyebrow.

**orchidectomy** Surgical removal of the testicles.

**orchiditis** See *orchitis*.

**orchiopexy** Surgery to bring down an undescended testicle.

**orchitis** Inflammation of the testis. Causes of orchitis include mumps and other infections; diseases, such as polyarteritis nodosa; and injury. Also called orchiditis.

**organic** 1 A chemical compound that contains carbon. 2 Related to an organ. 3 Grown or prepared without the use of chemicals or pesticides, as in organic food.

**organic brain syndrome** Psychiatric or neurological symptoms arising from damage to or disease in the brain. Also called organic mental disorder. See also *neurobiological disorders*.

**organic mental disorder** See *neurobiological disorders, organic brain syndrome*.

**Organisation Mondiale de la Santé** The World Health Organization (WHO).

**organotherapy** The use of extracts of animal glands or organs to treat disease.

**organs of reproduction, female** See *female organs of reproduction*. See also *ovary*.

**organs of reproduction, male** See *male gonad*.

**orgasm** A series of muscle contractions in the genital region, accompanied by sudden release of endorphins. Orgasm normally accompanies male ejaculation as a result of sexual stimulation, and also occurs in females as a result of sexual stimulation.

**orifice** An opening. For example, the mouth is an orifice.

**oromandibular dystonia** A condition affecting the muscles of the jaw, lips, and tongue. The jaw may be pulled open or shut, and speech and swallowing can be difficult.

**oropharynx** The area of the throat at the back of the mouth.

**orphan disease** A rare illness that has been inadequately researched, and for which no or few treatments exist.

**orphan drug** A drug that is not being produced, often a medication useful only to a small population of patients. Also, a drug available outside the US but not approved by the FDA for sale in the the US.

**ORS** Oral rehydration solution.

**ORT** Oral rehydration therapy.

**ortho-** Prefix meaning straight or erect. For example, orthodontics is the straightening of the teeth, and orthostatic is in an upright posture.

**orthodontic treatment** The use of devices, such as dental braces, to move teeth or adjust underlying bone. The ideal age for starting orthodontic treatment is between the ages of 3 to 12. Teeth can be moved by removable appliances or by fixed braces. Crowding of teeth can require extraction. Retainers may be necessary long after dental braces are placed, especially with orthodontic treatment of adults. Temporomandibular joint (TMJ) problems can be corrected with splinting or dental braces.

**orthodontics** The branch of dentistry that specializes in the diagnosis, prevention, and treatment of dental and facial irregularities. The practice of orthodontics involves the design, application, and control of corrective appliances, such as braces, to bring teeth, lips, and jaws into proper alignment and achieve facial balance.

**orthomolecular medicine** A form of alternative medicine originally based on the theories of Nobel prize winner Linus Pauling. Orthomolecular medical practitioners try to prevent and cure disease by using specific doses of vitamins, amino acids, fatty acids, trace minerals, electrolytes, and other natural substances.

**orthopaedics** The branch of surgery broadly concerned with the skeletal system. Sometimes spelled orthopedics.

**orthopaedist**  An orthopaedic surgeon, a doctor who corrects congenital or functional abnormalities of the bones with surgery, casting, and bracing. Orthopaedists also treat injuries to the bones. Sometimes spelled orthopedist.

**orthopedics**  See *orthopaedics*.

**orthopedist**  See *orthopaedist*.

**orthopnea**  The inability to breathe easily unless one is sitting up straight or standing erect.

**orthopod**  Slang term for an orthopaedist.

**orthoscopic**  Having correct vision, or producing it. Free from optical distortion, or designed to correct distorted vision.

**orthostatic hypotension**  See *hypotension, orthostatic*.

**os sacrum**  The large, heavy bone at the base of the spine. It is symmetrical and roughly triangular in shape. The female sacrum is wider and less curved than the male sacrum, to permit easier childbearing.

**Osgood-Schlatter disease**  A condition characterized by inflammation and sometimes tearing of ligaments within the knee and lower leg. Treatment is by rest, casting if necessary, and sometimes surgery. See also *osteochondrosis*.

**Osler nodes**  Small, tender, transient nodules in the pads of fingers and toes, and the palms and soles. They are a highly diagnostic sign of bacterial infection of the heart (subacute bacterial endocarditis).

**Osler-Rendu-Weber syndrome**  See *hereditary hemorrhagic telangectasia*.

**osseous**  Having to do with the bone, consisting of bone, or resembling bone.

**ossicle**  Any small bone, such as the tiny bones within the human ear.

**ossification**  **1** The normal process of bone growth. **2** Hardening, becoming bone-like.

**ossify**  To harden.

**osteitis**  Inflammation of the bone.

**osteitis fibrosa cystica**  A condition associated with hyperparathyroidism, in which bone tissue is gradually replaced by cysts and fibers.

**osteo-**  Prefix meaning bone. For example, osteosarcoma is cancer arising in the bone.

**osteoarthritis**  A type of arthritis caused by inflammation, breakdown, and eventual loss of cartilage in the joints.

**osteoblastoma**  A noncancerous tumor in bone tissue. Osteoblastomas are small, and are seen most frequently in children or young adults. Symptoms include pain and bone-mass reduction. Treatment is by surgery, sometimes followed by chemotherapy.

**osteochondritis dissecans**  A condition in which a fragment of bone in a joint is deprived of blood and separates from the rest of the bone, causing soreness and making the joint give way. Diagnosis is by X-ray. Treatment is usually by casting, although if the fragment has detached completely, arthroscopic surgery may be necessary. Abbreviated as OCD or OD.

**osteochondroma**  An abnormal, solitary, benign growth of bone and cartilage, typically at the end of a long bone. Osteochondromas are usually discovered in persons 15 to 25 years of age. They are typically detected when the area is injured, or when they become large. The condition can be hereditary, in which case it may be called hereditary multiple exostoses (HMS).

**osteochondromatosis**  The most common type of skeletal tumor (exostoses) disorder seen in childhood, osteochondromatosis is characterized by multiple projecting tumors. The tumors form most frequently on the long bones. In 2 to 10 percent of cases, an exostoses becomes malignant.

**osteochondrosis**  Any disease that affects the progress of bone growth by killing bone tissue. Osteochondrosis is seen only in children and teens whose bones are still growing.

**osteoclasia**  Destruction and reabsorption of bone tissue, as occurs when broken bones heal.

**osteoclasis**  The surgical destruction of bone tissue. Osteoclasis is performed to reconstruct a bone that is malformed, often a broken bone that healed improperly. The bone may be broken and then reshaped with the aid of metal pins, casting, and bracing.

**osteoclast**  A special type of large bone cell that appears when bones are growing or need to be repaired. Osteoclasts may also appear abnormally. See also *osteoclastoma*.

**osteoclastoma**  A tumor of the bone that begins in osteoclast cells, often osteoclasts that have formed abnormally. The tumor may be coated by new bony growth. It causes pain, restricts movement, and is usually cancerous. Treatment is by surgery, usually followed by chemotherapy.

**osteocyte**  A bone cell.

**osteodystrophy**  A bone disorder that adversely affects bone growth. See also *osteodystrophy, renal*.

**osteodystrophy, renal**  A bone-growth disorder caused by chronic kidney failure (renal disease). Also known as kidney osteodystrophy.

**osteogenesis**  The production of bone.

**osteogenesis imperfecta**  Brittle bone disease. A group of genetic diseases, all of which affect collagen in connective tissue in the body, and all of which result in fragile bones. The best known types are types I and II.

**osteogenesis imperfecta congenita**  See *osteogenesis imperfecta type II*.

**osteogenesis imperfecta tarda**  See *osteogenesis imperfecta type I*.

**osteogenesis imperfecta type I**  An inherited, generalized connective-tissue disorder featuring bone fragility and blue sclerae (blue whites of the eyes). Osteogenesis imperfecta type I is the classic, mild form of brittle bone disease. It is a dominant trait, so one copy of the mutant gene is sufficient to cause the disease, and both males and females can be affected. It is characterized by fragile bones, the onset after birth of growth deficiency, abnormal teeth that look as if they have been sandblasted, thin skin, blue sclerae, and overly extensible joints. Ten percent of patients have their first fractures noted at birth, about 25 percent in the first year, about 50 percent in the preschool years, and the balance in the early school years. The chance of fractures decreases after adolescence. Common problems include the development of bowed legs, curvature of the spine (scoliosis and kyphosis), umbilical and inguinal hernias, and mild mitral valve prolapse. Hearing impairment begins in the third decade due to otosclerosis, a disorder of the bones of the middle ear. OI I results from mutations that impair the production of type I collagen, a key component of connective tissue. Such mutations have been identified in both the COL1A1 gene on chromosome 17, and the COL1A2 gene on chromosome 7. Also known as osteogenesis imperfecta tarda, Lobstein disease.

**osteogenesis imperfecta type II**  An inherited connective-tissue disorder with very severe bone fragility. Osteogenesis imperfecta type II is the lethal form of brittle bone disease. It is a recessive trait, so two copies of the mutant gene are needed to cause the disease. Both males and females can be affected. The disease is characterized by short-limb dwarfism, thin skin, a soft skull, unusually large fontanels (soft spots), blue sclerae (bluish whites of the eyes), small nose, low nasal bridge, inguinal hernia, and numerous bone fractures at birth. There is bowing of limbs due to multiple fractures. Children with OI II are usually stillborn, or die of respiratory failure in early infancy. The condition results from mutations that impair the production of type I collagen, a key component of connective tissue. Mutations have been identified in both the COL1A1 gene on chromosome 17, and the COL1A2 gene on chromosome 7. Also known as osteogenesis imperfecta congenita, Vrolik disease.

**osteogenesis imperfecta with blue sclerae**  See *osteogenesis imperfecta type II*.

**osteogenesis, electrically stimulated**  Bone growth caused by implanting electrodes in an area of bone and sending electrical current to them. This procedure may be used to jump-start the healing process when a bone has been broken.

**osteogenic sarcoma**  See *osteosarcoma*.

**osteoid osteoma**  A benign tumor of bone tissue. It emerges most often in the teens or twenties, and is found most frequently in the femur and in males. Symptoms include pain, mostly at night. Diagnosis is by X-ray. Most cases do not require invasive treatment, but just the use of aspirin or nonaspirin analgesics for pain.

**osteomalacia**  Softening of the bone. It may be caused by poor diet or inadequate absorption of calcium and other minerals needed to harden bones. Treatment is by dietary change, and sometimes hormone supplements for postmenopausal women. See also *osteoporosis*.

**osteomyelitis**  Inflammation of the bone due to infection, for example, by the bacteria salmonella or staphylococcus. Osteomyelitis is sometimes a complication of surgery or injury, although infection can also reach bone tissue through the bloodstream. Both the bone and the bone marrow may be infected. Symptoms include deep pain and muscle spasms in the area of inflammation, and fever. Treatment is by bed rest, antibiotics (usually injected locally), and sometimes surgery to remove dead bone tissue.

**osteonecrosis**  Bone death resulting from poor blood supply to an area of bone. Also known as aseptic necrosis or avascular necrosis.

**osteopath**  An osteopathic physician; a Doctor of Osteopathy (DO). In most US states, osteopaths complete a course of study equivalent to that of an MD, and are licensed to practice medicine. They may prescribe medication and perform surgery, and they often use techniques similar to chiropractic or physical therapy.

**osteopathy**   A system of therapy founded in the 19th century, osteopathy is based on the concept that the body can formulate its own remedies against diseases when its parts are in a normal structural relationship, it has a normal environment, and it enjoys good nutrition. Although osteopathy takes a holistic approach to medical care, it also embraces modern medical knowledge, including medication, surgery, radiation, and chemotherapy when warranted. Osteopathy is particularly concerned with maintaining correct relationships between bones, muscles, and connective tissues. The practice of osteopathy often includes chiropractic-like adjustments of skeletal structures. Craniosacral therapy, a practice in which the bones and tissues of the head and neck are manipulated, also arose in osteopathy.

**osteopenia**   Mild thinning of the bone mass. Osteopenia represents a low bone mass, but is not as severe as osteoporosis. Osteopenia results when formation of new bone (osteod synthesis) is not sufficient to offset normal bone loss (lysis). Diminished bone calcification as visualized on plain X-ray film is referred to as osteopenia, whether or not osteoporosis is present.

**osteopetrosis**   Thickening of the bones. Also known as marble bones.

**osteoporosis**   Thinning of the bones with reduction in bone mass due to depletion of calcium and bone protein. Osteoporosis predisposes a person to fractures, which are often slow to heal and heal poorly. It is more common in older adults, particularly postmenopausal women; in patients on steroids; and in those who take steroidal drugs. Unchecked osteoporosis can lead to changes in posture, physical abnormality (particularly the form of hunched back known colloquially as "dowager's hump"), and decreased mobility. Treatment of osteoporosis includes ensuring that the diet contain adequate calcium and other minerals needed to promote new bone growth, and for postmenopausal women, estrogen or combination hormone supplements.

**osteosarcoma**   A cancer of the bone that is most common in children. Treatment is by surgery, usually followed by chemotherapy or radiation. Also called osteogenic sarcoma.

**osteotomy**   Taking out part or all of a bone, or cutting into or through bone.

**osteotomy, block**   Surgical removal of a section of bone.

**osteotomy, cuneiform**   Surgical removal of a triangular piece of bone.

**osteotomy, displacement**   Surgical reconfiguration of a bone by changing its physical relationship to other bones.

**ostomy**   An operation to create an opening from an area inside the body to the outside. An ostomy may be used to permit drainage of feces (colostomy) or urine from the body when the normal route is missing or blocked. It can be permanent or temporary. See also *colostomy*.

**OT**   Occupational therapist, or occupational therapy.

**Otahara syndrome**   A seizure disorder with very early onset, Otahara syndrome emerges within the first month of life. Patients may have many different types of seizures. Development is slowed, and the child can become progressively more impaired. Otahara syndrome is often due to underdevelopment of part of the brain, although it is due occasionally to a metabolic problem. An MRI scan can uncover brain underdevelopment; if none is found, metabolic testing should be done. Diagnosis is by observation and EEG. Treatment is by antispasmodic medication and educational and physical services aimed at enhancing development. Also known as early infantile epileptic encephalopathy.

**OTC**   Over-the-counter. OTC drugs are available without a prescription, in contrast to prescription drugs that require a doctor's order.

**otic barotrauma**   See *aerotitis, barotitis*.

**otitis**   Inflammation of the ear.

**otitis externa**   Inflammation of the external ear canal that leads inward to the eardrum (tympanic membrane). See *ear infection*.

**otitis interna**   Inflammation of the inner ear. See *ear infection*.

**otitis media, acute**   See *ear infection*.

**oto-**   Prefix meaning ear. For example, otitis is inflammation of the ear.

**otolaryngologist**   A doctor who specializes in treating diseases of the ear, nose, and throat.

**otology**   The study and medical care of the ear.

**otopharyngeal tube**   See *Eustachian tube*.

**otoplasty**   Plastic surgery to reshape the outer ear.

**otoscope**   Instrument for looking in the ear. Today, otoscopic or ophthalmoscopic heads can usually be attached to a single base, which supplies the electrical power, to look at the ears or eyes.

**ounce**   A measure of weight equal to 1/16 of a pound. Abbreviated as oz. An ounce of prevention is reputedly worth a pound of cure.

**outer ear**   See *ear, outer.*

**outpatient**   A patient who is not hospitalized, but instead comes to a doctor's office, clinic, or day surgery for treatment. Outpatient care is also known as ambulatory care.

**output, cardiac**   See *cardiac output.*

**ova**   Plural form of ovum.

**ovarian cancer**   See *cancer, ovarian.*

**ovarian carcinoma**   See *cancer, ovarian.*

**ovarian cyst**   See *cyst, ovarian.*

**ovarian disease, polycystic**   See *Stein-Leventhal syndrome.*

**ovarian teratoma**   An ovarian tumor, usually benign, that typically contains a diversity of tissues. It develops from a totipotential germ cell—a primary oocyte—that is retained within the ovary. Totipotential cells can give rise to all orders of cells necessary to form mature tissues and often recognizable structures, such as hair, bone, and sebaceous (oily) material, neural tissue, and teeth. Any of these tissues may be found in an ovarian teratoma. Such cysts may occur at any age, but the prime age of detection is in the childbearing years. Up to 15 percent of women with ovarian teratomas have them in both ovaries. They can range in size from less than 1/2 inch to about 17 inches in diameter. These cysts can cause the ovary to twist (torsion), imperiling its blood supply and requiring emergency surgery. The larger the dermoid cyst, the greater the risk of rupture. Spillage of its greasy contents can create problems, such as adhesions and pain. Although about 98 percent of these tumors are benign, the remaining fraction do become cancerous. Treatment is by surgical removal, which can be done by laparotomy (open surgery) or laparoscopy (with a scope). Also known as a dermoid cyst of the ovary. See also *cyst, ovarian.*

**ovary**   The female gonad, the ovary is one of a pair of reproductive glands in women. They are located in the pelvis, one on each side of the uterus. Each ovary is about the size and shape of an almond. The ovaries produce eggs (ova) and female hormones. During each monthly menstrual cycle, an egg is released from one ovary. The egg travels from the ovary through a Fallopian tube to the uterus. The ovaries are the main source of female hormones, which control the development of female body characteristics, such as the breasts, body shape, and body hair. They also regulate the menstrual cycle and pregnancy.

**ovary cyst, follicular**   See *cyst of the ovary, follicular.*

**ovary, dermoid cyst of the**   See *ovarian teratoma.*

**overgrowth**   Excessive growth.

**overgrowth syndromes**   Conditions with multiple abnormalities, including excessive growth. Early overgrowth syndromes that affect children include the Fragile X and Beckwith-Wiedemannn syndromes. Overactivity of the pituitary gland with overproduction of growth hormone causes overgrowth before adolescence, and a distinctive pattern of overgrowth called acromegaly.

**overload, iron**   See *iron excess.*

**over-the-counter drug**   See *OTC.*

**overweight**   See *obesity.*

**ovulation**   The release of the ripe egg from the ovary. The egg is released when the cavity surrounding it (the follicle) breaks open in response to a hormonal signal. Ovulation occurs around 14 or 15 days from the first day of the woman's last menstrual cycle. When ovulation occurs, the ovum moves into the Fallopian tube and becomes available for fertilization.

**ovum**   An egg within the ovary of the female. It can combine with sperm from a male to form a zygote.

**oximetry**   The process of determining the level of oxygenation in arterial blood, an important measure of whether the heart and lungs are working properly. Oximetry may be done continuously during certain medical treatments or surgery, or done sporadically to monitor a patient's health.

**oximetry catheter**   See *catheter, oximetry.*

**oxygen**   The odorless gas present in the air we breathe, and necessary to maintain life. Oxygen may be given in a medical setting, either to reduce the volume of other gases in the blood or as a vehicle for delivering anaesthetics in gas form. It can also be delivered via nasal tubes, an oxygen mask, or an oxygen tent. Patients with lung disease or damage may need to use portable oxygen devices on a temporary or permanent basis.

**oxygen mask**   A mask that covers the mouth and nose, and is hooked up to an oxygen tank. It delivers oxygen directly to the patient.

**oxygen tent**   A tent-like device used in a medical setting to deliver high levels of oxygen to a bedridden patient. The tent covers the entire head and upper body, and oxygen is pumped in from a tank.

**oxygen chamber, hyperbaric**   See *hyperbaric oxygen chamber.*

**oxygenation**   The process of treating a patient with oxygen, or of combining a medication or other substance with oxygen.

**oxymetholone**   A male hormone that stimulates production of the male hormone testosterone. It is sometimes given to treat hormonal imbalance in men or certain types of disease in both men and women.

**oxyuris**   A group of intestinal worms that includes pinworm.

**oz.**   Abbreviation for ounce.

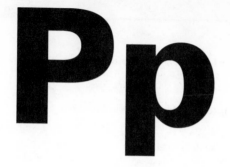

**p** **1** In biochemistry, the abbreviation for protein. For example, p53 is a protein that is 53 kilodaltons in size. **2** In population genetics, the frequency of the more common of two different alternative (allelic) versions of a gene. (The frequency of the less common allele is q.)

**p arm of a chromosome** The shorter of a chromosome's two arms. See *chromosome*.

**P-24 antibody** An antibody created by B cells in the immune system to fight the P-24 antigen. This antibody attaches to the foreign protein and sends a signal to T-4 cells to attack it. The presence of P-24 antibodies is a good sign in cases of HIV infection. See also *HIV, P-24 antigen*.

**P-24 antigen** A protein found only in the HIV virus, P-24 is considered a trend marker. In cases of HIV infection, tests for the level of P-24 antigen may be done to measure the progression of AIDS. These tests always return a positive value. On one blood test, the Coulter test, a score of 11 or less is considered negative (no disease progression), while a higher score may mean that the infection is progressing. On the Highly Sensitive (HS) blood test, the level of P-24 antigen can be detected more specifically. See also *Coulter test, HIV, HS test, P-24 antibody*.

**p.c.** Abbreviation meaning after meals. See also *Appendix A, "Prescription Abbreviations."*

**p.o.** Abbreviation meaning by mouth, orally. See also *Appendix A, "Prescription Abbreviations."*

**p.r.n.** Abbreviation meaning take as needed. See also *Appendix A, "Prescription Abbreviations."*

**p53** A protein, 53 kilodaltons in size, that is produced by a tumor-suppressor gene. Like other tumor-suppressor genes, the p53 gene normally controls cell growth. If p53 is physically lost or functionally inactivated, cells can grow without restraint.

**PA** **1** Physician assistant. **2** Posteroanterior.

**PA X-ray** An X-ray picture in which the beams pass from back to front (posteroanterior), as opposed to an AP (anteroposterior) film, in which the rays pass through the body from front to back.

**pacemaker** Usually, an artificial device that sends electrical impulses to the heart in order to set the heart rhythm. Although there are different types of pacemakers, all are designed to treat bradycardia, a heart rate that is too slow. Some pacemakers function continuously and stimulate the heart at a fixed rate or at an increased rate during exercise. A pacemaker can also be programmed to detect an overly long pause between heartbeats, and then stimulate the heart. See also *pacemaker, internal; pacemaker, natural*.

**pacemaker, internal** A pacemaker in which the electrodes into the heart, the electronic circuitry, and the power supply are all implanted internally, within the body. Also known as an implantable pacemaker, implantable artificial pacemaker.

**pacemaker, natural** The sinus node, one of the major elements in the cardiac conduction system.

**pachyonychia congenita with natal teeth** See *Jadassohn-Lewandowski syndrome*.

**pachyonychia congenita, Jadassohn-Lewandowski type** See *Jadassohn-Lewandowski syndrome*.

**pachyonychia congenita, type 1** See *Jadassohn-Lewandowski syndrome*.

**Paget disease** A condition of unknown cause in which the bone formation is out of synchrony with normal bone remodeling.

**pain** A sensation that can range from mild, localized discomfort to agony. Pain has both physical and emotional components. The physical part of pain results from nerve stimulation. Pain may be contained to a discrete area, as in an injury, or it can be more diffuse, as in disorders like fibromyalgia. See also *pain management*.

**pain management** The process of providing medical care that alleviates or reduces pain. Pain management is an extremely important part of health care, as patients forced to remain in severe pain often become agitated and/or depressed and have poorer treatment outcomes.

**pain, abdominal** Pain in the belly.

**pain, ankle** The ankle is a hinged joint that can be sprained fairly easily. Sprains are the most common cause of ankle pain. The severity of ankle sprains ranges from mild (resolving within a day or two) to severe (requiring surgical repair). Tendinitis of the ankle, another cause of ankle pain, can be caused by trauma or inflammatory arthritis.

**pain, back**   Pain in the low back can relate to the bony lumbar spine, discs between the vertebrae, ligaments around the spine and discs, spinal cord and nerves, muscles of the low back, internal organs of the pelvis and abdomen, or the skin covering the lumbar area. Causes can include injury, overstress, or disease. Pain in the upper back is more frequently muscular in nature, although it, too, can have a multitude of causes.

**pain, chest**   Chest pain has many causes, including angina, which results from inadequate oxygen supply to the heart muscle due to coronary artery disease or spasm of the coronary arteries. Treatment of angina includes rest, medication, angioplasty, and/or coronary artery bypass surgery. An incipient heart attack can also cause a type of chest pain that feels like a crushing pressure and may be preceded by tingling, numbness, or pain in an arm or the chest. Typical chest pain has more prosaic causes: heartburn, gastroesophageal reflux disease, asthma, and hyperventilation due to panic attacks are four of the most common reasons for emergency room visits due to chest pain.

**pain, elbow**   Elbow pain is most often the result of tendinitis, which can affect the inner or outer elbow. Treatment includes ice, rest, and medication for inflammation. Bacteria can infect the skin of a scraped (abraded) elbow and cause pain.

**pain, knee**   Causes of knee pain include injury, degeneration, arthritis, infrequently infection, and rarely bone tumors.

**pain, shingles**   Localized pain in the area of involvement of shingles, an inflammation of the nerves associated with the chicken pox virus in adults. When such pain persists beyond one month, it is referred to as postherpetic neuralgia. The pain can be severe and debilitating, and occurs primarily in persons over the age of 50. There is some evidence that treating shingles with steroids and antiviral agents can reduce the duration and occurrence of postherpetic neuralgia. However, the decrease is minimal. The pain of postherpetic neuralgia can be reduced by a number of medications. Tricyclic antidepressant medications like amitriptyline (brand name: Elavil), as well as antiseizure medications like gabapentin (brand name: Neurontin), have been used. Finally, capsaicin cream, a derivative of hot chili peppers, can be used topically after all blisters have healed. Acupuncture and electric nerve stimulation through the skin can be helpful for some patients.

**pains, growing**   See *growing pains*.

**palate**   The roof of the mouth. The bony front portion is called the hard palate, and the muscular back portion is the soft palate. See also *cleft palate*.

**palate, cleft**   See *cleft palate*.

**pale globe**   See *globus pallidus*.

**paleostriatum**   See *globus pallidus*.

**palilalia**   A speech disorder characterized by repetition of words or phrases, or of nonsense sounds. Palilalia may be seen in autistic spectrum disorders, Tourette syndrome, and sometimes other conditions.

**palindrome**   A word that reads the same in both directions as, for example, the names Eve and Anna. In genetics, a palindrome is a DNA or RNA sequence that reads the same in both directions. The sites of many restriction enzymes that cut (restrict) DNA are palindromes.

**palindromic rheumatism**   A form of joint inflammation whereby the joints involved appear to change periodically from one region of the body to another and back again.

**palladum**   See *globus pallidus*.

**palliate**   To treat a disease partially and insofar as possible, but not cure it completely. See *palliative care*.

**palliation**   See *palliative care*.

**palliative care**   **1** Medical or comfort care that reduces the severity of a disease or slows its progress rather than providing a cure. For incurable diseases, in cases where the cure is not recommended due to other health concerns, and when the patient does not wish to pursue a cure, palliative care becomes the focus of treatment. For example, if surgery cannot be performed to remove a tumor, radiation treatment might be tried to reduce its rate of growth, and pain management could help the patient manage physical symptoms. **2** In a negative sense, provision of only perfunctory health care when a cure is possible.

**Pallister-Killian syndrome**   A condition characterized by multiple malformations at birth, and mental retardation. It is due to isochromosome 12p mosaicism: the presence of an abnormal chromosome 12 in some cells.

**palmar surface**   The palm or grasping side of the hand.

**palpable**   Something that can be felt. A palpable growth is one that can be detected by touch.

**palpate**   To touch or feel. The liver's edge may be palpated.

**palpebra**   Medical term for eyelid. The plural is palpebrae.

**palpebral fissure**   The opening for the eyes between the eyelids.

**palpebral glands**   See *glands, Meibomian.*

**palpitations**   Unpleasant sensations of irregular and/or forceful beating of the heart. In some patients with palpitations, no heart disease or abnormal heart rhythms can be found. In others, palpitations result from abnormal heart rhythms (arrhythmias). Arrhythmias refer to heartbeats that are too slow, too rapid, irregular, or too early.

**palsy**   Paralysis, generally partial, whereby a local body area is incapable of voluntary movement. For example, Bell palsy is localized paralysis of the muscles on one side of the face.

**palsy, Bell**   See *Bell palsy.*

**palsy, cerebral**   See *cerebral palsy.*

**palsy, laryngeal**   See *laryngeal palsy.*

**palsy, laryngeal nerve**   See *laryngeal palsy.*

**paludism**   See *malaria.*

**panacea**   A universal remedy, a cure-all. The ancients sought—but never found—a panacea that would cure all disease.

**pancolitis**   See *colitis, universal; colitis, ulcerative.*

**pancreas**   A spongy, tube-shaped organ about six inches long, the pancreas is located in the back of the abdomen, behind the stomach. The head of the pancreas is on the right side of the abdomen. It is connected to the upper end of the small intestine. The narrow end of the pancreas, called the tail, extends to the left side of the body. The pancreas makes pancreatic juices and hormones, including insulin and secretin. Pancreatic juices, also called enzymes, help digest food in the small intestine. The pancreatic hormones are active in the digestive system, blood, and possibly the brain. Both enzymes and hormones are needed to keep the body working correctly. As pancreatic juices are made, they flow into the main pancreatic duct. This duct joins the common bile duct, which connects the pancreas to the liver and the gallbladder.

**pancreatic**   Having to do with the pancreas.

**pancreatic alpha cell**   See *alpha cell, pancreatic.*

**pancreatic beta cell**   See *beta cell, pancreatic.* See also *diabetes mellitus.*

**pancreatic cancer**   See *cancer, pancreatic.*

**pancreatic delta cell**   See *delta cell, pancreatic.*

**pancreatic insufficiency**   Not enough of the digestive enzymes normally secreted by the pancreas into the intestine. Pancreatic insufficiency is a hallmark of cystic fibrosis. See also *cystic fibrosis.*

**pancreatic juices**   Fluids made by the pancreas that contain digestive enzymes.

**pancreatitis**   Inflammation of the pancreas. Of the many diverse causes of pancreatitis, the most common are alcohol and gallstones.

**pancytopenia**   A shortage of all types of blood cells.

**pancytopenia, Fanconi**   See *anemia, Fanconi.*

**PANDAS**   Pediatric autoimmune disorders associated with strep. The sudden onset of symptoms like those of obsessive-compulsive disorder or Tourette syndrome following infection with streptococcus bacteria, caused by an autoimmune reaction that affects the basal ganglia in the brain. If tics are seen, they may or may not be choreaform like those of Sydenham chorea, a closely related condition that can follow a bout of rheumatic fever, which is caused by the streptococcus bacteria. Diagnosis is primarily by observation, although a blood marker for the disorder has been identified by researchers. Treatment is by plasmapheresis or intravenous immunoglobulin, prophylactic antibiotics, and/or medication for specific symptoms. See also *obsessive-compulsive disorder, streptococcus, Tourette syndrome.*

**pandemic**   An epidemic of disease that is very widespread, affecting a whole region, a continent, or the world.

**pandiculation**   One of the more wondrous medical words, pandiculation is the act of stretching and yawning.

**panencephalitis, subacute sclerosing**   See *subacute sclerosing panencephalitis.*

**pangamic acid**   See *dimethylglycine.*

**panic disorder**   An anxiety disorder characterized by sudden attacks of fear and panic. Panic attacks may occur without a known reason, but more frequently are triggered by fear-producing events or thoughts, such as taking an elevator or driving. Symptoms of panic attacks include rapid heartbeat, chest sensations, shortness of breath, dizziness, tingling, and anxiousness. Hyperventilation, agitation, and withdrawal are common results. Panic disorder is believed due to an abnormal activation of the body's hormonal system, causing a sudden "fight or flight" response. Treatment is by cognitive behavioral therapy using exposure to effect symptom reduction, and may be helped by medication.

**pantothenic acid** Vitamin B5. See *Appendix C, "Vitamins."*

**Panwarfin** See *warfarin.*

**Pap test** Microscopic examination of cells collected from the cervix, smeared on a slide, and specially stained. This test can reveal premalignant and malignant changes in the cells, as well as changes due to noncancerous conditions, such as inflammation. Also known as a Pap smear.

**papilla, fungiform** See *fungiform papillae.*

**papillary muscle** See *muscle, papillary.*

**papillary tumor** A tumor shaped like a small mushroom, with its stem attached to the inner lining of the bladder.

**papilledema** Swelling around the optic nerve, usually due to pressure on the nerve by a tumor.

**papilloma** A benign tumor that projects above the surface of the tissue from which it arises. Papillomas have clear-cut borders, and are usually small and fairly round.

**papilloma virus, human** See *human papilloma virus.*

**papilloma, cutaneous** A skin tag. See *skin tag.*

**papilloma, intraductal** See *intraductal papilloma.*

**papillomatosis** A disorder characterized by the growth of numerous papillomas (warts). For example, laryngeal papillomatosis is the presence of multiple papillomas on the vocal cords.

**papillomatosis, juvenile laryngeal** See *laryngeal papillomatosis, juvenile.*

**papillomatosis, laryngeal** See *laryngeal papillomatosis.*

**papillomatosis, recurrent respiratory** The appearance of numerous warty growths on the larynx or vocal cords, usually in children and young adults. A baby whose mother has vaginal warts can contract recurrent respiratory papillomatosis during birth. Treatment is usually by surgical excision. Recurrence is frequent, but remission may occur after several years.

**papule** A solid, rounded growth that is elevated from the skin. A papule is usually less than 1/2 inch across.

**para-** A prefix with many meanings, including alongside of, beside, near, resembling, beyond, apart from, and abnormal. For example, the parathyroid glands are adjacent to the thyroid, and paraumbilical is alongside the umbilicus.

**paracentric chromosome inversion** See *chromosome inversion, pericentric.*

**paradoxical embolism** See *embolism, paradoxical.*

**paralysis** Loss of voluntary movement (motor function). Paralysis that affects only one muscle or limb is partial paralysis, also known as palsy; paralysis of all muscles is total paralysis, as may occur in cases of botulism.

**paralysis, infantile** See *polio.*

**paralysis, laryngeal nerve** See *laryngeal paralysis.*

**paralysis, stomach** See *gastroparesis.*

**paralytic ileus** See *ileus.*

**paraneoplastic syndrome** A group of signs and symptoms caused by a substance produced by a tumor or in reaction to a tumor. Paraneoplastic syndromes can be due to a number of causes, including hormones or other biologically active products made by the tumor, blockade of the effect of a normal hormone, autoimmunity, immune-complex production, and immune suppression. By definition, a paraneoplastic syndrome is not produced by the primary tumor itself or by its metastases, nor is it caused by compression, infection, nutritional deficiency, or treatment of the tumor.

**paraphilia** One of several complex psychiatric disorders that are manifested as deviant sexual behavior. For example, in men the most common forms are pedophilia (sexual behavior or attraction toward children) and exhibitionism (exposing one's body in a public setting). Other paraphilias include compulsive sexual behavior (nymphomania and priapism), sadism, masochism, fetishism, bestiality (zoophilia), and necrophilia. Treatment may include cognitive behavioral therapy, psychotherapy, behavior modification, antidepressant medications, and medications that alter hormone production, particularly of testosterone. However, the cause and treatment of paraphilias are poorly understood, and treatment is rarely effective. In addition, many professionals prefer not to pathologize sexual behavior that involves only willing adults, even if the behavior might be deemed deviant in mainstream society. In cases where the behavior is potentially criminal, as in pedophilia, treatment is usually delivered within the penal system.

**paraphimosis** A condition in which the foreskin of the penis, once retracted, cannot return to its original location. The foreskin remains trapped behind the groove of the coronal sulcus between the shaft and the glans. This causes blood to pool in the veins behind the entrapment, leading to swelling and severe pain. The foreskin, with lubrication, can sometimes be reduced. This works only if the paraphimosis is discovered early, and requires a short-acting general anesthetic or heavy sedation. Circumcision can both prevent and cure paraphimosis.

**paraquat lung**   Paraquat, a weed killer, selectively accumulates in the lungs and is highly toxic. Once X-ray changes from paraquat are evident in the lungs, death is virtually certain. Paraquat lung emerged as a health concern in the 1970s, when the US government sprayed paraquat aerially over some illegal marijuana fields. Some of the sprayed plants survived and were sold, causing paraquat lung in purchasers who smoked the product.

**parasite**   A plant or animal organism that lives in or on another, and takes its nourishment from that other organism. Parasitic diseases include infections due to protozoa, helminths, or arthropods. For example, malaria is caused by plasmodium, a parasitic protozoa.

**parasitic**   Having to do with a parasite, as in a parasitic infection; or acting like a parasite by taking nourishment from another.

**parasympathetic nervous system**   The part of the nervous system that serves to slow the heart rate, increase intestinal and gland activity, and relax the sphincter muscles. The parasympathetic nervous system, together with the sympathetic nervous system, constitutes the autonomic nervous system.

**parathormone**   A hormone made by the parathyroid gland, parathormone is critical to maintaining calcium and phosphorus balance. Deficiency of parathormone results in abnormally low calcium in the blood (hypocalcemia). Also known as parathyrin.

**parathyrin**   See *parathormone*.

**parathyroid**   The gland that regulates calcium metabolism. The parathyroid gland is located behind the thyroid gland in the neck. It secretes a hormone called parathormone that is critical to calcium and phosphorus metabolism. Although the number of parathyroid glands can vary, most people have four, one above the other on each side. They are plastered against the back of the thyroid, and therefore are at risk for being accidentally removed during thyroidectomy.

**parathyroid hormone**   See *parathormone*.

**parathyroids, hypoplasia of the thymus and**   See *DiGeorge syndrome*.

**parenteral**   Not delivered via the intestinal tract. Something given by injection is parenteral.

**parenteral nutrition**   Intravenous feeding. Also known as parenteral alimentation.

**paresis**   Incomplete paralysis.

**paresis, general**   See *general paresis*.

**paresthesia**   An abnormal sensation of the body, such as numbness, tingling, or burning.

**parietal bone**   The side bone of the skull.

**parietal lobes**   A pair of lobes in the cerebral hemisphere that are involved in sensation, perception, memory, and integrating sensory input, primarily visual input.

**parietal pericardium**   The outer layer of the pericardium. See also *pericardium*.

**Parkinson disease**   An abnormal condition of the nervous system caused by degeneration of an area of the brain called the basal ganglia, and by low production of the neurotransmitter dopamine. The first gene connected to Parkinson was recently identified, but it is probably caused by a combination of genes and other factors. The disease results in rigidity of the muscles, slow body movement, and tremor. Most patients are over 50, but at least 10 percent are under 40. Treatment is by medication, such as levodopa (brand name: Larodopa) and carbidopa (brand name: Sinemet). A surgically implanted device that helps control the shaking has recently become available. In some cases, surgery on the globus pallidus or thalamus has proved helpful. A number of new and innovative therapies are currently under development. Also known as paralysis agitans and shaking palsy.

**parotid gland**   The largest of the three major salivary glands, the parotid gland is located in front of and below the ear, and behind the jawbone.

**parotids**   Salivary glands situated in front of the ears.

**parotitis**   Inflammation of the parotid glands, a classic feature of mumps.

**paroxysmal atrial tachycardia**   Bouts of rapid, regular heartbeating originating in the upper chamber of the heart (atrium). PAT is caused by abnormalities in the AV node that lead to rapid firing of electrical impulses from the atrium, bypassing the AV node under certain conditions. These conditions include alcohol excess, stress, caffeine, overactive thyroid or excessive thyroid hormone intake, and certain drugs. PAT is an example of an arrhythmia where the abnormality is in the electrical system of the heart, while the heart muscle and valves may be normal.

**parrot fever**   See *psittacosis*.

**Parry disease**   See *goiter, toxic multinodular*.

**parthenogenesis**   Development of a germ cell without fertilization. This is what happens in the formation of ovarian teratomas.

**partial hysterectomy**  See *hysterectomy, partial*.

**partial syndactyly**  See *syndactyly, partial*.

**parturition**  Childbirth.

**passage, nasal**  See *nasal passages*.

**Pasteur**  The French chemist and biologist Louis Pasteur (1822–1895) invented pasteurization, developed the germ theory, founded the field of bacteriology, and created the first vaccines against anthrax and rabies.

**pasteurization**  A method of treating food by heating it to a certain point, killing disease-causing organisms but keeping the flavor or quality of the food intact. Pasteurization is used with beer, milk, fruit juices, cheese, and egg products.

**PAT**  Paroxysmal atrial tachycardia.

**Patau syndrome**  A syndrome characterized by multiple malformations, commonly including scalp defects, hemangiomas (blood vessel malformations) of the face and nape of the neck, cleft lip and palate, malformations of the heart and abdominal organs, and flexed fingers with extra digits. Patients with Patau syndrome are also profoundly mentally retarded. This syndrome is due to the presence of an extra chromosome 13 (trisomy 13). The majority of trisomy 13 babies die soon after birth or in infancy. Also known as trisomy 13 syndrome.

**patella**  See *kneecap*. See also *knee*.

**patellectomy**  An operation to remove a shattered patella.

**patellofemoral joint**  The joint formed by the kneecap (patella) and the femur. See also *knee*.

**patellofemoral syndrome**  The most common cause of chronic knee pain, PFS characteristically results in vague discomfort of the inner knee area. It is aggravated by activity, such as running, jumping, climbing, or descending stairs, and also by prolonged sitting with the knees in a moderately bent position: the so-called "theater sign" of pain upon arising from a desk or theater seat. The knee may be mildly swollen. If chronic symptoms are ignored, the loss of quadriceps strength may cause the leg to "give out." PFS is caused by an abnormality in the way the kneecap slides over the lower end of the femur. Normally, the quadriceps muscle pulls the kneecap over the end of the femur in a straight line. In PFS, the kneecap is pulled toward the outer side of the femur. This off-kilter path permits the underside of the kneecap to grate along the femur, leading to chronic inflammation and pain. Females are at greater risk than males for PFS. Knock-kneed and flat-footed runners, and

persons with an unusually shaped patella, are also predisposed to PFS. Initial pain management is by icing, anti-inflammatory drugs such as ibuprofen, and avoiding motions that irritate the kneecap. Treatment and rehabilitation are designed to create a straighter pathway for the patella to follow during quadriceps contraction. Selective strengthening of the inner portion of the quadriceps muscle helps normalize its tracking. Occasionally, bracing with patellar centering devices is required. Also known as chondromalacia patella, housemaid's knee, secretary's knee.

**patent**  1 A legal device that gives exclusive control and possession of a device, invention, or procedure to an individual or corporation. Before the commercialization of biomedical inventions, the word patent had no place in a medical dictionary. Now the patent is the foundation of the biotechnology industry. Health-related items that may be patented include medical devices, surgical procedures, medications, and even cell lines.  2 Used as an adjective, patent means open, unobstructed, affording free passage. Thus, the bowel can be patent, as opposed to obstructed.

**patent ductus arteriosus**  See *ductus arteriosus*.

**patho-**  A prefix meaning suffering or disease. For example, a pathogen is a disease agent, and pathology is the study of disease.

**pathobiology**  The biology of disease.

**pathogen**  Agent of disease.

**pathogenesis**  The development of a disease, and the chain of events leading to that disease.

**pathogenic**  Capable of causing disease. Pathogenic E. coli are Escherishia coli bacteria that can make you ill.

**pathognomonic**  A sign or symptom that is so characteristic of a disease that it makes the diagnosis. For example, Koplik spots in the mouth opposite the first and second upper molars are pathognomonic of measles.

**pathologist**  A doctor who identifies diseases by studying cells and tissues under a microscope.

**pathology**  1 The study of disease. 2 Used incorrectly (but commonly) to mean disease. For example, "The doctor found no pathology" would mean he found no evidence of disease.

**-pathy**  Suffix indicating suffering or disease. For example, neuropathy is disease of the nervous system.

**Pavlov conditioning**  See *Pavlovian conditioning*.

**Pavlovian conditioning**  The Russian physiologist Ivan Petrovich Pavlov conditioned dogs to respond in what proved to be a predictable manner. For example, when he customarily rang a bell before feeding them, the dogs would begin to salivate whenever the bell rang. The principles of Pavlovian conditioning form the basis of much modern behavioral science.

**PCB**   Primary biliary cirrhosis. See *cirrhosis, primary biliary*.

**PCM**   Protein-calorie malnutrition. See *kwashiorkor*.

**PCO**   Polycystic ovarian disease. See *Stein-Leventhal syndrome*.

**PCO disease**   Polycystic ovarian disease. See *Stein-Leventhal syndrome*.

**PCP**   Pneumocystis carinii pneumonia.

**PCR**   Polymerase chain reaction.

**PDA**   Patent ductus arteriosus. See *ductus arteriosus*.

**PDR**   1 *Physicians' Desk Reference.* 2 Postdelivery room.

**pecs**   Slang term for the pectoral muscles.

**pectoral muscles**   Muscles of the front of the chest. Familiarly called the pecs.

**pectoralis muscle absence with syndactyly**   See *Poland syndrome*.

**pectus carinatum**   See *pigeon breast*.

**pectus excavatum**   See *funnel chest*.

**pediatric**   Pertaining to children.

**pediatric arthritis**   See *arthritis in children; arthritis, systemic-onset juvenile rheumatoid*.

**Pediatric Autoimmune Disorders Associated with Streptococcus**   See *PANDAS*.

**pediatric rheumatologist**   See *rheumatologist, pediatric*.

**pediatrics**   The medical specialty of care and treatment of childhood diseases.

**pediculosis**   See *head lice infestation*.

**pediculus humanus capitis**   See *head lice*.

**pedigree**   In medicine, a family health history diagrammed with a set of international symbols to indicate the individuals in the family, their relationships to one another, those with a disease, and other data. It can be used to track the transmission of hereditary conditions.

**pedodontics**   Children's dentistry.

**pedophilia**   Adult sexual interest in and activity with children. Pedophilia is a paraphilia, and if acted upon is legally defined as sexual child abuse. Pedophiles who have sexually abused children require intense psychological and pharmacological therapy prior to release into the community, because of the high rate of repeat offenders. Treatment is rarely effective, because the disorder is not yet well understood.

**peer review**   The process used by medical journals to screen articles submitted for publication. Peer-reviewed articles have been scrutinized by members of the biomedical community before publication.

**PEG**   See *gastrostomy, percutaneous endoscopic*.

**Peganone**   See *ethotoin*.

**pellagra**   Extreme niacin deficiency, characterized by a rash (dermatitis) on areas of the skin exposed to light, or trauma and ulcerations within the mouth, diarrhea, mental disorientation (dementia), confusion, delusions, and depression. Pellagra can end in death if untreated. A readily available B vitamin, niacin, both prevents and cures pellagra. See also *niacin*.

**pelvic**   Having to do with the pelvis.

**pelvic inflammatory disease**   Ascending infection of the female genital tract above the cervix, usually caused by bacteria. Symptoms include fever; foul-smelling discharge; extreme pain, including pain during intercourse; and bleeding. PID can scar the Fallopian tubes, leading to infertility. Treatment is with antibiotics, and should include the patient's sexual partners. Abbreviated as PID.

**pelvis**   The lower part of the abdomen that is located between the hip bones. Structures in the female pelvis include the uterus, vagina, ovaries, Fallopian tubes, bladder, and rectum. Structures in the male pelvis include the bladder, rectum, testicles, and penis.

**pelvis, android**   See *male pelvis*.

**pelvis, female**   See *female pelvis*.

**pelvis, gynecoid**   See *female pelvis*.

**pelvis, male**   See *male pelvis*.

**Pendred syndrome**   The hereditary association of congenital deafness and enlargement of the thyroid gland in the front of the neck (goiter) due to a defect in the making of thyroid hormone. The features of Pendred syndrome include congenital nerve deafness, defects in vestibular function, malformation of the balance portion of the ear (cochlea), a seemingly normal level of thyroid hormones (euthyroid) due to compensated hypothyroidism, swelling in front of neck, mental retardation due to congenital thyroid defect, possible increased risk of thyroid carcinoma, and evidence for defect in the making of thyroid hormone (thyroid hormone organification defect). Pendred syndrome is an autosomal recessive disorder, with both seemingly normal parents carrying a copy of the Pendred syndrome (PDS) gene. Each of their children has a 1 in 4 (25 percent) risk of inheriting both parental PDS genes and suffering from the syndrome. Also known as deafness with goiter, goiter-deafness syndrome, and thyroid hormone organification defect IIb.

**penetrance** The likelihood that a given gene will result in disease. For example, if 50 percent of people with the neurofibromatosis (NF) gene develop the disease NF, the penetrance of the NF gene would be 0.5.

**penicillin** Historically the most famous of antibiotics, penicillin kills most bacteria and some other microorganisms by attacking and destroying their cell walls. It is not effective against viruses, however, and specific penicillin types may be needed for certain bacteria. The different varieties of penicillin include amoxicillin, ampicillin, bacampicillin, carbenicillin, cloxicillin, dicloxicillin, nafcillin, oxacillin, penicillin G, and penicillin V. See also *antibiotic*.

**penicillin-resistant bacteria** A bacteria that is unaffected by penicillin. Such organisms can often be killed by using sulfa drugs, combinations of several medications, or other tactics, but some resistant infections cannot be treated successfully. The rise of penicillin-resistant bacteria is laid to overuse of penicillin drugs, including their ineffective but nonetheless frequent use against colds and viral infections.

**penile** Of or pertaining to the penis.

**penis** The external male sex organ. The penis contains two chambers, the corpora cavernosa, which run the length of the organ. These are filled with spongy tissue and surrounded by a membrane called the tunica albuginea. The spongy tissue contains smooth muscles, fibrous tissues, spaces, veins, and arteries. The urethra, which is the channel for urine and ejaculate, runs along the underside of the corpora cavernosa. The urethra emerges at the glans, the rounded tip of the penis.

**penis, cancer of the** See *cancer of the penis*.

**penis, erection of the** See *erection, penile*.

**penis, hypospadias of the** See *hypospadias*.

**penis, inflammation of the foreskin and glans** See *balanoposthitis*.

**penis, inflammation of the head of the** See *balanitis*.

**penis, small** See *micropenis*. See also *microorchidism*.

**peptic ulcer** See *ulcer, peptic*.

**percentile** The percentage of individuals in a group who have achieved a certain quantity, such as height, weight, or head circumference; or a developmental milestone. For example, the 50th percentile for walking well is 12 months of age.

**percutaneous** Through the skin, as in a percutaneous biopsy.

**percutaneous endoscopic gastrostomy** See *gastrostomy, percutaneous endoscopic*.

**percutaneous nephrolithotripsy** A technique for removing large, dense, and staghorn kidney stones. PNL is done via a port created by puncturing through the skin and into the kidney. This access port is then enlarged to about 3/8 inch in diameter. There is no surgical incision. PNL is done under anesthesia and with real-time, live X-ray control (fluoroscopy). Because X-rays are involved, a super-specialist in radiology, known as an interventional radiologist, may perform this part of the procedure. The urologist then inserts instruments into the kidney via the access port to break up the stone and to remove most of the debris from the stone.

**percutaneous transluminal coronary angioplasty** The use of a balloon-tipped catheter to enlarge a narrowed artery.

**percutaneous umbilical blood sampling** A procedure in which a needle is inserted through the mother's abdominal wall and then through the uterine wall. Blood can be withdrawn from the umbilical vein at the point where the umbilical cord inserts into the placenta. Blood may also be taken from the umbilical vein on its way to the fetal liver. PUBS is used both for prenatal diagnosis and prenatal treatment of the fetus.

**peri-** Prefix meaning around or about. For example, pericardial means around the heart, and periaortic lymph nodes are lymph nodes around the aorta.

**perianal** Located around the anus, the opening of the rectum to the outside of the body.

**perianal abscess** A local accumulation of pus that forms next to the anus, causing tender swelling in that area and pain on defecation.

**periaortic** Around the aorta: Periaortic lymph nodes are lymph nodes around the aorta.

**pericardial**   Referring to the pericardium, the sac of fibrous tissue that surrounds the heart.

**pericardial effusion**   Too much fluid within the pericardium that surrounds the heart. The pericardial sac normally contains a small amount of serous, pale yellow fluid.

**pericardial sac**   See *pericardium*.

**pericardial tamponade**   A life-threatening situation in which there is such a large amount of fluid, usually blood, inside the pericardial sac that it interferes with the performance of the heart. The end result, if untreated, is low blood pressure, shock, and death. The excess fluid in the pericardial sac acts to compress and constrict the heart. Pericardial tamponade can be due to excessive pericardial fluid, a wound to the heart, or rupture of the heart. Also called cardiac tamponade.

**pericarditis**   Inflammation of the lining around the heart (the pericardium) causing chest pain and accumulation of fluid around the heart (pericardial effusion).

**pericardium**   The conical sac of fibrous tissue that surrounds the heart and the roots of the great blood vessels. The pericardium's outer coat (the parietal pericardium) is tough and thickened, loosely cloaks the heart, and is attached to the central part of the diaphragm and the back of the breastbone. Its inner coat (the visceral pericardium, or epicardium) is double, with one layer closely adherent to the heart and the other lining the inner surface of the outer coat. The intervening space between these layers is filled with pericardial fluid. This small amount of fluid acts as a lubricant to allow normal heart movement within the chest.

**pericardium, parietal**   The tough, thickened outer layer of the pericardium. It loosely cloaks the heart, and is attached to the central part of the diaphragm and the back of the breastbone.

**pericardium, visceral**   The double inner layer of the pericardium. One layer of the visceral pericardium closely adheres to the heart, while the other lines the inner surface of the outer, or parietal, pericardium. The intervening space is filled with pericardial fluid. Also called the epicardium.

**pericentric chromosome inversion**   See *chromosome inversion, pericentric*.

**perichondrial**   Having to do with the perichondrium.

**perichondritis**   Inflammation of the perichondrium.

**perichondrium**   A dense membrane composed of fibrous connective tissue that closely wraps all cartilage,

except the cartilage in joints, which is covered by a synovial membrane.

**perichondroma**   A tumor arising from the perichondrium. Perichrondromas are benign.

**perimenopause**   See *menopause transition*. See also *menopause*.

**perinatal**   Pertaining to the period immediately before and after birth. The perinatal period is defined in diverse ways. Depending on the definition, it starts at the 20th to 28th week of gestation and ends 1 to 4 weeks after birth.

**perinatalogist**   An obstetrical subspecialist concerned with the care of the mother and fetus when there is a higher-than-normal risk of complications. Most perinatologist are obstetricians. A high-risk baby might be cared for by a perinatologist before birth and by a neonatologist after birth.

**perinatalogy**   A subspecialty of obstetrics concerned with the care of the mother and fetus when there is a higher-than-normal risk for complications.

**perineal surgery**   An operation to remove the prostate gland through an incision made between the scrotum and the anus.

**perineum**   The area between the anus and the scrotum in the male, or between the anus and the vulva in the female. The female perineum is sometimes known by the folk term taint. See also *episiotomy*.

**periodontal**   Having to do with the gums and supporting structures of the teeth.

**periodontal disease**   A bacterial infection that destroys the attachment fibers and supporting bone that hold the teeth in the mouth. Left untreated, these diseases can lead to tooth loss. The main cause of periodontal disease is bacterial plaque, a sticky, colorless film that constantly forms on teeth.

**periodontics**   The branch of dentistry concerned with prevention, diagnosis, and treatment of diseases affecting the gums and supporting structures of the teeth. Periodontists are also expert in the placement and maintenance of dental implants. Periodontics is one of the eight dental specialties recognized by the American Dental Association.

**periodontitis**   Gum disease with inflammation of the gums. See *periodontal disease*.

**periosteal**   Pertaining to the periosteum.

**periosteoma**   A benign tumor arising from the periosteum. Also called a periostoma.

**periosteum** A dense membrane composed of fibrous connective tissue that closely wraps all bone, except that of the articulating surfaces in joints, which are covered by a synovial membrane.

**periostitis** Inflammation of the periosteum.

**periostoma** A benign tumor arising from the periosteum.

**peripheral** Situated away from the center, as opposed to centrally located. For example, peripheral vision means the type of vision that allows one to see objects which are not in the center of one's visual field.

**peripheral blood stem cell transplantation** See *stem cell harvest, peripheral blood; stem cell transplantation.*

**peripheral nervous system** That portion of the nervous system that is outside the brain and spinal cord. The nerves in the peripheral nervous system (PNS) connect the central nervous system (CNS) to sensory organs, such as the eye and ear, and to other organs of the body, muscles, blood vessels, and glands. The peripheral nerves include the 12 cranial nerves, the spinal nerves and roots, and the autonomic nerves. The autonomic nerves are concerned with automatic functions of the body. Specifically, autonomic nerves are involved with the regulation of the heart muscle, the tiny muscles lining the walls of blood vessels, and glands.

**peripheral neuropathy** A problem with the functioning of the nerves outside the spinal cord. Symptoms may include numbness, weakness, burning pain (especially at night), and loss of reflexes.

**peripheral pulmonary stenosis with cholestasis** See *Alagille syndrome.*

**peripheral T cells** See *T cells, peripheral.*

**peristalsis** The rippling motion of muscles in the digestive tract. In the stomach, this motion mixes food with gastric juices, turning it into a thin liquid.

**peritoneal** Having to do with the peritoneum.

**peritoneal dialysis** A dialysis technique that uses the patient's own body tissues inside the abdominal cavity as a filter. A plastic tube called a dialysis catheter is placed through the abdominal wall into the abdominal cavity. A special fluid is then flushed into the abdominal cavity and washes around the intestines. The intestinal walls act as a filter between this fluid and the bloodstream. By using different types of solutions, waste products and excess water can be removed from the body.

**peritoneum** The membrane that lines the abdominal cavity and covers most of the abdominal organs.

**peritonitis** Inflammation of the peritoneum. Peritonitis can result from infection, as by bacteria or parasites; injury and bleeding; or diseases, such as systemic lupus erythematosus.

**peritonsillar abscess** A collection of pus behind the tonsils that pushes one of the tonsils toward the uvula. A peritonsillar abscess is generally very painful. It is usually associated with a decreased ability to open the mouth. If left untreated, the infection can spread deep in the neck, causing airway obstruction and life-threatening complications.

**pernicious anemia** See *anemia, pernicious.*

**pernicious vomiting of pregnancy** See *hyperemesis gravidarum.*

**perspiration** 1 The secretion of fluid by the sweat (sudoriferous) glands. These small, tubular glands are situated within the skin, as well as in the subcutaneous tissue under it. They discharge their fluid through tiny openings in the surface of the skin. Perspiration serves at least two purposes: the removal of waste products such as urea and ammonia, and cooling of the body as sweat evaporates. 2 The transparent, colorless, acidic fluid secreted by the sweat glands. It contains some fatty acids and mineral matter. Adult perspiration gains its characteristic odor from the waste products excreted. Also known as sweat.

**pertussis** Whooping cough, a communicable, potentially deadly illness characterized by fits of coughing followed by a noisy, "whooping" indrawn breath. It is caused by the bacteria Bordetella pertussis. The illness is most likely to affect young children, but sometimes appears in teenagers and adults, even those who have been previously immunized. Immunization with DPT (diphtheria-pertussis-tetanus) vaccine provides protection, although that immunity may wear off with age. When teenagers and adults get pertussis, it appears first as coughing spasms, and then as a stubborn dry cough that lasts up to eight weeks. Treatment is by supportive therapy, and young infants need hospitalization if the coughing becomes severe. See *DPT immunization, DTaP immunization.*

**pes** Latin word meaning foot.

**pes cavus** A foot with too high an arch.

**pes planum** Flat feet.

**pest** See *plague.*

**pestilence**   Originally referring to the bubonic plague, pestilence now refers to any epidemic disease that is highly contagious, infectious, virulent, and devastating. See also *plague*.

**pestis**   See *plague*.

**petechiae**   Tiny red spots in the skin that do not blanch when pressed upon. They result from red blood leaking from capillaries. They are not infrequently seen in the legs of patients taking aspirin, because of its mild blood-thinning effect.

**petit mal**   See *seizure, absence; seizure disorders*.

**Pfeiffer syndrome**   A form of craniosynostosis that results in multiple physical defects, including broad thumbs and great toes; depressed nasal bridge and generally flat profile; low-set, slanted ears; strabismus; and a prominent mandible. There may also be internal defects of the gallbladder, heart, inner ear, and other areas; and CNS abnormalities if there is a cloverleaf skull. Diagnosis is by comparison to similar syndromes, such as Alpert syndrome, and by chromosome analysis. Treatment is by surgery. See also *acrocephalosyndactyly, fibroblast growth factor receptor 2*.

**phacoemulsification**   A type of contemporary cataract surgery in which the lens with the cataract is broken up by ultrasound, irrigated, and suctioned out.

**phage**   See *bacteriophage*.

**phagedenic gingivitis**   See *acute membranous gingivitis*.

**phagocyte**   A cell that can engulf particles, such as bacteria and other microorganisms, or foreign matter. The principal phagocytes include the neutrophils and monocytes, both types of white blood cells.

**phalanges**   The bones of the fingers and of the toes. There are generally three phalanges (distal, middle, proximal) for each digit, except the thumbs and large toes. The singular of phalanges is phalanx.

**phalanx**   A general term for any one of the two or three bones in each finger or toe.

**phantom limb syndrome**   The perception of sensations, often including pain, in an arm or leg long after the limb has been amputated. Phantom limb syndrome is relatively common in amputees, especially in the early months and years after limb loss.

**phantom sensations**   Phenomena involving any of the senses that mimic the presence of sensory abilities no longer available. They are probably caused by abnormal firing of nerve impulses, although the mechanism for these sensations is not understood. For example, people who have lost much of their vision often experience visual phantoms. See also *phantom limb syndrome*.

**pharmacist**   A professional who fills prescriptions, and in the case of a compounding pharmacist, makes them. Pharmacists are very familiar with medication ingredients, interactions, cautions, and hints.

**pharmacogenetics**   The convergence of pharmacology and genetics, dealing with genetically determined responses to drugs. For example, after the administration of a muscle relaxant commonly used in surgery, a patient may remain apneic: incapable of breathing on his or her own for hours due to a genetically determined defect in metabolizing the muscle relaxant. The study of pharmacogenetics would seek to identify such patients and prevent the improper choice of that muscle relaxant. More prosaically, pharmacogenetics can find out about common differences in the metabolization of medications between children, adults, and senior citizens; men and women; and people with various medical conditions.

**pharmacologist**   A specialist in the science of drugs. A pharmacologist is usually especially knowledgeable about new and obscure medications that may be needed for hard-to-treat or rare illnesses, and about drug interactions and how to prevent them. Pharmacologists usually act as consultants to primary care physicians or specialists.

**pharmacology**   **1** The study of concocting and using medications. **2** The study of drugs, their sources, their nature, and their properties.

**pharmacopeia**   An official authoritative listing of drugs. Aspirin, for example, has long been in the pharmacopeia. Some countries, such as the UK, establish an official pharmacopeia, as do some medical groups and HMOs.

**pharmacy**   A location where prescription drugs are sold. A pharmacy is constantly supervised by a licensed pharmacist.

**pharmacy, compounding**   A place that both makes and sells prescription drugs. A compounding pharmacy can often concoct drug formulas that are specially tailored to patients: for example, liquid versions of medications normally available only in pill form, for patients who cannot swallow pills.

**pharyngeal**   Having to do with the throat (pharynx).

**pharyngitis**   Inflammation of the pharynx. Pharyngitis is a common cause for a sore throat.

**pharynx** The hollow tube about five inches long that starts behind the nose and ends at the top of the trachea (windpipe) and esophagus.

**phase, resting** See *interphase*.

**PhD** Doctor of Philosophy. PhDs are involved in clinical care, as in clinical psychology; biomedical research, as in the Genome Project; health administration, teaching, and other areas of medicine.

**phenocopy** A defect due to an environmental agent that imitates a defect produced by a specific gene.

**phenomenon, Babinski** See *Babinski reflex*.

**phenomenon, phantom limb** See *phantom limb syndrome*.

**phenomenon, Raynaud** See *Raynaud phenomenon*.

**phenotype** The appearance of an individual, which results from the interaction of the person's genetic makeup and his or her environment. By contrast, the genotype is merely the genetic constitution (genome) of an individual. For example, if a child's genotype includes the gene for osteogenesis imperfecta (brittle bone disease), minimal trauma can cause fractures. The gene is the genotype, and the brittle bones themselves are the phenotype.

**phenylketonuria** Inherited inability to process the amino acid phenylalanine. In the US, newborns are screened for PKU with a blood test. Treatment is a diet low in phenylalanine. Failure of treatment results in mental retardation, sometimes with autistic features. Abbreviated as PKU.

**Philadelphia chromosome** The hallmark of chronic myeloid leukemia (CML). The Philadelphia (Ph) chromosome is an abbreviated chromosome 22 that was shortchanged in an exchange with chromosome 9. This translocation occurs in a bone-marrow cell, and causes CML.

**Philippine hemorrhagic fever** See *dengue hemorrhagic fever*.

**philtrum** The area from below the nose to the upper lip. Normally the philtrum is grooved. In fetal alcohol syndrome, the philtrum is flat.

**phimosis** A condition in which the foreskin of the penis is too tight to be pulled back to reveal the glans. Circumcision prevents phimosis.

**phlebitis** Inflammation of a vein. With phlebitis, there is infiltration of the walls of the vein and, usually, the formation of a clot (thrombus) in the vein (thrombophlebitis). Phlebitis in a leg, for example, will cause the leg to swell with fluid (edema). The swollen leg will feel stiff and painful.

**phlebo-** Prefix meaning vein. For example, phlebitis is inflammation of the veins, and a phlebotomist is a person who draws blood from veins.

**phlebotomist** A person who draws blood. Most, but not all, phlebotomists are registered nurses (RNs).

**phlebotomy** Obtaining blood from a vein. This may be for diagnostic tests or treatment: for example, to relieve the iron overload in hemochromatosis.

**phobia** An unreasonable sort of fear that can cause avoidance and panic. Phobias are a relatively common type of anxiety disorder. Examples are extreme fear of spiders, called arachnophobia, and fear of being outside, which is known as agoraphobia. Phobias can be treated with cognitive behavioral therapy, using exposure and fear-reduction techniques. In many cases, antianxiety or antidepressant medication proves helpful, especially during the early stages of therapy.

**phocomelia** A birth defect in which the hands and feet are attached to abbreviated arms and legs. Phocomelia was one consequence of exposure of the developing fetus to the drug thalidomide.

**phosphatase, acid** See *acid phosphatase*.

**phosphatase, alkaline** See *alkaline phosphatase*.

**phosphate** A form of phosphoric acid. Phosphate may bind to other organic chemicals to form a variety of compounds. For example, calcium phosphate makes bones and teeth hard. See also *phosphorylation*.

**phosphorus** An essential element in the diet, and a major component of bone.

**phosphorylation** A biochemical process that involves the addition of phosphate to an organic compound. Examples include the addition of phosphate to glucose to produce glucose monophosphate, and the addition of phosphate to adenosine diphosphate (ADP) to form adenosine triphosphate (ATP). Phosphorylation is carried out through the action of enzymes known as phosphotransferases or kinases.

**photodynamic therapy** Treatment that destroys cancer cells with lasers, or with drugs that become active when exposed to light.

**photophobia** Painful oversensitivity to light. For example, photophobia is often seen in measles. Keeping the lights dim or the room darkened is helpful when a patient has photophobia. Sunglasses may also help.

**photorefractive keratectomy** A kind of laser eye surgery designed to change the shape of the cornea, potentially eliminating or reducing the need for glasses or contact lenses. The laser is used to remove the outer layer of the cornea and flatten the cornea. The flattening of the cornea is intended to correct myopia (nearsightedness) and astigmatism (uneven curvature of the cornea that distorts vision). PRK is done in the doctor's office with anesthesia via numbing eye drops. It takes about one minute to do, and about three days to heal. No eye patch need be worn after PRK.

**photosensitivity** The skin is oversensitive to light.

**phototherapy** Treatment with light. For example, a newborn with jaundice may be put under special lights that help reduce the amount of bilirubin pigment in the skin.

**PHS** Public Health Service.

**physiatrist** A physician specializing in physical medicine and rehabilitation. Physiatrists specialize in restoring optimal function to people with injuries to the muscles, bones, tissues, or nervous system, such as stroke victims.

**physical child abuse** See *child abuse*.

**physical map** A map of the locations of identifiable landmarks on chromosomes. Physical distance is measured in base pairs. The physical map differs from the genetic map, which is based purely on genetic linkage data. In the human genome, the lowest-resolution physical map is the banding patterns of the 24 different chromosomes. The highest-resolution physical map is the complete nucleotide sequence of all chromosomes.

**physical therapist** A person trained and certified by a state or accrediting body to design and implement physical therapy programs. Physical therapists may work in a hospital or clinic, in a school that provides assistance to special education students, or as an independent practitioner.

**physical therapy** A branch of rehabilitative health that uses specially designed exercises and equipment to help patients regain or improve their physical abilities. Physical therapists work with many types of patients, from infants born with musculoskeletal birth defects, to adults suffering from sciatica or the after-effects of injury, to elderly poststroke patients.

**physician** A person trained in the art of healing. Contemporary physicians express their skills by combining art with science. In the UK, a physician is a specialist in internal or general medicine, whereas in the US it is a more general term for a doctor of medicine. The term generally refers to a person who has earned a Doctor of Medicine (MD), Doctor of Osteopathy (DO), or Doctor of Naturopathy (ND) degree, and who is accepted as a practitioner of medicine under the laws of the state, province, and/or nation in which he or she practices.

**physician assistant** A midlevel medical practitioner who works under the supervision of a licensed doctor (MD), osteopathic physician (DO), or naturopathic doctor (ND). Although the physician need not be present during the time the PA performs his or her duties, there must be a method of contact between the supervising physician and the PA at all times.

***Physicians' Desk Reference*** A thick volume that provides a guide to all prescription drugs available in the United States. Although not exactly recommended for bedtime reading, it is a key reference to the American pharmacopeia. Abbreviated as PDR.

**physiologic** Something that is normal, neither due to anything pathologic nor significant in terms of causing illness.

**physiologic amenorrhea** See *amenorrhea, physiologic*.

**physiology** The study of how living organisms function, including such processes as nutrition, movement, and reproduction.

**phytanic acid storage disease** See *Refsum disease*.

**phytochemicals** Active health-protecting compounds that are components of plants. Antioxidant, immuneboosting, and other properties of active compounds in plants are being investigated. Phytochemicals that are being studied include terpenes, carotenoids, limonoids, and phytosterols. Also known as phytonutrients.

**phytonutrients** See *phytochemicals*.

**pia mater** One of the meninges, the pia mater is the delicate innermost membrane enveloping the brain and spinal cord. It is known informally as the pia.

**pianist's cramp** A dystonia that affects the muscles of the hand and sometimes the forearm, and only occurs when one plays the piano or another keyboard instrument. Similar focal dystonias have also been called writer's cramp, typist's cramp, musician's cramp, and golfer's cramp.

**pica** A craving for something not normally regarded as nutritive, such as dirt, clay, paper, or chalk. Pica is a classic clue to iron deficiency in children, and may also occur in zinc deficiency. Pica is also seen as a symptom in several neurobiological disorders, including autism and Tourette syndrome, and is sometimes seen during pregnancy.

**Pick disease**  A form of dementia characterized by a slowly progressive deterioration of social skills and changes in personality, leading to impairment of intellect, memory, and language. See also *dementia*.

**Pickwickian syndrome**  A syndrome characterized by the combination of obesity, somnolence, hypoventilation, and red face.

**PID**  Pelvic inflammatory disease.

**pigeon breast**  With a prominent breastbone and chest. Medically, pigeon breast is called pectus carinatum.

**pigment**  A substance that gives color to tissue. Pigments are responsible for the color of skin, eyes, and hair.

**piles**  See *hemorrhoids*.

**Pill, the**  Slang term for oral contraceptive pill.

**pilonidal cyst**  A special kind of abscess that occurs in the cleft between the buttocks. Pilonidal cysts are common in adolescence, often after long trips that involve sitting.

**pilonidal sinus**  A dimple in the crease between the buttocks.

**pimples**  Oil glands infected with bacteria, which results in an inflamed area with pus formation. Pimples are due to overactivity of the oil glands located at the base of the hair follicles, especially on the face, back, chest, and shoulders.

**pineal gland**  A small gland located deep within the brain. It is believed to secrete melatonin, and may therefore be part of the body's sleep-regulation apparatus.

**pineal region tumors**  A brain tumor on or near the pineal gland. There are at least 17 types of pineal gland tumors, most of which are not cancerous but can nonetheless cause extreme distress. They account for about 1 percent of brain tumors in adults, but up to 8 percent of such tumors in children. Symptoms include frozen upward gaze, hydrocephalus, and precocious puberty. Diagnosis is by biopsy of affected tissue. Treatment of benign pineal tumors is by surgery; malignant tumors are usually treated with radiation followed by chemotherapy.

**pineoblastoma**  A fast-growing brain tumor in the pineal gland that originates in germ cells. Also known as a pineal teratoma.

**pineocytoma**  A slow-growing type of brain tumor that arises in pineal cells.

**pinguecula**  A yellow spot on the white of the eye, usually toward the inside of the eye, associated with aging. It looks fatty, and is due to an accumulation of connective tissue.

**pinguicula**  Alternate spelling of pinguecula.

**pinkeye**  See *conjunctivitis*.

**pinna**  1 The ear. 2 The part of the ear that projects like a little wing from the head.

**pinworm infestation**  An infestation of the intestinal tract by a small, white worm: the pinworm or, more formally, Enterobius vermicularis. The pinworm is about the length of a staple, and lives for the most part within the rectum of humans. While a pinworm-infested person is asleep, female pinworms leave the intestines through the anus and deposit eggs on the skin around the anus. Most symptoms of pinworms are mild, such as anal itching, disturbed sleep, and irritability. If the infection is heavy, however, symptoms may include loss of appetite, restlessness, and insomnia. Pinworm is the most common worm infection in the United States. School-age children have the highest rates of pinworm infection, followed in frequency by preschoolers. Pinworms spread easily in day care centers, schools, and homes. Within a few hours of being deposited on the skin around the anus, pinworm eggs become capable of infesting another person. They can survive up to two weeks on clothing, bedding, or other objects. If pinworms are suspected, transparent adhesive tape or a pinworm paddle supplied by your health care provider is applied to the anal region. The eggs adhere to the sticky tape or paddle, and are identified by examination under a microscope. The test should be done as soon as you wake up in the morning, because bathing or having a bowel movement may remove eggs. Also known as enterobiasis.

**piriformis muscle**  See *muscle, piriformus*.

**piriformis syndrome**  Irritation of the sciatic nerve caused by compression of the nerve within the buttock by the piriformis muscle. Typically, the pain of piriformis syndrome is increased by contraction of the piriformis muscle, prolonged sitting, or direct pressure applied to the muscle. Buttock pain is common. The piriformis syndrome can cause difficulty walking due to pain in the buttock and lower extremity. The piriformis syndrome is one of the causes of sciatica. The doctor can often detect tenderness of the piriformis muscle during a rectal examination. Piriformis syndrome is treated with rest and measures to reduce inflammation of the muscle and its tendon. Treatments include piriformis stretching exercises, physical therapy, anti-inflammatory medications, and pain medications. With persistent symptoms, further treatment can include local injection of anesthetic and cortisone medication. Rarely, surgery is performed to relieve the pressure. During surgical operations, the piriformis muscle is thinned, elongated, divided, or removed.

**pit, ear**   See *ear pit*.

**pituitary adenoma**   A benign tumor of the pituitary, the master gland that controls other glands and influences numerous body functions, including growth. Although the tumor itself is not cancerous, it may affect pituitary function, and therefore may need to be removed. See also *pituitary gland; gigantism, pituitary*.

**pituitary dwarfism**   See *dwarfism, pituitary*.

**pituitary gigantism**   See *gigantism, pituitary*. See also *acromegaly*.

**pituitary gland**   The main endocrine gland, the pituitary gland produces hormones that control other glands and many body functions, especially growth.

**PKU**   Phenylketonuria.

**placebo**   A sugar pill or any other inactive substance given instead of medication. In a controlled clinical trial, one group may be given a medication and another group a placebo, to learn whether a difference in treatment response is due to the medication, the power of suggestion, or other factors. See also *placebo response*.

**placebo response**   A positive medical response to taking a placebo, as if it were an active medication. Up to one-third of patients given a placebo may respond with a reduction in symptoms, depending on the condition. Although this phenomenon is often laid to patients believing their symptoms have improved when in fact they have not, evidence is beginning to emerge that actual physiological changes can result from believing that one is receiving medical treatment.

**placenta**   A temporary organ joining the mother and fetus, the placenta transfers oxygen and nutrients from the mother to the fetus, and permits the release of carbon dioxide and waste products from the fetus. It is roughly disk-shaped, and at full term measures about seven inches in diameter and a bit less than two inches thick. The upper surface of the placenta is smooth, while the under surface is rough. The placenta is rich in blood vessels. The placenta is expelled with the fetal membranes during the birth process; together, these structures form the afterbirth.

**placenta accreta**   The abnormal adherence of the chorionic villi to the myometrium. Normally there is tissue intervening between the chorionic villi and the myometrium, but in placenta accreta, these vascular processes of the chorion grow directly in the myometrium. Placenta accreta can progress into placenta percreta.

**placenta percreta**   A placenta that invades the uterine wall. In placenta percreta, the vascular processes of the chorion (the chorionic villi), a fetal membrane that enters into the formation of the placenta, may invade the full thickness of the myometrium. This can cause an incomplete rupture of the uterus. The chorionic villi can go right on through both the myometrium and the outside covering of the uterus (serosa), causing complete and catastrophic rupture of the uterus.

**placenta previa**   A placenta implanted near the outlet of the uterus, so that at the time of delivery the placenta precedes the baby. Placenta praevia can cause painless bleeding in the last third of pregnancy, and may be a reason for a C-section. Also known as low placenta.

**placenta, accessory**   An extra placenta that is separate from the main placenta. Also known as a succenturiate or supernumerary placenta.

**placenta, low**   See *placenta previa*.

**placenta, succenturiate**   See *placenta, accessory*.

**placenta, supernumerary**   See *placenta, accessory*.

**placental chorioangioma**   A benign vascular (blood vessel) tumor of the placenta. Large chorioangiomas can cause complications, including excess amniotic fluid (polyhydramnios), maternal and fetal clotting problems (coagulopathies), premature delivery, toxemia, fetal heart failure, and hydrops (excess fluid) affecting the fetus. Chorioangiomas probably act as peripheral shunts between arteries and veins, leading to progressive heart failure of the fetus. Labor is usually induced once the fetus is viable. Fetal blood transfusion has also been used in fetuses found to be anemic. Alcohol injection into the placental chorioangioma is being tried as a new method of treatment.

**placental dystocia**   Difficulty in delivering the placenta. A number of techniques may be tried, including changing position, massage, nursing the newborn baby to induce uterine contractions, and in some cases medications that induce uterine contractions.

**placental stage of labor**   The part of labor that lasts from the birth of the baby until the placenta and fetal membranes are delivered. Also known as the third stage of labor.

**plague** An infectious disease caused by the bacteria Yersinia pestis. Y. pestis mainly infects rats and other rodents. Fleas function as the prime vectors for carrying the bacteria from one species to another. The fleas bite the rodents infected with Y. pestis, and then they bite people and so transmit the disease. Transmission of the plague to people can also occur from eating infected animals, such as squirrels. Once someone has the plague, he or she can transmit it to another person via aerosol droplets. The plague has been responsible for devastating epidemics. The disease occurs at a consistent but low level (endemically) in many countries, including the US. It can now be easily treated with antibiotics, if caught early enough. Also known as pest and pestis. See also *bubonic plague*.

**plague, black** In 14th century Europe, this name was used to describe the plague, in which victims had bleeding below the skin (subcutaneous hemorrhage) that darkened their bodies.

**plague, bubonic** The most common form of the plague, named for the characteristic buboes: enlarged, painful lymph nodes in the groin, armpits, neck, and elsewhere. Other features of the bubonic plague include headache, fever, chills, and weakness. Bubonic plague is caused by the bacteria Y. pestis, and can be treated with antibiotics. See also *plague*.

**Plague, Great** An epidemic that swept London in 1665. Today the Great Plague is believed to have been an epidemic of typhus, not of bubonic or other plague. See also *typhus, epidemic*.

**plague, sylvatic** Plague that is spread by ground squirrels and other wild rodents. It is sometimes seen in the western portion of the United States.

**plantar** Having to do with the sole of the foot.

**plantar fasciitis** See *fasciitis, plantar*.

**plantar response** See *Babinski reflex*.

**plantar warts** See *warts, plantar*.

**plaque** The white, semihardened substance that forms on the teeth as a result of bacterial action on food particles. Plaque formation provides an ideal environment for dental caries (cavities) to develop. To reduce the risk, plaque should be removed by daily brushing and flossing, and by regular dental cleanings.

**plaque, skin** A broad, raised area on the skin. By definition, a skin plaque has a greater surface than its elevation above the skin surface: it is broader than it is high.

**plasma** The liquid part of the blood and lymphatic fluid, which makes up about half its volume. Plasma is devoid of cells and, unlike serum, has not clotted. Blood plasma contains antibodies and other proteins. It is taken from donors and made into medications for a variety of blood-related conditions. Some blood plasma is also used in nonmedical products.

**plasma cells** Special white blood cells that produce antibodies.

**plasma donation** The donation or sale of blood plasma for use in medical or other products. Unlike blood donors, most plasma donors in the US are paid. The procedure is done in a walk-in facility, where whole blood is taken through an IV needle, and separated into plasma and blood cells. The blood cells are then returned intravenously to the donor. As long as the IV needles are disposable and not reused, there is no danger of infection for plasma donors.

**plasmacytoma** A tumor that is made up of cancerous plasma cells.

**plasmapheresis** A procedure in which whole blood is taken and separated into plasma and blood cells; the plasma is removed and replaced with another solution, such as saline, albumin, or specially prepared donor plasma; and the reconstituted solution is then returned to the patient. Plasmapheresis is used increasingly to treat autoimmune disorders, such as lupus, multiple sclerosis, and PANDAS. When the plasma is removed, it takes with it the antibodies that have been developed against self-tissue, hopefully stopping the attack on the patient's own body. Plasmapheresis carries with it the same risks as any intravenous procedure, but is otherwise generally safe. The risk of infection increases with the use of donor plasma, which may carry viral particles despite screening procedures. The procedure is done in a clinical or hospital setting. Topical numbing cream may be used to reduce discomfort.

**plasmid** A self-replicating (autonomous) circle of DNA that is distinct from the chromosomal genome of bacteria. A plasmid contains genes that normally are not essential for cell growth or survival. Some plasmids can integrate into the host genome, be artificially constructed in the laboratory, and serve as vectors for cloning.

**Plasmodium** The parasite guilty of causing malaria. Plasmodium is a type of protozoa, a single-celled organism able to divide only within a host cell.

**plastic surgeon** A surgeon who specializes in reducing scarring or disfigurement that may occur as a result of accidents, birth defects, or treatment for diseases, such as melanoma. Many plastic surgeons also perform cosmetic surgery that is unrelated to medical conditions, such as rhinoplasty to change the shape of the nose.

**plasticity, brain**   See *brain plasticity*.

**platelets**   Irregular, disc-shaped elements of the blood that assist in blood clotting. During normal blood clotting, the platelets group together (aggregate). Although platelets are often classed as blood cells, they are actually fragments of large cells called megakaryocytes. Also known as thrombocytes. See also *blood cell*.

**pleiotropic**   Producing or having multiple effects from a single gene. For example, the Marfan gene is pleiotropic, potentially causing long fingers and toes (arachnodactyly), dislocation of the lens of the eye, and dissecting aneurysm of the aorta.

**pleomorphic**   Many-formed. A tumor may be pleomorphic. Also known as protean.

**plethoric**   Florid, red-faced.

**pleura**   The thin covering that protects and cushions the lungs. The pleura is made up of two layers of tissue, which are separated by a small amount of fluid.

**pleural effusion**   Outpouring of fluid between the two layers of the pleural membranes that cover the lungs.

**pleural space**   The tiny area between the two layers of the pleura, which is normally filled with a small amount of fluid.

**pleurisy**   Pain as a result of inflammation of the pleural membrane that envelops the lungs. Pleurisy is typically noted as pain in the involved area of the chest, and is felt when the patient breathes.

**pleuritis**   Inflammation of the pleura. When the pleura becomes inflamed, it can produce more than the normal amount of fluid, causing a pleural effusion.

**pleurodynia**   See *Bornholm disease*.

**plumbism**   Lead poisoning.

**Plummer disease**   See *goiter, toxic multinodular*.

**PMR**   Polymyalgia rheumatica.

**PMS**   Premenstrual syndrome.

**pneumatic larynx**   A device that uses air to produce sound, helping a person whose larynx has been removed to talk.

**pneumo-**   Prefix pertaining to breathing, respiration, the lungs, pneumonia, or air.

**pneumococcal pneumonia immunization**   A vaccine that prevents one of the most common and severe forms of pneumonia. It is usually given only once in a lifetime, usually after the age of 55, to someone with ongoing lung problems such as chronic obstructive pulmonary disease or asthma, or to persons with other chronic diseases, including those involving the heart and kidneys. This vaccination is rarely given to children.

**pneumococcus**   See *Streptococcus pneumoniae*.

**pneumoconiosis**   Inflammation and irritation caused by deposition of particulate matter, such as asbestos and silicon, in the lungs.

**pneumocystis carinii pneumonia**   A parasitic infection of the lungs that is particularly common and life-threatening in immunosuppressed persons. Preventative treatment (prophylaxis) is available to prevent PCP in persons who are at special risk.

**pneumomediastinum**   Free air in the space between the lungs (mediastinum), which may give rise to pneumothorax or pneumopericardium, and compromise the lungs or heart.

**pneumonectomy**   An operation to remove an entire lung.

**pneumonia**   An infection that occurs when fluid and cells collect in the lungs.

**pneumonia, aspiration**   Inflammation of the lungs due to aspiration: the sucking in of food particles or fluids into the lungs.

**pneumonitis, radiation**   Inflammation of the lungs as a result of radiation. Although the radiation can be from various sources, including accidents, today it is usually from radiation therapy. Radiation pneumonitis typically occurs after radiation treatments for cancers within the chest or breast. Radiation pneumonitis usually manifests itself two weeks to six months after completion of radiation therapy. Symptoms include shortness of breath upon activity, cough, and fever. Radiation pneumonitis frequently is discovered serendipitously, as an incidental finding on a chest X-ray in patients who have no symptoms. Blood testing can indicate inflammation is present in the body. Abnormal white blood count and sedimentation rates are common. If radiation pneumonitis persists, it can lead to scarring of the lungs, referred to as radiation fibrosis. Radiation fibrosis typically occurs one year after the completion of radiation treatments. Radiation pneumonitis is often reversible with medications that reduce inflammation, such as cortisone drugs. Radiation fibrosis, however, is usually irreversible. See also *fibrosis, radiation*.

**pneumopericardium**   Air or other gas in the sac surrounding the heart (pericardium).

**pneumothorax**   Free air in the chest outside the lung. Pneumothorax can occur spontaneously, follow a fractured rib, occur in the wake of chest surgery, or be deliberately induced in order to collapse the lung.

**PNL**   Percutaneous nephrolithotripsy.

**PNS**   Peripheral nervous system.

**podiatrist**   A physician who specializes in the evaluation and treatment of diseases of the foot. The modern specialty of Podiatric Medicine and Surgery requires a minimum of three years of college education and completion of the Medical College Admission Test before an applicant will be considered for acceptance to one of the seven colleges of Podiatric Medicine. Training includes studies in the basic medical sciences, emphasizing the health and conditions affecting the lower extremities. Diagnosis and treatment skills, including surgery, are developed in the third and fourth years. A required National Board Examinations test is given prior to graduation. The graduate receives the degree of Doctor of Podiatric Medicine (DPM). Many states now require postdoctoral training in the form of a residency, usually one year's supervised work in hospital, before the state examination. In addition, continuing medical education credits are required annually to maintain state licensure as well as hospital staff privileges. Two optional Boards recognized by the American Podiatric Medical Association are the American Board of Podiatric Orthopedics and Primary Podiatric Care, and the American Board of Podiatric Surgery.

**poikiloderma atrophicans with cataract**   See *Rothmund-Thomson syndrome.*

**poikiloderma congenita**   See *Rothmund-Thomson syndrome.*

**point mutation**   A single nucleotide base change in the DNA as, for example, in sickle cell disease.

**point, McBurney**   See *McBurney point.*

**poison**   Any substance that can cause severe distress or death if ingested, breathed in, or absorbed through the skin. Many substances that normally cause no problems, including water and most vitamins, can be poisonous if taken in too large a quantity. Poison treatment depends on the substance: If there are treatment instructions on the substance's container and it contained no other item, follow those directions immediately. Always contact the nearest Poison Control Center with concerns about possible poison ingestion.

**Poison Control Centers**   Special information centers set up to inform Americans about how to respond to potential poisoning. These centers maintain a database of poisons and appropriate emergency treatment. Local Poison Control Centers should be listed with other community-service numbers in the front of the telephone book, and can also be reached immediately through any telephone operator.

**poison ivy**   Skin inflammation resulting from contact with the poison ivy vine. Chemicals produced by this vine cause an immune reaction, producing redness, itching, and blistering of the skin. Treatment is by topical medication, such as calamine lotion.

**poison oak**   Skin inflammation resulting from contact with the poison oak plant. Chemicals produced by this plant cause an immune reaction, producing redness, itching, and blistering of the skin. Treatment is by topical medication, such as calamine lotion.

**poisoning**   Taking a substance that is injurious to health or can cause death. Poisoning is still a major hazard to children, despite child-resistant (and sometimes adult-resistant) packaging and dose-limits per container. See also *poison, Poison Control Centers.*

**poisoning, silver**   See *argyria.*

**Poland anomaly**   See *Poland syndrome.*

**Poland sequence**   See *Poland syndrome.*

**Poland syndactyly**   See *Poland syndrome.*

**Poland syndrome**   A unique pattern of one-sided malformations characterized by a defect of the chest muscle (pectoralis) on one side of the body, and webbing and shortening of the fingers (cutaneous syndactyly) on the hand on the same side. The serratus anterior and latissimus dorsi muscles may also be absent, as may be the armpit (axillary) hair. In girls, the breast on the affected side is also usually absent. Usually the child is otherwise normal, although on rare occasions Poland syndrome is associated with more severe finger and arm involvement, or with vertebral or kidney problems. Intelligence is not impaired. Poland syndrome is right-sided three times more often than it is left-sided. It is not common, affecting 1 child in about 20,000. Poland syndrome is three times more frequent in boys than girls. Its cause is uncertain, although diminished blood flow through the subclavian artery that goes to the fetal arm has been blamed. The disorder is currently considered a nonspecific developmental field defect, occurring at about the sixth week of fetal development. The syndrome occurs sporadically and does not appear to run in families. Treatment has been by reconstructive surgery, but bioengineered cartilage may now be implanted to help give the chest a more normal look. Also known as Poland sequence, Poland anomaly, Poland syndactyly, absence of the pectoralis muscle with syndactyly.

**polio** Poliomyelitis, an acute and sometimes devastating viral disease. Man is the only natural host for poliovirus. The virus enters the mouth, and multiplies in lymphoid tissues in the pharynx and intestine. Small numbers of virus particles enter the blood and go to other sites, where the virus multiplies more extensively. Another round of virus in the bloodstream (viremia) leads to invasion of the spinal cord and brain, the target sites struck by the virus. When the central nervous system is inflamed, the anterior horn cells of the spinal cord and the brainstem are especially affected. Polio can be a minor illness, as it is in 80 to 90 percent of clinical infections. These appear chiefly in young children, and do not involve the central nervous system. Symptoms are slight fever, malaise, headache, sore throat, and vomiting three to five days after exposure. Recovery occurs in 24 to 72 hours. This is termed the abortive type of polio. As a major illness, polio may or may not be paralytic. Symptoms usually appear without prior illness, particularly in older children and adults, 7 to 14 days after exposure. Symptoms are fever, severe headache, stiff neck and back, deep muscle pain, and sometimes areas of increased sensation (hyperesthesia) or altered sensation (paresthesia). There may be no further progression from this picture of viral meningitis, or there may be loss of tendon reflexes, and weakness or paralysis of muscle groups. Recovery is complete in the abortive and nonparalytic forms of polio, although a set of symptoms known as postpolio syndrome may appear many years later. In paralytic polio, about 50 percent of patients recover with no residual paralysis, about 25 percent are left with mild disabilities, and the remaining patients have severe permanent disability. The greatest return of muscle function occurs in the first six months, but improvement may continue for up to two years. Physical therapy is the most important part of treatment of paralytic polio during convalescence. The ideal strategy with polio is clearly to prevent it by immunization against poliovirus. Also known as infantile paralysis.

**polio immunization** Two polio vaccines are available: oral polio vaccine (OPV) and inactivated polio vaccine (IPV). OPV is still the preferred vaccine for most children. As its name suggests, it is given by mouth. Infants and children should be given four doses of OPV. The doses are given at 2 months, 4 months, 6 to 18 months, and 4 to 6 years of age. Persons allergic to eggs or the drugs neomycin or streptomycin should receive OPV, not the injectable IPV. Conversely, IPV should be given if the vaccine recipient is on long-term steroid (cortisone) therapy, has cancer, or is on chemotherapy, or if a household member has AIDS or is an unimmunized adult. IPV is given as a shot in the arm or leg.

**polio vaccine, Salk** Vaccine against the virus that causes poliomyelitis. The Salk vaccine is named for Dr. Jonas Salk, who developed and introduced it in 1955. It was the first polio vaccine available, and was made by cultivating three strains of the virus separately in monkey tissue. The virus was separated from the tissue, stored for a week, and killed with formaldehyde. This killed-virus vaccine was given in four injections. The oral form of the vaccine, subsequently developed by Dr. Albert Sabin, is in standard use today.

**polio, abortive** A minor form of infection with poliovirus, abortive polio accounts for 80 to 90 percent of clinically apparent cases in the US, chiefly occurring in young children. The usual symptoms emerge three to five days after exposure to the virus, and include slight fever, malaise, headache, sore throat, and vomiting. Full recovery occurs in 24 to 72 hours. It does not involve the nervous system or cause permanent disabilities of any kind.

**poliomyelitis** See *polio*.

**pollen** Small, light, dry protein particles from trees, grasses, flowers, and weeds that may be spread by the wind. Pollen particles are usually the male sex cells of the plant, and are smaller than the tip of a pin. Pollen is a potent stimulator of allergic responses. It lodges in the mucous membranes that line the nose, and in other parts of the respiratory tract, causing irritation and histamine reactions.

**pollex** The thumb.

**poly-** 1 Prefix meaning much or many. For example, polycystic means characterized by many cysts. 2 Short form for polymorphonuclear leukocyte, a type of white blood cell.

**polyarteritis nodosa** An autoimmune disease characterized by spontaneous inflammation of the arteries (arteritis) of the body. Because arteries are involved, the disease can affect any organ of the body. It most commonly affects muscles, joints, intestines, nerves, kidneys, and skin.

**polyarticular** Involving many joints. As opposed to monoarticular, affecting just one joint.

**polycystic kidney disease** Genetic disorders characterized by the development of innumerable cysts in the kidneys. These cysts are filled with fluid, and replace much of the mass of the kidneys. This reduces kidney function, leading to kidney failure.

**polycystic ovarian disease**  See *Stein-Leventhal syndrome*.

**polycythemia**  The presence of too many red blood cells. Polycythemia formally exists when the hemoglobin, red blood cell (RBC) count, and total RBC volume are both above normal. For example, the percentage of red blood cells in whole blood (hematocrit) in polycythemia is significantly above 52 percent in men and above 48 percent in females. The normal hematocrit range is from about 42 to 52 percent in males, and from 37 to 48 percent in females. The opposite of anemia.

**polycythemia vera**  Overproduction of red blood cells due to bone marrow disease (myeloproferative disorder). PV tends to evolve into acute leukemia or a condition called myelofibrosis, in which the marrow is replaced by scar tissue. For a diagnosis of PV, there must be polycythemia. Abbreviated as PV. See also *polycythemia*.

**polydactyly**  More than the normal number of fingers or toes. Polydactyly is the opposite of oligodactyly, too few fingers or toes. See also *hexadactyly*.

**polydipsia**  Constant, excessive. Polydipsia occurs, for example, in untreated or poorly controlled diabetes mellitus.

**polygenes**  Many genes. Eye color is polygenically controlled.

**polygenic diseases**  Genetic disorders caused by the combined action of more than one gene. Examples of polygenic conditions include hypertension, coronary heart disease, and diabetes. Because such disorders depend on the simultaneous presence of several genes, they are not inherited as simply as single-gene diseases.

**polyhydramnios**  Too much amniotic fluid.

**polymerase chain reaction**  A key technique in molecular genetics that permits the analysis of any short sequence of DNA or RNA without having to clone it. PCR is used to amplify selected sections of DNA in only a few hours. The PCR technique has innumerable uses, from diagnosing genetic diseases, to DNA fingerprinting. PCR has become an essential tool for biologists, forensics labs, and scientists who wish to study genetic material.

**polymerase, DNA**  See *DNA polymerase*.

**polymerase, RNA**  See *RNA polymerase*.

**polymorphonuclear leukocyte**  See *leukocyte, polymorphonuclear*.

**polymyalgia rheumatica**  A disorder of the muscles and joints of older persons, characterized by pain and stiffness, affecting both sides of the body, and involving the shoulders, arms, neck, and buttock areas. Abbreviated as PMR.

**polymyositis**  An inflammatory disease of muscle that begins when white blood cells spontaneously invade muscles, especially those closest to the trunk or torso. This immune activity results in muscle pain, tenderness, and weakness.

**polyneuritis, acute idiopathic**  See *Guillain-Barre syndrome*.

**polyp**  A mass of tissue that develops on the inside wall of a hollow organ, such as the colon.

**polyploid**  Three or more full sets of chromosomes. A polyploid brain tumor cell might, for example, have 69 or 92 chromosomes.

**polypsis of the colon**  See *familial adenomatous polyposis*.

**polysomnography**  Electronic monitoring of a sleeping patient to look for abnormalities in sleep pattern and/or brain waves. Polysomnography correlates electroencephalogram readings with observation of the patient. Usually, respiration, oxygen saturation, body position, and other factors are also measured during polysomnography. See also *sleep apnea; sleep apnea, central; sleep apnea, obstructive; sleep disorders*.

**popliteal**  Adjective referring to the back of the knee.

**popliteal fossa**  The hollow behind the knee.

**popliteal pterygium syndrome**  An inherited condition characterized by a web (pterygium) behind the knee.

**pork tapeworm**  See *Taenia solium*.

**porphyria**  A varied series of hereditary diseases with increased formation and excretion of chemicals called porphyrins. One type of porphyria, acute intermittent porphyria, may have affected members of the House of Hanover in England, including "Mad" King George. The king may not have been mad, but rather may have suffered attacks of porphyria.

**portal vein**  A large vein formed by the union of the splenic and superior mesenteric veins. It conveys venous blood to the liver for detoxification before the blood is returned to the circulation via the hepatic veins.

**port-wine stain**  A mark on the skin whose rich, ruby-red color resembles that of port wine. Due to an abnormal aggregation of capillaries, a port-wine stain is a type of hemangioma. It can occur on the face as a sign of Sturge-Weber syndrome. See also *Sturge-Weber syndrome.*

**positive, false** See *false positive.*

**postnasal drip** Mucous accumulation in the back of the nose and throat, leading to or giving the sensation of mucus dripping down from the back of the nose.

**postpolio muscular atrophy** Belated muscle wasting that occurs as part of the postpolio syndrome. See *postpolio syndrome.*

**postpolio syndrome** A constellation of symptoms and signs that appear from 20 to 40 years after the initial polio infection, and at least 10 years after what was thought to be recovery from polio. It is estimated that 1.63 million Americans were struck by polio in the epidemics of the 1940s, '50s, and early '60s, and that 440,000 of the survivors suffer the effects of PPS. The typical features of PPS include unaccustomed weakness, muscle fatigue (and sometimes central fatigue), pain, breathing and/or swallowing difficulties, sleep disorders, muscle twitching (fasciculations), and gastrointestinal problems. The muscle problems in PPS can occur in previously affected muscles, or in muscles that were thought not to be affected at the onset of polio. The onset of PPS is usually gradual, but it is sometimes abrupt, with major loss of function suffered over several months or a couple of years. This process often seems to start after a physical or emotional trauma, an illness, or an accident. Complications of PPS may include neuropathies, nerve entrapments, arthritis, scoliosis, osteoporosis, and sometimes postpolio muscular atrophy (PPMA). Diagnosis is made by history, by clinical findings, and by ruling out other diseases that may mimic PPS. There are no specific tests to provide unquestionable confirmation of the diagnosis of PPS. The general rule is that those who were most seriously affected by the virus at initial onset and made the best recovery come to suffer the worst PPS symptoms years later. No clearcut cause for PPS has been found. There is known to be a failure at the neuromuscular junction. One idea is that nerves and muscles that have had to overwork prematurely fail, but this is unproven. There is also known to be impairment in the production of certain hormones and neurotransmitters, but whether these changes are the cause of PPS or its effect is unknown. Polio survivors tend to be hard-driving, type-A personalities, as compared to nondisabled control subjects—and the more driven polio survivors tend to have more PPS symptoms. Treatment may include slowing down to conserve strength and energy. Musculoskeletal problems can sometimes be helped by anti-inflammatory or pain medications, with or without surgical procedures.

**posterior** The back, as opposed to anterior (front). See also *Appendix B, "Anatomic Orientation Terms."*

**posterior cruciate ligament** The cross-shaped ligament that crosses behind the anterior cruciate ligament and within the knee joint. See also *knee.*

**posteroanterior** In anatomy, from back to front, as opposed to anteroposterior, from front to back. A chest X-ray taken with the chest against the film plate and the X-ray machine behind the patient is a posteroanterior (PA) view. See also *Appendix B, "Anatomic Orientation Terms."*

**postherpetic neuralgia** See *neuralgia, postherpetic.* See also *shingles.*

**posthitis** Inflammation of the foreskin of the penis. In the uncircumcised male, posthitis usually occurs together with balanitis, inflammation of the glans, as balanoposthitis. Circumcision prevents and cures posthitis. See also *balanitis, balanoposthitis.*

**postmature infant** A baby born seven days or more after the usual nine months of gestation. See also *postterm infant.*

**postmenopausal** After the menopause. Postmenopausal is defined as the period of time occurring after a woman has experienced 12 consecutive months without menstruation.

**postremission therapy** Chemotherapy to kill leukemia cells that survive after remission-induction therapy.

**post-term infant** A baby born 14 days or more after the usual 9 months of gestation, as calculated from the mother's last menstrual period (LMP). This is an important calculation, because if delivery is delayed 3 weeks beyond term, the possibility of infant mortality skyrockets to 3 times its normal rate.

**post-traumatic stress disorder** A psychological disorder that develops in some individuals who have had major traumatic experiences: for example, those who have experienced a serious accident, survived or witnessed an assault, or been through a war. Typically the person is emotionally numb at first, but later has symptoms that may include depression, excessive irritability, guilt for having survived if others were injured or died, recurrent nightmares, flashbacks to the traumatic scene, and overreactions to sudden noises. Although the name post-traumatic stress disorder is only two decades old, the condition is not. It was known as shell shock in World War I, and battle fatigue during World War II. Abbreviated as PTSD.

**postulates, Koch** See *Koch postulates.*

**postural hypotension**  See *hypotension, orthostatic*.

**Pott disease**  See *tuberculous diskitis*.

**pouch of Douglas**  An extension of the peritoneal cavity between the rectum and back wall of the uterus. Also known as the rectouterine pouch.

**pouch, rectouterine**  See *pouch of Douglas*.

**pound**  A measure of weight equal to 16 ounces or, metrically, 453.6 grams. Abbreviated as lb.

**power of attorney, durable**  See *durable power of attorney*.

**PPMA**  Postpolio muscular atrophy.

**PPS**  Postpolio syndrome.

**Prader-Willi syndrome**  A condition characterized by muscle floppiness (hypotonia), constant appetite that if unchecked leads to obesity, small hands and feet, mental retardation, and autistic tendencies. It is due to loss of part or all of chromosome 15, specifically the chromosome 15 from the father. This chromosomal change may cause metabolic as well as physical problems, although these have yet to be identified. There is currently no specific treatment or cure for Prader-Willi syndrome. Parents are advised to limit consumption of high-calorie foods, and to use techniques such as special education, speech therapy, and physical therapy to maximize the child's potential. In some cases, antidepressant or stimulant medication is tried, which may affect appetite, attention, and behavior.

**Prayer of Maimonides**  See *Daily Prayer of a Physician*.

**preauricular tag**  See *ear tag*.

**precancerous**  Adjective describing something that is not cancerous, but may become cancerous with time. Microscopic changes may be occurring in cells, or visible changes may be occurring in body tissues, that tend to indicate the later development of cancer.

**preclinical study**  A study to test a drug, procedure, or other medical treatment in animals. The aim is to collect data in support of safety. Preclinical studies are required before clinical trials in humans can be started.

**precocious puberty**  The onset of secondary sexual characteristics, such as breast buds in girls, growth of the penis and thinning of the scrotum in boys, and the appearance of pubic hair in both sexes, before the normal age of puberty. There is much normal variation in the age of puberty, but precocious puberty is generally defined as onset before the age of eight in girls or nine in boys.

**preconceptual**  Adjective meaning before conception.

**preconceptual counseling**  The interchange of information prior to pregnancy. Usually for pregnancy planning and care, but sometimes in the form of genetic counseling. See also *genetic counseling*.

**preeclampsia**  A condition characterized by a sharp rise in blood pressure during the third trimester of pregnancy. Hypertension may be accompanied by edema (swollen ankles), irritability, and kidney problems, as evidenced by protein in the urine. Although preeclampsia is relatively common, occurring in about 5 percent of all pregnancies and more frequently in first pregnancies, it can be a sign of serious problems. It may indicate that the placenta is detaching from the uterus, for example. In some cases, untreated preeclampsia can progress to eclampsia, a life-threatening situation for both mother and fetus characterized by coma and seizures. Treatment is by bed rest and sometimes medication. If treatment is ineffective, induced birth or a C-section may have to be considered. See also *eclampsia, HELLP syndrome*.

**pregnancy**  The state of carrying a developing embryo or fetus within the female body. This condition can be indicated by positive results on an over-the-counter urine test, and confirmed through a blood test, ultrasound, detection of fetal heartbeat, or an X-ray. Pregnancy lasts for about nine months, measured from the date of the woman's last menstrual period (LMP). It is conventionally divided into three trimesters, each roughly three months long. The most important tasks of basic fetal cell differentiation occur during the first trimester, so any harm done to the fetus during this period is most likely to result in miscarriage or serious disability. There is little to no chance that a first-trimester fetus can survive outside the womb, even with the best hospital care. Its systems are simply too undeveloped. This stage truly ends with the phenomenon of quickening: the mother's first perception of fetal movement. It is in the first trimester that some women experience morning sickness, a form of nausea on awaking that usually passes within an hour. The breasts also begin to prepare for nursing, and painful soreness from hardening milk glands may occur. As the pregnancy progresses, the mother may experience many physical and emotional changes, ranging from increased moodiness to darkening of the skin in various areas. During the second trimester, the fetus undergoes a remarkable series of developments. Its physical parts become fully distinct and at least somewhat operational. With the best medical care, a second-trimester fetus born prematurely has at least some chance of survival, although developmental delays and other handicaps may emerge later. As the fetus grows in size, the mother's pregnant state will begin to be obvious. In the third trimester, the fetus enters the final stage of preparation for birth. It increases rapidly in weight, as does the mother. As the end of the pregnancy nears, there may be discomfort as the fetus moves into position in the woman's lower abdomen. Edema (swelling of the ankles), back pain, and balance problems are sometimes experienced during this time. Most women are able to go about their usual activities, including nonimpact exercise and work, until the very last days or weeks of pregnancy. During the final days, some feel too much discomfort to continue at a full pace, although others report greatly increased energy just before the birth. Pregnancy ends when the birth process begins. See also *acute fatty liver of pregnancy; birth; birth defect; conception; eclampsia; ectopic pregnancy; fetal alcohol effect; fetal alcohol syndrome; HELLP syndrome; hyperemesis gravidarum; preeclampsia; pregnancy, tubal; prenatal care; prenatal development; teratogen.*

**pregnancy planning** Pregnancy planning addresses issues that may impact a woman's ability to carry a child to term, such as nutrition, vitamins, body weight, exercise, potentially harmful medications and illnesses, immunizations, and genetic counseling. A woman who plans to become pregnant should make lifestyle choices for optimal health in advance of the planned conception. See also *birth control, family planning.*

**pregnancy, acute fatty liver of** See *acute fatty liver of pregnancy.*

**pregnancy, alcohol during** See *fetal alcohol syndrome, fetal alcohol effect.*

**pregnancy, drugs during** See *teratogen.*

**pregnancy, ectopic** See *ectopic pregnancy.*

**pregnancy, extrauterine** See *ectopic pregnancy.*

**pregnancy, pernicious vomiting of** See *hyperemesis gravidarum.*

**pregnancy, tubal** An ectopic pregnancy that takes place in the Fallopian tube. Tubal pregnancies are due to the inability of the fertilized egg to make its way through the Fallopian tube into the uterus. Most tubal pregnancies occur in women 35 to 44 years of age. Tubal pregnancies account for 95 percent of all ectopic pregnancies. See *ectopic pregnancy.*

**preleukemia** See *leukemia, smoldering.*

**premature baby** A baby born before 37 weeks of gestation have passed since the mother's last menstrual period (LMP). A premature baby born very close to its due date may suffer few, if any, consequences. The earlier in development birth takes place, the greater the likelihood that life-support systems will be needed, and the greater the risk for birth defects and nonviability (death).

Colloquially known as a preemie. See also *pregnancy, premature birth.*

**premature birth** Birth before 37 weeks of gestation have passed. Premature birth carries greater risks the farther it occurs from that 37-week goal. Many procedures are available to prevent early birth, from bed rest to medications. If premature birth is medically necessary or inevitable, however, it may be accomplished via C-section to limit stress on the fetus. See also *pregnancy, premature baby.*

**premature contraction of the heart** A single heartbeat occurs earlier than normal. This phenomenon can be within normal limits, or may represent a medically significant arrhythmia.

**premature ventricular contractions** Contractions of the lower chambers of the heart, the ventricles, which occur earlier than usual because of abnormal electrical activity of the ventricles. The premature contraction is followed by a pause as the heart's electrical system resets itself; the contraction following the pause is usually more forceful than normal. These more forceful contractions are frequently perceived as palpitations.

**premenstrual syndrome** A combination of physical and mood disturbances that occur after ovulation and normally end with the onset of the menstrual flow. Premenstrual syndrome is believed to be a disorder of the neurotransmitters and other hormones. In its most severe form, it can be truly disabling for part of the month, and strongly resembles a type of bipolar disorder. Treatment of mild PMS may not be necessary, but treatment of moderate to severe PMS may involve exercise and medication, particularly antidepressants and/or mood stabilizers. Abbreviated as PMS.

**prenatal care** During pregnancy, women should receive regular health care from an obstetrician or midwife. Services needed include dietary and lifestyle advice, weighing to ensure proper weight gain, and examination for problems of pregnancy such as edema and preeclampsia. In cases where complications are likely, such as pregnancy after age 40 or in a women with diabetes, care may be sought from an experienced specialist.

**prenatal development** The process of growth and development within the womb, in which a single-cell zygote (the cell formed by the combination of a sperm and an egg) becomes an embryo, a fetus, and then a baby. The first two weeks of development are concerned with simple cell multiplication. This tiny mass of cells then adheres to the inside wall of the uterus. The next three weeks see intense cell differentiation, as the cell mass divides into separate primitive systems. At the end of eight weeks, the embryo has taken on a roughly human shape, and is called a fetus. For the next 20 weeks the fetus' primitive circulatory, nervous, pulmonary, and other systems become more mature, and it begins to move its limbs. At 28 weeks, fat begins to accumulate under the skin, toenails and fingernails appear, and downy hair sprouts on the body and scalp. The fetus may open its eyes periodically. For the remaining weeks of development, the fetus continues to gain weight, and its internal systems reach full development.

**prenatal diagnosis** Diagnosis before birth. Methods for prenatal diagnosis include ultrasound of the uterus, placenta, and/or developing fetus; chorionic villus sampling (CVS) to obtain tissue for chromosome or biochemical analysis; and amniocentesis to obtain amniotic fluid for the analysis of chromosomes, enzymes, or DNA. A growing number of birth defects and diseases can be diagnosed prenatally, and in some cases treated before birth. Also known as antenatal diagnosis.

**prepuce** The fold of skin that covers the head of the penis. Also known as the foreskin.

**prepuce, inflammation of the** See *posthitis*.

**prescription** A physician's order for the preparation and administration of a drug or device for a patient. A prescription has several parts. They include the superscription or heading, with the symbol **R** or **Rx**, which stands for the word recipe (Latin for to take); the inscription, which contains the names and quantities of the ingredients; the subscription or directions for compounding the drug; and the signature, often preceded by the sign **s.**, which stands for signa (Latin for mark), giving the directions to be marked on the container. See also *Appendix A, "Prescription Abbreviations."*

**prescription drug** A drug requiring a prescription, as opposed to an over-the-counter drug, which can be purchased without one.

**presentation, breech** Birth in which the buttocks present first.

**presentation, footling** Birth in which one or both feet present first. There are single-footling or double-footling presentations, depending on the number of feet emerging.

**presentation, vertex** Birth in which the top of the baby's head emerges first. This is the most common presentation.

**pressure, high blood** See *hypertension*.

**pressure, intraocular** See *intraocular pressure*. See also *glaucoma*.

**pressure, low blood** See *hypotension*.

**preventive medicine** Medical practices designed to avert and avoid disease. Screening for hypertension and treating it before it causes disease is good preventive medicine. Preventive medicine takes a proactive approach to patient care.

**priapism** Abnormally persistent erection of the penis in the absence of desire.

**primary amenorrhea** See *amenorrhea*.

**primary biliary cirrhosis** See *cirrhosis, primary biliary*.

**primary care** The patient's main source for regular medical care, ideally providing continuity and integration of health-care services. All family physicians, and most pediatricians and internists, are in primary care. The aims of primary care are to provide the patient with a broad spectrum of preventative and curative care over a period of time, and to coordinate all the care the patient receives.

**primary care provider** In insurance parlance, a physician chosen by or assigned to a patient, who both provides primary care and acts as a gatekeeper to control access to other medical services.

**primary dentition** See *primary teeth*.

**primary HIV infection** See *HIV infection, primary*.

**primary sclerosing cholangitis** A chronic disorder of the liver in which the ducts carrying bile from the liver to the intestine, and often the ducts carrying bile within the liver, become inflamed, thickened, scarred (sclerotic), and obstructed. This relentlessly progressive process can in time destroy the bile ducts and lead to cirrhosis. PSC can occur by itself or in association with other diseases, including inflammatory bowel disease, especially with ulcerative colitis; certain uncommon diseases, such as multifocal fibrosclerosis syndrome, Riedel struma, and pseudotumor of the orbit; and AIDS. Changes in the biliary tract are quite common in AIDS and are very much like those in PSC; however, in AIDS the changes in the biliary tract are probably due to infection with mycoplasma, cytomegalovirus, or other agents. PSC often triggers jaundice (yellowing), pruritus (generalized itching all over the body), upper abdominal pain, and infection. Later on, PSC progresses to cirrhosis of the liver and liver failure, creating a need for liver transplantation. Diagnosis is by clinical observation and routine laboratory tests, and is confirmed by demonstration of thickened bile ducts, using special radiologic tests called cholangiography. Treatment includes cholestyramine to diminish itching, antibiotics for infection, vitamin D and calcium to prevent bone loss (osteoporosis), sometimes balloon dilatation or surgery for obstructed ducts, and liver transplantation when necessary and possible. Prognosis depends on the age of the person, the degree of jaundice, the stage of PSC found via liver biopsy, and the size of the spleen. Most patients die within 10 years of diagnosis unless a liver transplant is performed. Also known as idiopathic sclerosing cholangitis.

**primary teeth** The first 20 teeth, which are shed and replaced by permanent teeth. The first primary tooth comes in (erupts) at about six months of age, and the last erupts at around two and a half years. Replacement with permanent teeth usually begins at about age six. Also known as baby teeth, milk teeth, primary dentition, temporary teeth, deciduous teeth.

**primitive neuroectodermal tumor** A type of brain tumor believed to originate in neural crest cells. Diagnosis is by biopsy. Treatment is by radiation and/or chemotherapy. Abbreviated as PNET.

**primitive neuroectodermal tumors, primitive** See *sarcoma, Ewing.*

**primum non nocere** Latin for "first do no harm," a fundamental medical precept and part of the Hippocratic oath.

**principal joints of the body** See *joints of the body, principal.* See also *joint.*

**Printzmetal angina** See *angina, Printzmetal.*

**prions** A newly discovered type of disease-causing agent, neither bacterial nor fungal nor viral, and containing no genetic material. A prion is a protein that occurs normally in a harmless form. By folding into an aberrant shape, the normal prion turns into a rogue agent. It then co-opts other normal prions to become rogue prions. Prions have been held responsible for a number of degenerative brain diseases, including mad cow disease, Creutzfeld-Jacob disease, fatal familial insomnia, kuru, an unusual form of hereditary dementia known as Gertsmann-Straeussler-Scheinker disease, and possibly some cases of Alzheimer disease.

**private mutation** A rare mutation usually found only in a single family or a small population. It is like a privately printed book.

**PRK** Photorefractive keratectomy.

**pro-** As a prefix, a combining form (from both Greek and Latin) with many meanings, including before, in front of, preceding, on behalf of, in place of, and the same as. Used as a word, pro of course means professional and, in medicine, is short for prothrombin.

**pro time** Short form for prothrombin time.

**probability** The likelihood that something will happen. For example, a probability of less than .05 indicates that the probability of something occurring by chance alone is less than 5 in 100, or 5 percent. This level of probability is usually taken as the level of biologic significance, so a higher incidence may be considered meaningful. Abbreviated as P.

**proband** The family member through whom a family's medical history comes to light. For example, a proband might be a baby with Down syndrome. The proband may also be called the index case, propositus (if male), or proposita (if female).

**probe** 1 In surgery, a slender, flexible rod with a blunt end, used to explore. For example, a probe might explore an opening to see where it goes. 2 In molecular genetics, a labeled bit of DNA or RNA used to find its complementary sequence or to locate a particular clone.

**probiotics** Substances that appear to replenish or support the growth of helpful bacteria in the intestinal tract. The most common probiotic is acidopholous in yogurt, acidopholous milk, or supplement form. As the name indicates, probiotics have been developed to counter one unfortunate effect of treatment with antibiotics: the decimation of helpful intestinal bacteria along with disease-causing bacteria. See also *Lactobacillus acidopholus.*

**PROC** Protein C.

**process** In anatomy, a projection from a structure. The process of the mandible is the part of the lower jaw that projects forward.

**proclivity** An inclination or predisposition toward something, especially a strong inherent inclination toward something objectionable. For example, a patient might be said to have a proclivity toward alcohol.

**proctitis** Inflammation of the rectum. This may be due to a considerable number of causes, among them infectious agents and ulcerative colitis. Infectious proctitis is often due to agents such as Chlamydia trachomatis, Neisseria gonorrheae, and herpes simplex virus, all of which can be acquired during receptive anoreceptive intercourse. Proctitis is also a hallmark of ulcerative colitis, in which case it may be accompanied by intermittent rectal bleeding, crampy abdominal pain, and diarrhea.

**proctitis, ulcerative** Ulcerative colitis that is limited to the rectum. See *colitis, ulcerative; proctitis.*

**proctology** A medical specialty that deals with disorders of the rectum and anus.

**proctosigmoidoscopy** An examination of the rectum and the lower part of the colon, using a thin, lighted instrument called a sigmoidoscope.

**product, gene** See *gene product*.

**progeria** A disorder characterized by premature aging. There is more than one type of progeria, and the mechanism behind these disorders is not yet known. Researchers have recently found dramatically lowered levels of antioxidant enzymes, particularly catalase and glutathione peroxidase, in patients with progeria. One theory is that lower levels of these enzymes permit cell damage by toxins and free radicals. There is currently no treatment for progeria, although gene therapy is being investigated.

**progesterone** A female hormone, progesterone is the principal hormone that prepares the uterus to receive and sustain the fertilized egg.

**prognathism** An overly prominent jaw.

**prognosis** The probable outcome or course of a disease; the patient's chance of recovery.

**progressive infantile poliodystrophy, Alpers** See *Alpers disease*.

**prokaryote** A cell lacking a discrete nucleus and other special subcellular compartments. Bacteria and viruses are prokaryotes. Humans are not prokaryotes, but rather eukaryotes.

**prominent vertebra** The seventh cervical (neck) vertebra, which has a long spinous process that projects out from the back of its vertebral body.

**prominentia laryngea** See *Adam's apple*.

**promoter** In molecular biology, a site on DNA to which the enzyme RNA polymerase can bind, initiating the transcription of DNA into RNA.

**pronation** Rotation of the arm or leg inward. In the case of the arm, the palm of the hand will face posteriorly. See also *Appendix B, "Anatomic Orientation Terms."*

**prone** With the front or ventral surface downward (lying face down), as opposed to supine. See also *Appendix B, "Anatomic Orientation Terms."*

**pronucleus** A cell nucleus with a haploid (halved) set of chromosomes—23 chromosomes in humans—resulting from germ-cell division (meiosis). The male pronucleus is the sperm nucleus after it has entered the ovum at fertilization, but before fusion with the female pronucleus. Similarly, the female pronucleus is the nucleus of the ovum before fusion with the male pronucleus.

**Propecia** See *finasteride*.

**prophylactic** **1** A medication or treatment given to prevent development of disease. For example, prophylactic antibiotics are often used after a bout of rheumatic fever to prevent the development of Sydenham chorea or PANDAS. **2** A drug or device for preventing pregnancy, particularly a condom.

**prophylactic cranial irradiation** Radiation therapy to the head, intended to prevent cancer from spreading to the brain.

**prophylaxis** The prevention of disease.

**propositus** See *proband*.

**propriception** The ability to sense stimuli arising within the body. Even if you are blindfolded, you know through propriception if your arm is above your head or hanging by your side. The sense of proprieception is disturbed in many neurological disorders. It can sometimes be improved through the use of sensory integration therapy, a type of specialized occupational therapy. See *sensory integration*.

**Proscar** See *finasteride*.

**prostate** See *prostate gland*.

**prostate acid phosphatase** An enzyme produced by the prostate that is elevated in some patients with prostate cancer.

**prostate cancer** An uncontrolled (malignant) growth of cells in the prostate gland. Prostate cancer is the second leading cause of death of males in the US. See also *prostate gland*.

**prostate enlargement** Overgrowth of the prostate gland, usually due to a common, benign, and very treatable condition known as benign prostatic hyperplasia (BPH). Far fewer cases of prostate enlargement are due to prostate cancer, but men over age 30 should have regular prostate examinations to lower their risk. See also *digital rectal exam; prostate cancer; prostate gland; prostate specific antigen test; prostatic hyperplasia, benign*.

**prostate gland** A gland in the male reproductive system located just below the bladder. It surrounds part of the urethra, the canal that empties the bladder. The prostate gland helps to control urination, and forms part of the semen.

**prostate specific antigen test**　A test used to screen for cancer of the prostate, and to monitor treatment. Prostate specific antigen (PSA) is a protein produced by the prostate gland. Although most PSA is carried out of the body in semen, a very small amount escapes into the blood stream. The PSA test is done on blood. PSA in blood can be by itself, as free PSA; or it can join with other substances in the blood, as bound PSA. Total PSA is the sum of free and bound forms. The PSA value used most frequently as the highest normal level is 4 ng/mL (nanograms per milliliter). However, since the prostate gland generally increases in size and produces more PSA with increasing age, it is normal to have lower levels in young men and higher levels in older men. Age-specific PSA levels are as follows: 2.5 for ages 40 to 49, 3.5 for ages 50 to 59, 4.5 for ages 60 to 69, and 6.5 for age 70 and older. The use of age-specific PSA ranges for the detection of prostate cancer is controversial. Not all studies have agreed that this is better than simply using a level of 4 ng/mL as the highest normal value. An abnormal result on the PSA test indicates the need for additional testing if it is being used as a screening measure. Levels above 4 ng/mL but less than 10 ng/mL are suspicious. However, most men who have this level of abnormality will actually not have prostate cancer. As levels increase above 10 ng/mL, the probability of prostate cancer increases dramatically. When the PSA is used as a monitoring test following therapy, an abnormal result indicates recurrence of prostate cancer. PSA is not specific to prostate cancer. Other diseases can cause an elevated PSA. The most frequent is benign prostatic hypertrophy (BPH), an increase in the size of the prostate that typically occurs with aging. Infection of the prostate gland (prostatitis) is another relatively common cause of an elevated PSA. Other conditions that can increase PSA include ischemia or infarction, urethral instrumentation, urinary retention, and prostate biopsy. Also, a small proportion of prostate cancers do not produce a detectable increase in blood PSA, even with advanced disease. Many early cancers will not produce enough PSA to cause a significantly abnormal blood level. It is therefore important not to rely only on blood PSA testing. The most useful additional test is a physical prostate exam known as the digital rectal exam (DRE). See also *digital rectal exam; prostate cancer; prostate gland; prostatic hyperplasia, benign.*

**prostate, nodular hyperplasia**　See *prostatic hyperplasia, benign.*

**prostatectomy**　Surgical removal of the prostate gland

**prostatectomy, retropubic**　Surgical removal of the prostate through an incision in the abdomen.

**prostatic hyperplasia, benign**　A common cause of prostate enlargement, benign prostatic hyperplasia (BPH)

generally begins in a man's 30s, evolves slowly, and only causes symptoms after age 50. In BPH, the normal elements of the prostate gland grow in size and number. Their sheer bulk may compress the urethra, which courses through the center of the prostate, and impede the flow of urine from the bladder through the urethra to the outside. This leads to urine retention and the need for frequent urination. If severe enough, complete blockage can occur. BPH is very common. Half of men over 50 develop symptoms of BPH, but only 10 percent need medical or surgical intervention. BPH is completely benign, and is *not* a sign of prostate cancer. Treatment of BPH is usually reserved for men with significant symptoms. Watchful waiting with medical monitoring once a year is appropriate for most men with BPH. Treatment options include drugs, such as finasteride (brand name: Proscar, Propecia) or terazosin (brand name: Hytrin). The prostate enlargement in BPH is directly dependent on DHT, the principal androgen hormone in the prostate. Finasteride blocks the enzyme needed to make DHT, lowering blood and tissue DHT levels and so reducing the size of the prostate. Terazosin, an alpha 1 blocker, relaxes the smooth muscles of the arteries, the prostate, and the bladder neck. Relaxing the smooth muscles of the arteries lowers blood pressure, while relaxing the smooth muscles around the bladder neck helps relieve urinary obstruction caused by an enlarged prostate. Prostate surgery has traditionally been seen as offering the most benefits for BPH, and also the most risks. Also known as benign prostatic hypertrophy, nodular hyperplasia of the prostate.

**prostatic hypertrophy, benign**　See *prostatic hyperplasia, benign.*

**prostatitis**　Inflammation of the prostate gland.

**prosthesis**　An artificial replacement of a part of the body, such as a tooth, a facial bone, the palate, or a joint. A prosthesis may be removable, as in the case of most prosthetic legs or a prosthetic breast form used after mastectomy. A person who uses a removable prosthesis—for example, an artificial hand—may want to have more than one available for different types of tasks. Other types of prosthetic devices, such as an artificial hip or tooth, are permanently implanted. And with advances in medical science, a few experimental prostheses have been integrated with body tissues, including the nervous system. These highly advanced devices can respond to commands from the central nervous system, more closely approximating normal movement and utility.

**prosthetics**　The art and science of developing artificial replacements for body parts. Depending on the type of prosthesis, prosthetics may be built and fitted/implanted in a hospital (as in the case of an artificial knee joint), or by an outside specialist. Postmastectomy prosthetics, for example, may be purchased and fitted by specialized lingerie shops.

**prosthodontist** A dentist with special training in making replacements for missing teeth or other structures of the oral cavity, restoring the patient's appearance, comfort, and/or health.

**protease** An enzyme that can split a protein into the peptides from whence it was originally created.

**protease inhibitor** An agent that can keep a protease from splitting a protein into peptides. Protease inhibitors include saquinavir (brand name: Invirase, Fortovase) and ritonavir (brand name: Norvir), and are used primarily in HIV/AIDS treatment. They are taken as part of a two- or three-drug cocktail, accompanied by one or more nucleoside antiviral drugs. These treatments are capable of lowering the level of HIV virus in the blood until it cannot be measured with current tools. Side effects associated with protease inhibitors include a lipodystrophy syndrome in which the face, arms and legs become thin due to loss of subcutaneous fat, the skin becomes dry, weight loss occurs, and abnormal deposits of fat occur. Some new strains of HIV may be resistant to protease inhibitors.

**protein** One of the three nutrients used as energy sources (calories) by the body. Proteins are essential components of the muscle, skin, and bones. Proteins and carbohydrates each provide 4 calories of energy per gram, whereas fats provide 9 calories per gram.

**protein C** A vitamin K–dependent protein in plasma that enters into the cascade of biochemical events, leading to the formation of a clot.

**protein C deficiency** A condition that results in thrombotic (clotting) disease, and excess platelets with recurrent inflammation of the vein that occurs when a clot forms (thrombophlebitis). The clot can break loose and travel through the blood stream (thromboembolism) to the lungs, causing a pulmonary embolism; to the brain, causing a stroke (cerebrovascular accident); to the heart, causing an early heart attack; to the skin, causing what in the newborn is called neonatal purpura fulminans; or to the adrenal gland, causing hemorrhage with abdominal pain, abnormally low blood pressure (hypotension), and salt loss. Protein C deficiency is due to possession of one gene (heterozygosity) in chromosome band 2q13-14. The possession of two such genes (homozygosity) is usually lethal.

**protein malnutrition** Insufficient intake of nitrogen-containing food (protein) to maintain a nitrogen balance or nitrogen equilibrium. Children are particularly prone to develop protein malnutrition. To grow, children have to consume enough nitrogen-containing food (protein) to maintain a positive nitrogen balance, whereas adults need only be in nitrogen equilibrium. See also *kwashiorkor.*

**protein, C-reactive** See *C-reactive protein.*

**protein-calorie malnutrition** See *kwashiorkor.*

**protein-losing enteropathy** Condition in which plasma protein is lost in excess to the intestine. This can be due to diverse causes, including gluten enteropathy, extensive ulceration of the intestine, intestinal lymphatic blockage, or infiltration of leukemic cells into the intestinal wall.

**proteins, acute-phase** Proteins whose plasma concentrations increase or decrease by 25 percent or more during certain inflammatory disorders. C-reactive protein (CRP) is perhaps the best known of acute-phase proteins.

**proteins, G** See *G proteins.*

**proteinuria** Excess protein in the urine. Some protein is normal in the urine. Too much means protein is leaking through the kidney, most often through the glomeruli. The main protein in human blood, and the key to the regulation of the osmotic pressure of blood, is albumin. Also known as albuminuria.

**Proteus syndrome** A disturbance of cell growth that causes benign tumors under the skin; overgrowth of the body, often more on one side than the other (hemihypertrophy); and overgrowth of fingers (macrodactyly). John Merrick, the 19th century Englishman known as the "elephant man," is thought to have had Proteus syndrome.

**prothrombin** A coagulation (clotting) factor is needed for the normal clotting of blood. A cascade of biochemical events leads to the formation of the final clot. In this cascade, prothrombin is a precursor to thrombin. Also known as thrombinogen. See also *prothrombin time.*

**prothrombin time** A test done to gauge the integrity of part of the clotting process. Prothrombin time is commonly used to monitor the accuracy of blood-thinning treatment (anticoagulation) with drugs like warfarin (brand names: Coumadin, Panwarfin, Sofarin). It measures the time needed for clot formation after a substance called thromboplastin and calcium are added to plasma. Familiarly known as pro time.

**proto-oncogene** A normal gene involved in cell division or proliferation that, when altered by mutation, becomes an oncogene that can contribute to cancer.

**protozoa** A parasitic single-cell organism that can only divide within a host organism. For example, malaria is caused by the protozoa Plasmodium.

**proximal**   The nearer of two or more items; toward the beginning. For example, the proximal end of the femur is part of the hip joint, and the shoulder is proximal to the elbow. The opposite of proximal is distal. See also *Appendix B, "Anatomic Orientation Terms."*

**proximal white subungual onychomycosis**   See *onychomycosis, proximal white subungual.*

**proxy, health care**   See *health care proxy.*

**pruritic**   Itchy. A scab may be pruritic.

**pruritus**   Itching. Pruritus can result from drug reaction, food allergy, kidney or liver disease, cancers, parasites, aging or dry skin, contact skin reaction (such as poison ivy), or for unknown reasons.

**pruritus ani**   See *anal itching.*

**PSA**   Prostate specific antigen.

**PSC**   Primary sclerosing cholangitis.

**pseudo-**   Prefix indicating a medical condition that resembles another condition, but appears to have different causes. For example, a pseudoseizure is a seizure-like episode that may not show up as unusual electrical activity in the brain.

**pseudodementia**   A severe form of depression resulting from a progressive brain disorder in which cognitive changes mimic those of dementia.

**pseudogout**   Inflammation of the joints caused by deposits of calcium pyrophosphate crystals, resulting in arthritis, most commonly of the knees, wrists, shoulders, hips, and ankles. Pseudogout usually affects only one or a few joints at a time. True gout is due to a different type of crystal, formed by the precipitation of uric acid.

**pseudo-Hurler polydystrophy**   A rare genetic disease that is passed on via an autosomal recessive gene. It is characterized by abnormal lysosomal enzyme transport in cells of mesenchymal origin, causing elevated lysosomal enzymes in body fluids and tissues. Diagnosis is by blood test. There is currently no treatment for this disorder. Also known as mucolipidosis III.

**pseudomembranous colitis**   See *colitis, pseudomembranous.*

**pseudomonas pseudomallei**   A bacteria that causes an infectious illness called melioidosis. See *melioidosis.*

**pseudo-obstruction, intestinal**   A group of chronic disorders that impair gastrointestinal motility, despite the absence of an actual obstruction. Symptoms include cramping and abdominal pain, malnutrition, nausea, and vomiting. Some forms of pseudo-obstruction appear to be genetically inherited. Diagnosis is by observation of symptoms, measuring pressure in the GI tract, and microscopic examination of the bowels. There is no specific treatment for this disorder, although medications can be used to relieve specific symptoms. Special diets, and sometimes tube-feeding, are sometimes necessary. Surgery is rarely effective.

**pseudo-obstruction, myopathic**   Intestinal pseudo-obstruction caused by damage to muscle cells in the walls of the bowel.

**pseudo-obstruction, neuropathic**   Intestinal pseudo-obstruction caused by damage to nerve cells in the walls of the bowel.

**pseudoparalysis, spastic**   See *Creutzfeldt-Jakob disease.*

**pseudorubella**   See *measles.*

**pseudotumor cerebri**   The presence of elevated levels of cerebrospinal fluid without the presence of a tumor. It can cause headache, ringing in the ears, double vision, loss of visual accuracy, and even complete blindness. It is most common in young to middle-aged women. Although its cause is usually not known, pseudotumor cerebri is sometimes linked to tetracycline, nalidixic acid, nitrofurantoin, phenytoin, lithium, amiodarone, or overuse of vitamin A. Diagnosis is by brain imaging and lumbar puncture. Treatment is by medication, diet if the patient is overweight, and sometimes a type of surgery called optic nerve sheath fenestration that allows the excess fluid to escape.

**pseudoxanthoma elasticum**   A rare disorder characterized by degeneration of the elastic fibers, with tiny areas of calcification in the skin, back of the eyes (retinae), and blood vessels. Pseudoxanthoma elasticum (PXE) can be inherited as an autosomal recessive or somal dominant trait. It typically causes small, yellow-white raised areas in the skin folds, often appearing in the second or third decades of life. These skin abnormalities frequently appear on the neck, armpits, and other areas that bend a great deal (flexure areas). The face is not affected by PXE. The doctor may see abnormalities in the back of the eye called angioid streaks; these tiny breaks in the elastin-filled tissue can lead to blindness. Other areas that can be affected include the heart, which can be affected by atherosclerosis and mitral valve prolapse. Small blood vessels are abnormally fragile in patients with PXE, because the blood-vessel walls contain elastin and are weakened. This can lead to abnormal bleeding in such areas as the bowel and, very rarely, the uterus. Impairment of circulation to the legs can lead to pains in the legs while walking (claudication).

**psittacosis** An infectious disease due to a bacteria (Chlamydia psittaci) contracted from psittacine birds, especially caged birds like parrots, parakeets, and lovebirds. It is also seen in turkey-processing plants. The bacteria enters the human body by inhalation of air that contains it, or by a bite from an infected bird. The incubation period is one to three weeks. Signs and symptoms include fever and chills, ill feeling (malaise), loss of appetite, cough, and shortness of breath. Diagnosis is by recovering the bacteria in the laboratory from the patient's blood or sputum. Treatment is by antibiotics, such as tetracycline. With early diagnosis and proper treatment, the disease is usually over in a week or two. To avoid psittacosis, avoid dust from bird feathers and cage contents, and do not handle a sick bird. Also known as parrot fever.

**psoriasis** A reddish, scaly rash, often located over the surfaces of the elbows, knees, scalp, and around or in the ears, navel, genitals, or buttocks. Approximately 10 to 15 percent of patients with psoriasis develop joint inflammation (inflammatory arthritis). It is caused by the body making too many skin cells, and in some cases it is believed to be an autoimmune condition. Treatment options include topical steroid creams, tar soap preparations, and exposure to ultraviolet light. See also *psoriasis, guttate; psoriasis, pustular; psoriatic arthritis*.

**psoriasis, guttate** A type of psoriasis characterized by red, scaly patches of inflamed skin on all parts of the body. It is associated with a lung infection in many cases.

**psoriasis, pustular** A type of recurring psoriasis characterized by the appearance of pus-filled pimples and sores in clusters. It can be intensely painful, and hospitalization may be necessary.

**psoriatic arthritis** Joint inflammation associated with psoriasis. Psoriatic arthritis is a potentially destructive and deforming form of arthritis that affects approximately 10 percent of persons with psoriasis.

**psyche** The mind.

**psychiatrist** A physician (MD) who specializes in the prevention, diagnosis, and treatment of mental illness. Psychiatrists must receive additional training and serve a supervised residency in their specialty. They may also have additional training in a psychiatric specialty, such as child psychiatry or neuropsychiatry. They can prescribe medication, which psychologists cannot do.

**psychogenic** Caused by the mind or emotions.

**psychological child abuse** See *child abuse, emotional*.

**psychologist** A professional who specializes in the diagnosis and treatment of diseases of the brain, emotional disturbance, and behavior problems. Psychologists can only use talk therapy as treatment; you must see a psychiatrist or other medical doctor to be treated with medication. Psychologists may have a master's degree (MA) or doctorate (PhD) in psychology. They may also have other qualifications, including Board certification and additional training in a type of therapy.

**psychosis** A thought disorder in which perception of reality is grossly impaired. Symptoms can include seeing, hearing, smelling, or tasting things that are not there; paranoia; and delusional thoughts. Depending on the condition underlying the psychotic symptoms, symptoms may be constant or they may come and go. Psychosis can occur as a result of brain injury or disease, and is seen particularly in schizophrenia and bipolar disorders. Psychotic symptoms can occur as a result of drug use, but this is not true psychosis. Diagnosis is by observation and interview. Treatment is with neuroleptic medication, either the newer, safer, atypical neuroleptics like risperadone (brand name: Risperdal) or the older neuroleptics like haloperidol (brand name: Haldol). In cases that do not respond to medication, electroshock therapy (ECT) is sometimes valuable.

**psychosis, ICU** See *ICU psychosis*.

**psychosomatic illness** An illness that has no physical basis.

**PTCA** Percutaneous transluminal coronary angioplasty.

**pterygium** A wing-like triangular membrane. Although a pterygium can be anywhere, including behind the knee, it commonly refers to a winglet of the conjunctiva. This pterygium may extend across the white of the eye toward the inner corner of the eye. It is caused by prolonged exposure of the eyes to wind and weather, or can be an inherited disorder caused by a single gene.

**ptosis** Downward displacement. Ptosis of the eyelids is drooping of the eyelids.

**ptosis of the eyelids, congenital** Drooping of the upper eyelids at birth. The lids may droop only slightly, or they may cover the pupils and restrict or even block vision. Moderate or severe pstrosis calls for treatment to permit normal vision development. If not corrected, amblyopia (lazy eye) may develop, which can lead to permanently poor vision. Ptosis at birth is often caused by poor development of the levator muscle, which lifts the eyelid. Children with ptosis may tip their heads back into a chin-up position to see underneath the eyelids, or raise their eyebrows in an attempt to lift up the lids. Congenital ptosis rarely improves with time. Treatment is usually surgery to tighten the levator muscles. If the levator is very weak, the lid can be attached or suspended from under the eyebrow so that the forehead muscles can do the lifting. Even after surgery, focusing problems can develop as the eyes grow and change shape. All children with ptosis, whether they have had surgery or not, should therefore be followed by an ophthalmologist. Usually, mild or moderate ptosis does not require surgery early in life.

**pubarche**  The age at which pubic hair first appears; puberty.

**puberty**  Adolescence, the period in which the human body first becomes capable of reproduction.

**pubic symphysis**  The joint between the pubic bones at the front of the pelvis.

**pubis**  The front center portion of the pelvis.

**public health**  **1** Medicine concerned with the health of the community as a whole. Community health. **2** In common use, a facility or government agency that provides low-income or free health care.

**Public Health Service, United States**  See *United States Public Health Service.*

**PUBS**  Percutaneous umbilical blood sampling.

**pueperal fever**  See *childbed fever.*

**pueperium**  The time immediately after the delivery of a baby.

**pulmonary**  Having to do with the lungs.

**pulmonary edema**  Fluid in the lungs.

**pulmonary embolism**  Sudden closure of a pulmonary artery or one of its branches, caused by a blood-borne clot or foreign material that plugs the vessel.

**pulmonary embolus**  A blood clot within the lung's pulmonary artery. An embolus causes an embolism. In this case, the embolus, a clot or foreign material, has been carried through the blood into the pulmonary artery or one of its branches, plugging the vessel.

**pulmonary hypertension**  High blood pressure in the pulmonary arteries. Normally, the pressure in the pulmonary arteries is low compared to that in the aorta. Pulmonary hypertension can irrevocably damage the lungs.

**pulmonary insufficiency**  A condition in which the valve between the right ventricle of the heart and the pulmonary artery is incompetent in its performance, allowing

blood to slosh back from the pulmonary artery into the right ventricle.

**pulmonary stenosis**  A condition in which the pulmonary valve is too tight, so that the flow of blood from the right ventricle of the heart into the pulmonary artery is impeded. This means that the right ventricle must pump harder than normal to overcome the obstruction. If the stenosis is severe in a baby, the infant may become blue (cyanotic). Older children often have no symptoms. Treatment is necessary if the pressure in the right ventricle is higher than normal. The obstruction can usually be relieved by a procedure called balloon valvuloplasty or by open heart surgery during which the stenotic valve is opened. The outlook after either procedure is favorable.

**pulmonary stenosis, peripheral, with cholestasis**  See *Alagille syndrome.*

**pulmonary syndrome, hantavirus**  See *hantavirus pulmonary syndrome.*

**pulmonary valve**  One of the four valves in the heart, the pulmonary valve stands at the opening from the right ventricle in the pulmonary artery trunk. It moves blood toward the lungs, and keeps it from sloshing back from the pulmonary artery into the heart.

**pulmonary vein**  One of four vessels that carry aerated blood from the lungs to the left atrium of the heart. The pulmonary veins are the only veins that carry bright-red oxygenated blood.

**pulse**  The rhythmic dilation of an artery resulting from beating of the heart. It is often measured by feeling the arteries of the wrist.

**pulse rate**  A measure of the number of pulsations in the radial artery each minute. It is usually taken at the wrist.

**pulse, Corrigan**  See *Corrigan pulse.*

**pulse, water-hammer**  See *Corrigan pulse.*

**pump-oxygenator**  See *heart-lung machine.*

**punch biopsy**  A biopsy performed by using a punch, an instrument for cutting and removing a disk of tissue. For example, a punch biopsy of the skin may be done to make the diagnosis of a malignancy.

**puncture wound**  An injury caused by a pointed object that pierces or penetrates the skin. Any puncture wound through tennis shoes (as with a nail) has a high risk of infection, because the foam in tennis shoes can harbor the bacteria Pseudomonas. Puncture wounds also carry a danger of tetanus.

**puncture, lumbar**   See *lumbar puncture.*

**pupil**   The opening of the iris. The pupil may appear to open (dilate) and close (constrict), but it is really the iris that is the prime mover; the pupil is merely the absence of iris. The pupil determines how much light is let into the eye. Both pupils are usually of equal size. If they are not, that condition is called anisocoria.

**purine**   One of the two classes of bases in DNA and RNA. The purine bases are guanine (G) and adenine (A). Uric acid, the offending substance in gout, is a purine end-product.

**purpura**   A hemorrhage area in the surface of the skin. The appearance of an individual area of purpura varies with the duration of the lesions. Early purpura is red and becomes darker, then purple, and brown-yellow as it fades.

**purpura, acute thrombocytopenic**   See *acute thrombocytopenic purpura.*

**purpura, anaphylactoid**   See *anaphylactoid purpura.*

**purpura, Henoch-Schonlein**   See *anaphylactoid purpura.*

**pus**   A thick, whitish-yellow fluid that results from the accumulation of white blood cells (WBCs), liquefied tissue, and cellular debris. Pus is commonly a sign of infection or foreign material in the body.

**pustulosis**   A highly inflammatory skin condition resulting in large, fluid-filled, blister-like areas (pustules). Pustulosis typically occurs on the palms of the hands and/or the soles of the feet. The skin of these areas peels and flakes (exfoliates).

**PV**   Polycythemia vera.

**PVC**   Premature ventricular contraction.

**PXE**   Pseudoxanthoma elasticum.

**pycnodysostosis**   An inherited disorder of the bone that causes short stature and abnormally dense brittle bones. Due to a defect in an enzyme cathepsin K. Sometimes spelled pyknodysostosis.

**pyelo**   See *pyelonephritis.*

**pyelogram**   X-ray study of the kidney, especially showing the pelvis (urine-collecting basin) of the kidney and the ureter.

**pyelonephritis**   Bacterial infection of the kidney. Pyelonephritis can be acute or chronic, and is most often due to the ascent of bacteria from the bladder up the ureters to infect the kidneys. Symptoms include flank (side) pain, fever, shaking chills, sometimes foul-smelling urine, frequent and urgent need to urinate, and general malaise. Tenderness is elicited on gently tapping over the kidney with a fist (percussion). Diagnosis is by urinalysis, which reveals white blood cells and bacteria in the urine. Usually there is also an increase in circulating white cells in the blood. Treatment involves appropriate antibiotics.

**pyloric stenosis**   Narrowing (stenosis) of the outlet of the stomach so that food cannot pass easily from it into the duodenum. This results in feeding problems and projectile vomiting. The obstruction can be corrected by a relatively simple surgical procedure.

**pylorus**   The outlet of the stomach.

**pyoderma gangrenosum**   An ulcerating condition of skin resulting in heaped borders with a typical appearance. Pyoderma gangrenosum appears to be mediated by the immune system, but the exact cause is unknown. The lesion usually begins as a soft nodule on the skin, which proceeds to ulcerate. The ulcer enlarges and the skin at the edge is purple-red. Ulcers can become quite large. This condition is associated with several other diseases, including ulcerative colitis, Crohn disease, rheumatoid arthritis, leukemia, and cryoglobulinemia. Pyoderma gangrenosum is usually responsive to corticosteroids.

**pyrexia**   See *fever.*

**pyrimidine**   One of the two classes of bases in DNA and RNA. The pyrimidine bases are thymine (T) and cytosine (C) in DNA, and thymine (T) and uracil (U) in RNA.

**pyuria**   Pus in the urine. Pyuria is a sign of inflammation, often related to infection.

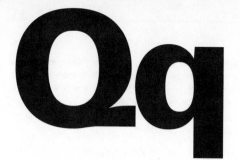

**q arm of a chromosome** The long arm of a chromosome.

**Q bands** The alternating bright and dull fluorescent bands seen on chromosomes under ultraviolet light after they are stained with quinacrine.

**Q fever** An acute, self-limited febrile illness first reported in Queensland, Australia. The Q stands for Query, as the cause of the disease was long a question mark. It is now known to be due to Coxiella burnetti, a rickettsia bacteria. Symptoms include fever, headache, malaise, and pneumonia (interstitial pneumonitis), but not rash.

**q in population genetics** The frequency of the less common of two alternative (allelic) versions of a gene. The frequency of the more common allele is p.

**q.d.** Seen on a prescription, one a day. Also known as quotid. See *Appendix A, "Prescription Abbreviations."*

**q.h.** On a prescription, every hour. See *Appendix A, "Prescription Abbreviations."*

**q.2h.** On a prescription, every two hours. See *Appendix A, "Prescription Abbreviations."*

**q.3h.** On a prescription, every three hours. See *Appendix A, "Prescription Abbreviations."*

**q.i.d.** On a prescription, four times daily. See *Appendix A, "Prescription Abbreviations."*

**q.n.s.** On a lab report, insufficient quantity of sample.

**QALY** Quality adjusted life year.

**QRS complex** The deflections in an electrocardiographic (EKG) tracing that represent the ventricular activity of the heart.

**QT syndrome, long** See *long QT syndrome.*

**q.s.** On a prescription, as needed. See *Appendix A, "Prescription Abbreviations."*

**quack** 1 A practitioner who suggests substances or devices for prevention or treatment of disease that are known to be ineffective. 2 Someone who pretends to be able to diagnose or heal people, but is unqualified and incompetent.

**quackery** Deliberate misrepresentation of the ability of a substance or device to prevent or treat disease.

**quadrant** A quarter. For example, the liver is in the right upper quadrant of the abdomen.

**quadriceps** 1 Any four-headed muscle. 2 The quadriceps muscle of the thigh, the large muscle that comes down the bone of the upper leg (femur) and over the kneecap (patella), and then anchors into the top of the big bone in the lower leg (tibia). The function of the quadriceps is to straighten (extend) the leg. Also known as the musculus quadriceps femoris, or quad.

**quadriparesis** Weakness of all four limbs, both arms and both legs. For example, muscular dystrophy can cause quadriparesis.

**quadriplegia** Paralysis of all four limbs, both arms and both legs, as from a high spinal cord accident or stroke.

**qualitative** Having to do with quality, in contrast to quantitative, which pertains strictly to quantity. The results of a qualitative analysis may vary from those of a quantitative analysis, even if the same event or procedure is being examined.

**quality adjusted life year** A year of life adjusted for its quality or its value. A year in perfect health is considered equal to 1.0 QALY. The value of a year in ill health would be discounted. For example, a year bedridden might have a value equal to 0.5 QALY.

**quality of life** An important consideration in medical care, quality of life refers to the patient's ability to enjoy normal life activities. Some medical treatments can seriously impair quality of life without providing appreciable benefit, while others greatly enhance quality of life.

**quantitative** Having to do with quantity or with the amount. See also *qualitative.*

**quarantine** A period of isolation decreed to control the spread of infectious disease. Before the era of antibiotics and the like, quarantine was one of the few available means for halting the reach of infectious diseases.

**quasi-** Prefix meaning seemingly. For example, quasidominant means seemingly dominant.

**quasidiploid** Describing a cell that seems to have the usual 2 full sets of 23 chromosomes, but does not. Many malignant cells are quasidiploid. Also called pseudodiploid.

**quasidominant**  Pattern of inheritance that seems due to a dominant trait but is in fact due to the mating of a person who has a recessive disorder (with two copies of a gene causing the disease) with someone who is an asymptomatic carrier (with one copy of the same gene, but no symptoms).

**Queensland tick typhus**  See *typhus, Queensland tick.*

**quickening**  The moment during pregnancy when the baby is first felt to move.

**quiescent**  Inactive, resting. Tuberculosis can be a quiescent (inactive) infection.

**quinacrine**  An antimalarial drug and, in cytogenetics, a fluorescent dye used to stain chromosomes. The Y chromosome stains brilliantly with quinacrine.

**Quincke disease**  See *angioedema, hereditary.*

**quinidine**  A medication (brand name: Cardioquin, Quinaglute, Quinalan, Quinidex, Quinora) prescribed to treat abnormal heart rhythms. It is derived from the same botanical source as quinine. Side effects may include nausea and diarrhea. Quinidine interacts with a number of other medications, particularly over-the-counter cold and cough remedies. Talk to your doctor before taking any other drug with quinidine.

**quinine**  A classic antimalarial agent.

**quinsy**  See *peritonsillar abscess.*

**Quintan fever**  See *trench fever.*

**quotid**  See *q.d.*

**quotidian**  Recurring each day, as in a fever that returns every day.

**quotient**  The result of mathematical division. For example, an Intelligence Quotient (I.Q.) can be derived from dividing a person's mental age as determined by the Stanford-Binet test by the person's chronological age, and multiplying by 100. If a six-year-old child scores at the eight-year-old level, the I.Q. is 8/6 multiplied by 100: 125.

# Rr

**R**   This much-used symbol has many meanings in medicine. They include **1** Respiration. A nurse's note of "R20" is shorthand for 20 respirations (breaths) per minute. **2** Right. A doctor's note of a burn on the "R digit 5" places the burn on the right little finger or toe. **3** Roentgen. **4** In chemistry, a radical. **5** On a prescription, R (or Rx), recipe, which is Latin for "to take."

**rabies**   A potentially fatal viral infection that attacks the central nervous system. Rabies is carried by wild animals (particularly bats and raccoons), and finds its way to humans either by direct contact or by contact with domestic animals that have contracted the virus. Most cases can be traced to animal bites, but cases have been documented where the virus was inhaled in bat caves, contracted in lab accidents, or received from transplanted donor tissue. Symptoms include fever, aching muscles, and headache, potentially progressing to inflammation of the brain, confusion, seizures, paralysis, coma, and death. There is no cure for rabies once it has settled in the brain, so immediate emergency care for any suspicious animal contact is a must. Rabies immunoglobulin (RIG) shots, antibiotics, and rabies vaccine may be used immediately after contact. To prevent rabies, vaccinate all pets against the virus, and avoid contact with wild or unknown animals. A human rabies vaccine is available, but is recommended only for those in high-risk occupations (game wardens, zookeepers, animal control officers, and so on).

**racemose**   A descriptive term for something that is in a cluster or bunch.

**racemose aneurysm**   An aneurysm that looks like a bunch of grapes.

**rad**   Radiation absorbed dose, a measure for a dose of ionizing radiation.

**radial**   Spreading from a central point. For example, the radial artery branches out from a central point in the forearm.

**radial aplasia-thrombocytopenia syndrome**   See *TAR syndrome.*

**radial artery**   A major artery that emerges through the neck of the radius in the crook of the elbow, and sends out 12 branches to various areas of the forearm, wrist, and hand.

**radiate**   To spread out from a central area. For example, sciatic pain may radiate outward from the lower back.

**radiation**   **1** Rays of energy. Gamma rays and X-rays are two types of energy waves often used in medicine. **2** The use of energy waves to diagnose or treat disease.

**radiation fibrosis**   See *fibrosis, radiation.*

**radiation menopause**   See *menopause, induced.*

**radiation oncologist**   A specialist in the use of radiation therapy as a treatment for cancer.

**radiation oncology**   The medical specialty involved with the use of radiation to treat cancer.

**radiation pneumonitis**   See *pneumonitis, radiation.*

**radiation therapy**   The use of high-energy rays to damage cancer cells, stopping them from growing and dividing. Like surgery, radiation therapy is a local treatment that affects cancer cells only in the treated area. Radiation can come from a machine (external radiation) or from a small container of radioactive material implanted directly into or near the tumor (internal radiation). Some patients receive both kinds of radiation therapy. External radiation therapy is usually given on an outpatient basis in a hospital or clinic, five days a week for several weeks. Patients are not radioactive during or after the treatment. For internal radiation therapy, the patient stays in the hospital for a few days. The implant may be temporary or permanent. Because the level of radiation is highest during the hospital stay, patients may not be able to have visitors, or may have visitors only for a short time. Once an implant is removed, there is no radioactivity in the body. The amount of radiation in a permanent implant goes down to a safe level before the patient leaves the hospital. Side effects of radiation therapy depend on the treatment dose and the part of the body treated. The most common side effects are fatigue, skin reactions (such as a rash or redness) in the treated area, and loss of appetite. Radiation therapy can cause inflammation of tissues and organs in and around the body site radiated. Radiation therapy can also cause a decrease in the number of white blood cells. Although the side effects of radiation therapy can be unpleasant, they can usually be treated or controlled. It also helps to know that, in most cases, they are not permanent.

**radiation therapy, external**   Radiation therapy in which the source of radiation is a machine outside the body.

**radiation therapy, internal** Radiation therapy in which a small container of radioactive material is implanted in the body, in or near the cancerous tumor.

**radiation therapy, interstitial** A form of radiotherapy in which tiny, radioactive "seeds" are permanently implanted directly in the affected tissue with a needle-like instrument. It has shown particular promise in treating prostate cancer.

**radiation therapy, stereotactic** The use of a number of precisely aimed beams of ionizing radiation, each coming from a different direction and meeting at a specific point, to deliver radiation treatment to that spot.

**radiation, seed** See *radiation therapy, interstitial*.

**radical dissection** Removal of not only affected tissue, but also of nearby tissue that may be covertly affected.

**radical mastectomy** See *mastectomy, radical*.

**radical, free** See *free radical*.

**radioactive** Emitting energy waves due to decaying atomic nuclei. Radioactive substances are used in medicine as tracers for diagnosis, and in treatment to kill cancerous cells.

**radioactive tracer** A radioactive molecule that can be sent through the body's circulatory or urinary system, with its progress followed by a radiation-sensitive machine.

**radioallergosorbent test** See *RAST*.

**radiograph** Medical term for an X-ray, or a film produced by X-ray.

**radiography** Film records (radiographs) of internal structures of the body. Radiography is made possible by X-rays passing through the body to act on a specially sensitized film.

**radioimmunoassay** A very sensitive, specific laboratory test (assay) using radiolabeled and unlabeled substances in an immunological (antibody-antigen) reaction.

**radioinsensitive** Not sensitive to X-rays and other forms of radiant energy. For example, a tumor may be radioinsensitive, and therefore cannot be successfully attacked using radiation therapy. The opposite of radiosensitive.

**radioiodine** A version (isotope) of the chemical element iodine that is radioactive. Radioiodine is used in diagnostic tests as well as in radiotherapy of the thyroid. For hyperthyroidism, radioiodine is administered in capsule form on a one-time basis. It directly radiates thyroid tissues, thereby destroying them. It takes 8 to 12 weeks

for the thyroid to become euthyroid (normal) after treatment. The majority of patients undergoing this treatment eventually become hypothyroid, which is easily treated using thyroid hormones (levothyroxine). Radioiodine should not be used during pregnancy and breast feeding. See also *Graves disease*.

**radioisotope** An alternate version (isotope) of a chemical element that has a different atomic mass, and is radioactive.

**radiologic** Having to do with radiology.

**radiology** The science of radiation, both ionizing radiation like X-rays and nonionizing radiation like ultrasound, and of how it can be applied to the diagnosis and treatment of disease. Also known as roentgenology.

**radiology, interventional** The use of image guidance methods to gain access to the deepest interior of most organs and organ systems. Through a galaxy of techniques, interventional radiologists can treat certain conditions through the skin (percutaneously) that might otherwise require surgery. The technology includes the use of balloons, catheters, microcatheters, stents, therapeutic embolization (deliberately clogging up a blood vessel), and more. The specialty of interventional radiology overlaps with other surgical arenas, including interventional cardiology, vascular surgery, endoscopy, laparoscopy, and other minimally invasive techniques, such as biopsies. Specialists performing interventional radiology procedures today include not only radiologists but also other types of doctors, such as general surgeons, vascular surgeons, cardiologists, gastroenterologists, gynecologists, and urologists.

**radiolucent** Permeable to one or another form of radiation, such as X-rays. Radiolucent objects do not block radiation, but let it pass. The opposite of radiolucent is radiopaque. Plastic is usually radiolucent.

**radionuclide scan** An exam that produces pictures (scans) of internal parts of the body. The patient is given an injection or swallows a small amount of radioactive material. A machine called a scanner then measures the radioactivity in certain organs.

**radiopaque** Opaque to one or another form of radiation, such as X-rays. Radiopaque objects block radiation rather than allowing it to pass through. Metal, for instance, is radiopaque, so metal objects that a patient may have swallowed are visible on X-rays. Radiopaque dyes are used in radiology to enhance X-ray pictures of internal anatomic structures. For example, an intravenous pyelogram (IVP) is an X-ray study of the kidneys that highlights the renal pelvis and the ureters. The opposite of radiopaque is radiolucent.

**radiosensitive**   Sensitive to X-rays and other forms of radiant energy. For example, a tumor may be radiosensitive, and therefore potentially treatable with radiation therapy. The opposite is radioinsensitive.

**radiotherapy**   See *radiation therapy*.

**radium**   The celebrated radioactive element discovered by Marie and Pierre Curie in 1898.

**radius**   The smaller of the two bones on the thumb's side of the forearm. Its larger companion is the ulna.

**radon**   A radioactive element formed as a gas during the breakdown of radium.

**Raeder syndrome**   See *cluster headache*.

**ragweed**   Any of several weedy composite herbs that produce a pollen. Of all allergy sufferers in the US, 75 percent are allergic to ragweed.

**RAI**   Radioiodine.

**rale**   An abnormal lung sound that can be heard through a stethoscope. Rales may be sibilant (whistling), dry (crackling), or wet (sloshy), depending on the amount and density of fluid refluxing back and forth in the air passages.

**Ramsey Hunt syndrome**   A herpes virus infection of the geniculate nerve ganglion, the Ramsey Hunt syndrome causes paralysis of the facial muscles on the same side of the face as the infection. It is usually associated with an unusual rash (vesicles or tiny water-filled bumps in the skin) in or around the ear, and sometimes on the roof of the mouth. Ramsey Hunt syndrome is commonly more painful and more debilitating than Bell palsy. Treatment with steroids and antiviral agents, such as acyclovir (brand name: Zovirax) may improve recovery and lessen pain.

**ramus**   In anatomy, a branch, such as a branch of a blood vessel or nerve. For example, the ramus acetabularis arteriae circumflexae femoris medialis is the branch of an artery that goes to the socket of the hip joint. The plural of ramus is rami.

**ramus of the mandible**   One of the two prominent, projecting back parts of the horseshoe-shaped lower jaw bone.

**random**   Determined solely by chance.

**random mating**   Totally haphazard mating, with no regard to the genetic makeup (genotype) of the mate, so that any sperm has an equal chance of fertilizing any egg.

This rarely if ever occurs, but the concept is important in population genetics. Also called panmixus.

**random sample**   A test group selected randomly, solely by chance.

**range**   In medicine and statistics, the difference between the lowest and highest numerical values. For example, if five premature infants are born weighing two, three, four, four, and five pounds respectively, the range of their birth weights is two to five pounds.

**range of motion**   The full movement potential of a joint, usually its range of flexion and extension. For example, a knee might lack 10 degrees of full extension due to an injury.

**range, normal**   See *normal range*.

**ranitidine**   A medication (brand name: Zantac) in the $H_2$ antagonist family that turns off the production of stomach acid and other secretions. It is used to treat the symptoms of ulcers and gastrointestinal reflux disease (GERD). Side effects may include depression, insomnia, dizziness, confusion, and thought disturbances. This remedy may be counteracted by antacids, and interacts with some other medications. Ranitidine is available in both prescription and over-the-counter forms. See also *ranitidine bismuth citrate*.

**ranitidine bismuth citrate**   A drug that combines the $H_2$ antagonist ranitidine with an antibacterial agent that can kill H. pylori, the bacteria involved in most ulcers. It treats both the symptoms and causes of ulcers.

**rapid eye movement sleep**   See *REM sleep*.

**rash**   Breaking out (eruption) of the skin. Rash can be caused by an underlying medical condition, hormonal cycles, allergies, or contact with irritating substances. Treatment depends on the underlying cause of the rash. Medically, a rash is referred to as an exanthem.

**rash, butterfly**   See *butterfly rash*. See also *lupus; lupus, discoid; lupus erythematosus, systemic; roseola*.

**rash, chicken pox**   See *chicken pox rash*.

**rash, maculopapular**   A red, raised rash.

**rash, malar**   See *butterfly rash*.

**rash, varicella**   See *chicken pox rash*.

**rash, vesicular**   A raised, blistery rash.

**Rasmussen syndrome**   A rare brain disorder caused by inflammation of brain cells in one hemisphere. Its cause is unknown. Rasmussen syndrome causes seizures, which can be difficult or impossible to control with medication, and eventually results in brain shrinkage (atrophy). Treatment is with surgery, if possible. The inflammation seems to stop of its own accord eventually, but the damage done is irreversible.

**RAST**   Radioallergosorbent test, an allergy test done on a sample of blood. RAST is used to check for allergic sensitivity to specific substances.

**rate, basal metabolic**   See *basal metabolic rate*.

**rate, birth**   See *birth rate*.

**rate, death**   See *death rate*.

**rate, erythrocyte sedimentation**   See *sedimentation rate*.

**rate, fetal mortality**   See *fetal mortality rate*.

**rate, heart**   See *heart rate*.

**rate, infant mortality**   See *infant mortality rate*.

**rate, maternal mortality**   See *maternal mortality rate*.

**rate, neonatal mortality**   See *neonatal mortality rate*.

**rate, pulse**   See *pulse rate*.

**rate, respiratory**   See *respiratory rate*.

**rate, sed**   See *sedimentation rate*.

**rate, sedimentation**   See *sedimentation rate*.

**rat-flea typhus**   See *typhus, murine*.

**rattlesnake bite**   A poisonous bite from a member of the pit viper family. All rattlesnakes are venomous and secrete poisonous venom, and they are the main culprit in deaths from snakebites in the US. Emergency treatment is essential: With proper care, rattlesnake bites are rarely fatal. The affected part should be kept immobile and below the level of the heart, and the bite victim should be taken to the nearest hospital. Do not use a tourniquet or bandage, and do not attempt to suction out the wound by mouth. Treatment is with antivenom, as well as care for the puncture wound itself and any symptoms that emerge, such as respiratory distress. See also *snakebite*.

**Raynaud disease**   A condition resulting in discoloration of the skin on the fingers and/or toes when a person is exposed to changes in temperature or to emotional events. It can occur alone or as part of another disease,

such as rheumatoid arthritis. When it occurs alone, it is referred to as Raynaud disease or primary Raynaud phenomenon. When it accompanies other diseases, it is called Raynaud phenomenon or secondary Raynaud phenomenon. The skin discoloration occurs because an abnormal spasm of the blood vessels causes a diminished blood supply. Initially, the digits involved turn white because of diminished blood supply, then blue because of prolonged lack of oxygen. Finally the blood vessels reopen, causing flushing that turns the digits red.

**Raynaud phenomenon**   A condition resulting in discoloration of fingers and/or toes when a person is exposed to changes in temperature or emotional events. Raynaud phenomenon occurs with a number of conditions, including rheumatic diseases like scleroderma, rheumatoid arthritis, and systemic lupus erythematosus; hormone imbalance, including hypothyroidism and carcinoid imbalances; trauma, such as from frostbite or the use of vibrating tools; medications, particularly propranolol (brand name: Inderal), estrogens, nicotine, and bleomycin; and, uncommonly, cancer. When it occurs alone, it is called Raynaud disease. See also *Raynaud disease*.

**reabsorption**   Absorbing again. For example, the kidney selectively reabsorbs substances already secreted into the renal tubules, such as glucose, proteins, and sodium. These reabsorbed substances return to the blood.

**reaction kinetics**   The rate of change in a biochemical (or other) reaction.

**reaction, allergic**   See *allergic reaction*.

**reaction, chemical**   See *chemical reaction*.

**reaction, desmoplastic**   See *desmoplastic reaction*.

**reaction, hibernation**   See *seasonal affective disorder*. See also *bipolar disorders*.

**reaction, polymerase chain**   See *polymerase chain reaction*.

**reaction, vasovagal**   See *vasovagal reaction*. See also *syncope*.

**reactive arthritis**   See *Reiter syndrome*.

**reading frame**   One of the three possible ways to read a nucleotide sequence in DNA, depending on whether reading starts with the first, second, or third base in a triplet.

**reading frame, open**   A reading frame in DNA that has no termination codon: no signal to stop reading the nucleotide sequence. This allows the reading frame to be translated into protein.

**reading retardation**   Impaired ability to read. It may reflect mental retardation, cultural deprivation, or learning disability. See also *dyslexia*.

**reagent**   A substance used to produce a chemical reaction that allows researchers to detect, measure, produce, or change other substances.

**rebound**   The reversal of response upon withdrawal of the stimulus.

**rebound effect**   The production of increased negative symptoms when the effect of the drug has passed, or the patient no longer responds to it. If a drug produces a rebound effect, the condition it was used to treat may come back even stronger when it is discontinued or loses effectiveness.

**recalcitrant**   Stubborn. For example, a recalcitrant case of pneumonia stubbornly resists treatment.

**recent memory**   See *memory, short-term*.

**receptor**   **1** In cell biology, a structure on the surface of a cell or inside a cell that selectively receives and binds a specific substance. For example, there are insulin receptors, low-density lipoprotein (LDL) receptors. **2** In neurology, a receptor may also be the terminal of a sensory nerve that receives and responds to stimuli.

**receptor, chemokine**   See *chemokine receptor*. See also *chemokine*.

**receptor, visual**   The layer of rods and cones, the visual cells, of the retina.

**recessive**   A gene that expresses itself only when there is no other type of gene present at that spot on the chromosome (locus). For example, cystic fibrosis (CF) is a recessive disorder. A child with cystic fibrosis has the CF gene on both copies of chromosome 7.

**recessive, autosomal**   A gene on a nonsex chromosome (autosome) that expresses itself only when there is no different gene present at that spot on the chromosome (locus). For example, cystic fibrosis (CF) is an autosomal recessive disorder.

**recessive, X-linked**   A gene on the X chromosome that expresses itself only when there is no different gene present at that spot on the chromosome (locus). For example, Duchenne muscular dystrophy (DMD) is an X-linked recessive disorder. A boy with DMD has the DMD gene on his sole X chromosome. Although it is much rarer, a girl could have the DMD gene on both her X chromosomes.

**recipient**   In medicine, someone who is given something, such as a blood transfusion or an organ transplant, derived from another person (the donor).

**reciprocal translocation**   Mutual exchange of chromosome segments between two nonhomologous chromosomes (chromosomes that do not belong to the same pair).

**recombinant**   A person with a new combination of genes, a combination not present in either parent, due to parental recombination of those genes.

**recombinant clones**   Clones containing recombinant DNA molecules.

**recombinant DNA molecules**   A combination of DNA molecules of different origin that are joined, using recombinant DNA technology.

**recombinant DNA technology**   A series of procedures used to join together (recombine) DNA segments. A recombinant DNA molecule is constructed from segments of two or more different DNA molecules. Under certain conditions, a recombinant DNA molecule can enter a cell and replicate there, either on its own or after it has been integrated into a chromosome.

**recombination**   The trading of fragments of genetic material between chromosomes before the egg and sperm cells are created. Key features of recombination include the point-to-point association of paired chromosomes (synapsis), followed by the visible exchange of segments (crossing over) at X-shaped crosspoints (chiasmata). Recombination is the principal way of creating genetic diversity between generations. By shuffling the genetic deck of cards, recombination ensures that children are dealt a different genetic hand than their parents.

**Recombivax-HB**   A vaccine that stimulates the body's immune system to produce antibodies against the hepatitis B virus. See also *hepatitis B, hepatitis B immunization*.

**recrudescence**   Reappearance, as of a rash or arthritis.

**rectal**   Having to do with the rectum.

**rectal cancer**   See *cancer, rectal*.

**rectouterine pouch**   See *pouch of Douglas*.

**rectum**   The last six to eight inches of the large intestine. The rectum stores solid waste until it leaves the body through the anus.

**rectus**   See *rectus abdominis*.

**rectus abdominis** A large muscle in the front of the abdomen. It assists in regular breathing movements, supports the muscles of the spine while a person lifts something, and keeps the intestines and other abdominal organs in place.

**recuperate** To recover health and strength. To recuperate is to convalesce.

**recur** To occur again; to return. Any symptom, sign, or disease can recur.

**recurrence** The return of a sign, symptom, or disease after a remission. The reappearance of cancer cells at the same site or in another location is, unfortunately, a familiar form of recurrence.

**recurrence risk** In medical genetics, the chance that an inherited disease present in a family will recur in that family, affecting another person or persons.

**recurrent** Back again. A recurrent fever is a fever that has returned after an intermission, a recrudescent fever.

**recurrent aural vertigo** See *Ménière disease*.

**recurrent laryngeal nerve** One of the best-known branches of the vagus nerve, a long and important nerve that originates in the brain stem and runs down to the colon. After the recurrent laryngeal nerve leaves the vagus nerve, it goes down into the chest, and then loops back up to supply the larynx. Damage to the recurrent laryngeal nerve can result from diseases inside the chest (intrathoracic diseases), such as a tumor or an aneurysm of the arch of the aorta or the left atrium of the heart. The consequence of damage to the recurrent laryngeal nerve is laryngeal palsy on the affected side. Laryngeal palsy can also be caused by damage to the vagus nerve before it gives off the recurrent laryngeal nerve.

**recurrent respiratory papillomatosis** See *laryngeal papillomatosis; laryngeal papillomatosis, juvenile*.

**red blood cells** Cells that carry oxygen in the blood. A decrease in the number of red blood cells is anemia. Also known as erythrocytes, red cells, red corpuscles. Abbreviated as RBCs. See also *anemia, erythrocyte*.

**red cells** See *red blood cells*.

**red corpuscles** See *red blood cells*.

**red-green colorblindness** A form of colorblindness in which red and green are perceived as identical. It is thought to be caused by aberrant functioning of the retina, and is the most common type of colorblindness. Also known as deuteranomaly, deuteranopia, Daltonism. See also *colorblindness*.

**reduction division** The first cell division in meiosis, the process by which germ cells are formed. A unique event in which the chromosome number is reduced from diploid (46 chromosomes) to haploid (23 chromosomes). Also known as first meiotic division or first meiosis.

**Reed-Sternberg cell** A type of cell that appears in patients with Hodgkin disease. The number of these cells increases as the disease advances.

**referral** The recommendation of a medical or paramedical professional. If you get a referral to ophthalmology, for example, you are being sent to the eye doctor. In HMOs and other managed-care schemes, a referral is usually necessary to see any practitioner or specialist other than your primary care physician (PCP), if you want the service to be covered. The referral is obtained from your PCP, who may require a telephone or office consultation first. The term "referral" can pertain both to the act of sending a patient to another doctor or therapist, and to the actual paper authorizing the visit.

**reflex** An involuntary reaction. For example, the corneal reflex is the blink that occurs with irritation of the eye.

**reflex sympathetic dystrophy syndrome** A condition that features a group of typical symptoms, including pain (often perceived as burning pain), tenderness, and swelling of an extremity. It is associated with varying degrees of sweating, warmth and/or coolness, flushing, discoloration, and shiny skin.

**reflex, Babinski** See *Babinski reflex*.

**reflux** The term used when liquid backs up into the esophagus from the stomach.

**reflux disease, gastroesophageal** See *gastroesophageal reflux*.

**reflux laryngitis** See *laryngitis, reflux*. See also *reflux*.

**reflux, esophageal** See *gastroesophageal reflux*.

**refraction** In opthalmology, the bending of light that takes place within the human eye. Refractive errors include nearsightedness (myopia), farsightedness (hyperopia), and astigmatism. Lenses can be used to control the amount of refraction, correcting those errors.

**refractory** Not yielding, at least not yielding readily, to treatment.

**refractory anemia**   Shortage of red blood cells that is unresponsive to treatment.

**Refsum disease**   A genetic disorder affecting metabolism of the fatty acid phytanic acid. When phytanic acid accumulates, it causes a number of progressive problems, including inflammation of numerous nerves (polyneuritis), diminishing vision due to retinitis pigmentosa, and wobbliness (ataxia) caused by damage to the cerebellar portion of the brain. Also known as phytanic acid storage disease.

**regenerate**   To reproduce or renew something lost. For example, after an injury, the liver has the capacity to regenerate.

**regimen**   A plan or regulated course, such as a diet, exercise, or treatment, designed to give a good result. A low-salt diet is one type of dietary regimen.

**region, regulatory**   See *regulatory sequence*.

**regional enteritis**   See *Crohn disease*.

**regional lymphadenitis**   See *cat scratch fever*.

**registry**   A collection of information. A registry is usually organized so that the data can be analyzed. For example, analysis of data in a tumor registry maintained at a hospital may show a rise in lung cancer among women.

**regress**   To return or go back, particularly to return to a pattern of behavior or level of skill characteristic of a younger age. For example, if a three-year-old child begins to regress by losing the ability to control his bowels or speak, that is a cause for medical concern.

**regulatory gene**   A gene that regulates the expression of other genes.

**regulatory region**   See *regulatory sequence*.

**regulatory sequence**   A sequence of bases in DNA that controls gene expression.

**regurgitation**   A backward flowing. For example, vomiting is a regurgitation of food from the stomach, and the sloshing of blood back into the heart when a heart valve is incompetent is a regurgitation of blood.

**rehab**   Short for rehabilitation.

**rehabilitation**   The process of helping a person who has suffered an illness or injury restore lost skills and so regain maximum self-sufficiency. For example, rehabilitation work after a stroke may help the patient walk and speak clearly again.

**rehydrate**   To restore lost water to the body tissues and fluids. Prompt rehydration is imperative whenever dehydration occurs, whether from diarrhea, exposure, lack of drinking water, or medication use. Rehydration can be by oral or IV administration of fluids.

**Reiter syndrome**   A chronic form of inflammatory arthritis that combines arthritis, inflammation of the eyes (conjunctivitis), and inflammation of the genital, urinary, or gastrointestinal systems. Reiter syndrome is a systemic rheumatic disease, meaning that it can and does affect organs as well as the joints. It can cause inflammation in many areas, including the eyes, mouth, lungs, kidneys, heart, and skin. See also *arthritis; arthritis, Reiter; keratodermia blennorrhagicum*.

**rejection**   In transplantation biology, the body's refusal to accept transplanted cells, tissues, or organs. For example, a transplanted kidney may be rejected.

**relapse**   The return of signs and symptoms of a disease after a remission.

**relaxant**   Something that relaxes, relieves, or reduces tension. For example, a muscle relaxant is often administered during abdominal surgery to relax the diaphragm and keep it from moving during the surgery.

**release, carpal tunnel**   See *carpal tunnel release*. See also *carpal tunnel syndrome*.

**rem**   **1** In radiation, Roentgen equivalent for man: an international unit of X-ray or gamma-ray radiation adjusted for the atomic makeup of the human body. **2** In ophthalmology, rapid eye movement. See also *REM sleep*.

**REM sleep**   The portion of sleep during which rapid eye movements (REMs) occur. Dreams occur during REM sleep, and people typically have three to five periods of REM sleep per night. They occur at intervals of one to two hours, and can vary in length from five minutes to over an hour. REM sleep is also characterized by rapid, low-voltage brain waves detectable on the electroencephalographic (EEG) recording; irregular breathing and heart rate; and involuntary muscle jerks. See also *NREM sleep*.

**remedy**   Something that consistently helps treat or cures a disease.

**remission**   Disappearance of the signs and symptoms of cancer or other disease. When this happens, the disease is said to be in remission. A remission can be temporary or permanent.

**remission induction chemotherapy**   The initial chemotherapy a patient with acute leukemia receives to bring about a remission.

**renal**  Having to do with the kidney.

**renal aneurysm**  An aneurysm involving the kidney.

**renal calculi**  See *kidney stone*. See also *cystine kidney stones*.

**renal cancer**  See *cancer, kidney*.

**renal capsule**  The fibrous connective tissue that surrounds each kidney.

**renal cell cancer**  See *cancer, renal cell*.

**renal cell carcinoma**  See *cancer, renal cell*.

**renal osteodystrophy**  See *osteodystrophy, renal*.

**renal pelvis**  The area at the center of the kidney. Urine collects here and is funneled into the ureter.

**renal stone**  See *kidney stone*. See also *cystine kidney stones*.

**renal syndrome with hemorrhagic fever**  See *hemorrhagic fever with renal syndrome*. See also *arborvirus, Ebola virus, hantavirus*.

**renal tubules**  Small structures in the kidney that filter the blood and produce urine.

**Rendu-Osler-Weber syndrome**  See *hereditary hemorrhagic telangectasia*.

**rep**  Roentgen equivalent physical, a unit of absorbed radiation approximately equivalent to one roentgen.

**repair, DNA**  See *DNA repair*.

**reperfusion**  The restoration of blood flow to an organ or tissue. After a heart attack, an immediate goal is to quickly open blocked arteries and reperfuse the heart muscles. Early reperfusion minimizes the extent of heart muscle damage, and preserves the pumping function of the heart.

**repetitive DNA**  See *DNA, repetitive*.

**replacement therapy, estrogen**  See *estrogen replacement therapy*. See also *hormone replacement therapy*.

**replacement therapy, hormone**  See *hormone replacement therapy*. See also *estrogen replacement therapy*.

**replication**  A turning back, repetition, duplication, or reproduction. See also *DNA replication*.

**replication, DNA**  See *DNA replication*.

**reporting, named**  See *named reporting*.

**reporting, unique identifier**  See *unique identifier reporting*.

**reproduction**  The production of offspring. Reproduction need not be sexual: Yeast can reproduce by budding.

**reproductive cells**  The eggs and sperm. Each mature reproductive cell is haploid, in that it has a single set of 23 chromosomes and so contains half the usual amount of DNA.

**reproductive organs, female**  See *female internal genitalia, ovary*.

**reproductive organs, male**  See *male gonad*.

**reproductive system**  In women, the organs that are directly involved in producing eggs and in conceiving and carrying babies. In men, the organs directly involved in creating, storing, and delivering sperm to fertilize an egg.

**research, clinical**  A study of a treatment, procedure, or medication done in a medical setting. See also *clinical research trials*.

**research, controlled**  A study that compares results from a treated group and a control group. The control group may receive no treatment, a placebo, or a different treatment. See also *blinded study*, *double-blinded study*.

**resection**  Surgical removal of part of an organ.

**reservoir, Ommaya**  A device implanted under the scalp that delivers anticancer drugs to the fluid surrounding the brain and spinal cord.

**residual**  Something left behind. If there is residual disease, the disease has not been fully eradicated.

**resin, bile acid**  See *bile acid resin*.

**resistance**  Opposition to something, or the ability to withstand it. For example, some forms of staphylococcus are resistant to treatment with antibiotics.

**resistance, antibiotic**  See *antibiotic resistance*. See also *penicillin-resistant bacteria*.

**resistance, pulmonary**  Opposition of the respiratory system to air flow.

**resistance, vascular**  Opposition to the flow of blood by a blood vessel.

**resolution** In genetics, the degree of molecular detail on a physical map of DNA. Resolution may range from low to high.

**resorb** Literally, to absorb again. To lose substance. Some of a tooth may be resorbed.

**resorption** The process of losing substance. When bone is surgically reshaped, it undergoes both new formation and resorption.

**respiration** The act of inhaling and exhaling air in order to exchange oxygen for carbon dioxide.

**respiratory** Having to do with respiration.

**respiratory distress** See *airway obstruction*.

**respiratory distress syndrome, acute** See *acute respiratory distress syndrome*.

**respiratory papillomatosis, recurrent** See *laryngeal papillomatosis; laryngeal papillomatosis, juvenile*.

**respiratory rate** The number of breaths per minute or, more formally, the number of movements indicative of inspiration and expiration per unit time. In practice, the respiratory rate is usually determined by counting the number of times the chest rises or falls per minute. The aim of measuring respiratory rate is to determine whether the respirations are normal, abnormally fast (tachypnea), abnormally slow (bradypnea), or nonexistent (apnea).

**respiratory syncytial virus** A virus that causes mild respiratory infections, colds, and coughs in adults, but can produce severe respiratory problems, including bronchitis and pneumonia, in young children. Effective immunity against RSV requires a continuous, solid level of antibodies against the virus. There is particular concern about RSV occurring in premature babies, because their immune systems lack maturity and antibodies.

**respiratory system** The organs involved in breathing, including the nose, throat, larynx, trachea, bronchi, and lungs. Also known as the respiratory tree.

**respiratory therapy** Exercises and treatments that help patients recover lung function, such as after surgery.

**response, Babinski** See *Babinski reflex*.

**response, plantar** See *Babinski reflex*.

**resting phase** See *interphase*.

**restitution** In cytogenetics, the spontaneous rejoining of broken chromosomes to reconstitute the original chromosome configuration.

**restriction endonuclease** See *restriction enzyme*.

**restriction enzyme** An enzyme from bacteria that can recognize specific base sequences in DNA and cut (restrict) the DNA at that site. Also known as a restriction endonuclease.

**restriction fragment length polymorphism** A difference in DNA between people that can be recognized by the use of a restriction enzyme.

**restriction map** An array of sites in DNA that is susceptible to cleavage by diverse restriction enzymes.

**restriction site** A sequence in DNA that can be recognized and cut by a specific restriction enzyme.

**retardation, mental** See *mental retardation*.

**retardation, reading** See *reading retardation*.

**Retin-A** Trademark for a drug (tretinoin) used to treat acne and other skin conditions.

**retina** The nerve layer that lines the back of the eye, senses light, and creates impulses that travel through the optic nerve to the brain. A small area called the macula in the retina contains special light-sensitive cells. The macula allows the clear perception of fine details. The retina is also filled with tiny blood vessels. See also *eye*.

**retinal vasculitis** Inflammation of the tiny blood vessels of the retina. Retinal vasculitis ranges in severity from mild to severe. Damage to the blood vessels of the retina can cause minimal, partial, or even complete blindness. Retinal vasculitis by itself is painless, but many of the diseases that cause it can also cause painful inflammation elsewhere, as in the joints. Signs of retinal vasculitis can be observed by a doctor using an ophthalmoscope. Further definition of the blood-vessel condition can be determined by a special X-ray dye test (angiogram) of the retina. Diseases that cause retinal vasculitis include Behcet syndrome, systemic lupus erythematosus, antiphospholipid antibody syndrome, systemic necrotizing vasculitis, Wegener granulomatosus, Takayasu vasculitis, and giant cell arteritis. Treatment typically involves high doses of cortisone-related medications, such as prednisone. Additionally, some related diseases require immune suppression with medication, such as cyclosporine, chlorambucil, and cyclophosphamide.

**retinoblastoma** A malignant eye tumor caused by the loss of a pair of tumor-suppressor genes. An inherited form of retinoblastoma typically appears at birth, leads to multiple tumors, and affects both eyes. It is due to a transmissible mutation followed by an acquired mutation. The sporadic form of retinoblastoma has later onset and leads to a single tumor in one eye. It is due to acquired mutations of both tumor-suppressor genes. When the tumor is detected at an early stage, it can sometimes be treated locally, but it often requires removal of the eye (enucleation).

**retinol**   Vitamin A. See also *Appendix C, "Vitamins."*

**retrograde intrarenal surgery**   A procedure for performing surgery within the kidney, using a viewing tube called a fiberoptic endoscope. In retrograde intrarenal surgery (RIRS), the scope is placed through the urethra into the bladder, and then through the ureter into the urine-collecting part of the kidney. The scope is thus moved in a retrograde direction—up the urinary tract system, through which urine normally flows outward—to a position within the kidney (intrarenal). RIRS may be done to remove a stone. The stone can be seen through the scope, manipulated or crushed by an ultrasound probe, evaporated by a laser probe, or grabbed by small forceps. RIRS is performed by a specialist, a urologist (endourologist) with special expertise in RIRS. The procedure is usually done under general or spinal anesthesia. The advantages of RIRS over open surgery include a quicker solution of the problem, the elimination of prolonged pain after surgery, and much faster recovery. Also known as kidney scoping.

**retropubic prostatectomy**   Surgical removal of the prostate through an incision in the abdomen.

**retrosternal**   Behind the sternum (breastbone).

**retrovirus**   A virus composed not of DNA, but of RNA. Retroviruses have an enzyme, called reverse transcriptase, that gives them the unique property of transcribing their RNA into DNA. The retroviral DNA can then integrate into the chromosomal DNA of the host cell, to be expressed there. The human immunodeficiency virus (HIV), the cause of AIDS, is a retrovirus.

**Rett syndrome**   A condition, probably of genetic origin, that is characterized by hand-wringing movements; shaking of the torso and limbs; wobbly, rigid gait; difficulty with breathing and eating; small stature; microcephaly; retardation that ranges from severe to profound; and autistic-like behavior. About 80 percent of Rett syndrome patients also have epilepsy. Rett syndrome usually emerges after the age of six months. It is believed to affect girls only, although a few boys have shown very similar symptoms. A very few girls with Rett syndrome gain or recover near-normal function, although these patients usually retain their autistic behaviors. See also *autism, seizure disorders*.

**reversal of organs, total**   Complete transposition of the thoracic and abdominal organs from right to left,

placing the heart in the right side of the chest, and so on. Organs appear as if in mirror image when examined or X-rayed. Total organ reversal has been estimated to occur once in about 6,000 to 8,000 births. It also occurs in a rare, abnormal congenital condition called Kartagener syndrome. Also known as situs inversus totalis. See also *dextrocardia, Kartagener syndrome*.

**reverse genetics**   In classic genetics, the traditional approach was to find a gene product and then try to identify the gene itself. In molecular genetics, the reverse has been done by identifying genes purely on the basis of their position in the genome, with no knowledge whatsoever of the gene product. This revolutionary approach is reverse genetics. Also known as positional cloning.

**reverse transcriptase**   An enzyme that permits DNA to be made, using RNA as the template. A retrovirus, such as the HIV virus implicated in AIDS, can propagate itself by converting its RNA into DNA with reverse transcriptase.

**Reye syndrome**   A sudden and sometimes fatal disease of the brain (encephalopathy) with degeneration of the liver. Reye syndrome usually occurs in children between the ages of 4 and 12, comes after infection with chicken pox (varicella) or an influenza-type illness, and is also associated with taking medications containing aspirin. The child with Reye syndrome first tends to be unusually quiet, lethargic (stuporous), and sleepy. Vomiting may occur. In the second stage, the lethargy deepens, and the child becomes confused, combative, and delirious. This stage is followed by decreasing consciousness, coma, seizures, and eventually death. Early diagnosis and control of the increased intracranial pressure can prevent death or brain damage. Reye syndrome is a good reason to have your child immunized against chicken pox. It is also why doctors no longer recommend giving children aspirin for fever.

**RF**   Rheumatoid factor.

**RFLP**   Restriction fragment length polymorphism.

**Rh+**   Rh positive. See *Rh factor*.

**Rh−**   Rh negative. See *Rh factor*.

**Rh factor**   An antigen found in the red blood cells of most people: Those who have Rh factor are said to be Rh positive (Rh+), while those who do not are Rh negative (Rh−). Blood used in transfusions must match donors for Rh status as well as for ABO blood group, as Rh− patients will develop anemia if given R+ blood. Rh typing is also important during abortion, miscarriage, pregnancy, and birth, as mother and fetus may not be Rh-compatible. Rh stands for rhesus monkeys, in whose blood this antigen was first found. See also *RhoGAM, Rh incompatibility*.

**Rh incompatibility** The state of mother and fetus having different Rh status. An Rh+ fetus may be attacked by antibodies in an Rh– mother's blood. Treatment is with $Rh_o(D)$ immune globulin (brand name: RhoGAM).

**Rh negative** See *Rh factor*.

**Rh positive** See *Rh factor*.

**rhabdomyolysis** A condition in which skeletal muscle is broken down, releasing muscle enzymes and electrolytes from inside the muscle cells. Risks include muscle breakdown and kidney failure, as the cellular component myoglobin is toxic to the kidneys. Rhabdomyolysis is relatively uncommon, but most often occurs as the result of extensive muscle damage as, for example, in crush injury or electrical shock. Drugs or toxins, particularly some the cholesterol-lowering medications, may cause this disorder. Underlying diseases that can also lead to rhabdomyolysis include collagen vascular diseases, such as systemic lupus erythematosus.

**rhabdomyosarcoma** A fast-growing cancer that emerges in the soft tissues, particularly in the pelvic area, head, and neck. It is seen primarily in children. See also *sarcoma, sarcoma botryoides*.

**rheumatic fever** An illness that occurs in the wake of a streptococcus infection (strep throat, or related conditions) or scarlet fever, primarily in children. Symptoms include fever, pain in the joints, nausea, stomach cramps, and vomiting. Rheumatic fever can cause long-lasting effects in the joints, heart, brain, and skin. Rheumatic fever may be followed by Sydenham chorea and by symptoms characteristic of obsessive-compulsive disorder or a tic disorder. Diagnosis is by observation: A blood marker has recently been found for rheumatic fever, but a test is not yet commercially available. Treatment is usually by prophylactic antibiotics, as reoccurrence is common and can cause further damage to body tissues. See also *Sydenham chorea*.

**rheumatic heart disease** Heart damage caused by rheumatic fever. Treatment is by preventing reinfection, and with heart drugs as needed.

**rheumatism** An older term used to describe a number of painful conditions of muscles, tendons, joints, and bones. Rheumatic conditions have been classified as localized, regional, or generalized.

**rheumatism, generalized** Rheumatism affecting many and diverse parts of the body, such as fibromyalgia.

**rheumatism, localized** Rheumatism confined to a specific location, such as bursitis and tendinitis.

**rheumatism, psychogenic** Rheumatism in which the patient reports inconsistent pains of muscles and joints that do not correspond to true anatomy and physiology. The patient is felt to have underlying psychological causes for these symptoms.

**rheumatism, regional** Rheumatism in a larger region, such as chest wall pain, temporomandibular joint pain, and myofascial pain syndromes.

**rheumatoid arthritis** See *arthritis, rheumatoid*.

**rheumatoid arthritis, systemic-onset juvenile** See *arthritis, systemic-onset juvenile rheumatoid*.

**rheumatoid factor** An antibody that is measurable in the blood. Measures of rheumatoid factor are commonly taken with a blood test, and used to diagnose rheumatoid arthritis. Rheumatoid factor is present in about 80 percent of adults, but a much lower proportion of children, with rheumatoid arthritis. It is also present in patients with other connective-tissue diseases, such as systemic lupus erythematosus, and in some with infectious diseases, such as infectious hepatitis.

**rheumatoid nodules** Firm lumps in the skin of patients with rheumatoid arthritis. They usually occur in pressure points of the body, most commonly the elbows.

**rheumatologist** A specialist in the treatment of rheumatic illnesses, especially forms of arthritis. Classical rheumatology training includes four years of medical school, one year of internship in internal medicine, two years of internal medicine residency, and two years of rheumatology fellowship. There is a subspecialty board for rheumatology certification, the American College of Rheumatology, which can offer board certification to approved rheumatologists. See also *rheumatologist, pediatric; rheumatology*.

**rheumatologist, pediatric** A rheumatologist who specializes in caring for children with rheumatic diseases. Pediatric rheumatologists are pediatricians who have completed an additional two to three years of specialized training in pediatric rheumatology, and are usually Board-certified in pediatric rheumatology. They have special interests in unexplained rash, fever, arthritis, anemia, weakness, weight loss, fatigue, muscle pain, autoimmune disease, and anorexia. They are skilled in the evaluation of juvenile arthritis, spondylitis, systemic lupus erythematosus, antiphospholipid syndrome, dermatomyositis, Sjogren syndrome, vasculitis, scleroderma, mixed connective-tissue disease, sarcoidosis, Lyme disease, osteomyelitis, relapsing polychondritis, Henoch-Schonlein purpura, serum sickness, reactive arthritis, Kawasaki disease, fibromyalgia, erythromelalgia, Raynaud disease, growing pains, iritis, and osteoporosis in children.

**rheumatology** A subspecialty of internal medicine that involves the nonsurgical evaluation and treatment of rheumatic diseases and conditions. Rheumatic diseases and conditions are characterized by symptoms involving the musculoskeletal system; many also feature immune system abnormalities.

**rhinitis** Irritation of the nose.

**rhinitis, acute** Inflammation of the nose that occurs for only a few days. Typically, this is caused by a virus (a cold). If rhinitis continues longer than a week, it is probably bacterial.

**rhinitis, allergic** The medical term for hay fever. Symptoms include nasal congestion, a clear runny nose, sneezing, nose and eye itching, and tearing eyes. Postnasal dripping of clear mucus frequently occurs, and causes a cough. Loss of smell is common, and loss of taste occasionally happens. The nose may bleed if the condition is severe. Eye-itching, redness, and tearing frequently accompany the nasal symptoms.

**rhinitis, allergic, perennial** Allergic rhinitis that occurs throughout the year.

**rhinitis, allergic, seasonal** Allergic rhinitis that occurs during a specific season.

**rhinitis, chronic** Inflammation of the nose that goes on for weeks to months. It may be caused by bacterial infection, allergy, nasal irritants, structural issues, or physiological problems.

**rhinitis, vasomotor** Inflammation of the nose due to abnormal neuronal (nerve) control of the blood vessels in the nose. Vasomotor rhinitis is not allergic rhinitis.

**rhinophyma** A condition characterized by a bulbous, enlarged red nose and puffy cheeks. There may also be thick bumps on the lower half of the nose and the nearby cheek areas. It occurs mainly in men. Rhinophyma is a complication of rosacea. See also *rosacea*.

**rhinoplasty** Plastic surgery on the nose, known familiarly as a nose job. Rhinoplasty is a facial cosmetic procedure, usually performed to enhance the appearance of the nose. During this type of rhinoplasty, the nasal cartilage and bones are modified, or tissue is added. Rhinoplasty is also performed to repair nasal fractures or other structural problems. In these cases, the goal is to restore preinjury appearance or to create a normal appearance.

**rhinorrhea** Medical term for a runny nose.

**RhoGAM** Rh$_0$(D) immune globulin, an injectable drug used to protect an Rh+ fetus from antibodies in an Rh– mother's blood, and to prevent Rh allergy in the mother.

**rib** One of the 12 paired arches of bone that form the skeletal structure of the chest wall (the rib cage). The ribs attach to the vertebrae of the spine in the back. The 12 pairs of ribs consist of 7 pairs of ribs that attach to the sternum in the front, and are known as true or sternal ribs; and 5 pairs of lower ribs that do not connect directly to the sternum, and are known as false ribs. The upper 3 false ribs connect to the costal cartilages of the ribs just above them. The last 2 false ribs usually have no anchor in front, and are known as floating, fluctuating, or vertebral ribs.

**rib, cervical** A extra rib that arises from the seventh cervical vertebra. It is located above the normal first rib. A cervical rib is present in only about 1 in 200 people. It may cause nerve and artery problems.

**rib, false** One of the last 5 pairs of ribs, which do not attach to the sternum.

**rib, floating** See *rib, false*.

**rib, fluctuating** See *rib, false*.

**rib, sternal** See *rib, true*.

**rib, true** One of the first seven pairs of ribs, which attach to the sternum.

**rib, vertebral** See *rib, false*.

**ribonucleic acid** RNA, a chemical (specifically, a nucleic acid) similar to DNA, but containing ribose rather than deoxyribose. RNA is in fact formed upon a DNA template. The several classes of RNA molecules play important roles in protein synthesis and other cell activities. See also *RNA, messenger; RNA, ribosomal; RNA, transfer*.

**ribosomes** Structures composed of RNA and protein, the ribosomes are situated outside the nucleus in the cytoplasm of the cell, where the cell uses messenger RNA to make up polypeptides. Also known as organelles.

**rickets** A disease of infants and children that disturbs normal bone formation (ossification). Rickets is a failure to mineralize bone. This softens bone, producing osteomalacia, and permits marked bending and distortion of bones. Other signs and symptoms include softness of the infant's skull (craniotabes), enlargement of the front end of the ribs (creating the "rachitic rosary"), thickening of the wrists and ankles, lateral curving of the spine (scoliosis), abnormal forward-backward curving of the spine (kyphosis and lumbar lordosis), and deforming and narrowing of the pelvis, which in females interferes later with vaginal childbirth. As the child begins to walk, the weight on the soft shafts of the legs results in knock-knees or, more often, bowlegs. The deformities of the spine, pelvis, and legs reduce height, leading to short stature. The spinal deformities also impair posture and gait. Until the first third of the 20th century, rickets was usually due to lack of direct exposure to sunlight, or to lack of vitamin D, calcium, and phosphorus. Sunlight provides the necessary ultraviolet rays, and thanks to improved diets, vitamin D supplements, and enriched food products, nutritional rickets has become relatively rare in industrialized nations. It still occurs sometimes in breast-fed babies whose mothers are underexposed to sunlight, and in dark-skinned babies who are not given vitamin D supplements. In unindustrialized countries, vitamin D–deficiency rickets continues to be a problem. Rickets in North America and Europe is usually now due to other causes, such as disorders that create vitamin D deficiency by interfering with the absorption of vitamin D through the intestines; diseases of the liver, kidney, or other organs that impair the normal metabolic conversion and activation of vitamin D; and conditions that disrupt the normal balance in the body (homeostasis) between calcium and phosphorus.

**rickets, celiac**  Rickets caused by failure of the intestines to absorb calcium and fat from foods. See also *celiac sprue*.

**rickets, hypophosphatemic**  A rare type of rickets in which phosphate collects abnormally in the kidneys. Treatment is with oral phosphate and vitamin D supplements.

**rickets, renal**  Rickets-like bone malformations caused by prolonged inflammation of the kidneys.

**rickets, vitamin D resistant**  A rickets-like condition caused by an inborn defect of metabolism, usually in males. Vitamin D cannot be absorbed, and so does not work to treat the illness.

**Rickettsia**  A member of genus Rickettsia, a family of microorganisms that, like viruses, require other living cells for growth, but also resemble bacteria in that they use oxygen, have metabolic enzymes and cell walls, and are susceptible to antibiotics. Rickettsiae cause a series of diseases, including Rocky Mountain spotted fever, typhus, and trench fever. See *rickettsial diseases*.

**rickettsial diseases**  Infectious diseases caused by the Rickettsiae fall into four groups: typhus, including epidemic typhus, Brill-Zinsser disease, murine (endemic) typhus, and scrub typhus; spotted fever, including Rocky Mountain spotted fever, Eastern tick-borne rickettsioses, and rickettsialpox; Q fever; and trench fever.

**rickettsialpox**  A mild infectious disease first observed in New York City. It is caused by Rickettsia akari, transmitted from its mouse host by chigger or adult mite bites.

There is fever, a dark spot that becomes a small ulcer at the site of the bite, swollen glands (lymphadenopathy) in that region, and a raised, blistery (vesicular) rash. Also known as vesicular rickettsiosis.

**rickettsioses**  See *rickettsial diseases*.

**rickettsioses of the eastern hemisphere, tick-borne**  North Asian tick-borne rickettsiosis, Queensland tick typhus, and African tick typhus (fièvre boutonneuse).

**rickettsiosis, North Asian tick-borne**  One of the tick-borne rickettsial diseases of the eastern hemisphere, similar to Rocky Mountain spotted fever but less severe. Symptoms include fever, a small ulcer (eschar) at the site of the tick bite, swollen glands nearby (satellite lymphadenopathy), and a red, raised (maculopapular) rash.

**rickettsiosis, vesicular**  See *rickettsialpox*.

**right heart**  The right atrium, which receives deoxygenated blood from the body; and the right ventricle, which pumps it to the lungs. The right heart is a low-pressure system.

**right ventricle**  The chamber of the heart that receives blood from the right atrium and pumps it under low pressure into the lungs via the pulmonary artery.

**ring chromosome**  A structurally abnormal chromosome in which the end of each chromosome arm has been lost, and the broken arms have been reunited in ring formation. A ring chromosome is denoted by the symbol r.

**ring, intrastromal corneal**  See *intrastromal corneal ring*.

**ringworm of the nails**  See *dermatophytic onychomycosis*.

**RIRS**  Retrograde intrarenal surgery.

**risk factor**  Something that increases a person's chances of developing a disease.

**risk of recurrence**  See *recurrence risk*.

**risks, obesity-related**  See *obesity-related diseases*.

**ritonavir**  A medication (brand name: Norvir) in the protease inhibitor family, ritonavir is used to treat HIV infection (AIDS). See also *protease inhibitor*.

**Ritter disease**  See *staphylococcal scalded skin syndrome*.

**RLL**  Right lower lobe (of the lung).

**RLQ** Right lower quadrant (quarter) of the abdomen.

**RML** Right middle lobe (of the lung).

**RMSF** Rocky Mountain spotted fever.

**RNA** Ribonucleic acid.

**RNA polymerase** A unique enzyme that makes (synthesizes) the large-molecule (macromolecule) RNA by joining together many smaller molecules (monomers), using DNA as a template.

**RNA, messenger** A class of RNA that is the template upon which polypeptides are put together. Abbreviated as mRNA.

**RNA, ribosomal** A component of ribosomes, ribosomal RNA functions as a nonspecific site for making polypeptides. Abbreviated as rRNA.

**RNA, transfer** In cooperation with the ribosomes, transfer RNA brings (transfers) activated amino acids into position along the messenger RNA template. Abbreviated as tRNA.

**Rochalimaea quintana** See *Bartonella quintana*. See also *trench fever*.

**Rocky Mountain spotted fever** An acute febrile (feverish) disease initially recognized in the Rocky Mountain states. It is caused by Rickettsia rickettsii, transmitted by hard-shelled (ixodid) ticks, and occurs only in the western hemisphere. Anyone frequenting tick-infested areas is at risk for RMSF. Onset of symptoms is abrupt, with headache, high fever, chills, muscle pain, and then a rash. The rickettsiae grow within damaged cells lining blood vessels, which may become blocked by clots. Blood vessel inflammation (vasculitis) is widespread. Early recognition of RMSF and prompt antibiotic treatment is important to prevent death. Also known as spotted fever, tick fever, and tick typhus.

**roentgen** An international unit of X-ray or gamma-ray radiation.

**roentgenology** Radiology.

**rooting reflex** A relex seen in normal newborn babies, who automatically turn the face toward the stimulus and make sucking (rooting) motions with the mouth when the cheek or lip is touched. The rooting reflex helps to ensure breast-feeding.

**rosacea** A chronic skin disease that causes persistent redness over the areas of the face and nose that normally blush: mainly the forehead, the chin, and the lower half of the nose. The tiny blood vessels in these areas enlarge (dilate) and become more visible through the skin, appearing like tiny red lines (telangiectasias). Pimples that look like teenage acne can occur. Unlike acne, rosacea occurs most often in adults between the ages of 30 and 50, especially those with fair skin. It affects both sexes, and although it tends to be more common in women, it is often worse in men. Unlike acne, there are no blackheads or whiteheads in rosacea. When rosacea first develops, it may come and go. However, in time the skin fails to return to its normal color, and the enlarged blood vessels and pimples arrive. Rosacea rarely reverses itself, and will worsen if untreated. Untreated rosacea can cause a condition called rhinophyma, characterized by a bulbous, enlarged red nose and puffy cheeks. There may also be thick bumps on the lower half of the nose and the nearby cheek areas. Rhinophyma occurs mainly in men. Another complication of advanced rosacea affects the eyes. About half of all people with rosacea feel burning and grittiness of the eyes (conjunctivitis). If this is not treated, the complications of what is called rosacea keratitis may impair vision. Rosacea can be treated but not cured. Topical antibiotics such as metronidazole, and oral antibiotics such as tetracycline, are often used. Short-term topical cortisone (steroid) preparations of the right strength may also be used to reduce local inflammation. Over-the-counter medications for acne can irritate the skin in rosacea, however. Avoiding smoking and food and drink that cause flushing (such as spicy food, hot beverages, and alcoholic drinks) helps minimize the blood-vessel enlargement. Limiting exposure to sunlight and to extreme hot and cold temperatures also helps relieve rosacea. Rubbing the face tends to irritate the reddened skin. Some cosmetics and hair sprays may aggravate redness and swelling. Facial products such as soap, moisturizers, and sunscreens should be free of alcohol and other irritating ingredients. Moisturizers should be applied very gently after any topical medication has dried. Outdoors, sunscreens with an SPF of 15 or higher are needed. Cosmetics can be used to cover the telangiectasias, or they can be treated with a small electric needle, a laser, or surgery to close off the dilated blood vessels. Rhinophymas are treated by surgery. The excess tissue is removed with a scalpel, laser, or electrosurgery. Dermabrasion can help improve the look of the scar tissue.

**rosacea keratitis** A condition affecting the eyes in about half of all cases of rosacea. It is characterized by burning and grittiness of the eyes (conjunctivitis). If this is not treated, inflammation of the cornea may impair vision.

**roseola** See *measles*.

**roseola infantilis** See *measles*.

**roseola infantum** See *measles*.

**rotator cuff** A group of four tendons that stabilize the shoulder joint. Each of these tendons hooks up to a muscle that moves the shoulder in a specific direction. The four muscles whose tendons form the rotator cuff are the subscapularis muscle, which moves the arm by turning it inward (internal rotation); the supraspinatus muscle, which is responsible for elevating the arm and moving it away from the body; the infraspinatus muscle, which assists the lifting of the arm during outward turning (external rotation) of the arm; and the teres minor muscle, which also helps in the outward turning (external rotation) of the arm. Damage to the rotator cuff is one of the most common causes of shoulder pain.

**rotator cuff disease** Damage to the rotator cuff. It can be due to trauma, as from falling and injuring the shoulder; overuse in sports, particularly those that involve repetitive overhead motions; inflammation, as from tendinitis, bursitis, or arthritis of the shoulder; or degeneration, as from aging. The main symptom of rotator cuff disease is shoulder pain of gradual or sudden onset, typically located to the front and side of the shoulder, and increasing when the shoulder is moved away from the body. A person with torn rotator cuff tendons may not be able to hold the arm up because of pain. With very severe tears, the arm falls because of weakness—this is called the positive drop sign. Diagnosis is by observation, and can be confirmed by X-rays showing bony injuries; an arthrogram in which contrast dye is injected into the shoulder joint to detect leakage out of the injured rotator cuff; or an MRI, which can provide more information than either an X-ray or an arthrogram. Treatment depends on severity. Mild rotator cuff disease is treated with ice, rest, and anti-inflammatory medications, such as ibuprofen. Persistent pain and motion limitation may benefit by a cortisone injection in the rotator cuff, and by exercises specifically designed to strengthen the rotator cuff. More severe rotator cuff disease may require arthroscopic or open surgical repair. Subacromial decompression, the removal of a small portion of the bone (acromion) that overlies the rotator cuff, can relieve pressure on the rotator cuff and promote healing. Very severe, complete full-thickness rotator cuff tears require surgery to mend the torn rotator cuff. Without treatment, including exercise, the outlook is guarded. Scarring around the shoulder (adhesive capsulitis) can lead to marked limitation of range of shoulder motion, a condition called a frozen shoulder. Some patients never recover full use of the shoulder joint.

**rotavirus** A leading cause of severe winter diarrhea in young children, RV each year causes an estimated 500,000 doctor visits and 50,000 hospital admissions in the United States. Almost everyone catches RV before entering school but, with rehydration and good nutrition, nearly all recover fully. However, in poor countries it is estimated that there are at least 600,000 deaths of children under the age of five from RV diarrhea and dehydration. Aside from causing acute infantile gastroenteritis and diarrhea in young children, RV infection is typically accompanied by low-grade fever.

**rotavirus immunization** A vaccine against rotavirus, which was approved in 1998. Use of the rotavirus vaccine was suspended by the Centers for Disease Control in July 1999 after reports of negative responses, including deaths due to bowel obstruction, following vaccination. As of October 1999, the CDC no longer recommended its use in US infants.

**Rothmund-Thomson syndrome** An hereditary disease characterized by progressive degeneration (atrophy), and effects on multiple parts of the body, including skin (premature aging, excess pigmentation, dilated blood vessels), eyes (juvenile cataract), nose (depressed nasal bridge), teeth (maldeveloped), skeletal system (congenital bone defects), hair (abnormal), gonads (underdevelopment), limbs (soft tissue contractures), growth (short stature), blood (anemia), and a tendency to develop a type of bone cancer (osteogenic sarcoma). Rothmund-Thomson syndrome (RTS) is inherited as an autosomal recessive trait. A child born to two parents with the RTS gene stands a 25 percent chance of receiving both RTS genes and the disease. The RTS gene has been mapped to chromosome 8. The outlook for survival is generally fairly good. Also known as poikiloderma congenita and poikiloderma atrophicans with cataract.

**RPR test** Rapid plasma reagin, a blood test for syphilis. See *syphilis test, RPR*. See also *measles immunization, MMR*.

**RSV** 1 Respiratory syncytial virus. 2 Rous sarcoma virus.

**RTS** Rothmund-Thomson syndrome.

**rubella** German measles, a contagious viral disease caused by human papillomavirus 77 (HPV77). Symptoms include upper respiratory tract infection, fever, swollen lymph glands, and a rash with small spots. Exposure of a pregnant woman to rubella during early pregnancy can cause a syndrome of congenital malformations, including cataracts, heart problems, and mental retardation. The virus persists throughout pregnancy, is still present at birth, and continues to be shed by the infected child for many months after birth. Even if the child born with rubella looks normal, the child can be contagious and infect caregivers.

**rubella immunization**   See *measles immunization, MMR.*

**RUL**   Right upper lobe (of the lung).

**runny nose**   Rhinorrhea is the medical term for this common problem.

**ruptured spleen**   See *spleen, ruptured.*

**RUQ**   Right upper quadrant (quarter).

**RV**   Abbreviation for rotavirus.

**Rx**   **1** On a prescription, abbreviation for recipe (Latin for "to take"). See also *Appendix A, "Prescription Abbreviations."* **2** In a pharmacological catalog, an indicator that one will need a prescription to buy a listed item.

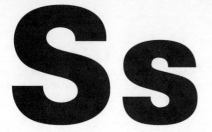

**SA node** Sinoatrial node.

**Sabin vaccine** See *polio immunization*.

**sac, egg** See *ovary*.

**sac, pericardial** See *pericardium*.

**saccular** Like a small pouch. For example, the alveolar saccules are little air pouches within the lungs.

**saccular aneurysm** See *aneurysm, saccular*. See also *aneurysm, brain*.

**sacral agenesis** Absence of all or part of the sacrum. See also *caudal regression syndrome, sacrum*.

**sacral vertebrae** The five vertebral bones situated between the lumbar vertebrae and the coccyx (the lowest segment of the vertebral column). By adulthood, the sacral vertebrae normally are fused to form the sacrum. They are represented by the symbols S1 through S5. See also *vertebra, vertebral column*.

**sacrum** The large, heavy bone at the base of the spine, which is made up of fused sacral vertebrae. The sacrum is located in the vertebral column, between the lumbar vertebrae and the coccyx. It is roughly triangular in shape, and makes up the back wall of the pelvis. The female sacrum is wider and less curved than the male. See also *pelvis, vertebral column, sacral vertebrae*.

**SAD** Seasonal affective disorder.

**safe sex** Sexual practices that do not involve the exchange of bodily fluids, including blood, sperm, vaginal secretions, and saliva, to avoid AIDS and other sexually transmitted diseases. Generally used to mean sex without penetration, or sex using condoms and Nonoxynol-9 spermacide, and/or vaginal dams, with consistency. In reality, "safer sex" is a better term.

**sagittal** A vertical plane passing through the body, dividing it into left and right sides. The midsagittal, or median plane, splits the body into left and right halves. See also *Appendix B, "Anatomic Orientation Terms."*

**salivary glands** Glands in the mouth that produce saliva. The salivary glands can become inflamed, as in Sjogren syndrome and mumps.

**Salk vaccine** See *polio immunization*.

**Salmonella** A group of bacteria that cause typhoid fever and other illnesses, including food poisoning, gastroenteritis, and enteric fever from contaminated food products. See also *food poisoning, Salmonellosis*.

**Salmonellosis** Infection with bacteria belonging to the genus Salmonella. Salmonellosis is particularly dangerous for people with immunodeficiency diseases and sickle cell disease. Symptoms usually begin within 12 to 24 hours after exposure, and may include stomach cramps, diarrhea, fever, and sometimes vomiting. Diagnosis can be confirmed by examination of a stool sample for Salmonella bacteria. Most people exposed to Salmonella will feel fine within a few days, and do not require treatment other than extra fluids. Some will need antibiotics, and a few will need hospitalization. See also *food poisoning*.

**salpingo-oophorectomy** Removal of the Fallopian tubes and ovaries. See also *hysterectomy*.

**Salter-Harris fracture** See *fracture, Salter-Harris*.

**salvage therapy** A final treatment for people who are not responsive to or cannot tolerate other available therapies for a particular condition.

**sample, random** See *random sample*.

**Sandhoff disease** A ganglioside disorder with symptoms that are very similar to those of Tay-Sachs disease, and that is characterized by accumulation of fatty material called GM2 ganglioside in the nerve cells of the brain. Symptoms begin around six months of age with motor weakness, and progress to include difficulties with swallowing and breathing. Death usually occurs by the age of three. It is an autosomal recessive disorder caused by a mutation to chromosome 5. Unlike Tay-Sachs, it is more common in the non-Jewish population. See also *Tay-Sachs disease*.

**Sanfilippo syndrome** A hereditary lysosomal storage disorder with onset between the ages of two and six. Sanfilippo syndrome is characterized by accumulation of heparin sulfate in the central nervous system and other tissue. Also known as mucopolysaccharidosis Type III (MPS III).

**sanguine** 1 Having a ruddy (reddish) complexion. 2 Cheerful, hopeful, confident, and optimistic; impulsive.

**saphenous vein, great** The larger of the two saphenous veins, the great saphenous vein goes from the foot all the way up to the saphenous opening, an oval aperture in the broad fascia of the thigh. The vein passes through this fibrous membrane. Also known as the large saphenous vein.

**saphenous vein, large** See *saphenous vein, great*. See also *saphenous veins*.

**saphenous vein, small** The smaller of the two saphenous veins, the small saphenous vein runs behind the outer malleolus (the protuberance on the outside of the ankle joint), comes up the back of the leg, and joins the popliteal vein in the space behind the knee (the popliteal space). See also *saphenous veins*.

**saphenous veins** The two saphenous veins—the great and the small saphenous veins—serve as the principal veins running near the surface (superficially) up the leg. They carry deoxygenated blood from the feet and legs toward the heart. See *saphenous vein, great; saphenous vein, small*.

**SAPHO syndrome** A condition characterized by a combination of synovitis, acne, pustulosis, hyperostosis, and osteitis. Symptoms include warmth, tenderness, pain, swelling, and stiffness of involved joints (arthritis); fluid-filled blister-like areas (pustules), typically on the palms of the hands and/or the soles of the feet, and peeling and flaking of skin in those areas; abnormal, excessive growth of bone, frequently at the points of the bone where tendons attach; and inflammation of the sacroiliac joints (sacroiliitis), as well as inflammation of the spine (spondylitis), leading to stiffness and pain of the neck and back. SAPHO syndrome is thought to be related to other arthritic conditions that typically affect the spine, including ankylosing spondylitis and reactive arthritis.

**sapphism** Female homosexuality, lesbianism.

**saquinavir** A protease inhibitor medication (brand name: Invirase, Fortovase) prescribed to treat AIDS. Saquinavir is taken along with antiviral drugs. Common side effects include nausea and diarrhea. See also *protease inhibitor*.

**sarcoma** A type of cancer that starts in bone or connective tissue. The first sign of sarcoma is usually a soft, painless swelling in the affected area. Most sarcomas are fast-growing. Different types of cells may be found in a sarcoma, and the type of cell (such as spindle cell, clear cell, osteoblast) may be used to describe the cancer. Treatment of sarcoma is usually aggressive, and may include radiation, chemotherapy, and sometimes surgery. See also *angiosarcoma; chondrosarcoma; chordoma; desmoid tumor; fibrosarcoma; liposarcoma; osteosarcoma; rhabdomyosarcoma; sarcoma botryoides; sarcoma, Ewing; sarcoma, metastatic; sarcoma, soft-tissue; sarcoma, synovial*.

**sarcoma botryoides** A muscle-cell sarcoma that affects the vagina, bladder, or nearby areas. Unlike other sarcomas, this form usually does cause pain. It is fast-growing, and affects primarily children. See also *rhabdomyosarcoma; sarcoma; sarcoma, soft-tissue*.

**sarcoma, Ewing** A type of sarcoma that arises in bone or soft tissue, and usually occurs in children or teenagers. The most common areas to find Ewing sarcoma are the legs, arms, ribs, or pelvis. Diagnosis is by observation of symptoms and X-rays or imaging, and can be confirmed by biopsy. Treatment is by chemotherapy, radiation, and/or surgery. Also known as peripheral primitive neuroectodermal tumors (PNET) of bone.

**sarcoma, Kaposi** See *Kaposi sarcoma*.

**sarcoma, metastatic** A sarcoma that is spreading into other body tissues through the lymphatic system. The most common site for metastatic sarcoma is the lungs, and there are usually multiple lesions. Treatment is by chemotherapy and surgery, but prognosis is poor.

**sarcoma, osteogenic** See *osteosarcoma*.

**sarcoma, soft-tissue** A sarcoma that begins in the muscle, fat, fibrous tissue, blood vessels, or other supporting tissue of the body. See also *sarcoma*.

**sarcoma, synovial** A soft-tissue sarcoma that usually emerges in adolescence or young adulthood. Synovial sarcomas usually arise near a joint (particularly the knee joint), and are made up of cells similar to the synovial cells that normally line a joint. Most synovial sarcomas are slow-growing, and escape notice until they cause pain. They sometimes spread to the lungs. Diagnosis is by X-ray or imaging, and can be confirmed by biopsy. Treatment is by chemotherapy, radiation, and/or surgery.

**sartorius muscle** The long band of muscle that stretches from the calf to the pelvis. It moves the thigh and, by extension, the leg.

**satellite DNA** See *DNA, satellite*.

**scabicide** A medication used to treat scabies. Although they were the most effective treatment, pyrethrin-based medications such as the lindane solution Qwell contain benzene, and are no longer generally recommended for use.

**scabies** Infestation of the skin by the human itch mite, Sarcaptes scabies. The initial symptom of scabies are red, raised bumps that are intensely itchy. A magnifying glass will reveal short, wavy lines of red skin, which are the burrows made by the mites. Treatment is with any of several scabicide medications.

**scabies, crusted** A severe form of scabies caused by delayed treatment of the initial infestation, characterized by mite-filled lesions covered with scabs. These lesions often fall victim to secondary infections, as with staphylococcus bacteria. Crusted scabies is most common in people with immune-system problems, including AIDS, diabetes, and lupus. Also known as keratotic scabies, Norwegian scabies.

**scalded skin syndrome** See *staphylococcal scalded skin syndrome.*

**scapula** The shoulder blade: the familiar flat triangular bone at the back of the shoulder.

**SCFE** Slipped capital femoral epiphysis.

**Scheuermann disease** A skeletal disease that usually begins in adolescence and results in a hunched back. Treatment with casting and a back brace is successful if undertaken early. Also known as juvenile kyphosis, curvature of the spine.

**schistosoma haematobium** A species of trematode worm that parasitizes humans and causes urinary tract disease. See *bilharzia.*

**schistosoma japonicum** A species of trematode worm that parasitizes humans and causes liver and gastrointestinal tract disease. See *bilharzia.*

**schistosoma mansoni** A species of trematode worm that parasitizes humans and causes liver and gastrointestinal tract disease. See *bilharzia.*

**schistosomiasis** See *bilharzia.* See also *bilharziasis.*

**schizoaffective disorder** A mood disorder that is coupled with some symptoms resembling those of schizophrenia, particularly loss of personality (flat affect) and/or social withdrawal.

**schizoid** Having symptoms similar to those of schizophrenia. See *schizophrenia.*

**schizophrenia** One of several brain diseases whose symptoms may include loss of personality (flat affect), agitation, catatonia, confusion, psychosis, unusual behavior, and withdrawal. The illness usually begins in early adulthood. The cause of schizophrenia is not yet known, but there appear to be both genetic (inherited) and environmental components, possibly including metabolic defects or viral infection. Schizophrenia is not caused by abuse or poor parenting practices. Treatment is with neuroleptic medication and supportive interpersonal therapy. The prognosis is currently fairly good, with two-thirds of those diagnosed recovering significantly.

**schizophrenia, childhood** The onset of schizophrenia before adulthood. This condition is very rare in young children, but occurs with more frequency in the teenage years. Autism was once known as childhood schizophrenia, but is a completely different disorder. See also *autism, childhood disintegrative disorder, developmental disorder, schizophrenia.*

**schizotypal personality disorder** A personality type characterized by unusual patterns of speech and behavior, and social withdrawal. See also *Asperger syndrome.*

**sciatic nerve** The largest nerve in the body, the sciatic nerve begins from nerve roots in the lumbar spinal cord in the low back (the sacrum) and extends through the buttock area, sending nerve endings down through the legs and knees. See also *sciatica.*

**sciatica** Pain resulting from irritation of the sciatic nerve, typically felt at the back of the thigh. Although sciatica can result from a herniated disc pressing directly on the nerve, any cause of irritation or inflammation of this nerve can reproduce the painful symptoms of sciatica. Diagnosis is by observation of symptoms, physical and nerve tests, and sometimes by X-ray or MRI if a herniated disk is suspected. Treatment options include avoiding movements that further irritate the condition, medication, physical therapy, and sometimes surgery.

**science, cognitive** See *cognitive science.*

**scintigraphy** A diagnostic test in which a two-dimensional picture of a body radiation source is obtained by the use of radioisotopes. For example, scintigraphy of the biliary system (cholescintigraphy) is done to diagnose obstruction of the bile ducts by a gallstone, tumor, or other problem; disease of the gallbladder; and bile leaks. For cholescintigraphy, a radioactive chemical is injected intravenously into the patient. The chemical is removed from the blood by the liver, and secreted into the bile that the liver makes. The chemical then goes everywhere that the bile goes: into the bile ducts, the gallbladder, and the intestine. By placing a camera that senses radioactivity over the patient's abdomen, a picture of the liver, bile ducts, and gallbladder may be obtained that corresponds to where the radioactivity is within the bile-filled liver, ducts, and gallbladder.

**scintimammography** A scintigraphic imaging technique that uses the radioisotope technetium tetrofosmin (Tc-99 tetrofosmin) to detect breast cancer. It can sometimes work better than standard mammography in situations where there is considerable uncertainty, as in women who have especially dense breast tissue.

**sclerencephaly** A general term for scarring and shrinkage of the substance of the brain. Sclerencephaly occurs because of chronic inflammation of the brain matter.

**sclerosing cholangitis** See *primary sclerosing cholangitis*.

**sclerosing panencephalitis, subacute** See *subacute sclerosing panencephalitis*.

**sclerosis, multiple** See *multiple sclerosis*.

**SCN** Severe congenital neutropenia.

**scoliosis** Sideways (lateral) curvature of the spine, giving the back an "S" shape. Scoliosis is usually an incidental and harmless finding. It appears most frequently in teenagers, and is a more serious matter when it appears in younger children. Severe scoliosis can often be improved by bracing, casting, physical therapy, and/or surgical correction.

**scoliosis, acquired** Curvature of the spine due to disease, accident, or surgery gone awry.

**scoliosis, congenital** Curvature of the spine as a result of a musculoskeletal disorder that is present at birth.

**scoliosis, idiopathic** Curvature of the spine due to unknown causes. This is the most common type of scoliosis.

**score, Apgar** See *Apgar score*.

**scrape** An abrasion or cut caused by something rubbing roughly against the skin. To treat scrape, wash the area with soap and water, and keep it clean and dry. Alcohol, hydrogen peroxide, and iodine can delay healing and should be avoided. Seek medical care if you think you might need stitches, as any delay can increase the rate of wound infection. Redness, swelling, increased pain, or pus indicate an infection that requires professional care.

**scratch test for allergy** See *allergy skin test*.

**scrotum** A pouch of skin that contains the testes, epididymides, and lower portions of the spermatic cords.

**scrub typhus** See *typhus, scrub*.

**scurvy** A disorder caused by lack of vitamin C. Symptoms include anemia; soft, bleeding gums; and bumps under the skin near muscles. Scurvy in early childhood can cause musculoskeletal problems. Treatment is by including foods high in vitamin C in the diet, and vitamin C supplements if necessary.

**seasonal affective disorder** Depression that tends to occur (and recur) as the days grow shorter in the fall and winter. Affected persons may react adversely to decreasing amounts of light or colder temperatures, which affect the production of neurotransmitters in the brain. Also known as winter blues, winter depression, the hibernation reaction. See *bipolar disorders*.

**sebaceous cyst** See *cyst, sebaceous*.

**sebaceous glands** See *glands, sebaceous*.

**seborrhea** An accumulation of scales of greasy skin, often on the scalp (dandruff). Treatment is with gentle washing, avoiding the use of harsh or perfumed soaps that can further irritate the oil glands. Coal-tar soap and similar preparations may also be useful.

**seborrheic keratosis** See *keratosis, seborrheic*.

**sebum** An oily secretion of the sebaceous glands, which helps to preserve the flexibility of the hair and retain moisture in the skin. Sebum is also secreted by the Meibomian glands of the eyes.

**Seckel syndrome** An inherited birth-defect syndrome characterized by severely short stature (dwarfism) and, characteristically, low birth weight, microcephaly, receding forehead, large eyes, low ears, prominent beak-like protrusion of the nose, and smallish chin. Defects of bones in the arms and legs, dislocations of the elbow and hip, and inability to straighten the knees are all common, as is (in boys) failure of the testes to descend into the scrotum (cryptorchidism). Underproduction of all types of blood cells (pancytopenia) occurs in some patients, as does chromosome instability. Due to microcephaly, there is usually developmental delay and mental retardation. About half of Seckel children have IQs below 50. Most children with Seckel syndrome are described as having a good disposition, despite hyperactivity and distractibility. Seckel syndrome is an autosomal recessive disorder, so both parents must carry the gene to pass it on to their offspring. Each of their children runs a one-in-four risk of receiving the Seckel gene from both parents, and so having Seckel syndrome. Also known as birdheaded dwarfism, microcephalic primordial dwarfism, nanocephalic dwarfism, Seckel-type dwarfism. See also *dwarfism*.

**second cranial nerve** See *optic nerve*.

**second stage of labor** The part of labor that lasts from the full dilatation of the cervix until the baby is completely out of the birth canal. Also known as the stage of expulsion. See also *labor*.

**secondary amenorrhea** See *amenorrhea, secondary*. See also *amenorrhea*.

**secretary's knee** See *patellofemoral syndrome*.

**secretin** A hormone made by glands in the small intestine, secretin stimulates pancreatic secretion and may have other effects as well. It is often administered as part of the endoscopy process. In 1999, several research centers began studies of secretin as a treatment for autism. Commercially available secretin is either porcine (from pigs) or a synthesized form of human secretin.

**section** 1 In anatomy, a slice of tissue. A biopsy obtained by surgery is usually sectioned (sliced), and these sections are inspected under a microscope. 2 In obstetrics, short for Caesarian section. 3 In surgery, the division of tissue during an operation.

**section, Caesarian** See *Caesarian section.*

**section, cross** A transverse cut through a structure. The opposite is a longitudinal section.

**section, longitudinal** A cut along the long axis of a structure. The opposite is a cross section.

**section, lower segment Caesarian** See *Caesarian section, lower segment.*

**sedative** A drug that calms a patient, easing agitation and permitting sleep. Sedatives generally work by modulating signals within the central nervous system. These sedatives, if misused or accidentally combined, as in the case of combining prescription sedatives with alcohol, can dangerously depress important signals needed to maintain heart and lung function. Most sedatives also have addictive potential. For these reasons, sedatives should be used under supervision, and only as necessary.

**sedimentation rate** A blood test that detects and monitors inflammation in the body. It measures the rate at which red blood cells (RBCs) in a test tube separate from blood serum over time, becoming sediment at the bottom of the test tube. The sedimentation rate increases with more inflammation. Abbreviated as sed rate.

**Segawa dystonia** See *dopa-responsive dystonia.*

**seizure** Uncontrolled electrical activity in the brain, which may produce a physical convulsion, minor physical signs, thought disturbances, or a combination of symptoms. The type of symptoms and seizures experienced depend on where the abnormal electrical activity takes place in the brain, what its root cause is, and such factors as the patient's age and general state of health. Seizures can be caused by head injuries, brain tumors, lead poisoning, maldevelopment of the brain, genetic and infectious illnesses, and fevers. In fully half the patients with seizures, no cause can yet be found. See specific seizure types below. See also *epilepsy, seizure disorders.*

**seizure disorders** One of a great many medical conditions that are characterized by episodes of uncontrolled electrical activity in the brain (seizures). Some seizure disorders are hereditary, but others are caused by birth defects or environmental hazards, such as lead poisoning. Seizure disorders are more likely to develop in patients who have other neurological disorders, psychiatric conditions, or immune-system problems. In some cases, uncontrolled seizures can cause brain damage, lowered intelligence, and permanent mental and physical impairment. Diagnosis is by observation, neurological examination, electroencephalogram (EEG), and in some cases, more advanced brain-imaging techniques. Treatment is usually by medication, although in difficult cases a special diet (see *ketogenic diet*) or brain surgery may be tried. See also *Aicardis syndrome, epilepsy, Landau-Kleffner syndrome, Lennox-Gastaut syndrome, Otahara syndrome, Ramsey Hunt syndrome, Rasmussen syndrome, Rett syndrome, seizure, Sturge-Weber syndrome, Tassinari syndrome,* as well as the following list of seizure types.

**seizure, absence** A seizure that takes the form of a staring spell: The person suddenly seems to be "absent."

**seizure, atonic** A seizure in which the person suddenly loses muscle tone and cannot sit or stand upright. Also called drop attacks or drop seizures.

**seizure, complex partial** A form of partial seizure during which the person loses awareness. The patient does not actually become unconscious, and may carry out actions as complex as walking, talking, or driving. There may be physical, sensory, and thought disturbances. When the seizure ends, there will be no memory of these actions. See also *seizure, partial; fugue state.*

**seizure, drop** See *seizure, atonic.*

**seizure, febrile** A convulsion that occurs in association with a fever. Febrile seizures are common in infants and young children and are usually of no lasting importance.

**seizure, focal** See *seizure, partial.*

**seizure, grand mal** See *seizure, tonic-clonic.*

**seizure, Jacksonian** See *seizure, partial.*

**seizure, local** See *seizure, partial.*

**seizure, myoclonic** A seizure characterized by jerking (myoclonic) movements of a muscle or muscle group, without loss of consciousness.

**seizure, partial** A seizure that affects only one part of the brain. Symptoms will depend on which part is affected: One part of the body, or multiple body parts confined to one side of the body, may start to twitch uncontrollably. Partial seizures may involve head turning, eye movements, lip smacking, mouth movements, drooling, rhythmic muscle contractions in a part of the body, apparently purposeful movements, abnormal numbness, tingling, and a crawling sensation over the skin. Partial seizures can also include sensory disturbances, such as smelling or hearing things that are not there, or having a sudden flood of emotions. Although the patient may feel confused, consciousness is not lost. Also known as focal or local seizures. See also *seizure, complex partial*.

**seizure, petit mal**   See *seizure, absence*.

**seizure, tonic-clonic**   The most obvious type of seizure. There are two parts to a tonic-clonic seizure. In the tonic phase the body becomes rigid, and in the clonic phase there is uncontrolled jerking. Tonic-clonic seizures may or may not be preceded by an aura, and are often followed by headache, confusion, and sleep. They may last for mere seconds, or continue for several minutes. If a tonic-clonic seizure does not resolve or if such seizures follow each other in rapid succession, seek emergency help. The person could be in a life-threatening state known as status epilepticus. Also known as grand mal seizures. See also *status epilepticus*.

**selective estrogen-receptor modulator**   A "designer estrogen" that possesses some, but not all, of the actions of estrogen. For example, raloxifene (brand name: Evista) prevents bone loss and lowers serum cholesterol as estrogen does, but unlike estrogen, it does not stimulate the endometrial lining of the uterus. Abbreviated as SERM. See also *designer estrogen*.

**selective mutism**   An inability to speak in certain situations. See also *apraxia, autism, elective mutism, mutism, social phobia*.

**selective serotonin reuptake inhibitor**   See *SSRI*.

**selenium**   An essential mineral that is a component of a key antioxidant enzyme, glutathione reductase, in tissue respiration. The National Academy of Sciences' recommended dietary allowance of selenium is 70 mg per day for men and 55 mg per day for women. Food sources of selenium include seafoods; some meats, such as kidney and liver; and some grains and seeds. Too much selenium may cause reversible balding and changes in the nails, give a garlic odor to the breath, and cause intestinal distress, weakness, and slowed mental functioning. Deficiency of selenium causes Keshan disease.

**selenium deficiency**   See *Keshan disease*.

**seminal vesicles**   Two structures about 5 cm long that are located behind the bladder and above the prostate gland. The seminal vesicles contribute fluid to the ejaculate.

**sensory integration**   A form of occupational therapy in which special exercises are used to strengthen the patient's sense of touch (tactile), sense of balance (vestibular), and sense of where the body and its parts are in space (proprioceptive). It appears to be effective for helping patients with movement disorders or severe under- or oversensitivity to sensory input. See also *occupational therapy*.

**sentinel lymph node**   See *lymph node, sentinel*.

**sentinel-lymph–node biopsy**   See *biopsy, sentinel-lymph–node*.

**sepsis**   The presence of bacteria (bacteremia), other infectious organisms, or toxins created by infectious organisms in the blood (septicemia) or in other tissues of the body. Sepsis may be associated with clinical symptoms of systemic illness, such as fever, chills, malaise, low blood pressure, and mental-status changes. Sepsis can be a serious situation, a life-threatening disease calling for urgent and comprehensive care. Treatment depends on the type of infection, but usually begins with antibiotics or similar medications. Also known as blood poisoning, septicemia.

**sepsis, neonatal**   A serious blood bacterial infection in an infant less than four weeks of age. Babies with sepsis may be listless, overly sleepy, floppy, weak, and very pale.

**septal defect, atrial**   See *atrial septal defect*.

**septal defect, ventricular**   See *ventricular septal defect*.

**septate**   Divided. A septate uterus is one that is divided.

**septate vagina**   See *vagina, septate*.

**septic**   Infected, or denoting infection. For example, septic shock is shock caused by infection.

**septic arthritis**   See *arthritis, septic*.

**septic bursitis**   See *bursitis, septic*.

**septicemia**   Infection of the blood, blood poisoning. See *sepsis*.

**septorhinoplasty**   A surgical procedure done on the nose and the nasal septum. It is performed for patients who have nasal obstruction. Septorhinoplasty not only improves the appearance of the nose, but also removes any internal obstructions that may be blocking breathing through the nose. See also *rhinoplasty*.

**septum**   A dividing wall or enclosure. For example, the septum of the nose is the thin cartilage that divides its left and right chambers from each other.

**septum, atrial**   The wall between the right and left atria of the heart.

**septum, cardiac**   The dividing wall between the right and left sides of the heart. That portion of the septum that separates the right and left atria of the heart is termed the atrial (or interatrial) septum. The portion of the septum that lies between the right and left ventricles of the heart is called the ventricular (or interventricular) septum.

**septum, heart**   See *septum, cardiac*.

**septum, interatrial**   See *septum, atrial*.

**septum, interventricular**   See *septum, ventricular*. See also *septum, cardiac*.

**septum, nasal**   The dividing wall that runs down the middle of the nose, creating two nasal passages, each ending in a nostril.

**septum, ventricular**   The wall between the two lower chambers (ventricles) of the heart.

**sequence, complementary**   See *complementary sequence*.

**sequence, conserved**   See *conserved sequence*.

**sequence, regulatory**   See *regulatory sequence*.

**sequencing**   Learning the order of nucleotides (base sequences) in a DNA or RNA molecule, or the order of amino acids in a protein.

**SERM**   Selective estrogen-receptor modulator.

**seroconversion**   The development of detectable antibodies in the blood directed against an infectious agent. It normally takes some time for antibodies to develop after the initial exposure to the agent. Following seroconversion, a person tests positive for the antibody when given tests based on the presence of antibodies, such as the ELISA blot.

**serositis**   Inflammation of the serous tissues of the body: the tissues that line the lungs, heart, abdomen, and inner abdominal organs.

**serotonin**   A neurotransmitter involved in the transmission of nerve impulses. Serotonin can trigger the release of substances in the blood vessels of the brain that in turn cause the pain of migraine. Serotonin is also key to mood regulation; pain perception; gastrointestinal function, including hunger and satiety; and other physical functions.

**serotype**   The kind of microorganism characterized, through serologic typing of its surface, by recognizable antigens.

**sertraline**   An antidepressant medication (brand name: Zoloft) in the selective serotonin reuptake inhibitor (SSRI) family. Sertraline is prescribed to treat depression and obsessive-compulsive disorder. The most common side effects of sertraline include dry mouth, nausea, malaise, insomnia, dizziness, and sexual dysfunction.

**serum**   **1** The clear liquid that can be separated from clotted blood. Serum differs from plasma, the liquid portion of normal unclotted blood, which contains the red cells, white cells, and platelets. It is the clot that makes the difference between serum and plasma. **2** Any normal or pathological fluid that resembles serum as, for example, the fluid in a blister.

**serum glutamic oxaloacetic transaminase**   See *aspartate aminotransferase*.

**serum glutamic pyruvic transaminase**   See *alanine aminotransferase*.

**serum hepatitis**   Hepatitis B.

**sesamoid bone**   A little bone embedded in a joint capsule or tendon. The kneecap (patella) is a sesamoid bone.

**seven-day measles**   See *measles*.

**seventh cranial nerve**   See *facial nerve*.

**seventh cranial nerve paralysis**   See *Bell palsy*.

**Sever condition**   See *apophysitis calcaneus*.

**severe congenital neutropenia**   A condition characterized by a lack of neutrophils, a type of white blood cell important in fighting infection. It is usually, but not always, hereditary. Children with severe congenital neutropenia (SCN) suffer frequent infections from bacteria, which in the past led to death before 3 years of age in 75 percent of cases. Children with SCN have no special problems with viral or fungal infections, but they do have an increased risk of developing acute myelogenous leukemia or myelodysplasia, a bone-marrow disorder. Aside from agranulocytosis, the bone marrow and blood show a number of other abnormalities, and the gamma globulin level in blood is low. Hereditary SCN is an autosomal recessive disorder, so both parents must carry an SCN gene to transmit the disease. Each child of two parents with the SCN gene has a 25 percent risk of receiving both SCN genes, and therefore the disease. Treatment with recombinant human granulocyte colony–stimulating factor (GCSF) elevates the granulocyte counts, helps resolve preexisting infections, diminishes the number of new infections, and results in significant improvements in survival and quality of life. Some patients have developed leukemia or myelodysplastic syndrome following treatment with GCSF, however. Also known as Kostmann disease or syndrome, infantile genetic agranulocytosis, genetic infantile agranulocytosis.

**sexual child abuse**  See *child abuse, sexual.*

**sexually transmitted disease**  Any disease transmitted by sexual contact; caused by microorganisms that survive on the skin or mucous membranes of the genital area; or transmitted via semen, vaginal secretions, or blood during intercourse. Because the genital areas provide a moist, warm environment that is especially conducive to the proliferation of bacteria, viruses, and yeasts, a great many diseases can be transmitted this way. They include AIDS, chlamydia, genital herpes, genital warts, gonorrhea, syphilis, yeast infections, and some forms of hepatitis. Also known as a morbus venereus or venereal disease. Abbreviated as STD. See also *sexually transmitted diseases in men, sexually transmitted diseases in women.*

**sexually transmitted diseases in men**  Men can contract all the venereal diseases, but may have no symptoms, or have different symptoms than women do. For example, most men who have chlamydia have no symptoms at all, but can easily pass the infection on to their sexual partners. The only sure protection against STDs is sexual abstinence. For sexually active men, the use of nonpenetrative sex practices (safe sex), condoms, dental dams, and spermicide with Nonoxynol-9 offers some protection.

**sexually transmitted diseases in women**  Women can contract all the venereal diseases, but may have no symptoms, or have different symptoms than men do. For example, women infected with gonorrhea may not have any symptoms, but may have a severe pelvic infection later, and can pass the disease on to their sexual partners. The only sure protection against STDs is sexual abstinence.

**SGA**  Small for gestational age.

**SGOT**  Serum glutamic oxaloacetic transaminase. See *aspartate aminotransferase.*

**SGPT**  Serum glutamic pyruvic transaminase. See *alanine aminotransferase.*

**sharp**  Medical slang for a needle or similar pointed object.

**shell shock**  See *post-traumatic stress disorder.*

**shigella**  A group of bacteria that normally inhabit the intestinal tract and cause infantile gastroenteritis, summer diarrhea of childhood, and various forms of dysentery, including epidemic and opportunistic bacillary dysentery.

**shigellosis**  Epidemic and opportunistic dysentery due to infection with the shigella bacteria. It is a particular hazard for people with AIDS or other immunodeficiency states.

**shinbone**  The larger of the two bones in the lower leg, the shinbone is anatomically known as the tibia. Its smaller companion is the fibula. See *tibia.*

**shinbone fever**  See *trench fever.* See also *Bartonella quintana, rickettsial diseases.*

**shingles**  An acute infection caused by the virus herpes zoster, which also causes chicken pox. Shingles usually emerges in adulthood after exposure to chicken pox or reactivation of the chicken pox virus, which can remain latent in body tissues for years until the immune system is weakened. It is an extraordinarily painful condition that involves inflammation of sensory nerves. Treatment is by antiviral medication and pain medication. See also *neuralgia, postherpetic.*

**shock**  In medicine, a critical condition brought on by a sudden drop in blood flow through the body. The circulatory system fails to maintain adequate blood flow, sharply curtailing the delivery of oxygen and nutrients to vital organs. It also compromises the kidneys, and so curtails the removal of wastes from the body. Shock can be due to a number of different mechanisms, including not enough blood volume and not enough output of blood by the heart. The signs and symptoms of shock include low blood pressure (hypotension); overbreathing (hyperventilation); a weak, rapid pulse; cold, clammy, grayish-bluish (cyanotic) skin; decreased urine flow (oliguria); and a sense of great anxiety and foreboding, confusion, and sometimes, combativeness. Shock is a major medical emergency. Shock is common after serious injury. Emergency care for shock involves keeping the patient warm and giving fluids by mouth or, preferably, intravenously.

**shock syndrome, dengue**  See *dengue hemorrhagic fever.*

**shock therapy**  See *electroconvulsive therapy.*

**shock treatment**  See *electroconvulsive therapy.*

**shock, anaphylactic**  See *anaphylactic shock*. See also *allergic reaction*.

**shock, cardiogenic**  Shock due to low blood output by the heart, most often seen in conjunction with heart failure or heart attack (myocardial infarction). The heart fails to pump blood effectively. For example, a heart attack (a myocardial infarction) can cause an abnormal, ineffectual heartbeat (an arrhythmia) with very slow, rapid, or irregular contractions of the heart, impairing the heart's ability to pump blood, lowering the volume of blood going to vital organs. Cardiogenic shock can also be due to drugs that reduce heart function, or an abnormally low level of oxygen in the blood (hypoxemia) caused, for instance, by lung disease. Whatever the cause, the blood vessels constrict and adrenaline-like substances are secreted into the bloodstream, increasing the heart rate. Treatment of cardiogenic shock is aimed at improving the heart's function. Shock after a heart attack is extremely serious. The mortality rate is over 80 percent.

**shock, diabetic**  See *insulin shock*.

**shock, electric**  See *electric shock*.

**shock, hemorrhagic**  Shock due to serious loss of blood. See also *shock, hypovolemic; shock, secondary*.

**shock, hypovolemic**  Shock due to a decrease in blood volume. This is the most frequent cause of shock. It can be due to loss of blood from bleeding, loss of blood plasma through severe burns, and dehydration. The primary treatment is prompt intravenous administration of fluid. See also *shock, secondary*.

**shock, insulin**  See *insulin shock*.

**shock, primary**  Sudden loss of blood pressure due to fear or pain. See also *syncope, situational*.

**shock, psychological**  See *post-traumatic stress disorder*.

**shock, secondary**  Shock that occurs as a side effect of another problem, such as a crushing injury or heart attack.

**shock, septic**  Shock caused by infection. See also *septicemia*.

**shock, shell**  See *post-traumatic stress disorder*.

**shock, spinal**  Shock caused by injury to the spinal cord.

**shock, toxic**  See *toxic shock syndrome*.

**shock, vasogenic**  Shock caused by widening of the blood vessels, usually from medication.

**short arm of a chromosome**  The short arm of a human chromosome, also known as the p arm. See *chromosome*.

**short-term memory**  See *memory, short-term*.

**shot, flu**  See *influenza vaccine, Haemophilus influenzae type B immunization*.

**shots, allergy**  See *allergy desensitization*.

**shoulder**  A structure made up of two main bones: the scapula (shoulder blade) and the humerus (the long bone of the upper arm). The end of the scapula, called the glenoid, is a socket into which the head of the humerus fits, forming a flexible ball-and-socket joint. The scapula is an unusually shaped bone. It extends up and around the shoulder joint at the rear to create a roof called the acromion, and around the shoulder joint at the front to constitute the coracoid process. See also *shoulder joint*.

**shoulder blade**  The familiar flat, triangular bone at the back of the shoulder. Known familiarly as the wingbone or, medically, as the scapula.

**shoulder bursitis**  Infection of one or both of the two major bursae (fluid-filled sacs) in the shoulder. Treatment of noninfectious bursitis includes rest, ice, and medications for inflammation and pain. Infectious bursitis is treated with antibiotics, aspiration, and surgery.

**shoulder joint**  The flexible ball-and-socket joint formed by the junction of the humerus and the scapula. This joint is cushioned by cartilage that covers the face of the glenoid socket and head of the humerus. The joint is stabilized by a ring of fibrous cartilage (the labrum) around the glenoid socket. Ligaments connect the bones of the shoulder, and tendons join these bones to surrounding muscles. The biceps tendon attaches the biceps muscle to the shoulder and helps stabilize the joint. Four short muscles that originate on the scapula pass around the shoulder, where their tendons fuse together to form the rotator cuff. See also *shoulder*.

**shoulder, frozen**  Permanent severe limitation of the range of motion of the shoulder due to scarring around the shoulder joint (adhesive capsulitis). Frozen shoulder is an unwanted consequence of rotator cuff disease, which can be due to trauma, inflammation, or degeneration. See *rotator cuff, rotator cuff disease*.

**show**  An appearance.

**show, bloody**  Literally, the appearance of blood. The bloody show consists of blood-tinged mucus created by extrusion and passage of the mucous plug that filled the cervical canal during pregnancy. It is a classic sign of impending labor.

**Shprintzen syndrome** See *velo-cardio-facial syndrome*.

**Shulman syndrome** See *eosinophilic fasciitis*.

**shunt** 1 To move a body fluid, such as cerebrospinal fluid, from one place to another. 2 A catheter (tube) that carries cerebrospinal fluid from a ventricle in the brain to another area of the body. A shunt may be placed to relieve pressure from hydrocephalus, for example.

**shunt, triculoperitoneal** A shunt that drains fluid from the cerebral ventricle into the abdomen.

**shunt, ventriculoatrial** A shunt that drains fluid from the cerebral ventricle into the right atrium of the heart.

**shunt, ventriculopleural** A shunt that drains fluid from the cerebral ventricle into the chest cavity.

**sialidosis** A form of mucolipidosis characterized by deficiency of acid alpha-N-acetyl-neuraminidase (sialidase). Also known as mucolipidosis I (ML I). See *mucolipidosis*. See also *mucopolysaccharidosis*.

**sib** Sibling.

**sibling** A brother or sister.

**sibship** The total number of children born to a set of parents. Siblings belong to a sibship.

**sicca syndrome** See *Sjogren syndrome*.

**sick sinus syndrome** Symptoms of dizziness, confusion, fainting, and heart failure due to a problem with the sinus node of the heart, which acts as the body's natural pacemaker. If the sinus node is not functioning normally, that is reflected in an abnormally slow heart rate (bradycardia). This can cause poor pumping by the heart, which can impair the circulation. Diagnosis is usually by electrocardiogram (EKG). Treatment includes medications, such as the class of drugs called calcium antagonists.

**sickle cell disease** See *anemia, sickle cell*.

**sickle cell trait** The condition in which a person has one copy of the gene for sickle cell (and is called a sickle heterozygote) but does not have sickle cell disease (which requires two copies of the sickle cell gene). If two people with sickle cell trait mate and have children together, each of their children has a one in four (25 percent) chance of having sickle cell disease.

**sickness, acute mountain** See *acute mountain sickness*.

**sickness, altitude** See *altitude sickness*.

**sickness, mountain** See *altitude sickness*.

**side effects** Problems that occur when treatment affects healthy cells. For example, common side effects of cancer treatment are fatigue, nausea, vomiting, decreased blood cell counts, hair loss, and mouth sores. Drug manufacturers are required to list all known side effects of their products, regardless of how small the probability that a user will experience these effects. When side effects of necessary medication are severe, sometimes a second medication, lifestyle change, dietary change, or other measure can help to minimize them.

**SIDS** Sudden infant death syndrome.

**sight, day** See *nyctanopia*.

**sigmoidoscope** A lighted instrument used to view the inside of the lower colon.

**sigmoidoscopy** A procedure in which a doctor inserts a viewing tube (sigmoidoscope) into the rectum for the purpose of inspecting the lower colon and rectum. If an abnormal area is detected, a biopsy can be performed.

**sign** Any abnormality that indicates a disease process, such as a change in appearance, sensation, or function, which is observed by a physician during evaluation of a patient.

**sign, Babinski** See *Babinski reflex*.

**sign, Kernig** See *Kernig sign*.

**sign, Macewen** See *Macewen sign*.

**sign, toe** See *Babinski reflex*.

**signature** 1 That part of the prescription that contains the doctor's directions to the patient. For example, the signature might say "take twice daily with food." Also known as the sig. 2 The outward appearance of a natural object, which was once taken as a token of its special properties. This ancient doctrine of signatures led some to conclude that the walnut, which looks something like a tiny brain, could be used to heal brain problems; the liverwort plant, which has a three-lobed liver-like leaf, was useful in treating liver disease; and so on. Not too many physicians accept such fanciful ideas today.

**silver** A metal used in some medications and in many natural remedies, as well as in silver amalgam for filling cavities in teeth. Silver has antibiotic properties. However, overuse of silver, or use of products containing silver by people with certain health conditions, can result in silver poisoning (argyria). See also *argyria*.

**silver poisoning** See *argyria*.

**single-gene diseases**   Hereditary disorders caused by a change (mutation) in a single gene. There are thousands of single-gene diseases, including achondroplastic dwarfism, Huntington disease, cystic fibrosis, sickle cell disease, Duchenne muscular dystrophy, and hemophilia. Single-gene diseases typically feature classic, simple Mendelian patterns of inheritance, whether they are caused by autosomal dominant, autosomal recessive, or X-linked traits. By comparison, polygenic diseases (genetic disorders caused by a combination of two or more genes) tend to have a more complex and varied expression.

**singultus**   A rarely used medical word for an ordinary hiccough. See *hiccough.*

**sinoatrial node**   One of the major elements in the cardiac conduction system, the system that controls the heart rate. This stunningly designed system generates electrical impulses and conducts them throughout the muscle of the heart, stimulating the heart to contract and pump blood. The sinoatrial (SA) node is the heart's natural pacemaker. It consists of a cluster of cells that are situated in the upper part of the wall of the heart's right atrium, where the electrical impulses are generated. An electrical signal generated by the SA node moves from cell to cell down through the heart until it reaches the atrioventricular (AV) node, a cluster of cells situated in the center of the heart between the atria and ventricles. The AV node serves as a gate, slowing the electrical current before the signal is permitted to pass down to the ventricles. This delay ensures that the atria have a chance to fully contract before the ventricles are stimulated. After passing the AV node, the electrical current travels to the ventricles along special fibers embedded in the walls of the lower part of the heart. The autonomic nervous system controls the firing of the SA node to trigger the start of this cardiac cycle. The autonomic nervous system can transmit a message quickly to the SA node, so it in turn can increase the heart rate to twice normal within only three to five seconds. This rapid response is important during exercise, when the heart has to increase its beating speed to keep up with the body's heightened demand for oxygen. Also known as the sinus node.

**sinus barotrauma**   See *aerosinusitis.*

**sinus node**   See *sinoatrial node.*

**sinus tachycardia**   Fast heartbeat (tachycardia) occurring because of overly rapid firing by the SA node. Sinus tachycardia is usually a rapid contraction of a normal heart in response to a condition, drug, or disease as, for example, pain, fever, excessive thyroid hormone, exertion, excitement, low blood oxygen level (hypoxia), or stimulant drugs, such as caffeine, cocaine, and amphetamines. However, in some cases it can be a sign of heart failure, heart valve disease, or other illness.

**sinus, cavernous**   See *cavernous sinus.*

**sinusitis**   Inflammation of the lining membrane in any of the hollow areas (sinuses) of the skull around the nose. The sinuses are made of bone, and are directly connected to the nasal cavities.

**situational syncope**   See *syncope, situational.* See also *vasovagal reaction.*

**situs inversus totalis**   See *reversal of organs, total.* See also *dextrocardia, Kartagener syndrome.*

**six fingers or toes**   See *hexadactyly.*

**sixth cranial nerve**   See *abducent nerve.*

**sixth disease**   See *measles.*

**Sjogren syndrome**   An autoimmune disease that classically combines dry eyes, dry mouth, and another disease of the connective tissues, commonly rheumatoid arthritis, but sometimes lupus, scleroderma, polymyositis, or some other autoimmune condition. Sjogren syndrome is an inflammatory disease of glands and other tissues of the body. Inflammation of the glands that produce tears (the lacrimal glands) leads to decreased tears and dry eyes. Inflammation of the glands that produce saliva in the mouth (salivary glands, including the parotid glands) leads to dry mouth. Sjogren syndrome can consequently be complicated by infections of the eyes, breathing passages, and mouth. About 90 percent of Sjogren syndrome patients are female, usually middle aged or older. Diagnostic clues include the presence of antibodies that are directed against a variety of body tissues (autoantibodies). Diagnosis can be aided by biopsy of an affected gland. Treatment is directed toward the particular areas of the body involved, and to complications, such as infection. Also known as keratoconjunctivitis sicca, sicca syndrome.

**Sjogren-Larsson syndrome**   An inherited disease, usually characterized by a triad of clinical findings: ichthyosis (thickened, fish-like skin); spastic paraplegia (spasticity of the legs); and mental retardation. The skin changes seen in Sjogren-Larsson syndrome are similar to those in congenital ichthyosiform erythroderma, a genetic disease that results in fish-like, reddened skin. Hyperkeratosis (thickening of the skin) is a regular feature. Ecchymoses (bruises) are present at birth or soon after. Sweating is normal. Spasticity can affect the arms as well as the legs, resulting in spastic paraplegia. The mental retardation is significant. Most of the patients never walk; about half have seizures. Eye problems also are part of the syndrome, with about half of the patients experiencing pigmentary degeneration of the retina. Glistening white dots on the retina are characteristic. People with Sjogren-Larsson syndrome tend to be unusually short. The gene for Sjogren-Larsson syndrome has been found situated on chromosome number 17, in band 17p11.2, and is also known as the FALDH10 because it codes for an enzyme called fatty aldehyde dehydrogenase 10. It is an autosomal recessive disorder: One copy of the gene is harmless, but if two gene carriers mate, each of their children has a 25 percent risk of receiving both Sjogren-Larsson genes, and having the syndrome. Diagnosis is by testing for the FALDH10 enzyme. The syndrome's symptoms are caused by a deficit of FALDH10. Some clinical improvement has been reported to occur with fat restriction in the diet and supplementation with medium-chain triglycerides. At one time the Sjogren-Larsson syndrome was thought to affect only those of Swedish descent, but a similar constellation of symptoms has been seen in other Europeans, as well as in people of Arab and Native American descent. It is possible that more than one type of mutation on the FALDH gene can cause Sjogren-Larsson syndrome. Abbreviated as SLS. Also known as ichthyosis, spastic neurologic disorder and oligophrenia syndrome; fatty alcohol: NAD+ oxidoreductase deficiency (FAO deficiency); fatty aldehyde dehydrogenase deficiency (FALDH deficiency); fatty aldehyde dehydrogenase 10 deficiency (FALDH10 deficiency).

**skeletal dysplasia** One of a large contingent of genetic diseases in which the bony skeleton forms abnormally during fetal development. Achondroplasia is one form of skeletal dysplasia.

**skeletal muscle** One of three types of muscle tissue in the body (the other two are smooth and cardiac), skeletal muscle represents the majority of muscular tissue. It is the type of muscle that powers movement of the skeleton, as in walking and lifting.

**skeleton** The framework of the body, which is composed of 206 bones. See *bones of the arm, wrist, and hand; bones of the head; bones of the leg, ankle, and foot; bones of the trunk.*

**skin** The body's outer covering. It protects against heat and light, injury, and infection. It regulates body temperature, and stores water, fat, and vitamin D. Weighing about six pounds, the skin is the body's largest organ. It is made up of two main layers: the epidermis and the dermis. The outer layer of the skin (the epidermis) is mostly made up of flat, scale-like cells called squamous cells. Under the squamous cells are round cells called basal cells. The deepest part of the epidermis also contains melanocytes. These cells produce melanin, which gives the skin its color. The inner layer of skin (the dermis) contains blood and lymph vessels, hair follicles, and glands. These glands produce sweat, which helps regulate body temperature, and sebum, an oily substance that helps keep the skin from drying out. Sweat and sebum reach the skin's surface through tiny openings called pores.

**skin biopsy** Removal of a piece of skin for the purpose of microscopic examination in the laboratory. Skin biopsy most frequently is done to diagnose a skin growth, such as a mole, or a skin condition, such as a rash. Different techniques are used in different situations. A shave biopsy takes a thin slice, and can be used to remove superficial lesions. A punch biopsy takes a core, and can be used to remove small lesions, and to diagnose rashes and other conditions. Excisional biopsies are generally larger and deeper, and are used to completely remove an abnormal area of skin (lesion), such as a skin cancer.

**Skin Diseases, National Institute of Arthritis and Musculoskeletal and** See *National Institutes of Health.*

**skin graft** Skin used to cover an area where the patient's skin has been lost due to a burn, injury, or surgery. The most effective skin grafts involve moving the patient's own skin from one part of the body to another. The second most effective type are skin grafts between identical twins. Beyond these two procedures, there is a strong chance that the body will reject the new skin, although the graft may give the body time to grow new skin of its own. A skin-graft site should be protected and kept moist. Patients should consult with their physicians about topical medications and bandaging, if any, that may be appropriate for the type of graft they receive.

**skin graft, allogenic** A graft using donor skin.

**skin graft, autogenic** A graft using the patient's own skin. Also known as an autologous graft.

**skin graft, composite** A graft technique in which both the patient's own skin and donor skin are used together.

**skin graft, full-thickness** A graft technique in which sheets of skin containing both the epidermis and the dermis are used.

**skin graft, mesh** A graft technique in which multiple pieces of skin are carefully arranged to cover an area. This technique is used most frequently when a large area needs protection.

**skin graft, pedicle** A graft technique in which a piece of skin from a nearby area remains attached at one of its corners, while the main part of the piece is reattached over the area in need of coverage.

**skin graft, pinch** A graft technique in which very small squares of skin are attached to the area needing coverage, in hopes that they will start to grow and cover it.

**skin graft, porcine** A skin graft in which pig skin is used. Like grafts from human donors, porcine grafts are usually just a short-term protective measure.

**skin graft, split-thickness** A graft technique in which sheets of skin containing the epidermis and part of the dermis are used.

**skin plaque** See *plaque, skin*.

**skin tag** A small tag of skin that may have a stalk (peduncle). Skin tags appear almost anywhere, although their favorite locales are the eyelids, neck, armpits (axillae), upper chest, and groin. Invariably benign, these tiny tumors of the skin usually cause no symptoms unless repeatedly irritated as, for example, by the collar. Treatment may be by freezing with liquid nitrogen, or by cutting off with a scalpel or scissors if the skin tag is irritating or cosmetically unwanted. Also known as an acrochordon or cutaneous papilloma.

**skin test for allergy** See *allergy skin test*.

**skin test for immunity** A method of evaluating whether a person has developed an immune response to certain infections. A substance is injected into the deep layer of the skin (dermis), and will cause a reaction if the immune system recognizes it. One of the most common skin tests is the tuberculin test, which reveals whether a person has been exposed to tuberculosis. The injection is placed on the inside of the forearm. A positive reaction results in a firm area of skin within two days.

**skin, scalded, syndrome** See *staphylococcal scalded skin syndrome*.

**skull** A collection of bones that encase the brain and give form to the head and face. These bones include the frontal, parietal, occipital, temporal, sphenoid, ethmoid, zygomatic, maxilla, nasal, vomer, palatine, inferior concha, and mandible. See also *bones of the head*.

**slanted ear** See *ear, slanted*.

**SLE** Systemic lupus erythematosus.

**sleep** The body's rest cycle. Sleep is triggered by a complex group of hormones that respond to cues from the body itself and the environment. About 80 percent of sleep is dreamless, and is known as non-rapid eye movement (NREM) sleep. During NREM sleep, the breathing and heart rate are slow and regular, the blood pressure is low, and the sleeper is relatively still. NREM sleep is divided into four stages of increasing depth of sleep: Level 1 sleep is a transition period between sleep and wakefulness; Level 2 sleep features significant slowing of heartbeat and breathing, and makes up about 50 percent of all sleep; and Levels 3 and 4 (Delta) sleep are marked by very slow respiration and heartbeat. Level 4 sleep leads to rapid eye movement (REM) sleep, also known as Level 5 sleep. Dreams occur during three to five periods of REM sleep each night. REM sleep occurs at intervals of one to two hours, and is variable in length. REM sleep is characterized by irregular breathing and heart rate, and involuntary muscle jerks. Most adults need around 8 hours of sleep on a regular schedule to function well, although some require less, and others more. Children, particularly teenagers, often need 9 or 10 hours for optimal functioning. See also *NREM sleep, REM sleep*.

**sleep apnea** Temporary stoppage of breathing during sleep, often resulting in daytime sleepiness. See *sleep apnea, central; sleep apnea, obstructive; sleep disorders*.

**sleep apnea, central** A breathing disorder characterized by brief interruptions of breathing during sleep. Central sleep apnea occurs when the brain fails to send the appropriate signals to the breathing muscles to initiate respiration. Central sleep apnea is less common than obstructive sleep apnea. Diagnosis is by observation, patient history, and polysomnography. Treatment depends on the patient's medical history and the cause of sleep apnea. Options include lifestyle changes, dental appliances, continuous positive airway pressure (CPAP), and various types of surgery to correct physical defects that contribute to sleep apnea.

**sleep apnea, obstructive** A breathing disorder characterized by brief interruptions of breathing during sleep. Obstructive sleep apnea occurs when air cannot flow in or out of the person's nose or mouth, although efforts to breathe continue. The problem may involve structures in the mouth, such as enlarged tonsils, or structures in the nose. Obstructive sleep apnea is much more common than central sleep apnea.

**sleep disorders** Any disorder that affects, disrupts, or involves sleep. The most common sleep disorder is probably snoring, although it usually is not medically significant. Insomnia, sleep apnea, restless leg syndrome, and sleepwalking are also sleep disorders. Most large medical centers have diagnostic and treatment facilities dedicated to sleep disorders. See also *sleep apnea, sleepwalking, snoring*.

**sleep, non-rapid eye movement** See *NREM sleep*.

**sleep, NREM** See *NREM sleep*.

**sleep, rapid eye movement** See *REM sleep*.

**sleep, REM**  See *REM sleep*.

**sleepwalking**  Purposeful moving, usually but not always including walking, while in a deep stage of sleep. Sleepwalking occurs most frequently in children, particularly boys. Sedatives tend to exacerbate rather than cure sleepwalking. The best measures are preventative: Ensure that the sleepwalker is in a safe room for walking, and cannot accidentally fall through an open window or down stairs. Some types of sleepwalking are related to seizure disorders, bipolar disorders, or other neurological conditions, but most cases are transitory and due to unknown causes.

**slipped capital femoral epiphysis**  A condition in which the growth plate of the femur is pushed out of position, causing hip pain, stiff gait, and sometimes knee pain. It is most common in overweight teenagers. Treatment is by orthopedic surgery to bring the bone back into alignment. Abbreviated as SCFE.

**slipped disk**  See *herniated disk*.

**slow virus**  A virus that spreads extremely slowly through body tissue. Slow viruses have been suggested as the cause of several unexplained disorders of the central nervous system, including Alzheimer disease, although the theory has not been proven. However, Creutzfeldt-Jakob disease and kuru, previously said to be caused by slow viruses, are now believed to be due to smaller virus-like particles called prions.

**SLP**  Speech-language pathologist.

**SLS**  Sjogren-Larsson syndrome.

**sludge, biliary**  See *biliary sludge*.

**Sly syndrome**  An inherited disorder characterized by accumulation of dermatan, heparan, and chondroitin sulfates in the central nervous system and peripheral tissues. Signs include macrocephaly and coarse facial features. Sly syndrome is an autosomal recessive disorder. Also known as mucopolysaccharidosis Type VIII. See also *mucopolysaccharidosis*.

**small for gestational age**  In a full-term infant, weighing 2,500 g or less at birth. Such infants are considered to have intrauterine growth retardation (IUGR), given their gestational age. By contrast, an infant may weigh 2,500 g or less simply because of prematurity.

**small intestine**  See *intestine, small*.

**small saphenous vein**  See *saphenous vein, small*. See also *saphenous veins*.

**small-cell lung cancer**  See *oat-cell lung cancer*.

**smallpox**  A highly contagious and frequently fatal viral disease characterized by a biphasic fever and a distinctive skin rash that left pock marks in its wake. Smallpox is one of the success stories of medicine. Thanks to vaccination, smallpox has been eradicated. Also known as variola.

**smear, Pap**  See *Pap test*.

**smell**  The sense that provides information about an object's scent, often giving clues to the palatability of food, the safety of air, and other matters. The organs of smell are made up of patches of tissue (the olfactory membranes) about the size of a postage stamp. These membranes are located in a pair of clefts just under the bridge of the nose. Most air breathed in normally flows through the nose, but only a small part reaches the olfactory clefts—just enough to get a response to an odor. When a person sniffs to detect a smell, air moves faster through the nose, increasing the flow to the olfactory clefts and carrying more odor to these sensory organs.

**smoldering leukemia**  See *leukemia, smoldering*.

**smooth muscle**  One of the three types of muscle tissue in the body (the other two are skeletal and cardiac). Smooth muscle generally forms the supporting tissue of blood vessels and hollow internal organs, such as the stomach, intestine, and bladder. It is considered smooth because it does not have the microscopic lines (cross-striations) seen in the other two types of muscle.

**snake stick**  See *Aesculapius*.

**snakebite**  Most snakes are not poisonous, but their bites can nonetheless cause a painful puncture wound that requires treatment. If you know a snake was poisonous, or if you did not see or recognize the snake, immediately seek emergency treatment for the victim. The affected part should be kept immobile and below the level of the heart, and the bite victim should be taken to the nearest hospital. Do not use a tourniquet or bandage, and do not attempt to suction out the wound by mouth. Treatment is with antivenom, as well as care for the puncture wound itself and any symptoms that emerge, such as respiratory distress. See also *rattlesnake bite*.

**Snellen's chart**  See *chart, Snellen's*.

**snoring**  A sound created by vibrations of the uvula and soft palate during sleep. During normal breathing, air passing through the throat en route to the lungs travels by the tongue, soft palate, uvula, and tonsils. When a person is awake, the muscles in the back of the throat tighten to hold these structures in place and prevent them fromcollapsing and vibrating in the airway. Sometimes snoring can be a sign of obstructive sleep apnea or have repairable physical causes, in which case medical treatment may be necessary. Otherwise, patients who snore may want to try different sleep positions, nose clips, or similar steps to prevent unwanted snoring. See also *sleep apnea, obstructive; somnoplasty.*

**social phobia**  A paralyzing fear of interacting with others. Social phobia appears to have physical, rather than primarily environmental, causes. It can occur in very young children, or emerge in adulthood like any other phobia. Treatment is with cognitive-behavioral therapy, using exposure-response techniques, and sometimes by medication.

**social worker**  A health professional who assists individuals and families with social or emotional issues. Within the medical system, a social worker might help insured families who need medical care find help, work with grieving parents or spouses, provide individual therapy, or help patients find resources to meet their needs for personal and community support. Social workers may have a BA or master's in social work (MSW).

**socialization**  The learning process a child goes through as he or she learns how to interact appropriately with other people.

**socialized medicine**  A medical system like that of a socialist country, in which medical facilities and payments are under government, rather than private, control. Most industrialized nations, including the US, have medical systems under some combination of state and private control.

**soft palate**  The muscular part of the roof of the mouth. The soft palate is directly behind the hard palate, and lacks bone.

**somatization**  The normal, unconscious process by which psychological distress is expressed as physical symptoms. For example, a person with clinical depression may instead complain of stomach pains that, upon examination, appear to have no physical cause.

**somnoplasty**  A surgical treatment for snoring. Somnoplasty uses heat energy to remove tissues of the uvula and soft palate. It is usually done as an office procedure with local anesthesia. It is not indicated for the treatment of sleep apnea. See also *snoring.*

**Southeast Asian hemorrhagic fever**  See *dengue hemorrhagic fever.*

**span, memory**  See *memory span.*

**spasm**  A brief, automatic jerking movement. A muscle spasm can be quite painful, with the muscle clenching tightly. A spasm of the coronary artery can cause angina.

Spasms in various types of tissue may be caused by stress, medication, overexercise, or other factors.

**spasm, coronary artery**  See *coronary artery spasm.*

**spasmodic dysphonia**  See *dysphonia, spasmodic.*

**spastic dysphonia**  See *dystonia, laryngeal.*

**spastic pseudoparalysis**  See *Creutzfeldt-Jakob disease.*

**SPD calcinosis**  See *cerebral calcification, nonarteriosclerotic.*

**specific developmental disorders**  Developmental disorders that affect one area of development only, as opposed to pervasive developmental disorders, dyspraxias that affect multiple systems, cerebral palsy, and metabolic disorders. For example, dysgraphia is a disorder of the ability to write (and perhaps draw) legibly. See also *developmental disorder, dysarthria, dyscalculia, dyslexia.*

**specific-pathogen free**  A term applied to animals reared for use in laboratory experiments; it indicates that the animals are known to be free of germs that can cause disease.

**speckled iris**  See *Brushfield spots.*

**speculum**  An instrument used to widen the opening of the vagina so that the cervix is more easily visible.

**speech disorders**  Disorders of the ability to produce normal speech. Speech disorders may affect articulation (phonetic or phonological disorders), fluency (stuttering or cluttering), and/or voice (tone, pitch, volume, or speed). Most speech disorders have their roots in oral-motor differences, although some involve language processing problems. Diagnosis is by testing by a speech pathologist. Treatment is by speech therapy. See also *aphasia, apraxia of speech, articulation disorder, cluttering, stuttering.*

**speech therapist**  An older term for a speech-language pathologist.

**speech therapy**  The treatment of speech and communication disorders. The approach used depends on the disorder. It may include physical exercises to strengthen the muscles used in speech (oral-motor work), speech drills to improve clarity, or sound production–practice to improve articulation. See also *communication disorders, speech disorders, speech-language pathologist.*

**speech-language pathologist** A specialist who evaluates and treats people with communication and swallowing problems. Speech pathologists have an MA or doctorate in their specialty, as well as a Certificate of Clinical Competence (CCC) earned by working under supervision. Some states also require a state license. Abbreviated as SLP. See also *speech therapy*.

**sperm** The male gamete, or sex cell. The sperm has an oval head that contains its genetic matter, and is propelled by a flagellating tail. It is carried into the female reproductive tract within the semen (ejaculate). If the sperm is able to travel up into the Fallopian tubes, it must break through the cell wall of the egg (the female gamete, or ovum) to fertilize the egg and form a zygote. This formation process is called fertilization. See also *fertilization, ovulation, ovum*.

**spermatic cord** A group of structures that go through the inguinal canal to the testis. These structures include the vas deferens, arteries, veins, lymphatic vessels, and nerves.

**SPF** **1** Sun protection factor. **2** Specific-pathogen free, a term for laboratory animals known to be free of bacteria, viruses, and other disease-producing microorganisms.

**spherocytosis, hereditary** A genetic disorder of the red blood cell membrane. It is characterized by anemia, jaundice, and enlargement of the spleen (splenomegaly). In hereditary spherocytosis (HS) the red cells are smaller, rounder, and more fragile than normal. They have a spherical shape rather than the biconcave-disk shape of normal red cells. These rotund red cells (spherocytes) are osmotically fragile and less flexible than normal red cells, and they tend to get trapped in narrow blood passages, particularly in the spleen. If this occurs, they break up (hemolyze) where they have lodged, leading to hemolytic anemia. The clogging of the spleen with red cells almost invariably causes splenomegaly. The breakup of the red cells releases hemoglobin, and the heme part gives rise to bilirubin, the pigment of jaundice. This excess bilirubin leads to the formation of gallstones, even in childhood. Often there is also iron overload due to the excess destruction of iron-rich red cells. The disorder often appears in infancy or early childhood, causing anemia and jaundice. The bone marrow has to work extra hard to make more red cells, so if in the course of an ordinary viral illness the bone marrow stops making red cells, the anemia can quickly become profound. This is termed an aplastic crisis. HS is due to a deficiency of a blood cell membrane protein called erythrocytic ankyrin (ankyrin-R, ankyrin-1, or ANK1). Diagnosis is by laboratory study of the blood, which will show evidence not only of many and distinctively shaped spherocytes, but also increased numbers of young red blood cells (reticulocytes). Hereditary spherocytosis is most common in people of northern European ancestry. The HS gene, which codes for production of ANK1, has been mapped to chromosome 8 in band 8p11.2. It is a dominant trait, so any child of a person with HS has a 50 percent chance of inheriting the gene and the disorder. Treatment is by removing the spleen (splenectomy). Although the red cell defect persists after splenectomy, the hemolysis ceases. However, because splenectomy puts young children at increased risk for overwhelming bloodstream infection (sepsis), particularly with the pneumococcus bacteria, it is usually postponed, if possible, until the age of three years. Before having a splenectomy, anyone with HS should have the pneumococcal vaccine. Persons with HS or another cause of brisk, ongoing hemolysis should take supplemental folic acid. The prognosis after splenectomy is for a normal life, and a normal life expectancy. Also known as congenital hemolytic jaundice, severe atypical spherocytosis, spherocytosis type II, ankyrin deficiency, erythrocyte ankyrin deficiency, ankyrin-R deficiency, and ankyrin1 deficiency.

**sphingomyelinosis** See *histiocytosis, lipid*.

**spider bites** Bites from most spiders are irritating but not poisonous. Localized reddening and swelling are not unusual, and should pass within a few days. A few spiders are poisonous, notably the black widow and brown recluse (brown fiddler) in the US. Bites from these spiders require emergency treatment, especially for children.

**spider telangiectasia** See *spider veins*.

**spider veins** A group of widened veins that can be seen through the surface of the skin. Their wheel-and-spoke shape resembles a spider. Also known as a nevus araneus or spider telangiectasia.

**spina bifida** A bony defect in the vertebral column caused by the failure of the neural tube to close during its embryonic stage. The neural tube is the structure that gives rise to the brain and spinal cord. The risk of spina bifida and other neural-tube defects can be decreased by ample intake of folic acid during pregnancy.

**spina bifida cystica** A bony defect in the vertebral column that causes a cleft in that column. The meningeal membranes that cover the spinal cord, and part of the spinal cord itself, protrude through this cleft and are clearly visible. The opening can be surgically repaired, usually shortly after birth. Some children will also need treatment for related problems, such as hydrocephalus. Also known as meningomyelocele.

**spina bifida occulta** A bony defect in the vertebral column that causes a cleft in that column. The cleft remains covered by skin. Treatment is usually not required.

**spinal column**  See *spine, vertebral column*.

**spiral fracture**  See *fracture, torsion*. See also *fracture, toddler's*.

**spinal stenosis**  Narrowing of the vertebral canal, often affecting the spinal cord.

**spinal tap**  See *lumbar puncture*.

**spine**  **1** The column of bone known as the vertebral column, which surrounds and protects the spinal cord. The spine can be categorized according to level of the body: cervical spine (neck), thoracic spine (upper and middle back), and lumbar spine (lower back). See also *vertebral column*. **2** Any short prominence of bone. The spines of the vertebrae protrude at the base of the back of the neck and in the middle of the back. These spines protect the spinal cord from injury from behind.

**spirochete**  A microscopic bacterial organism in the Spirochaeta family. Spirochetes have a worm-like, spiral-shaped form, and wiggle vigorously when viewed under a microscope. Treponema pallidum, the cause of syphilis, is a particularly well-known spirochete.

**spleen**  The blood vessel–filled organ located in the upper left abdominal cavity. It is a storage organ for red blood cells, and contains many specialized white blood cells (macrophages) that filter blood.

**spleen, ruptured**  Rupture of the capsule of the spleen is a potential catastrophe that requires immediate medical and surgical attention. Splenic rupture permits large amounts of blood to leak into the abdominal cavity, and is severely painful and life-threatening. Shock, and ultimately death, can result. Patients typically require immediate surgery. Rupture of a normal spleen can be caused by trauma, such as an accident. If an individual's spleen is enlarged, as is frequent in mononucleosis, most physicians will not allow major contact sports or other activities where injury to the abdomen could be catastrophic.

**splenectomy**  An operation to remove the spleen.

**splenic artery**  The large artery within the abdomen. It arises from an arterial vessel called the celiac trunk, which emerges from the aorta. The splenic artery supplies blood not only to the spleen, but also to the esophagus, stomach, duodenum, liver, and pancreas. See also *artery*.

**splenic fever**  See *anthrax*.

**splenomegaly**  Enlargement of the spleen.

**split personality**  See *dissociation, dissociative disorder*.

**spondylitis, ankylosing**  See *ankylosing spondylitis*.

**spondylolisthesis**  Forward movement of one building block of the spine (vertebra) in relation to an adjacent vertebra.

**spondylolysis**  The breaking down (dissolution) of a portion of a vertebra. The affected portion of the vertebra is a bone segment called the pars interarticularis, which can separate. Spondylolysis can be a cause of abnormal movement of the spine (spondylolisthesis) and lead to localized back pain.

**spongy degeneration of the central nervous system**  See *Canavan disease*.

**spots in front of the eyes**  Spots due to deposits of protein drifting about in the vitreous humor—the clear, jelly-like substance that fills the middle of the eye. Also known as floaters.

**spots, Brushfield**  See *Brushfield spots*.

**spots, Koplik**  See *Koplik spots*. See also *measles*.

**spotted fever**  See *Rocky Mountain spotted fever*.

**sprue, nontropical**  See *celiac sprue*.

**spur, heel**  See *heel spur*.

**sputum**  Mucous material from the lungs that is produced by coughing.

**squamous cell carcinoma**  See *carcinoma, squamous cell*. See also *carcinoma in situ, squamous cell*.

**squamous cell carcinoma in situ**  See *carcinoma in situ, squamous cell*.

**squamous cells**  Flat cells that look like fish scales. Squamous cells make up most of the outer layer of the skin (epidermis). They also line the hollow organs of the body, and the passages of the respiratory and digestive tracts.

**squamous intraepithelial lesion**  Abnormal growth of squamous cells on the surface of the cervix. The changes in the cells are described as low grade or high grade, depending on how much of the cervix is affected and how abnormal the cells are. Abbreviated as SIL.

**SSPE**  Subacute sclerosing panencephalitis.

**SSRI**  Selective serotonin reuptake inhibitor, one of a family of antidepressant medications (brand names: Celexa, Luvox, Paxil, Prozac, Zoloft) that affect the neurotransmitter serotonin.

**St. Anthony's fire** **1** An intensely painful burning sensation in the limbs and extremities caused by a fungus (Claviceps purpurea) that can contaminate rye and wheat. The fungus produces alkaloid substances known as ergotamines, which constrict blood vessels and cause the muscle of the uterus to contract. In excess, ergotamines are highly toxic and cause symptoms such as hallucinations, severe gastrointestinal upset, and a type of dry gangrene. Chronic ergot poisoning (ergotism) was rife during the Middle Ages due to the consumption of contaminated rye. **2** Erysipelas, a type of spreading hot, bright-red strep skin infection.

**staff of Aesculapius** See *Aesculapius*.

**stage** The extent of a cancer, and especially whether the disease has spread from the original site to other parts of the body. See also *staging*.

**stage of dilatation** The part of labor during which the cervix dilates fully to 10 cm. Also known as the first stage of labor. See also *labor*.

**stage of expulsion** See *second stage of labor*. See also *labor*.

**staging** Doing exams and tests to learn the extent of a cancer, especially whether it has spread from its original site to other parts of the body. The following stages are typically used:

**Stage I:** Cancer cells are found only on the surface of the affected organ or area.

**Stage II:** Cancer cells are found in the deeper tissues of the organ or area and have spread.

**Stage III:** Cancer cells are found in even deeper tissues, and have spread to nearby lymph nodes or other nearby area.

**Stage IV:** Cancer cells are found throughout the organ or area, and in nearby the lymph nodes, and/or have spread to other parts of the body.

**staph** Shortened form of staphylococcus. See *staphylococcus*.

**staph infection** See *staphylococcal infection*.

**staphylococcal infection** Infection with one of the staphylococcal bacteria. Staph infection can cause pus-filled abscesses on the skin or internal organs, and can migrate through the blood to infect the heart, meninges, and other areas. Treatment is with antibiotics and drainage of abscesses as necessary. See also *staphylococcal scalded skin syndrome, staphylococcus*.

**staphylococcal scalded skin syndrome** An infection of the skin with group II staphylococcus aurea bacteria. The bacteria release toxins, causing inflamed, scaling skin that looks as though it has been burned. It is more common in children than in adults, but is more likely to cause death when it does occur in adults. Rehydration and intravenous antibiotics are the most common treatments. Steroids will worsen the condition, and should not be used. Abbreviated as SSSS. See also *staphylococcus*.

**staphylococcus** A group of bacteria that cause a multitude of diseases. Under a microscope, staphylococcus bacteria are round and bunched together. They can cause illness directly by infection, or indirectly through products they make, such as the toxins responsible for food poisoning and toxic shock syndrome. The best known member of the staphylococcus family is staphylococcus aurea. Staphylococci are the main culprit in hospital-acquired infections, and cause thousands of deaths every year.

**staphylococcus, antibiotic-resistant** A form of staphylococcus bacteria that is unaffected by commonly used antibiotics. Antibiotic-resistant staphylococcus is a growing problem, particularly in hospitals where staph infections can run rampant. Treatment is with "super-antibiotics" when possible, although this type of infection can prove to be untreatable and deadly.

**startle disease** See *hyperexplexia*.

**startle reflex** A reflex seen in normal infants in response to a loud noise. The infant will make a sudden body movement, bringing the legs and arms toward the chest.

**STAT** A common medical abbreviation (from the Latin word *statum:* immediately), meaning urgent or rush.

**state, hypercoagulable** See *hypercoagulable state*. See also *estrogen-associated hypercoagulability*.

**statins** A class of drugs that lower cholesterol. Currently, six statin drugs are on the market in the US: lovastatin (brand name: Mevacor), simvastatin (Zocor), pravastatin (Pravachol), fluvastatin (Lescol), atorvastatin (Lipitor), and cerivastatin (Baycol). The major effect of the statins is that they lower LDL-cholesterol levels; in fact, they lower LDL-cholesterol more than other type of drugs. Statins inhibit an enzyme, HMG-CoA reductase, that controls the rate of cholesterol production in the body. This slows the production of cholesterol. They also increase the liver's ability to remove the LDL-cholesterol already in the blood. Studies have reported 20 to 60 percent lower LDL-cholesterol levels in patients on these drugs, as well as modest increases in HDL-cholesterol, and reduced triglyceride levels. Such reductions should prevent many heart attacks and deaths from heart disease. The statins are usually given in a single dose at the evening meal or at bedtime, taking advantage of the fact that the body makes more cholesterol at night than during the day. Results should be seen after several weeks, with a maximum effect in four to six weeks. Serious side effects are rare, but a few patients will experience an upset stomach, gas, constipation, and abdominal pain or cramps. These symptoms usually are mild to moderate in severity, and generally go away as the body adjusts. Rarely, a patient will develop liver blood test abnormalities, or will develop muscle soreness, pain, and weakness as a side effect of muscle problems.

**status epilepticus**  An epileptic seizure that lasts more than 30 minutes; a constant or near-constant state of having seizures. Status epilepticus is a health crisis, and requires immediate treatment. See also *epilepsy, seizure disorders*.

**STD**  Sexually transmitted disease.

**STDs in men**  See *sexually transmitted diseases in men*.

**STDs in women**  See *sexually transmitted diseases in women*.

**Stein-Leventhal syndrome**  A hormonal problem, also known as polycystic ovarian disease (PCO), that causes women to have symptoms that include irregular or no menstruation, acne, obesity, and excess hair growth. Women with PCO do not ovulate (release an egg for fertilization) every month. They are at a higher risk for high blood pressure, diabetes, heart disease, and cancer of the uterus (endometrial cancer). Much of this risk can be reversed by exercise and weight loss. Medication is generally prescribed to induce regular menstruation, thereby reducing the cancer risk. For acne and excess hair growth, the diuretic medication spironolactone (brand name: Aldactazide) can help. Clomiphene (brand name: Clomid) can be used to induce ovulation if pregnancy is desired. A type of surgery called a wedge resection, in which a piece of the ovary is removed, seems to help some women. No one is sure what causes PCO, but the ovaries of women with PCO contain a number of small cysts.

**stem cell**  Small, round cells with a squat nucleus and scant surrounding cytoplasm. They are a special type of cell that can reproduce forever. A stem cell can forgo immortality and turn into an ordinary blood cell, a red blood cell (an erythrocyte), a white blood cell (a leukocyte), or a large cell (a megakaryocyte) that fragments into the platelets necessary for blood to clot. A limited number of stem cells can miraculously repopulate the whole bone marrow, providing an endless supply of stem cells, reconstituting the entire repertory of blood cells, and restoring the immune system.

**stem cell harvest**  The taking of stem cells for use in cancer or other treatment. Usually these cells are taken from the patient's own bone marrow. The procedure ordinarily involves use of a general anesthetic and an overnight hospital stay. Small cuts are made over the hipbones to allow entrance for the large needles used to puncture the bones and draw out the marrow. The marrow is frozen for later use. In some cases, stem cells from a donor are used.

**stem cell harvest, peripheral blood**  A technique for obtaining stem cells from the patient's blood for use in bone marrow transplantation. The stem cells are lured out of the bone marrow by a special regimen of drugs. The blood is then filtered through a machine, and the stem cells skimmed off. They can be used right away or stored in liquid nitrogen until needed. Also known as apheresis.

**stem cell transplantation**  The use of stem cells as a treatment for cancer or other illness. The stem cells are removed (or obtained from a donor) first. Before the transplant is done, the patient receives high-dose chemotherapy and/or radiation therapy to destroy diseased cells. Then the stem cells are returned to the patient, where they can produce new blood and immune cells, and replace the cells destroyed by the treatment. The stem-cell preparation is infused into a vein and, once in the bloodstream, the stem cells act like homing pigeons by heading straight for the bone marrow space.

**stenosis**  A narrowing. For example, aortic stenosis is a narrowing of the aortic valve in the heart.

**stenosis, aortic**  See *aortic stenosis*.

**stenosis, pulmonary**  See *pulmonary stenosis*. See also *Alagille syndrome*.

**stenosis, subaortic**  See *subaortic stenosis*. See also *idiopathic hypertrophic subaortic stenosis*.

**stent**  A tiny tube. Stents are often inserted in diseased coronary arteries to help keep them open after balloon angioplasty. The stent allows normal flow of blood and oxygen to the heart. Stents placed in narrowed carotid arteries appear useful for treating patients at elevated risk for stroke.

**stereotactic**  Adjective referring to precise positioning in three-dimensional space. For example, biopsies, surgery, or radiation therapy can be done stereotactically.

**stereotactic needle biopsy**  A biopsy in which the spot to be biopsied is located three-dimensionally, the information is entered into a computer, and the computer calculates the information and positions a needle to remove the biopsy sample.

**stereotactic radiotherapy**  Radiation therapy in which a number of precisely aimed beams of ionizing radiation coming from different directions meet at a specific point, delivering the radiation treatment to that spot.

**stereotactic surgery**  Surgery in which a system of three-dimensional coordinates is used to locate the site to be operated on.

**stereotaxis**  Use of a computer and scanning devices to create three-dimensional pictures. This method can be used to direct a biopsy, external radiation, or the insertion of radiation implants.

**sternal rib**  See *rib, true.*

**sternum**  The wide, flat bone that runs down the middle of the chest, and to which most of the ribs are attached. Also known as the breastbone.

**steroid**  One of a large group of chemical substances classified by chemical structure. Steroids include drugs used to relieve swelling and inflammation, such as prednisone; vitamin D; and some sex hormones, such as testosterone.

**steroid abuse**  Use of substances containing steroids to increase muscle mass. Steroids can have many side effects when misused, including psychiatric problems, liver tumors, reduction in the size of male genitals, sterility, and heart damage.

**stiff baby syndrome**  See *hyperexplexia.*

**Still disease**  A form of arthritis characterized by systemic (bodywide) illness, including high intermittent fever, a salmon-colored skin rash, swollen lymph glands, enlargement of the liver and spleen, and inflammation of the lungs (pleuritis) and the area around the heart (pericarditis). The arthritis may not be immediately apparent, but it does appear in time, and may persist after the systemic symptoms are gone. Although Still disease was first described in children, it is known to occur in adults. Also known as systemic-onset juvenile rheumatoid arthritis and systemic-onset juvenile chronic arthritis.

**stings, Africanized bee**  See *bee stings, Africanized.* See also *bee stings.*

**stings, bee**  See *bee stings.*

**stings, insect**  See *insect stings.*

**stoma**  An opening into the body from the outside, created by a surgeon.

**stomach**  The digestive organ located in the upper abdomen, under the ribs. The upper part of the stomach connects to the esophagus, and the lower part leads into the small intestine. When food enters the stomach, muscles in the stomach wall create a rippling motion (peristalsis) that mixes and mashes the food. At the same time, juices made by glands in the lining of the stomach help digest the food. After about three hours, the food becomes a liquid and moves into the small intestine, where digestion continues.

**stomach cancer**  See *cancer, gastric.*

**stomach emptying study**  See *gastric emptying study.*

**stomach flu**  See *flu, stomach.*

**stomach paralysis**  See *gastroparesis.*

**stomatitis, Vincent**  See *acute membraneous gingivitis.*

**stone, kidney**  See *kidney stone.*

**stone, renal**  See *kidney stone.*

**stone, tonsil**  See *tonsillolith.*

**stones, cystine kidney**  See *cystine kidney stones.* See also *cystinuria.*

**stool**  The solid matter discharged in a bowel movement.

**stool test**  See *fecal occult blood test.*

**storm supplies kit**  See *disaster supplies.*

**strep**  Shortened form of streptococcus. See *streptococcus.*

**strep throat**  An infection caused by group A streptococcus bacteria, which can lead to serious complications if not adequately treated. Treatment is usually with antibiotics. See *streptococcus.*

**streptococcus**  A group of bacteria that cause a multitude of diseases. Under a microscope, strep bacteria look like a twisted bunch of little round berries. Illnesses caused by strep include strep throat, strep pneumonia, scarlet fever, rheumatic fever (and rheumatic heart valve damage), glomerulonephritis, the skin disorder erysipelas, and PANDAS. Familiarly known as strep. See also *streptococcus faecalis, streptococcus haemolyticus, streptococcus pneumoniae, streptococcus pyogenes.*

**streptococcus faecalis** A form of strep bacteria that usually are passed to a new host through fecal matter.

**streptococcus haemolyticus** Strep bacteria that produce substances which can destroy red blood cells.

**streptococcus pneumoniae** The most common cause of bacterial pneumonia and middle ear infection (otitis media), and the third most frequent cause of bacterial meningitis. Also known as pneumococcus.

**streptococcus pyogenes** The bacterial cause of strep throat (streptococcal pharyngitis), impetigo, rheumatic fever, scarlet fever, glomerulonephritis, invasive fasciitis, strep skin infections, and rheumatic fever. Autoimmune reactions to this strain of streptococcus have also been associated recently with a number of disorders, including gutate psoriasis (cradle cap), Sydenham chorea (a movement disorder related to rheumatic fever), obsessive-compulsive disorder, Tourette syndrome, autistic spectrum disorders, and anorexia. See also *PANDAS, rheumatic fever, strep throat, streptococcus, Sydenham chorea.*

**streptococcus, group A** See *streptococcus pyogenes.*

**streptococcus, group B** A major cause of infections, including those involving the pregnant woman and her newborn infant. Strep B can infect the mother's uterus, placenta, and urinary tract; in fact, it is present in the vagina of 10 to 25 percent of all pregnant women. Infections in the infant can be localized, or may involve the entire body. In babies, strep infections are divided into early-onset and late-onset disease. Early-onset disease presents within the first six days of life with breathing difficulty, shock, pneumonia, and occasionally infection of the spinal fluid and brain (meningitis). Late-onset disease presents between the seventh day and the third month of age with a bloodstream infection (bacteremia) or meningitis. The bacteria can also infect an area of bone; a joint, like the knee or hip; or the skin. Group B strep infection in the newborn is a serious and potentially life-threatening event, particularly because fever and warning signs are often minimal or absent, and because the newborn's immune system is not mature. Early signs of infection can be as subtle as poor feeding, lethargy, or poor temperature control. Women with vaginal group B strep can transmit it to the infant before birth, after the membranes are ruptured, or during the delivery. These babies have a .5 to 1 percent chance of contracting the early-onset type of infection. The risk rises with premature infants; infants born more than 18 hours after the amniotic membranes have ruptured; and infants whose mothers had fever, evidence of infection of the uterus lining, or infection of the urinary tract during labor and delivery. Because many infants today are discharged less than 24 hours after birth, there is growing pressure to culture all women during pregnancy for group B step. Antibiotic treatment can be considered for culture-positive women before delivery. A positive culture permits the infant's doctor to be especially alert to early signs of problems. Group B strep infection of the newborn is treated aggressively with antibiotics, usually in a neonatal intensive care unit, but the disease still carries a significant mortality rate. Prevention and early detection are critically important.

**stricture of the esophagus, acute** See *esophageal stricture, acute.*

**stricture of the esophagus, chronic** See *esophageal stricture, chronic.*

**striopallidodentate calcinosis** See *cerebral calcification, nonarteriosclerotic.*

**stroke** The sudden death of brain cells due to lack of oxygen, caused by blockage of blood flow or rupture of an artery to the brain. Sudden weakness or paralysis of one side of the body can be a symptom. A suspected stroke can be confirmed by scanning the brain with special X-ray tests, such as CAT scanning. Prevention involves minimizing risk factors, such as by controlling high blood pressure and diabetes. Also known as cerebrovascular accident.

**stroke prevention** If a person has a transient ischemic attack (TIA), a neurological event with the symptoms of a stroke, the symptoms go away within a short period of time. TIAs are often caused by narrowing or ulceration of the carotid arteries, however, and if this is not treated, there is a high risk of major stroke in the future. If you suspect a TIA, you should seek medical attention right away. An operation called a carotid endarterectomy can clean out the carotid artery and restore normal blood flow through the artery, markedly reducing the incidence of a subsequent stroke. In other cases, when a person has a narrowed carotid artery but no symptoms, the risk of stroke can be reduced with medications like aspirin and ticlopidine (brand name: Ticlid). These medications act by partially blocking the blood-clotting function of the platelets in the patient's blood. Controlling other factors that contribute to strokes, such as high blood pressure and diabetes, is also important for stroke prevention.

**stroke volume** The amount of blood pumped by the left ventricle of the heart in one contraction. The stroke volume is not all the blood contained in the left ventricle: normally, only about two-thirds of the blood in the ventricle is expelled with each beat. Together with the heart rate, the stroke volume determines the output of blood by the heart per minute (cardiac output).

**STS**  Sequence tagged site.

**study, antro-duodenal motility**  See *antro-duodenal motility study*.

**study, crossover**  See *crossover study*.

**study, cross-sectional**  See *cross-sectional study*.

**study, diachronic**  See *longitudinal study*.

**study, gastric emptying**  See *gastric emptying study*.

**study, longitudinal**  See *longitudinal study*.

**study, preclinical**  See *preclinical study*.

**study, stomach emptying**  See *gastric emptying study*.

**study, synchronic**  See *cross-sectional study*.

**Sturge-Weber syndrome**  A congenital, but not inherited, disorder that affects the skin, the neurological system, and sometimes the eyes and internal organs. The main sign of Sturge-Weber syndrome is a port wine–stain birthmark. Neurological symptoms may include seizures and developmental delay. Also known as encephelotrigeminal angiomatosi. See also *port-wine stain*.

**stuttering**  A speech disorder characterized by repetition of the first sound of a word. Stuttering can usually be eliminated or significantly modified with speech therapy. See also *cluttering, communication disorders, speech disorders*.

**subacute**  Rather recent onset or somewhat rapid change. In contrast to acute, which indicates very sudden onset or rapid change, and chronic, which indicates indefinite duration or virtually no change.

**subacute sclerosing panencephalitis**  A chronic brain disease of children and adolescents that occurs months to often years after an attack of measles, causing convulsions, motor abnormalities, mental retardation, and usually death. Abbreviated as SSPE.

**subaortic stenosis**  Narrowing of the left ventricle of the heart just below the aortic valve through which blood must pass on its way up into the aorta. The narrowing cuts the flow of blood. Subaortic stenosis may be present at birth (congenital) or acquired as part of a specific form of heart disease known as idiopathic hypertrophic subaortic stenosis (IHSS). Treatment options include drugs and surgery. See also *idiopathic hypertrophic subaortic stenosis*.

**subclinical disease**  An illness that stays below the surface of clinical detection. A subclinical disease has no recognizable clinical findings. It is distinct from a clinical disease, which has signs and symptoms that can be recognized. Many diseases, including diabetes, hypothyroidism, and rheumatoid arthritis, are subclinical before they surface as clinical diseases.

**subcu**  Abbreviation for subcutaneous.

**subcutaneous**  Under the skin. With a subcutaneous injection, a needle is inserted just under the skin. A drug can then be delivered into the tissues below the skin. After the injection, the drug moves into small blood vessels and the bloodstream. The subcutaneous route is used with many protein and polypeptide drugs such as insulin which, if given by mouth, would be broken down and digested in the intestinal tract.

**subglottis**  The lower part of the larynx; the area from just below the vocal cords down to the top of the trachea.

**sublingual**  Underneath the tongue. A sublingual medication is a type of lozenge that is dissolved under the tongue.

**sublingual gland**  The smallest of the three major salivary glands, it lies under the floor of the mouth, close to the midline.

**subluxation**  Partial dislocation of a joint. A complete dislocation is a luxation.

**submandibular gland**  The second largest of the three major salivary glands, it is located deep under the mandible (jawbone).

**submaxillary gland**  See *submandibular gland*.

**subq**  Abbreviation for subcutaneous.

**subscapular**  Under the scapula, like the subscapularis muscle, which originates beneath the scapula.

**subscapularis muscle**  A muscle that moves the arm by turning it inward (internal rotation). The tendon of the subscapularis muscle is one of four tendons that stabilize the shoulder joint and constitute the rotator cuff. Each of these four tendons hooks up to a muscle that moves the shoulder in a specific direction.

**subtotal hysterectomy**  See *hysterectomy, partial*.

**subungual onychomycosis, proximal white**  See *onychomycosis, proximal white subungual*.

**succenturiate**  Substituting for or accessory to an organ.

**succenturiate placenta**  See *placenta, accessory*.

**suction-assisted lipectomy**　See *liposuction*.

**sudden infant death syndrome (SIDS)**　The sudden and unexpected death of a baby with no known illness, typically affecting sleeping infants between the ages of two weeks to six months. Infants with a brother or sister who died of SIDS; babies whose mothers used heroin, methadone, or cocaine during pregnancy; infants born weighing less than 4.4 pounds; children with an abnormal breathing pattern that includes long periods without taking a breath (apnea); and babies who sleep on their stomachs are at elevated risk for SIDS. Since babies who sleep on their stomachs are at least three times more likely to die of SIDS than babies who sleep on their backs, children's health authorities recommend always placing infants on their backs to sleep.

**sudoriferous glands**　Small, tubular structures situated within and under the skin that discharge sweat through tiny openings in the surface of the skin. Also known as sweat glands. See also *perspiration*.

**sulcus**　From the Latin for a groove, furrow, or trench; the plural of sulcus is sulci. In medicine, there are many sulci; an example is the superior pulmonary sulcus.

**sulfa drugs**　See *sulfonamides*.

**sulfatidosis**　A condition characterized by low or absent production of several sulfatidase enzymes, resulting in proliferation and storage of waste substances in the body. The brain and nervous system degenerate as a result, and there may be physical deformities as well. Like related diseases, sulfatidosis is believed to be an autosomal recessive genetic disorder. Also known as mucosulfatidosis, multiple sulfatidase deficiency. See also *mucopolysaccharidosis*.

**sulfonamides**　The sulfa-related group of antibiotics, which are used to treat bacterial infection and some fungal infections. The sulfonamide family includes sulfadiazine, sulfamethizole (brand name: Thiosulfil Forte), sulfamethoxazole (Gantanal), sulfasalazine (Azulfidine), sulfisoxazole (Gantrisin), and various high-strength combinations of three sulfonamides. Sulfa drugs kill bacteria and fungi by interfering with cell metabolism. They were the wonder drugs before penicillin, and are still used today. Because sulfa drugs concentrate in the urine before being excreted, treatment of urinary tract infections is one of their most common uses. Sulfa drugs can have a number of potentially dangerous interactions with prescription and over-the-counter drugs (including PABA sunscreens), and are not appropriate for patients with some health conditions. Before taking sulfonamides, be sure your doctor knows about any other medications you take and your full health history.

**sumatriptin**　A medication (brand name: Imitrex) prescribed to treat migraine attacks. It is available as a pill or a shot. Never take sumatriptin with another drug that affects serotonin, such as antidepressants.

**summer cold**　See *hay fever*. See also *allergic rhinitis*.

**sun protection factor**　A measurement of a sunscreen's potency, expressed on a scale from two upward. Sunscreens with an SPF of 15 or higher provide the best protection from the sun's harmful rays.

**sunscreen**　A substance that blocks the effect of the sun's harmful rays. Using of lotions that contain sunscreen can reduce the risk of skin cancer, including melanoma.

**superaspirin**　See *cox-2 inhibitor*.

**superficial**　On the surface or shallow, as opposed to deep. The skin is superficial to the muscles. The cornea is on the superficial surface of the eye. See also *Appendix B, "Anatomic Orientation Terms."*

**superior**　Above, as opposed to inferior. The heart is superior to the stomach. The superior surface of the tongue rests against the palate. See also *Appendix B, "Anatomic Orientation Terms."*

**superior vena cava syndrome**　Symptoms that result from compression of the large vein that carries blood down to the heart. Compression may be caused by disease of any of the structures or lymph nodes surrounding this vein. The syndrome is characterized by swelling of the face, neck, and/or arms, with visible widening (dilation) of the veins of the neck. Patients often have a persistent cough and shortness of breath. Other symptoms may include hoarseness, swelling around the eyes, fatigue, chest pain, headaches, and dizziness. Causes of superior vena cava syndrome include cancer and several benign conditions. Common forms of cancer that can cause superior vena cava syndrome are lung cancer, cancer of the lymph nodes (lymphoma), and cancer that has spread (metastasized) to the chest, most commonly breast and testicular cancer. Noncancerous causes include infections, such as tuberculosis, fungus, and syphilis; benign tumors, such as teratomas, thymomas, and dermoid cysts; aortic aneurysm; pericarditis; sarcoidosis; irradiation treatment to the chest; air in the chest (pneumothorax); and complications of central line catheters and congenital heart surgery. Diagnosis is by observation of typical findings, and is supported by identifying a cause for the superior vena cava syndrome, a procedure that typically requires X-ray imaging or CAT or MRI scanning. Treatment is directed toward the underlying cause, and therefore might include radiation, antibiotics, chemotherapy, clot-busting (thrombolytic) drugs, blood thinners (anticoagulants), balloon angioplasty, and even surgery.

The outlook for patients with superior vena cava syndrome depends on the underlying cause. See also *vena cava, superior*.

**supernumerary** Beyond the normal number. Anything supernumerary is extra. A supernumerary chromosome is an extra one beyond the usual number of 46; a supernumerary digit is an extra finger or toe.

**supernumerary digit** An extra finger or toe.

**supernumerary nipple** An extra nipple.

**supernumerary placenta** See *placenta, accessory*.

**supertaster** A person who has an unusually large density of taste buds, each surrounded by pain fibers.

**supination** Rotation of the arm or leg outward. In the case of the arm, the palm of the hand will face forward.

**supine** With the back or dorsal surface downward; lying face up, as opposed to prone. See also *Appendix B, "Anatomic Orientation Terms."*

**supplies kit, disaster** See *disaster supplies*.

**supplies kit, emergency** See *disaster supplies*.

**supportive care** Treatment given to prevent, control, or relieve complications and side effects, and to improve the patient's comfort and quality of life.

**suppressant, cough** See *cough suppressant*.

**suppressor T cells** See *T-suppressor cells*.

**supraglottis** The upper part of the larynx, including the epiglottis; the area above the vocal cords.

**suprarenal gland** See *adrenal glands*.

**supraspinatus muscle** The muscle that elevates the arm and moves it away from the body. The tendon of the supraspinatus muscle is one of four tendons that stabilize the shoulder joint and constitute the rotator cuff.

**suprasternal notch** The V-shaped notch at the top of the breastbone (sternum).

**Suprax** See *cefixime*.

**surgery** The branch of medicine that employs operations in the treatment of disease or injury. Surgery can involve cutting, abrading, suturing, or otherwise physically changing body tissues and organs.

**surgery, cataract** See *cataract surgery*.

**surgery, retrograde intrarenal** See *retrograde intrarenal surgery*.

**surgery, stereotactic** See *stereotactic surgery*.

**surgery, Yag laser** See *Yag laser surgery*.

**surgical menopause** See *menopause, induced*.

**susceptibility genes, breast cancer** See *breast cancer susceptibility genes*. See also *BRCA1; BRCA1 breast cancer susceptibility gene; BRCA2; BRCA2 breast cancer susceptibility gene; breast cancer, familial*.

**suture** 1 A type of bone joint where two bones are held tightly together by fibrous tissue, as in the skull. 2 Threadlike material used to sew tissue. 3 To stitch a wound closed.

**swallowing syncope** The temporary loss of consciousness upon swallowing. See *syncope, situational; vasovagal reaction*.

**sweat** See *perspiration*.

**sweat chloride test** See *sweat test*.

**sweat gland** See *sudoriferous glands*. See also *perspiration*.

**sweat gland tumor** See *syringoma*.

**sweat test** A simple test used to evaluate a patient who is suspected of having cystic fibrosis (CF). The goal of the test is to painlessly stimulate the patient's skin to produce a certain amount of sweat, which may then be absorbed by a special filter paper and analyzed for chloride content. In a technique called iontophoresis, a minute, painless electric current is applied to the forearm or back, allowing penetration of a medication that maximizes sweat stimulation. Normal sweat chloride values are 10 to 35 milliequivalents per liter; patients with CF usually have a value greater than 60 milliequivalents per liter. Intermediate values (between 35 and 60) may be seen in some CF patients, and in some normal children. In those cases, the sweat test should be repeated in the very near future. In a severely malnourished patient with CF, the sweat chloride may be normal; once the malnutrition is corrected, however, the test will become positive. A few rare conditions that produce a false positive test include diseases of adrenal, thyroid, or pituitary glands; rare lipid storage diseases, and infection of the pancreas. Generally, children with these conditions are easily differentiated from patients with CF by their clinical condition, and molecular tests for CF can be done to clarify the situation. Also known as the sweat chloride test. See also *cystic fibrosis*.

**sweating** The act of secreting fluid from the skin by the sudoriferous (sweat) glands. See also *sudoriferous glands, perspiration.*

**sweating, gustatory** Sweating on the forehead, face, scalp, and neck occurring soon after ingesting food. Some gustatory sweating is normal after eating hot, spicy foods. Otherwise, gustatory sweating is most commonly a result of damage to a nerve that goes to the parotid gland, the large salivary gland in the cheek. In this setting, referred to as Frey syndrome, the sweating is usually on one side of the head. Gustatory sweating is also a rare complication of diabetes mellitus. In this case, sweating may occur on both sides of the head, with mild or substantial severity. This distressing problem can be difficult to treat. Treatments used include oxybutynin chloride, propantheline bromide, and clonidine (brand name: Catapres). Recently, some success has been reported in the using of topical applications of glycopyrrolate: the lotion was applied to the skin of the forehead and face, sparing the eyes and mouth. See also *Frey syndrome, diabetes mellitus.*

**sweats, night** See *night sweats.*

**swimming pool granuloma** See *granuloma, fish bowl.*

**Sydenham chorea** A disorder that emerges after a bout of rheumatic fever, and is most frequently seen in children. The choreaform movements are twisting. Sydenham chorea can be treated with medication. See also *PANDAS, rheumatic fever.*

**sylvatic plague** See *plague, sylvatic.*

**Sylvius, aqueduct of** See *aqueduct of Sylvius.*

**symmetric lipomatosis, multiple** See *cephalothoracic lipodystrophy.*

**sympathetic nervous system** A part of the nervous system that serves to accelerate the heart rate, constrict blood vessels, and raise blood pressure. The sympathetic nervous system and the parasympathetic nervous system constitute the autonomic nervous system.

**symphysiotomy** A surgical procedure to effect an immediate dramatic increase in the size of the pelvic outlet to permit delivery of a baby. The cartilage of the area where the pubic bones come together (the symphysis pubis) is surgically divided, which can be a life-saver for the baby.

**symphysis pubis** The area in the front of the pelvis where the pubic bones meet.

**symptom** Any abnormal change in appearance, sensation, or function experienced by a patient, that indicates a disease process.

**synapse** A specialized junction at which a neural cell (neuron) communicates with a target cell. At a synapse, a neuron releases a chemical transmitter that diffuses across a small gap and activates special sites called receptors on the target cell. The target cell may be another neuron, or a specialized region of a muscle or secretory cell. Neurons can also communicate through direct electrical connections (electrical synapses).

**synchronic study** A study done at a single point in time rather than over the course of a period of time (longitudinally).

**syncope** Partial or complete loss of consciousness with interruption of awareness of self and surroundings. When the loss of consciousness is temporary and there is spontaneous recovery, it is referred to as syncope or, in nonmedical parlance, fainting. Syncope accounts for 1 in every 30 visits to an emergency room. Syncope is due to a temporary reduction in blood flow, and therefore a shortage of oxygen to the brain. This leads to lightheadedness or a "blackout" episode: a loss of consciousness. Temporary impairment of the blood supply to the brain can be caused by heart conditions, and by conditions that do not directly involve the heart. Heart conditions that can cause syncope or fainting include abnormal heart rhythms (heart beating too fast or too slow), abnormalities of the heart valves (aortic stenosis or pulmonic valve stenosis), high blood pressure in the arteries supplying the lungs (pulmonary artery hypertension), tears in the aorta (aortic dissection), and widespread disease of the heart muscle (cardiomyopathy). However, syncope is most commonly caused by conditions that do not directly involve the heart. These conditions include postural (orthostatic) hypotension, a drop in blood pressure due to changing body position to a more vertical position after lying or sitting; dehydration, which can cause a decrease in blood volume; blood pressure medications that lead to overly low blood pressure; diseases of the nerves to the legs in older people, especially those with diabetes or Parkinson disease, in which poor tone of the nerves of the legs draws blood into the legs from the brain; high altitude; brain stroke or "near-stroke" (transient ischemic attack); and a migraine attack. Another common form of noncardiac syncope is known as situational syncope, because the fainting occurs after certain situations. Triggers for situational syncope include having blood drawn, urinating (micturition syncope), defecating (defecation syncope), swallowing (swallowing syncope), and coughing (cough syncope). In some individuals, one or more of these situations can trigger a reflex of the involuntary nervous system called the vasovagal reaction, which slows the heart, dilates blood vessels in the legs, and causes the person to feel nausea, sweating, or weakness just before fainting. Many causes of temporary loss of consciousness can be detected by taking a careful history. In an older person, dizziness after standing up suggests postural hypotension. Temporary loss of consciousness after urinating, defecating, or coughing suggests situational syncope. Cardiac causes of temporary loss of consciousness, such as aortic stenosis or cardiomyopathy, are suggested by the occurrence of the event during exercise. Signs of weakness localized to certain areas of the body with temporary loss of consciousness suggest stroke. To diagnose the cause of syncope, the blood pressure and pulse are tested in lying, sitting, and standing positions. Unequal blood pressures in each arm is a sign of aortic dissection. The heart is examined with a stethoscope to listen for sounds that indicate valve abnormalities. The nervous system is tested for sensation, reflexes, and motor function to detect conditions of the nerves and brain. An EKG is done to check for abnormal heart rhythms. Other tests may include echocardiograms, rhythm monitoring tests (heart event recorders), and electrophysiologic testing for abnormalities of the heart's electrical system. When heart conditions are not suspected, tilt-table testing can be used. No treatment is needed for many noncardiac causes of syncope, as the person regains consciousness by simply sitting or lying down. The person is thereafter advised to avoid trigger situations. Older people should have their medications reviewed, and be cautioned to slow the process of changing positions. This simple technique allows the body to adjust to the new position, as the nerves and circulation of the legs adjust slower in older persons than in younger ones. See also *syncope, situational; tilt-table test; vasovagal reaction.*

**syncope, coughing** The temporary loss of consciousness upon coughing. See *syncope, situational.* See also *syncope, vasovagal reaction.*

**syncope, defecation** The temporary loss of consciousness upon defecating (having a bowel movement). See *syncope, situational.* See also *syncope, vasovagal reaction.*

**syncope, micturition** The temporary loss of consciousness upon urinating (micturation). See *syncope, situational.* See also *syncope, vasovagal reaction.*

**syncope, situational** The temporary loss of consciousness in a particular kind of situation. The situations that trigger this reaction are diverse, and include having blood drawn, straining while urinating or defecating, and coughing. The reaction can be caused also by emotional stress, fear, or pain. When experiencing the trigger condition, the person often becomes pale and feels nauseated, sweaty, and weak just before losing consciousness.

Situational syncope is caused by a reflex of the involuntary nervous system called the vasovagal reaction. The vasovagal reaction leads the heart to slow down (bradycardia), while at the same time leading the nerves that serve the blood vessels in the legs to permit those vessels to dilate (widen). The result is that the heart puts out less blood, blood pressure drops, and circulating blood tends to go into the legs rather than to the head. The brain is deprived of oxygen, and the fainting episode occurs. Situational syncope is also known as vasovagal syncope, vasodepressor syncope, and Gower syndrome. See also *syncope, vasovagal reaction.*

**syncope, swallowing** The temporary loss of consciousness upon swallowing. See *syncope, situational.* See also *syncope, vasovagal reaction.*

**syncope, vasodepressor** See *syncope, situational.* See also *syncope, vasovagal reaction.*

**syncope, vasovagal** See *syncope, situational.* See also *syncope, vasovagal reaction.*

**syndactyly** A condition in which fingers or toes are joined together. Syndactyly can involve the bones (bony syndactyly) or just the skin (cutaneous syndactyly, or webbing).

**syndactyly, bony** A condition in which the bones of fingers or toes are joined together. Bony syndactyly is the opposite of cutaneous syndactyly, in which the bones are normal but skin between the digits is webbed.

**syndactyly, complete** A condition in which fingers or toes are completely joined together, with the connection extending from the base to the tip of the involved digits. Complete syndactyly is the opposite of partial syndactyly, in which the connection extends only partway up from the base of the involved digits.

**syndactyly, cutaneous** A condition in which fingers or toes are joined together, and the joining involves only the skin, not the bones. Cutaneous syndactyly is the opposite of bony syndactyly, in which the bones of the digits are joined.

**syndactyly, partial** A condition in which fingers or toes are partially joined together. Syndactyly can involve the bones or just the skin. With partial syndactyly, the connection extends from the base only partway up the involved digits. Partial syndactyly is the opposite of complete syndactyly, in which the connection extends from the base to the tip of the involved digits.

**syndactyly, Poland** See *Poland syndrome.*

**syndromatic hepatic ductular hypoplasia** See *Alagille syndrome.*

**syndrome**   A combination of symptoms and signs that together represent a disease process. For specific syndromes, please see their alphabetical listings.

**synesthesia**   A condition in which the normal separation between the senses appears to have broken down. In synesthesia, sight may mingle with sound, taste with touch, and so on. People with synesthesia are six times more likely to be female than male. Most find their unusual sensory abilities enjoyable. People with synesthesia often report that one or more of their family members also had synesthesia, so it may in some cases be an inherited condition. Synesthesia can be induced by certain hallucinogenic drugs, and can also occur in some types of seizure disorders.

**synovia**   See *synovial fluid*.

**synovial cyst, popliteal**   See *Baker cyst*.

**synovial fluid**   The slippery fluid that lubricates joints. Also known as the synovia.

**synovial lining**   The lining of the joints.

**synovitis**   Inflammation of the synovial membrane, the lining of the joints.

**Synthroid**   See *levothyroxine sodium*.

**syphilis**   A sexually transmitted disease caused by Treponema pallidum, a microscopic organism called a spirochete. This worm-like, spiral-shaped organism infects people by burrowing into the moist mucous membranes of the mouth or genitals. From there, the spirochete produces a nonpainful ulcer known as a chancre. There are three stages of syphilis. The first (primary) stage is formation of the chancre, and can last from one to five weeks. At this stage, syphilis is highly contagious. The disease can be transmitted from any contact with one of the ulcers, which are teeming with spirochetes. If the ulcer is outside the vagina or on the scrotum, the use of condoms may not help in preventing transmission. Likewise, if the ulcer is in the mouth, merely kissing the infected individual can spread syphilis. Even without treatment, the early infection resolves on its own in most women. However, 25 percent will proceed to the secondary stage of syphilis, which lasts from four to six weeks. This phase can include hair loss; a sore throat; white patches in the nose, mouth, and vagina; fever; headaches; and a skin rash. There can be lesions on the genitals that look like genital warts, but are caused by spirochetes rather than the wart virus. These wart-like lesions, as well as the skin rash, are highly contagious. The rash can occur on the palms of the hands, and the infection can be transmitted by casual contact. The third (tertiary) stage of the disease involves the brain and heart,

and usually is no longer contagious. At this point, however, the infection can cause extensive damage to the internal organs and the brain, and can lead to death. Diagnosis is by blood test, either the rapid plasma reagin (RPR) or Venereal Disease Research Laboratory (VDRL) test. Treatment is with antibiotics. See also *chancre; spirochete; syphilis, congenital; syphilis test, RPR; syphilis test, VDRL*.

**syphilis test, RPR**   Rapid plasma reagin, a blood test for syphilis that looks for an antibody which is present in the bloodstream when a patient has syphilis. A negative (nonreactive) RPR is compatible with a person not having syphilis, but in the early stages of the disease, the RPR often gives false-negative results. Conversely, a false-positive RPR can be encountered in infectious mononucleosis, lupus, antiphospholipid antibody syndrome, hepatitis A, leprosy, malaria and, occasionally, pregnancy. See also *syphilis; syphilis test, VDRL*.

**syphilis test, VDRL**   A blood test for syphilis (VDRL stands for Venereal Disease Research Laboratory) that looks for an antibody which is present in the bloodstream when a patient has syphilis. A negative (nonreactive) VDRL is compatible with a person not having syphilis, but in the early stages of the disease, the VDRL often gives false-negative results. Conversely, a false-positive VDRL can be encountered in infectious mononucleosis, lupus, antiphospholipid antibody syndrome, hepatitis A, leprosy, malaria and, occasionally, pregnancy. See also *syphilis; syphilis test, RPR*.

**syphilis, congenital**   Infection of a fetus or newborn with syphilis. Syphilis in a fetus can cause deformity, particularly of the long bones, or death. Syphilis infection acquired at birth is also dangerous. See also *TORCH infection*.

**syphilis, tertiary**   The third stage of syphilis, in which the syphilis spirochetes infect the brain and other organs of the body. Dementia is a common outcome. Tertiary syphilis can develop many years after an initial untreated infection. The spirochetes can cause extensive damage in the body, sometimes leading to death.

**syringe**   A medical device used to inject fluid into, or withdraw fluid from, the body. Medical syringes consist of a needle attached to a hollow cylinder that is fitted with a sliding plunger. The downward movement of the plunger injects fluid; upward movement withdraws fluid. Medical syringes were once made of metal or glass, and required cleaning and sterilization before they could be used again. Now most syringes used in medicine are plastic and disposable.

**syringoma**   A benign (noncancerous) skin tumor that derives from eccrine cells, specialized cells related to sweat glands. The skin lesions usually appear during puberty or adult life, and consist of small bumps 1 to 3 mm in diameter that form under the surface of the skin. The most frequent site is the eyelids and around the eyes, but other areas of the body can also be affected. There may be only one or a few lesions in a localized area, or numerous lesions may cover a wide area. Syringomas more frequently affect women and do have an hereditary basis in some, but not all, cases. They are also associated with Down syndrome, Marfan syndrome, and Ehlers-Danlos syndrome. Treatment of syringomas can be a problem, depending on their number and location. One method that seems to be effective and creates minimal scarring is the use of a hair-removal electric needle; another promising technique uses a CO2 laser.

**system, autonomic nervous**  See *autonomic nervous system*.

**system, cardiac conduction**  See *cardiac conduction system*.

**system, central nervous**  See *central nervous system*.

**system, locomotive**  See *locomotive system*.

**system, parasympathetic nervous**  See *parasympathetic nervous system*.

**system, peripheral nervous**  See *peripheral nervous system*.

**system, sympathetic nervous**  See *sympathetic nervous system*.

**systemic lupus erythematosus**  See *lupus erythematosus, systemic*. See also *lupus*.

**systemic therapy**  Treatment that reaches cells throughout the body by traveling through the bloodstream.

**systemic-onset juvenile chronic arthritis**  See *arthritis, systemic-onset juvenile chronic; Still disease*.

**systemic-onset juvenile rheumatoid arthritis**  See *arthritis, systemic-onset juvenile rheumatoid; Still disease*.

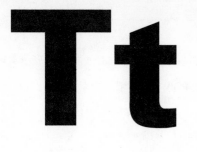

**T**   Thymine, one member of the adenine-thymine (A-T) base pair in DNA.

**T cells**   A type of white blood cells made in the bone marrow. Immature T cells (T-stem cells) migrate to the thymus gland, where they mature, differentiate into various types of T cells, and become active in the immune system in response to a hormone called thymosin and other factors. T cells that are potentially activated against the body's own tissues are normally killed or changed (down-regulated) during this maturation process. There are several types of mature T cells, and not all of their functions are known. T cells can produce cytokines, such as the interleukins, which in turn further stimulate the immune response. T-cell activation is measured as a way to assess the health of patients with the HIV virus (AIDS). T-cell activity is examined less frequently in other disorders, but as we learn more about how the immune system works, it is becoming part of the routine process for assessing autoimmune conditions and some types of cancer. Also known as T lymphocytes. See *natural killer cells; T-4 cells; T-4 count; T lymphocytes, cytotoxic; T-suppressor cells; T-suppressor count.*

**T cells, CD4+**   See *T-4 cells.*

**T cells, CD8+**   See *T lymphocytes, cytotoxic; T-suppressor cells.*

**T cells, peripheral**   T cells found in the peripheral blood rather than in the lymphatic system.

**T lymphocytes, cytotoxic**   T cells that express the CD8 transmembrane glycoprotein (CD8+ T cells). They are antigen-specific: able to search out and kill specific types of infected cells. When they find cells carrying the viral peptide they are looking for, they induce these cells to secrete proteins that attract nearby macrophages (white blood cells). These macrophages then surround and destroy the infected cells. Cytotoxic T cells are particularly important in the body's response to viruses and cancer. Abbreviated as CTL. Also known as $T_c$ cells. See also *CD8, T cells, T-suppressor cells.*

**T1–T12**   Symbols that represent the 12 thoracic vertebrae.

**T-4 cells**   T cells that express the CD4 transmembrane glycoprotein (CD4+ T cells). They are active in the body's immune response, helping to turn on this system when it is challenged by an infection or by foreign matter in the body. The HIV virus attacks T-4 cells, knocking out the body's ability to defend itself against infections. There are at least two types of T-4 cells. Also known as T-helper cells, $T_H$ cells. See also *CD4, T cells.*

**T-4 count**   A test that counts the number of T-4 cells in the blood, usually to assess the immune status of a patient with the HIV virus (AIDS). It's important to note that there are also T-4 cells in the lymphatic system, and they may be more severely affected there than in the bloodstream. Of the various ways to read this test, the best indicator of health may be the absolute T-4 count. Also known as T-helper count. See also *helper/suppressor ratio, T cells.*

**T-8 cells**   See *T-suppressor cells.*

**T-cell receptor**   A method used by T cells for recognizing specific antigens. T cells have receptors that are only activated by the target antigen(s).

**T-helper cells**   See *T-4 cells.*

**T-suppressor cells**   T cells that express the CD8 transmembrane glycoprotein (CD8+ T cells). They close down the immune response after invading organisms are destroyed. Suppressor T cells are sensitive to high concentrations of circulating lymphokine hormones, and release their own lymphokines after an immune response has achieved its goal. This signals all other immune-system participants to cease their attack. Some memory B-cells remain after this signal to ward off a repeat attack by the invading organism. Also known as T-8 cells. See also *CD8, T cells; T lymphocytes, cytotoxic.*

**T-suppressor count**   A test that counts the number of T-suppressor (T-8) cells in the bloodstream. It appears that some T-8 cells secrete a substance that can kill the HIV virus, so a high count is believed to be a good indicator for people with HIV (AIDS). See also *helper/ suppressor ratio, T-suppressor cells.*

**t.i.d.**   Seen on a prescription, three times a day. See also *Appendix A, "Prescription Abbreviations."*

**tabes dorsalis**   See *neurosyphilis, tabes.*

**tablespoon**   An old-fashioned but convenient household measure of capacity. A tablespoon holds about 15 cc of liquid.

**tache noire**   French for "black spot," used to describe a small ulcer covered with a black crust at the site of a tick bite. A tache noire is characteristic of several tick-borne rickettsial diseases. See *rickettsial diseases.*

**tachycardia**   A rapid heart rate, usually defined as greater than 100 beats per minute. See also *paroxysmal atrial tachycardia.*

**tachycardia, paroxysmal atrial**  See *paroxysmal atrial tachycardia.*

**tachycardia, sinus**  See *sinus tachycardia.*

**tachycardia, ventricular**  See *ventricular tachycardia.* See also *ventricular arrhythmias.*

**tachypnea**  Abnormally fast breathing.

**tactile**  Having to do with touch.

**taenia**  **1** In medicine, a genus of large tapeworms some of which are parasitic in humans. **2** In anatomy, a band or a structural line; specifically, several bands and lines of nervous matter in the brain. Also spelled tenia.

**Taenia saginata**  The beef tapeworm. The most common of the big tapeworms that parasitizes people, it can be contracted from infected raw or rare beef.

**Taenia solium**  The pork tapeworm, which can parasitize people. It can be contracted from undercooked or infested pork. Also known as the armed tapeworm and the measly tapeworm.

**tag, ear**  See *ear tag.*

**tag, preauricular**  See *ear tag.*

**tag, skin**  See *skin tag.*

**taint**  **1** To poison, infect, or spoil. **2** Folk term for the female perineum. See *perineum.*

**talipes**  See *clubfoot.*

**talipes equinovarus**  The most common (classic) form of clubfoot. See *clubfoot.*

**talus**  The ankle bone, or the ankle itself. The ankle joint is formed by the talus and the bottom of the tibia and fibula that rest upon it.

**tampon**  A pack or pad used to stop or collect the flow of blood or other fluids. The tampon may be made of cotton, sponge, or another material. Tampons serve in surgery to control bleeding, and are used to stop severe nosebleeds. Vaginal tampons collect the flow of menstrual blood.

**tamponade, balloon**  See *balloon tamponade.*

**tamponade, cardiac**  See *cardiac tamponade.*

**tamponade, chronic**  See *chronic tamponade.*

**tamponade, esophagogastric**  See *balloon tamponade.*

**tamponade, pericardial**  See *cardiac tamponade.*

**tap, joint**  See *arthrocentesis.*

**tap, spinal**  See *lumbar puncture.*

**Tapazol**  See *methimazole.*

**tapeworm**  A worm that is flattened like a tape measure and functions as an intestinal parasite, unable to live freely on its own but able to do so within an animal's gut.

**tapeworm, African**  See *Taenia saginata.*

**tapeworm, armed**  See *Taenia solium.*

**tapeworm, beef**  See *Taenia saginata.*

**tapeworm, measly**  See *Taenia solium.*

**tapeworm, pork**  See *Taenia solium.*

**TAR syndrome**  Acronym for thrombocytopenia (low blood platelets) and aplasia (absence) of the radius. TAR syndrome features phocomelia (flipper-limb), with the thumbs always present. The smaller bone in the lower leg (fibula) is often absent. The risk of bleeding from too few platelets is high in early infancy, but lessens with age. The condition is inherited as an autosomal recessive trait, with one gene on a nonsex chromosome coming from each parent to the TAR child. Also known as thrombocytopenia-absent radius syndrome, radial aplasia-thrombocytopenia syndrome, and tetraphocomelia-thrombocytopenia syndrome.

**tarsal cyst**  See *cyst, Meibomian.*

**tarsal glands**  See *glands, Meibomian.*

**tarsus, bony**  See *bony tarsus.*

**tartar**  The hardened product of minerals from saliva and foods, which accumulate in plaque around the teeth. Dental plaque and tartar cause periodontal disease, inflammation of the bone surrounding the teeth. Tartar can become as hard as rock, and then can require a dentist or dental hygienist with special tools to remove it. Antitartar toothpastes and mouthwashes are sometimes recommended to prevent tartar buildup.

**Tassinari syndrome**  A form of epilepsy that emerges around the age of four. The first signs are slowed learning, and receptive and/or expressive dysphasia. Absence, myoclonic, and focal seizures may be seen. The cause of Tassinari syndrome is unknown. Treatment is with antiseizure medications. This condition usually improves significantly by adulthood. See also *epilepsy, seizure disorders.*

**tattoo** The permanent insertion of ink below the skin, using a sharp instrument. Humans have done tattooing for cosmetic and ritual purposes since at least the Neolithic era. Today the practice can be made safer through the use of nonreactive pigments; sterile, disposable needles; and sterile work conditions. Without these refinements, inks may cause inflammation, and infection is an ever-present danger. Persons who are prone to keloid scarring should be aware that tattoos can keloid. Ink lines may also spread or change color over the years, a fact of special concern for those interested in so-called "permanent cosmetics" (tattooed lip color, eyebrows, eyeliner, and the like). Tattooed skin requires some special care. Fresh tattoos should be kept clean, dry, and covered for the first day, and antibiotic ointment should be used for several days to promote healing and prevent infection. Once healed, tattooed skin should be protected from UV rays with sunscreen to prevent fading and skin damage.

**tattoo removal** Those who regret getting a tattoo have three choices: hide it, cover it with a better tattoo, or have it removed. The most effective form of tattoo removal is the use of lasers to destroy the ink itself. Multiple treatments may be necessary, depending on the size of the piece and the inks used. Some tattoos cannot be completely removed with lasers, and lasers may scar some types of skin. One's best choice is prevention: Don't get a tattoo one can't live with forever.

**Tay-Sachs disease** An inherited metabolic disorder caused by deficiency of the enzyme hexosaminidase A (hex-A), resulting in failure to process GM2 ganglioside, a lipid (fat) that then accumulates and is deposited in the nerve cells of the brain and other tissues. The classic form of TSD begins in infancy. The child usually develops normally for the first few months, although an exaggerated startle reaction may be noted. Head control is lost by six to eight months of age; the infant cannot roll over or sit up, spasticity and rigidity develop, and excessive drooling and convulsions become evident. Blindness and head enlargement set in by the second year. TSD worsens with time as the central nervous system progressively deteriorates. After age two, constant nursing care is needed. Death is due usually to cachexia (wasting away) or aspiration pneumonia. There are also forms of TSD, juvenile TSD and adult TSD, in which the person has somewhat more hex-A and hence later onset. The classic infantile form of Tay-Sachs disease is usually fatal by age five. The autosomal recessive Tay-Sachs gene is found on chromosome 15q23-q24. Two copies of the gene, one from each parent, are necessary to cause the illness. The frequency of TSD is much higher in Ashkenazi Jews (Jews of European origin). Knowledge of the biochemical basis of TSD now permits screening for carrier status and prenatal diagnosis. Also known as amaurotic familial idiocy,

type 1 GM2-gangliosidosis, B variant GM2-gangliosidosis, hexosaminidase A deficiency, hex-A deficiency. See also *Sandhoff disease*.

**TB** Tuberculosis.

**TC-99 tetrofosmin scintimammography** See *scintimammography*.

**Td** Adult diphtheria and tetanus toxoids. See *Td immunization*.

**Td immunization** The vaccine given to children over the age of six and to adults as a booster for immunity to diphtheria and tetanus.

**teaspoon** An old-fashioned but convenient household measure. A teaspoon holds about 5 cc of liquid.

**technetium tetrofosmin scintimammography** See *scintimammography*.

**technology, recombinant DNA** See *recombinant DNA technology*.

**teeth** The structures within the mouth that allow for biting and chewing. Teeth have different shapes, depending on their purpose. The sharp canine and frontal teeth allow for biting, while the flattened, thick molars in the back of the mouth provide grinding surfaces for masticating food. All teeth have essentially the same structure: a hard crown above the gum line, which is attached to two or four roots by a portion called the neck. The roots are covered with a very thin layer of bone, and keep the tooth embedded in the bones of the jaw. The exposed exterior of the tooth is covered with tough enamel. Under the enamel is a thick layer of dentin, and in the center is the pulp, which contains blood vessels and nerves.

**telangiectasia, hereditary hemorrhagic** See *hereditary hemorrhagic telangectasia*.

**telomere** The end of a chromosome. The ends of chromosomes are specialized structures, and are involved in the replication and stability of DNA molecules.

**temperature** The specific degree of hotness or coldness of the body. It is usually measured with a thermometer.

**temporal arteritis** See *arteritis, cranial*.

**temporary loss of consciousness** See *syncope*.

**temporomandibular joint** The joint that hinges the lower jaw (mandible) to the temporal bone of the skull. It is one of the most frequently used joints in the entire body, moving whenever a person eats, drinks, or talks.

**temporomandibular joint syndrome**   A disorder of the temporomandibular joint(s) that causes pain, usually in front of the ear(s), sometimes in the form of a headache. Pain in the TMJ can be due to trauma, such as a blow to the face; inflammatory or degenerative arthritis; or poor dental work or structural defects that push the mandible back toward the ears whenever the patient chews or swallows. Grinding or clenching the teeth due to stress is a frequent culprit. Sometimes muscles around the TMJ used for chewing can go into spasm, causing head and neck pain, and difficulty opening the mouth normally. Treatment depends on the cause and severity of the problem, and can range from a mouth guard or medication to prevent nighttime tooth-grinding, to surgery.

**ten-day measles**   See *measles*.

**tendo Achilles**   See *Achilles tendon*.

**tendo calcaneus**   See *Achilles tendon*.

**tendon**   The soft tissue by which muscle attaches to bone. It is somewhat flexible, but tough. When a tendon becomes inflamed, the condition is referred to as tendinitis or tendonitis.

**tendon, Achilles**   See *Achilles tendon*.

**tenia**   See *taenia*.

**tension**   **1** The pressure within a vessel, such as blood pressure: the pressure within the blood vessels. **2** Stress, especially stress that is translated into clenched muscles and bottled-up emotions. This is the type of tension blamed for tension headaches.

**tension headache**   See *headache, tension*.

**tension, arterial**   See *arterial tension*.

**tension, intraocular**   See *intraocular pressure*.

**tension, intravenous**   See *intravenous tension*.

**tenth cranial nerve**   See *vagus nerve*.

**teratogen**   Any agent that can disturb the development of an embryo or fetus. Teratogens halt the pregnancy by causing a miscarriage, or cause a birth defect in the child. Classes of teratogens include radiation, maternal infections, chemicals, and drugs. Drugs known to be capable of acting as teratogens include, but are by no means limited to, ACE inhibitors like benazepril (brand name: Lotensin), captopril (Capoten), enalapril (Vasotec), fosinopril sodium (Monopril), lisinopril (Zestril, Prinivil), lisinopril and hydrochlorothiazide (Zestoretic, Prinzide), quinapril (Accupril), and ramipril (Altace); the acne medication isotretinoin (Accutane, Retin-A); alcohol, whether ingested chronically or in binges; androgens (male hormones); the antibiotics tetracycline (Achromycin), doxycycline (Vibramycin), and streptomycin; blood-thinners, such as warfarin (Coumadin); seizure medications, including phenytoin (Dilantin), valproic acid (Depakene, Depakote, Valprotate), trimethadione (Tridione), paramethadione (Paradione), and carbamazepine (Tegretol); the antidepressant/antimanic drug lithium (Eskalith, Lithotab); antimetabolite/anticancer drugs methotrexate (Rheumatrex) and aminopterin; the antirheumatic agent and chelator penicillamine (Ciprimene, Depen); antithyroid drugs, such as thiouracil/propylthiouracil and carbimazole/methimazole; cocaine; DES (diethylstilbestrol), a hormone; and thalidomide (Thalomid). Obviously, alcohol and illegal or unnecessary drugs should never be used by women who are pregnant, or who plan to get pregnant. However, sometimes a medication necessary for health is also a teratogen: thyroid medication, blood thinners, and lithium are just a few examples. In these cases, female patients should work carefully with their doctors to determine whether an alternative treatment is possible before and during pregnancy. In some cases the danger of birth defects is limited to a certain part of the pregnancy, and medication can be started again after that period has passed. Other medications can be safely restarted with the baby's birth. Some medications also pass through breast milk, however, and if they cannot be avoided the mother may need to choose formula feeding instead.

**teratoma, ovarian**   See *ovarian teratoma*. See also *cyst, ovarian*.

**teres minor muscle**   A muscle that assists the lifting of the arm during outward turning (external rotation). The tendon of the teres minor muscle is one of four tendons that stabilize the shoulder joint and constitute the rotator cuff.

**terminal ileitis**   See *Crohn disease*.

**test, allergy scratch**   See *allergy skin test*.

**test, allergy skin**   See *allergy skin test*.

**test, CA 125**   See *CA 125 test*. See also *CA 125*.

**test, carcinoembryonic antigen**   See *carcinoembryonic antigen test*.

**test, CEA**   See *carcinoembryonic antigen test*.

**test, EPO**   See *EPO test*. See also *erythropoietin*.

**test, erythropoietin**   See *EPO test*. See also *erythropoietin*.

**test, eye chart**   See *eye chart test.* See also *chart, Snellen's.*

**test, eye drop**   See *eye drop test.* See also *pupil dilation test.*

**test, Fisher's exact**   See *Fisher's exact test.*

**test, glucose tolerance**   See *glucose tolerance test.*

**test, NSE**   See *neuron-specific enolase test.* See also *neuron-specific enolase.*

**test, ovarian cancer**   See *CA 125 test.*

**test, Pap**   See *Pap test.*

**test, prostate specific antigen**   See *prostate-specific antigen test.*

**test, PSA**   See *prostate-specific antigen test.*

**test, pupil dilation**   See *pupil dilation test.*

**test, RPR**   See *syphilis test, RPR.*

**test, sweat**   See *sweat test.*

**test, sweat chloride**   See *sweat test.*

**test, syphilis**   See *syphilis test, RPR; syphilis test, VDRL.*

**test, tilt-table**   See *tilt-table test.*

**test, triglyceride**   See *triglyceride test.*

**test, VDRL**   See *syphilis test, VDRL.*

**test, visual acuity**   See *eye chart test.* See also *chart, Snellen's.*

**test, visual field**   See *visual field test.*

**testes**   The male sex glands, which are located behind the penis in a pouch of skin called the scrotum. The testes produce and store sperm, and are also the body's main source of male hormones, such as testosterone. These hormones control the development of the reproductive organs and other male characteristics, such as body and facial hair, low voice, and wide shoulders. Also known as the testicles.

**testicles**   See *testes.*

**testicular cancer**   See *cancer, testicular.*

**testicular self-examination**   A monthly procedure for detecting the early signs of testicular cancer. Men should check the testes visually for new swelling or other changes on the skin of the scrotum, roll each testicle between thumb and fingers to detect internal growths, and check the cord (epididymis) on the top and back of each testicle for growths. A warm bath or shower will relax the scrotum, making examination easier. Early detection of testicular cancer greatly improves the likelihood of successful treatment. See also *cancer, testicular.*

**testis**   See *testes.*

**testosterone**   A sex hormone produced by the male testes, testosterone stimulates the hormones known as androgens. Androgens cause male sex characteristics, such as a deep voice, to develop; they also strengthen muscle and bone mass. High levels of testosterone appear to promote good health in men, lowering the risk of high blood pressure and heart attack, for example. High testosterone levels also correlate with risky behavior, however, including increased aggressiveness and smoking, which may cancel out these health benefits. Testosterone may be given to treat medical conditions, including female (but not male) breast cancer. See also *androgen, testosterone replacement therapy.*

**testosterone replacement therapy**   The practice of giving testosterone to treat conditions in which the testes produce a deficient amount due to absence, injury, or disease. Testosterone is available in oral, IV, and patch forms. As with estrogen replacement therapy for women, dosing must be carefully calibrated to gain the greatest benefits without unwanted side effects. See also *testosterone.*

**tetanus**   An often fatal infectious disease caused by the bacteria Clostridium tetani, which usually enters the body through a puncture, cut, or open wound. Tetanus leads to profound painful spasms of muscles, including "locking" of the jaw so that the mouth cannot open (lockjaw), and death. The C. tetani bacteria releases a toxin that affects the motor nerves, which stimulate the muscles. Prevention is by immediately cleaning and covering any open wound, and by vaccination. The DPT, DTaP, DT, and Td vaccines all protect against tetanus. Regular boosters are necessary to ensure immunity. Unvaccinated people who get a puncture wound or cut should get tetanus immunoglobulin and a series of tetanus shots immediately; those who have been immunized but are unsure of the date of their last tetanus shot should get a booster.

**tetraphocomelia-thrombocytopenia    syndrome**   See *TAR syndrome.*

**Thai hemorrhagic fever**   See *dengue hemorrhagic fever.*

**thalassemia** A complex group of genetic disorders that involve underproduction of hemoglobin, the indispensable molecule in red blood cells that carries oxygen. All forms of hemoglobin are made up of two molecules: heme and globin. The globin part of hemoglobin is made up of four polypeptide chains. In normal adult hemoglobin (Hb A), the predominant type of hemoglobin after the first year of life, two of the globin chains are identical to each other and are called the alpha chains. The other two chains, which are also identical to each other but are different from the alpha chains, are termed the beta chains. In fetal hemoglobin (Hb F), the predominant hemoglobin during fetal development, there are two alpha chains and two different chains called gamma chains. In thalassemia, there is a mutation (change) in one or both of the alpha or beta globin chains. Depending on which globin chain is affected, the mutation leads to underproduction or absence of that globin chain, a deficiency of hemoglobin, and anemia.

**thalassemia major** The most serious form of thalassemia, in which there is a mutation in both beta globin chains. This leads to underproduction or absence of beta chains, underproduction of hemoglobin, and profound anemia. Children with thalassemia major seem entirely normal at birth, because at birth they still have predominantly fetal hemoglobin, which does not contain beta chains. The anemia emerges in the first few months of life and becomes progressively more severe, leading to pallor, fatigue, failure to thrive, bouts of fever due to infections, and diarrhea. The gene for beta thalassemia is relatively frequent in people of Mediterranean origin. Children with thalassemia major inherit one thalassemia gene from each parent. People with just one thalassemia gene are said to have thalassemia minor and are essentially normal, although they can transmit the gene to their offspring. Treatment based on blood transfusions is helpful but not curative. Gene therapy will, it is hoped, be applicable to this disease. Also known as beta thalassemia, Cooley anemia, Mediterranean anemia.

**thalassemia minor** Also called thalassemia trait, thalassemia minor is the carrier state for thalassemia major (beta thalassemia). People who are carriers have just one thalassemia gene and are essentially normal.

**thalassemia, alpha** A form of thalassemia in which the alpha chain is involved. If a fetus inherits two genes for alpha thalassemia, one from each parent, the disorder is lethal before birth: No alpha chains can be made, and without alpha chains, there can be no fetal hemoglobin. If the fetus inherits only one alpha thalassemia gene, it will survive and have no or few symptoms as a child, as there is another gene still able to make alpha chains.

**thalassemia, beta** See *thalassemia major*.

**thalidomide** A drug (Thalomid) that was once prescribed for morning sickness in pregnancy, with tragic results. When taken by pregnant women, it causes a syndrome of serious, deforming defects in the developing fetus. Thalidomide was taken off the market in 1962, but was reapproved by the FDA in 1997 for the treatment of a complication of leprosy (erythema nodosum leprosum). It also appears to have other beneficial uses, including treatment of several different types of cancer, and HIV-related ulcers. Side effects may include peripheral neuritis. Obviously, this medication is a potent teratogen, and should never be taken by women who are or could become pregnant.

**thalidomide baby** An infant affected by prenatal exposure to the drug thalidomide. This medication was prescribed to pregnant women for treatment of morning sickness until removal from the market in 1962. It causes a wide variety of serious birth defects, including short, flipper-like limbs. Most thalidomide babies have lived into adulthood. This population is now reaching middle age, and in some cases new health problems are emerging.

**therapy, adjuvant** See *adjuvant therapy, adjuvent chemotherapy*.

**therapy, biological** See *biological therapy*. See also *biological response modifiers*.

**therapy, estrogen replacement** See *estrogen replacement therapy*.

**therapy, fever** See *fever therapy*.

**therapy, gene** See *gene therapy*.

**therapy, hormone replacement** See *hormone replacement therapy*.

**therapy, occupational** See *occupational therapy*.

**therapy, physical** See *physical therapy*.

**therapy, salvage** See *salvage therapy*.

**therapy, speech** See *speech therapy*.

**thermally induced asthma** See *asthma, exercise-induced*.

**thiamine** Vitamin B1. Thiamine acts as a coenzyme in the metabolism of carbohydrates into blood sugar. Deficiency of thiamine leads to beriberi, a disease affecting the heart and nervous system. See also *Appendix C, "Vitamins."*

**thigh** The thick, muscular portion of the leg that extends from the hip to the knee. The thigh has only one bone, the femur, which is the largest bone in the human body.

**thighbone**  See *femur*.

**third and fourth pharyngeal pouch syndrome**  See *DiGeorge syndrome*.

**third cranial nerve**  See *oculomotor nerve*.

**third stage of labor**  The part of labor from the birth of the baby until the placenta (afterbirth) and fetal membranes are delivered. Also known as the placental stage.

**third ventricle**  One cavity in a system of four communicating cavities within the brain that are continuous with the central canal of the spinal cord. The third ventricle is a median (midline) cavity in the brain, and is bounded by the thalamus and hypothalamus on either side. It communicates anteriorly (in front) with the lateral ventricles, and posteriorly (in back) with what is called the aqueduct of the midbrain, also known as the aqueduct of Sylvius. All the ventricles are filled with cerebrospinal fluid, which is formed by structures, called choroid plexuses, located in the walls and roofs of the ventricles.

**thoracentesis**  Removal through a needle of fluid from the membranes surrounding the lungs (the pleura).

**thoracic**  Pertaining to the chest.

**thoracic aneurysm**  See *aneurysm, thoracic*. See also *aneurysm, aortic*.

**thoracic aorta**  A section of the aorta within the chest. It starts after the arch of the aorta, and runs down to the diaphragm, the great muscle that separates the chest from the abdomen. The thoracic aorta gives off numerous branches that supply oxygenated blood to the chest cage and the organs within the chest. Also known as the aorta thoracica, the aorta thoracalis, and the pars thoracalis aortae. See also *aorta*.

**thoracic duct**  A vascular structure that recirculates lymph into the bloodstream. It begins in the abdomen, tracks alongside the aorta and esophagus, and eventually joins with the left brachiocephalic vein.

**thoracic outlet syndrome**  A condition due to compromise of blood vessels or nerve fibers between the armpit (axilla) and base of the neck, usually due to compression of nerves or blood vessels between the neck and shoulders. Symptoms include pain, arm weakness, and numbness in the hands and fingers. Thoracic outlet syndrome can be caused by overstress from some types of manual work or exercise, injury, or malformation. Treatment is by physical therapy and anti-inflammatory medication, and sometimes by surgery.

**thoracic vertebrae**  The 12 vertebrae situated between the cervical (neck) vertebrae and the lumbar vertebrae. The thoracic vertebrae provide attachment for the ribs and make up part of the back of the thorax (chest). Represented by the symbols T1 through T12. See also *vertebra, vertebral column*.

**thoracotomy**  An operation to open the chest.

**thorax**  The area of the body located between the abdomen and the neck. Within the thorax are the lungs, heart, and first section of the aorta. Also known as the chest.

**thrive, failure to**  See *failure to thrive*.

**thrombectomy**  Procedure to remove a clot (thrombus).

**thrombi**  The plural of thrombus. See *thrombus*.

**thrombin**  A key clot promoter, thrombin is an enzyme that presides over the conversion of a substance called fibrinogen to fibrin, the right stuff for a clot.

**thrombinogen**  See *prothrombin*.

**thrombocytes**  See *platelets*.

**thrombocytopenia-absent radius syndrome**  See *TAR syndrome*.

**thrombocytopenic purpura, acute**  See *acute thrombocytopenic purpura*.

**thrombolytic agents**  Medications, such as plasminogen-activator (t-PA) and streptokinase, that are effective in dissolving clots and reopening arteries. Thrombolytic agents are used in the treatment of heart attacks, thrombosis, and related disorders.

**thrombophlebitis**  Inflammation of a vein that occurs when a blood clot forms.

**thrombosis, cavernous sinus**  See *cavernous sinus thrombosis*. See also *cavernous sinus syndrome*.

**thrombosis, deep vein**  See *deep vein thrombosis*.

**thrombotic disease due to protein C deficiency**  See *Protein C deficiency*.

**thrombus**  A clot in a blood vessel or within the heart.

**thrush**  A yeast infection of the mucous membranes within the throat and mouth. It looks like a light or white coating on the affected tissue, and may cause irritation. Seen most often in infants, young children, elderly people (especially those who wear dentures or take medications that lower output of saliva), and people with compromised immune systems. Diagnosis is by observation, and can be confirmed by culturing a saliva sample or cheek scraping. Treatment is with oral antifungal medications. See also *yeast, yeast infection*.

**thymine** One member of the base pair A-T (adenine-thymine) in DNA.

**thymus** An organ in which lymphocytes mature and multiply. It lies behind the breastbone.

**thymus and parathyroids, hypoplasia of** See *DiGeorge syndrome*.

**thyroglobulin** A protein found in the thyroid gland. Some thyroglobulin can be found in the blood, and this amount may be measured after thyroid surgery to determine whether thyroid cancer has recurred. Thyroglobulin derived from pig thyroid glands is sometimes given to treat thyroid dysfunction. Abbreviated as Tg.

**thyroglossal cyst** See *cyst, thyroglossal*.

**thyroid binding globulin** A blood protein that binds with the thyroid hormone thyroxine (T4).

**thyroid gland** See *gland, thyroid*.

**thyroid hormone organification defect IIb** See *Pendred syndrome*.

**thyroid hormones** Chemical substances made by the thyroid gland, which is located in the front of the neck. This gland uses iodine to make thyroid hormones, which are essential for the function of every cell in the body. They help regulate growth and the rate of chemical reactions (metabolism), and are involved in the circadian rhythms that govern sleep, among other essential functions. The two most important thyroid hormones are thyroxine (T4) and triiodothyronine (T3). The thyroid also makes calcitonin, which is involved in calcium metabolization and bone strength, and other substances. Thyroid stimulating hormone (TSH), which is produced by the pituitary gland, acts to stimulate hormone production by the thyroid gland. The pituitary gland is stimulated to make TSH by the hypothalamus gland in the brain. See *calcitonin, thyroxine, triiodothyronine*.

**thyroid scan** An image taken of the thyroid gland after radioactive iodine or technetium is taken by mouth. The image shows the thyroid gland in action as it accumulates radioactive material. Thyroid scanning is used to determine how active thyroid tissue is in manufacturing thyroid hormone. This can determine whether inflammation of the thyroid gland (thyroiditis) is present. It can also detect the presence and degree of overactivity of the gland

(hyperthyroidism). Thyroid scanning is especially helpful in evaluating thyroid nodules, particularly after a fine-needle aspiration biopsy has failed to provide a diagnosis. A scan will reveal whether a thyroid nodule is functioning. A functioning nodule is actively taking up iodine to produce thyroid hormone, and so produces a localized "hot" area on the image. A nonfunctioning nodule does not take up iodine, and produces a localized "cold" area. Functioning nodules are rarely from cancer, as nearly all thyroid cancers are nonfunctioning—and even among "cold" nodules, cancer is present in less than 5 percent of cases.

**thyroid stimulating hormone** A hormone produced by the pituitary gland at the base of the brain in response to signals from the hypothalamus gland in the brain. TSH promotes the growth of the thyroid gland in the neck and stimulates it to produce more thyroid hormones. When the amount of thyroid hormones is excessive, the pituitary gland stops producing TSH, thus reducing thyroid hormone production. This mechanism maintains a relatively constant level of thyroid hormones circulating in the blood. Also known as thyrotropin.

**thyroid stimulating immunoglobulin** A form of immunoglobulin G (IgG) that can bind to thyrotropin (TSH) receptors on the thyroid gland. TSIs mimic the action of TSH, causing excess secretion of thyroxine and triiodothyronine. The TSI level is abnormally high in persons with hyperthyroidism due to Graves disease.

**thyroidectomy** Surgery to remove part or all of the thyroid gland. This might be done to remove a tumor, or to treat hyperthyroidism or goiter (enlarged thyroid gland). The complications of surgery can include vocal cord paralysis and accidental removal of the parathyroid glands, which are located behind the thyroid gland. As the parathyroid glands regulate calcium metabolism, their removal can result in low calcium levels.

**thyroiditis** Inflammation of the thyroid gland. The inflamed thyroid gland can release an excess of thyroid hormones into the bloodstream, resulting in a temporary hyperthyroid state. Once the thyroid gland is depleted of thyroid hormones, the patient commonly goes through a hypothyroid (low thyroid) phase. This phase can last for three to six months, until the thyroid gland fully recovers. Thyroiditis can be diagnosed by a thyroid scan.

**thyroiditis, autoimmune** See *Hashimoto disease*.

**thyroiditis, Hashimoto** See *Hashimoto disease*.

**thyroiditis, postpartum** Inflammation of the thyroid gland after pregnancy.

**thyroiditis, subacute** Inflammation of the thyroid gland after a viral illness.

**thyrolingual cyst** See *cyst, thyroglossal*.

**thyrotropin** See *thyroid stimulating hormone*.

**thyroxine** A hormone made by the thyroid gland. Thyroxine is one of the most important thyroid hormones. Four iodine molecules are attached to its molecular structure. Along with the more powerful thyroid hormone triiodothyronine (T4), thyroxine affects almost every process in the body, including body temperature, growth, and heart rate. Also known as T4.

**tibia** The larger of the two bones in the lower leg, the tibia is familiarly known as the shinbone.

**tibia vara** A condition characterized by disturbance of normal growth in the inner part of the upper tibia. Tibia vara causes a bowlegged gait, and can impair the knees significantly. It is most common in children of African descent. Treatment is usually by surgery, although a knee-ankle–foot orthosis (KAFO) brace may be tried. Also known as Blount disease.

**tibial bowing** Improper growth of the tibia in the leg, causing bowlegs or other leg problems. The tibia may bow anteriorly (in the front) or posteriorly (in the back). See also *tibia vara*.

**tic** A repetitive movement that is difficult, if not impossible, to control. Tics can affect any group of muscles. The most common are facial tics, such as eye-blinking, nose-twitching, or grimacing. Tics that affect the muscles used to produce speech are known as vocal tics, and can range from grunts or whistles to the repetition of complete words or phrases. Complex motor tics involve multiple, sequenced movements, and can include behaviors such as twirling in place, tapping a certain number of times, or stooping to touch the ground. Tics are believed to arise in differences in or damage to the basal ganglia, a structure deep within the brain that controls automatic movements and that also affects impulsivity. See also *coprolalia, echolalia, palilalia, tic disorder, Tourette syndrome*.

**tic disorder** A disorder characterized by the presence of tics. If both motor and vocal tics are present for more than six months, the diagnosis of Tourette syndrome may be made. Diagnosis is by observation. Treatment is not usually recommended for minor tics that are not bothersome to the patient. When treatment is desired, medication choices include the blood-pressure drugs guanfacine (brand name: Tenex) and catapres (brand name: Clonadine), or one of the atypical or older neuroleptics. See also *tic, Tourette syndrome*.

**tick bite** A bite from a bloodsucking, parasitic insect that punctures the skin with a sharp beak. The tick burrows into the skin with its head. Tick bites can carry serious illness, including Rocky Mountain spotted fever, other forms of tick typhus, and Lyme disease.

**tick fever** See *Rocky Mountain spotted fever*. See also *Rickettsia, rickettsial diseases*.

**tick typhus** See *typhus, tick*. See also *Rickettsia, rickettsial diseases*.

**tick typhus, African** See *typhus, African tick*. See also *Rickettsia, rickettsial diseases*.

**tick typhus, Queensland** See *typhus, Queensland tick*. See also *Rickettsia, rickettsial diseases*.

**tick-borne rickettsioses of the eastern hemisphere** See *rickettsioses of the eastern hemisphere, tick-borne*. See also *Rickettsia, rickettsial diseases*.

**tick-borne rickettsiosis, north Asian** See *rickettsiosis, North Asian tick-borne*. See also *Rickettsia, rickettsial diseases*.

**tight foreskin** See *phimosis*.

**tilt-table test** A test that involves placing the patient on a table with a foot-support, tilting the table upward, and measuring the blood pressure and pulse. Symptoms are recorded with the patient in diverse positions. The tilt-table test is designed to detect postural hypotension (orthostatic hypotension), a condition caused by changing body position from a prone, supine, or sitting position to a more vertical position. Poor tone of the nerves of the legs can cause a disproportionate distribution of blood to the legs, instead of to the brain, so a person feels light-headed and may even faint. Tilt-table testing may be done when heart disease is not suspected of being responsible for an attack of syncope (fainting) or near-syncope. Depending on the presence or absence of symptoms during the tilt-table test, persons with certain forms of temporary loss of consciousness may be admitted to the hospital for observation and further testing. See also *syncope; syncope, situational; vasovagal reaction*.

**time, prothrombin** See *prothrombin time*.

**Tinea unguium** See *dermatophytic onychomycosis*.

**tinnitus** Ringing in the ears. Tinnitus has many causes, such as medications (including aspirin and other anti-inflammatory drugs), aging, and ear trauma.

**tissue** A group or layer of cells that perform specific functions. For example, muscle tissue is a layer of muscle cells.

**TMA** Trimethylaminuria. See *fish-odor syndrome*.

**TMJ** Temporomandibular joint.

**TMJ syndrome** See *temporomandibular joint syndrome*.

**toc-, toco-** Prefix meaning childbirth. For example, tocolysis is the slowing or halting of labor. Sometimes spelled tok-, toko-.

**tocolysis** The inhibition or delaying of labor during the birth process.

**tocolytic** Relating to the inhibition of labor, delaying or halting labor.

**tocophobia** Fear of childbirth.

**tocus** Labor, childbirth.

**toddler's fracture** See *fracture, toddler's*. See also *fracture*.

**toe sign** See *Babinski reflex*.

**toenail** A tough, protective plate produced by living skin cells in the toe. A toenail consists of several parts, including the nail plate (the visible part of the nail), the nail bed (the skin beneath the nail plate), the cuticle (the tissue that overlaps the plate and rims the base of the nail), the nail folds (the skin that enfolds the frame and supports the nail on three sides), the lunula (the whitish half-moon at the base of the nail), and the matrix (the hidden part of the nail unit under the cuticle). Toenails grow from the matrix. They are composed largely of keratin, a hardened protein also found in fingernails, skin, and hair. As new cells grow in the matrix, the older cells are pushed out and compacted, taking on the flattened, hardened form of the toenail. The average growth rate for toenails is .1 mm per day. The exact rate of nail growth depends on numerous factors, including the age and sex of the individual, and the time of year. Toenails generally grow faster in young people, in males, and in the summer. Toenails grow more slowly than fingernails. See also *nail, nail care*.

**toenail, ingrown** A common disorder, particularly on the big (great) toe. The corner of the nail curves down into the skin because of mistrimming of the nail, or because of shoes that are too tight. An ingrown toenail can be painful and lead to infection. Sometimes simply removing the corner of the nail from the skin is enough to cure this problem, although you may need to have this done by a doctor, podiatrist, or foot-care specialist. If infection is present, that also requires treatment. In some cases the entire nail must be removed. If ingrown toenails are caused by congenital nail malformations, the nail bed can be treated to permanently prevent regrowth.

**toes, six** See *hexadactyly*. See also *polydactyly*.

**tok-, toko-** See *toc-, toco-*.

**tongue** A strong muscle anchored to the floor of the mouth. It is covered by the lingual membrane, which has special areas to detect different types of tastes. The tongue muscles are attached to the lower jaw and to the hyoid bone, a small, U-shaped bone that lies deep in the muscles at the back of the tongue and above the larynx. On the top surface of the tongue are small nodules, called papillae, that give the tongue its rough texture. Between the papillae, at the sides and base of the tongue, are the taste buds, which are small bulb-like structures. The muscle fibers of the tongue are heavily supplied with nerves. Babies have more taste buds than adults, and they have them almost everywhere in the mouth, including the cheeks. The tongue aids in the formation of the sounds of speech, and coordinates its movements to aid in swallowing.

**tonsil** See *tonsils*.

**tonsil stone** See *tonsillolith*.

**tonsillectomy** The surgical removal of both tonsils. A tonsillectomy may be performed in cases of recurrent tonsillitis, or to treat sleep apnea and some speech disorders.

**tonsillitis** Inflammation of one or both tonsils, typically as a result of infection by a virus or bacteria.

**tonsillolith** A tiny stone (calculus) in the tonsils. Such stones are found within little pockets (crypts) in the tonsils. These pockets typically form in chronic recurrent tonsillitis, and harbor bacteria. Tonsilloliths are foul-smelling, as they tend to contain high quantities of sulfa. When crushed, they give off a characteristic rotten-egg smell, and can cause bad breath. Tonsilloliths may also give the sense of something caught in the back of the throat.

**tonsils** Small masses of lymphoid tissue at either side of the back of the throat. Like other lymphatic tissue, they are part of the immune system.

**tooth** See *teeth*.

**tooth root** The lower two-thirds of a tooth. The roots are normally buried in bone, and serve to anchor the tooth in position. They are covered with a thin layer of bone, and insert into sockets in the bone of the jaw.

**tooth root sensitivity** When the roots of a tooth are no longer protected by healthy gum and bone, they may become oversensitive to cold, hot, and sour foods. Chronic gum disease contributes to toothache due to root sensitivities. The bacterial toxins dissolve the bone around the roots and cause the gum and the bone to recede. Tooth root sensitivity may be so severe that the person avoids many foods. Treatment is by addressing the underlying gum disease and improving oral hygiene.

**tooth, cracked, syndrome**  See *cracked-tooth syndrome*.

**tooth, wisdom**  Large molars in the very back of the jaw. The human jaw has changed in size over the course of evolution, but these teeth continue to erupt in many individuals. If the jaw is too small to accommodate them, they may cause pain or crowd other teeth out of position. The wisdom teeth may need to be surgically removed.

**toothache**  A pain in the tooth or gum. The most common cause of a toothache is a cavity or injury to a tooth that exposes the pulp, which is heavily supplied by nerves.

**tophaceous gout**  See *gout, tophaceous*. See also *gout*.

**tophi**  The plural of tophus. Tophi are characteristically deposited in different soft-tissue areas of the body in chronic (tophaceous) gout. Even though tophi are most commonly found as hard nodules around the fingers, at the tips of the elbows, and around the big toe, they can appear anywhere in the body. They have been reported in unexpected areas such as in the ears, vocal cords, or around the spinal cord.

**tophus**  A nodular mass of uric acid crystals. See also *tophi*.

**TORCH infection**  An acronym for the infections Toxoplasma gondii, other viruses (HIV, measles, syphilis, and more), rubella, cytomegalovirus, and herpes, all of which are capable of causing birth defects.

**tornado supplies kit**  See *disaster supplies*.

**torsion dystonia**  See *dystonia, torsion*.

**torsion fracture**  See *fracture, torsion*. See also *fracture, toddler's*.

**torticollis**  The most common of the focal dystonias, torticollis is a state of excessive or inadequate muscle tone in the muscles in the neck that control the position of the head. It can cause the head to twist and turn to one side, and the head may also be pulled forward or backward. Torticollis can occur at any age, although most individuals first experience symptoms in middle age. It often begins slowly, and usually reaches a plateau. About 10 to 20 percent of those with torticollis experience a spontaneous remission, but unfortunately the remission may not be long-lasting. Also known as spasmodic torticollis.

**torticollis, congenital**  A deformity of the neck that is evident at birth. It is due to shortening of the neck muscles. Congenital torticollis tilts the head to the side on which the neck muscles are shortened, so that the chin points to the other side. The shortened neck muscles are principally supplied by the spinal accessory nerve. Also known as wryneck.

**torticollis, spasmodic**  See *torticollis*.

**torus fracture**  See *fracture, torus*. See also *fracture*.

**total hysterectomy**  See *hysterectomy, total*.

**Tourette syndrome**  A genetically transmitted tic disorder characterized by the presence of chronic vocal and motor tics, and probably based in differences in or damage to the basal ganglia of the brain. Tourette syndrome usually emerges between the ages of 6 and 18, and is somewhat more common in persons with ADHD, obsessive-compulsive disorder, or an autistic spectrum disorder than in the general population. Tics may be minor or debilitating, and their type, severity, and frequency tend to wax and wane. Infection, particularly with streptococcus bacteria, can exacerbate and sometimes start Tourette syndrome. Emotional distress and stress also appear to influence the frequency of tics. People with this disorder tend to have an impulsive, quick, and frequently humorous disposition. Some, particularly those with co-morbid disorders, experience episodes of rage that are difficult to control. Diagnosis is by observation. Treatment with medication is not usually recommended unless the tics are self-injurious or embarrassing to the patient, or in cases in which rage is a problem. When treatment is desired, medication choices include the blood-pressure drugs guanfacine (brand name: Tenex) and catapres (brand name: Clonadine), or one of the atypical or older neuroleptics. Some patients have also found the nicotine patch to be useful as an adjunct to other medications. Therapy can help the patient develop social coping strategies and maintain a positive self-image. See also *tic, tic disorder*.

**toxemia**  See *eclampsia*.

**toxic multinodular goiter**  See *goiter, toxic multinodular*.

**toxic shock syndrome**  A grave condition occurring predominantly in menstruating women using tampons, toxic shock is characterized by sudden high fever, vomiting, diarrhea, and muscle aches, followed by low blood pressure (hypotension), which can lead to shock and death. There may be a rash resembling sunburn, with peeling of skin. The condition is caused by a toxin produced by staphylococcus aureus bacteria growing under conditions with little or no oxygen. See also *staphylococcus*.

**toxins**   Poisons produced by certain animals, plants, or bacteria.

**trachea**   A tube-like portion of the respiratory tract that connects the larynx with the bronchial parts of the lungs. Also known as the windpipe.

**tracheoesophageal puncture**   A small opening made by a surgeon between the esophagus and the trachea. A valve is inserted to keep food out of the trachea but allow air into the esophagus to permit esophageal speech.

**tracheostomy**   Surgery to create an opening (stoma) into the windpipe. The opening itself may also be called a tracheostomy. A tracheostomy may be made as an emergency measure in cases of airway blockage.

**tracheostomy button**   A 1/2-inch- to 1 1/2-inch-long plastic tube placed in the stoma to keep it open.

**tracheostomy tube**   A 2-inch to 3-inch metal or plastic tube that keeps the stoma and trachea open. Also called a trach (trake) tube.

**traction**   In medicine, a procedure for manually pulling a part of the body to a beneficial effect. See *orthopedic traction*.

**tranquilizer**   In pharmacology, a drug that calms and relieves anxiety. The first tranquilizer, chlordiazepoxide-hydrochloride (brand name: Librium) received FDA approval in 1960. Tranquilizers range in potency from mild to major, with increasing levels of drowsiness occurring as potency increases. They are prescribed for a wide variety of conditions, but are used primarily to treat anxiety and insomnia. Most tranquilizers are potentially addictive, particularly those in the benzodiazepine family. See *benzodiazepine tranquilizer*.

**trans-**   Prefix meaning across, over, or beyond. For example, a transplant operation takes an organ from one person and reinstalls it over in another person.

**transaminase, serum glutamic oxaloacetic**   An enzyme that normally is present in liver and heart cells, and is released into the blood when the liver or heart is damaged. Blood SGOT levels are thus elevated with liver damage (for example, from viral hepatitis) or with an insult to the heart (for example, from a heart attack). Some medications can also raise SGOT levels. Interpretation of elevated SGOT levels depends on the context, and can necessitate additional clinical and laboratory information. Also known as aspartate aminotransferase (AST).

**transaminase, serum glutamic pyruvic**   An enzyme that normally is present in liver and heart cells, and is released into the blood when the liver or heart is damaged. Blood SGPT levels are thus elevated with liver damage (for example, from viral hepatitis) or with an insult to the heart (for example, from a heart attack). Some medications can also raise SGPT levels. Interpretation of elevated SGPT levels depends on the context, and can necessitate additional clinical and laboratory information. Also known as alanine aminotransferase (ALT).

**transcription**   Making an RNA copy from a sequence of DNA (a gene). Transcription is the first step in gene expression.

**transfer RNA**   See *RNA, transfer*.

**transfusion**   The transfer of blood or blood products from one person (the donor) into the bloodstream of another person (the recipient). In most situations, this is done as a lifesaving maneuver to replace blood cells or blood products lost through severe bleeding. Transfusion of one's own blood (autologous transfusion) is the safest method, but requires planning ahead, and not all patients are eligible. Directed donor blood allows the patient to receive blood from known donors. Volunteer donor blood is usually most readily available and, when properly tested, has a low incidence of adverse events.

**transfusion medicine**   The practice of blood transfusion and blood conservation. These are complementary activities that ensure the best balance between safety and convenience during emergency care or surgery.

**transition, menopause**   See *menopause transition*. See also *menopause*.

**transitional cell carcinoma**   See *carcinoma, transitional cell*.

**translation**   The process by which the genetic code carried by messenger RNA (mRNA) directs the production of proteins from amino acids.

**transmission, perinatal**   See *vertical transmission*.

**transmission, vertical**   See *vertical transmission*.

**transplant**   The grafting of a tissue from one place to another, just as in botany a bud from one plant might be grafted onto the stem of another. The transplanting of tissue can be from one part of the patient to another (autologous transplantation), as in the case of a skin graft using the patient's own skin; or from one patient to another (allogenic transplantation), as in the case of transplanting a donor kidney into a recipient.

**transplant, bone marrow**   See *bone marrow transplantation*.

**transplant, heart**　See *heart transplant*.

**transplant, kidney**　See *kidney transplant*.

**transplant, lung**　See *lung transplant*.

**transplantation, peripheral blood stem cell**　See *peripheral blood stem cell transplantation*.

**transport disease, cystine**　See *cystinuria*. See also *cystine kidney stones*.

**transsexual**　A person who desires or has achieved transsexualism. See *transsexualism*.

**transsexualism**　Consistently strong desire to change one's anatomical gender. Some transsexuals were misassigned gender at birth (for example, being anatomically male but raised as female), either on purpose or due to indistinct anatomy. Most, however, are perfectly normal physically. Transsexuals may dress and behave as individuals of the opposite sex, and may choose to use hormones or surgery to develop desired secondary sex characteristics. Surgery to change the appearance of the external genitals is known as sex reassignment surgery. Surgery and hormonal treatments for gender reassignment are available for both male and female transsexuals. Transsexualism is distinct from transvestitism (cross-dressing), and does not always indicate a change in the individual's sexual preference.

**transurethral resection**　Surgery performed with a special instrument inserted through the urethra. Abbreviated as TUR.

**transvaginal ultrasound**　The creation of a picture called a sonogram by sending sound waves out through a probe inserted in the vagina. The waves bounce off the ovaries, and a computer uses the echoes to create the sonogram. Abbreviated as TVS.

**transverse**　A horizontal plane passing through the standing body parallel to the ground. See also *Appendix B, "Anatomic Orientation Terms."*

**transverse fracture**　See *fracture, transverse*.

**transvestite**　A person who dresses in the clothing of the opposite sex.

**transvestitism**　Dressing in the clothing of the opposite sex. Transvestitism is distinct from both transexualism and homosexuality. In psychiatry, it can be considered a paraphilia. Also known as cross-dressing.

**trauma**　A physical or emotional injury.

**trauma center**　A specialized hospital facility designed to provide diagnostic and therapeutic services for patients with injuries.

**traumatic alopecia**　See *alopecia, traumatic*.

**traumatology**　The branch of surgery that deals with injured patients, usually on an emergency basis. Patients who have suffered significant physical trauma, as from a car accident, may be cared for in a trauma center.

**travelers' diarrhea**　Diarrhea that results from infections acquired while traveling to another country. Among the causes of travelers' diarrhea are enterotoxigenic E. coli, and a variety of viruses.

**treadmill, exercise**　See *exercise treadmill*.

**tremor**　An abnormal, repetitive shaking movement of the body. Tremors have many causes, and can be inherited, related to illnesses (such as thyroid disease), or caused by fever, hypothermia, drugs, or fear.

**trench fever**　A disease borne by body lice that was first recognized in the trenches of World War I, when it is estimated to have affected more than a million people. Trench fever is still seen endemically in Mexico, Africa, Eastern Europe, and elsewhere. Urban trench fever occurs among homeless people and street alcoholics. Outbreaks have been documented, for example, in Seattle, Baltimore, Marseilles, and Burundi. The cause of trench fever is Bartonella quintana (also called Rochalimaea quintana), an unusual rickettsial organism that multiplies in the gut of the body louse. Transmission to people can occur by rubbing infected louse feces into abraded (scuffed) skin or into the whites of the eyes. The disease is classically a five-day fever, characterized by the sudden onset of high fever, severe headache, back pain and leg pain, and a fleeting rash. Recovery takes a month or more, and relapses are common. Also known as Wolhynia fever, shinbone fever, quintan fever, five-day fever, Meuse fever, His' disease, His-Werner disease, Werner-His disease. See also *Bartonella quintana, rickettsial diseases*.

**trench foot**　A painful condition caused by exposure of the foot for several days. It was common during trench warfare in World War I and World War II, when soldiers stood for days and weeks in wet, muddy ditches without being able to change their footwear; today it is seen most frequently in urban homeless people. The feet become numb, turn red and then blue, develop blisters, and become infected. Gangrene may set in. Untreated trench foot can lead to amputation due to gangrene, and even to death.

**trench mouth**　See *acute membranous gingivitis*.

**Treponema pallidum**  The cause of syphilis, T. pallidum is a spirochete, a worm-like, spiral-shaped bacteria that wiggles vigorously when viewed under a microscope.

**triceps**  The triceps muscle extends (straightens) the forearm. It can be felt as the tense muscle in the back of the upper arm while one is doing push-ups. The triceps has three heads, or origins. Its full name is the triceps brachii.

**Trichinella spiralis**  The worm that causes trichinosis. Trichinella spiralis larvae can infest pigs and wild game, hibernating in muscle tissue within a protective cyst. When a human or an animal eats meat that contains infective Trichinella cysts, the acid in the stomach dissolves the hard covering of the cyst and releases the worms. The worms pass into the small intestine and become mature within a day or two. After mating, adult females lay eggs. Eggs develop into immature worms, travel through the arteries, and are transported to muscles. Within the muscles, the worms curl into a ball and encyst (become enclosed in a capsule). Infection occurs when these encysted worms are consumed in meat, continuing the cycle. See also *trichinosis*.

**trichinellosis**  See *trichinosis*.

**trichinosis**  A disease that comes from eating raw or undercooked pork or wild game that is infected with Trichinella spiralis larvae. Initial symptoms are abdominal discomfort, nausea, diarrhea, vomiting, fatigue, and fever. Next usually come headaches, fevers, chills, cough, eye swelling, aching joints, muscle pains, itchy skin, diarrhea, or constipation. With heavy infection, patients may experience difficulty coordinating movements, and have heart and breathing problems. In severe cases, death can occur. The severity of symptoms depends on the number of infectious worms consumed in meat. To avoid trichinosis, cook meat until the juices run clear, or to an internal temperature of 170°F; freeze any piece of pork less than six inches thick for 20 days at 5°F to kill any worms; cook wild game meat thoroughly—freezing wild game may not effectively kill all worms; cook all meat fed to pigs or other wild animals; clean meat grinders thoroughly if you prepare your own ground meats; remember that curing (salting), drying, smoking, or microwaving meat does not consistently kill infective worms. If you think you may have trichinosis, seek medical attention. Also known as trichinellosis.

**trichobezoar**  A wad of swallowed hair and food. Trichobezoars can sometimes cause blockage of the digestive system, especially at the exit of the stomach. See also *bezoar*.

**tricuspid**  Having three flaps or cusps. The aortic valve and tricuspid valve in the heart have three cusps.

**tricuspid valve**  One of the four heart valves, the tricuspid valve is the first one that blood encounters as it enters the heart. It stands between the right atrium and right ventricle, and allows blood to flow only from the atrium into the ventricle.

**tricyclic antidepressant**  One of a family of medications that affect the neurotransmitters norepinephrine, serotonin, and acetylcholine. The tricyclics amitriptyline (brand name: Elavil; also sold in combination with other drugs), amoxapine (brand name: Asendin), desipramine (brand name: Norpramin), doxepan (brand name: Sinequan), imipramine (brand name: Tofranil), nortriptyline (brand name: Aventyl, Pamelor), protriptyline (brand name: Vivactil), and trimipramine (brand name: Surmontil) are prescribed to counteract clinical depression, anxiety and panic disorders, migraines, eating disorders, bedwetting, and herpes lesions, among many other conditions. The tricyclic clomipramine (brand name: Anafranil) is prescribed to treat obsessive-compulsive disorder. The tricyclics can be very effective but do carry some risk of side effects, some of them very serious. Patients should be sure to discuss with their doctors any preexisting health conditions they may have, as well as any other medications they take. The most common side effects are sedation and anticholinergic actions. See also *anticholinergic side effects*.

**trigeminal nerve**  The chief nerve of sensation for the face, which is also the motor nerve controlling the muscles used for chewing. Problems with the sensory part of the trigeminal nerve result in pain or loss of sensation in the face. Problems with the motor root of the trigeminal nerve result in deviation of the jaw toward the affected side, and trouble chewing. The trigeminal nerve is the fifth cranial nerve.

**triglyceride test**  A simple blood test to measure the level of triglycerides in the blood. Triglyceride levels are influenced by recent fat and alcohol intake, so you should fast from food for at least 12 hours, and abstain from alcohol for at least 24 hours before being tested. The normal level of triglyerides depends on the age and sex of the individual. Mild to moderate triglyceride increases occur in many conditions, including alcohol abuse, obstruction of the bile ducts, and diabetes. High levels of triglycerides (greater than 200mg/dl) are associated with a heightened risk of coronary heart disease. Markedly high triglyceride levels (greater than 500mg/dl) can cause inflammation of the pancreas (pancreatitis). See also *triglycerides*.

**triglycerides**  The major form of fat. A triglyceride consists of three molecules of fatty acid combined with one molecule of the alcohol glycerol. Triglycerides serve as the backbone of many types of lipids (fats). Triglycerides come from the food we eat, and are also produced by the body. See also *triglyceride test*.

**trihexosylceramidosis** See *Anderson-Fabry disease*. See also *glycosphingolipidoses*.

**triiodothyronine** A hormone made by the thyroid gland. It has three iodine molecules attached to its molecular structure. It is the most powerful thyroid hormone, and affects almost every process in the body, including body temperature, growth, and heart rate. Also known as T3, liothyronine.

**trimester** The nine months of pregnancy are traditionally divided into three trimesters, distinct periods of roughly three months each, in which different phases of fetal development take place. The first trimester is a time of basic cell differentiation. It is said to truly end at the mother's first perception of fetal movement, which usually occurs around the end of the third month. The second trimester is a period of rapid growth and maturation of body systems. A second-trimester fetus born prematurely may be viable, given the best hospital care possible. The third trimester marks the final stage of fetal growth, in which systems are completed, fat accumulates under the soon-to-be-born baby's skin, and the fetus at last moves into position for birth. This trimester ends, of course, with the birth itself.

**trimethylaminuria** See *fish-odor syndrome*.

**trismus pseudocamptodactyly syndrome** See *Hecht syndrome*.

**trisomy 13 syndrome** The presence of three copies of chromosome 13, rather than two. See *Patau syndrome*.

**trisomy 18 syndrome** The presence of three copies of chromosome 18, rather than the normal two. See *Edwards syndrome*.

**trisomy 21 syndrome** The presence of three copies of chromosome 21, rather than two. See *Down syndrome*.

**tRNA** Transfer RNA.

**trochlear nerve** The nerve that controls the superior oblique muscle of the eye, one of the muscles that move the eye (extraocular muscles). Paralysis of the trochlear nerve results in rotation of the eyeball upward and outward (and, therefore, in double vision). The trochlear nerve is the fourth cranial nerve, and the only cranial nerve that arises from the back of the brain stem. It follows the longest course within the skull of any of the cranial nerves.

**tropical typhus** See *typhus, scrub*.

**true rib** See *rib, true*. See also *rib*.

**trunk bones** See *bones of the trunk*.

**Trypanosoma cruzi** The microorganism that causes Chagas disease. See *Chagas disease*.

**trypanosomiasis, American** See *Chagas disease*.

**TSH** Thyroid stimulating hormone.

**TSI** Thyroid stimulating immunoglobulin.

**Tsutsugamushi disease** See *typhus, scrub*.

**tubal pregnancy** See *pregnancy, tubal*. See also *ectopic pregnancy*.

**tube** A long, hollow cylinder. There are many tube-like structures in the human body, such as the Eustachean tube in the ear.

**tube, auditory** See *Eustachian tube*.

**tube, ear** See *ear tubes*.

**tube, endotracheal** See *endotracheal tube*.

**tube, Eustachian** See *Eustachian tube*.

**tube, Fallopian** See *Fallopian tubes*.

**tube, nasogastric** See *nasogastric tube*.

**tube, NG** See *nasogastric tube*.

**tube, otopharygeal** See *Eustachian tube*.

**tube, tympanostomy** See *ear tubes*.

**tuber** A lump or bump. The backward protrusion of the heel is called the tuber calcanei or, alternatively, the tuberosity of the calcaneus. Small tubers are a characteristic finding in tuberculosis, and tubers in the brain are seen in tuberous sclerosis.

**tubercle** A small tuber; a small lump or bump.

**tuberculosis** A highly contagious infection caused by the bacteria Mycobacterium tuberculosis. Tubercles (tiny lumps) are a characteristic finding. Diagnosis is by skin test, which if positive will be followed by a chest X-ray to determine the status (active or dormant) of the infection. Tuberculosis is more common in people with immune-system problems, including AIDS, than in others. Treatment of active tuberculosis is mandatory by law in the US, and should be available at no cost to the patient through the public health system. It involves a course of antibiotics and vitamins that lasts about six months. It is important to finish the entire treatment, both to prevent reoccurrence and to prevent the development of antibiotic-resistant tuberculosis. Most patients with tuberculosis do not need to be quarantined, but it is sometimes necessary. Abbreviated as TB. See also *tuberculosis, active; tuberculosis, antibiotic-resistant; tuberculosis, dormant; tuberculosis, miliary*.

**tuberculosis vaccination**   A vaccination for TB is available, but it is rarely used in the US. Known as BCG, it may not provide full immunity against infection.

**tuberculosis, active**   The presence of Mycobacterium tuberculosis infection with a positive chest X-ray. Treatment of active tuberculosis is mandatory by law in the US. See also *directly observed therapy, tuberculosis*.

**tuberculosis, antibiotic-resistant**   A variant of TB that is not affected by one or more of the antibiotics normally used to treat it. If the strain of TB is unaffected by more than one medication, it is called multidrug-resistant (MDR) TB. A person with any form of drug-resistant TB will need care from a specialist who knows how to use stronger medications. These forms of TB are particularly contagious. Family members and other contacts of diagnosed patients may also need to take medications as a preventative measure.

**tuberculosis, dormant**   The presence of Mycobacterium tuberculosis infection without a positive chest X-ray. Treatment is not mandatory, as with active tuberculosis, but is a good idea because the bacteria could become active later. Treatment is with a short course of antibiotics and vitamins.

**tuberculosis, extrapulmonary**   TB that occurs outside the lungs. For example, TB can also be active in the lymph nodes or kidneys.

**tuberculosis, MDR**   See *tuberculosis, antibiotic-resistant*.

**tuberculosis, miliary**   The presence of numerous sites of tuberculosis infection, each of which is minute. It is caused by dissemination of infected material through the bloodstream in a process somewhat like the metastatis of a malignancy.

**tuberculosis, pulmonary**   TB in the lungs. This is the most common form of active tuberculosis. It can be easily transmitted to others when the patient coughs.

**tuberculous diskitis**   An infection of the spine, seen most often in children. The main symptom is back pain. Untreated tuberculous diskitis can lead to inward or outward curvature of the spine. Imaging of the spine will find abscesses, some of which may have ossified (hardened). Also known as Pott disease.

**tuberous sclerosis**   A genetic disorder characterized by seizures, skin differences, benign tumors (tubers) that harden as the patient gets older, and developmental delays. Many children with tuberous sclerosis have autistic-like symptoms. Diagnosis is by observation of symptoms, particularly seizures combined with white spots on the skin that are most easily seen under ultraviolet light. Two genes associated with tuberous sclerosis have been found, one on chromosome 9, and one on chromosome 16, but genetic testing is not yet available. No treatment specifically for tuberous sclerosis is available, but surgery and medication can minimize associated problems.

**tubes**   See *Fallopian tubes*.

**tubule**   A small tube.

**tumescent**   Swelling; slightly swollen. For example, tumescent liposuction involves pumping a solution beneath the skin, swelling it to facilitate suctioning out fat.

**tumescent liposuction**   See *liposuction, tumescent*. See also *liposuction*.

**tumor**   An abnormal mass of tissue. Tumors are a classic sign of inflammation, and can be benign or malignant (cancerous). There are dozens of different types of tumors. Their names usually reflect the kind of tissue they arise in, and may also tell you something about their shape or how they grow. For example, a medullablastoma is a tumor that arises from embryonic cells (a blastoma) in the inner part of the brain (the medulla). Diagnosis depends on the type and location of the tumor. Tumor marker tests and imaging may be used; some tumors can be seen (for example, tumors on the exterior of the skin) or felt (palpated with the hands). Treatment is also specific to the location and type of the tumor. Benign tumors can sometimes simply be ignored, or they may be reduced in size (debulked) or removed entirely via surgery. For cancerous tumors, options include chemotherapy, radiation, and surgery. See also *blastoma, carcinoembryonic antigen test, desmoid tumor, ear tumor, epidermoid carcinoma, epithelial carcinoma, esophageal cancer, fibroid, syringoma, tumor marker*.

**tumor debulking**   Surgically removing as much of a tumor as possible.

**tumor marker**   Substances that can be detected in higher-than-normal amounts in the blood, urine, or body tissues of some patients with certain types of cancer. A tumor marker may be made by a tumor itself, or made by the body in response to the tumor. Tumor-marker tests are not used alone to detect and diagnose cancer because most tumor markers can be elevated in patients who don't have a tumor; because no tumor marker is entirely specific to a particular type of cancer; and because not every cancer patient has an elevated tumor-marker level, especially in the early stages of cancer, when tumor-marker levels are usually still normal. Although tumor markers are typically imperfect as screening tests to detect occult (hidden) cancers, once a particular tumor has been found with a marker, the marker can be a means of monitoring the success or failure of treatment. The tumor-marker level may also reflect the extent (stage) of the disease, indicate how quickly the cancer is likely to progress, and so help determine the outlook. Examples of tumor markers include alpha-fetoprotein (AFP), carcinoembryonic antigen (CEA), human chorionic gonadotropin (HCG), lactate dehydrogenase (LDH), and neuron-specific enolase (NSE).

**tumor marker, CEA**  See *carcinoembryonic antigen test*.

**tumor marker, NSE**  See *neuron-specific enolase*.

**tumor registry**  Recorded information about the status of patients with tumors. Although a registry was originally the place (like Registry House in Edinburgh) where information was collected (in registers), the word registry has also come to mean the collection itself. A tumor registry is organized so that the data can be analyzed. For example, analysis of data in a tumor registry maintained at a hospital may show a rise in lung cancer among women.

**tumor, desmoid**  See *desmoid tumor*.

**tumor, ear**  See *ear tumor*.

**tumor, sweat gland**  See *syringoma*.

**tunica albuginea**  The whitish membrane within the penis that surrounds the spongy chambers (corpora cavernosa). It helps to trap the blood in the corpora cavernosa, thereby sustaining erection of the penis.

**Turner syndrome**  A genetic disorder affecting only females, in which the patient has one X chromosome in some or all cells; or has two X chromosomes, but one is damaged. Signs include short stature, delayed growth of the skeleton, shortened fourth and fifth fingers, broad chest, and sometimes heart abnormalities. Women with Turner syndrome are usually infertile due to ovarian failure. Diagnosis is by blood test (karyotype). Treatment may include human growth hormone and estrogen replacement therapy.

**Turner-Kieser syndrome**  See *Fong disease*.

**twelfth cranial nerve**  See *hypoglossal nerve*.

**twin**  One of two children born during the same birth.

**tympanic membrane**  The eardrum.

**tympanites**  See *tympany*.

**tympano-**  Prefix indicating a relationship to the eardrum (tympanum). For example, tympanometry is a test that measures the function of the middle ear.

**tympanometry**  A test that measures the function of the middle ear. Tympanometry works by varying the pressure within the ear canal and measuring the movement of the eardrum (tympanic membrane).

**tympanoplasty**  A surgical operation to correct damage to the middle ear and restore the integrity of the eardrum.

**tympanostomy tube**  See *ear tubes*. See also *tympanoplasty*.

**tympanum**  The cavity of the middle ear, which is separated from the outer ear by the eardrum.

**tympany**  A hollow drum-like sound produced when a gas-containing cavity is tapped sharply. Tympany is heard if the chest contains free air (pneumothorax) or the abdomen is distended with gas. Also known as tympanites.

**type I error**  The statistical error (said to be "of the first kind," or alpha error) made in testing an hypothesis when it is concluded that a treatment or intervention is effective but it really is not. Sometimes referred to as a false positive.

**type II error**  The statistical error (said to be "of the second kind," or beta error) made in testing an hypothesis when it is concluded that a treatment or intervention is not effective but it really is. Sometimes referred to as a false negative.

**type 1 GM2-gangliosidosis**  See *Tay-Sachs disease*.

**typhoon supplies kit**  See *disaster supplies*.

**typhus, African tick**  One of the tick-borne rickettsial diseases of the eastern hemisphere, similar to Rocky Mountain spotted fever but less severe. Symptoms include fever, a small ulcer (tache noire) at the site of the tick bite, swollen glands nearby (satellite lymphadenopathy), and a red, raised (maculopapular) rash. Also known as fièvre boutonneuse. See also *rickettsial diseases*.

**typhus, classic**  See *typhus, epidemic*.

**typhus, endemic**  See *typhus, murine*.

**typhus, epidemic**  A severe, acute disease with prolonged high fever up to 104°F, intractable headache, and a pink-to-red raised rash. The cause is a microorganism called Rickettsia prowazekii. It is found worldwide, and is transmitted by lice. The lice become infected on typhus patients, and transmit illness to other people. The mortality increases with age, and over half of untreated persons age 50 or more die. Also known as European, classic, or louse-borne typhus; jail fever. See also *rickettsial diseases*.

**typhus, European**   See *typhus, epidemic*.

**typhus, louse-borne**   See *typhus, epidemic*.

**typhus, mite-borne**   See *typhus, scrub*.

**typhus, murine**   An acute infectious disease with fever, headache, and rash that are similar to, but milder than, epidemic typhus. It is caused by a related microorganism, Rickettsia typhi (mooseri), and transmitted to humans by rat fleas (Xenopsylla cheopis). The animal reservoir includes rats, mice, and other rodents. Murine typhus occurs sporadically worldwide, but is more prevalent in congested, rat-infested urban areas. Also known as endemic typhus, rat-flea typhus, and urban typhus of Malaya. See also *rickettsial diseases*.

**typhus, Queensland tick**   One of the tick-borne rickettsial diseases of the eastern hemisphere, similar to Rocky Mountain spotted fever but less severe. Symptoms include fever, a small ulcer (eschar) at the site of the tick bite, swollen glands nearby (satellite lymphadenopathy),

and a red, raised (maculopapular) rash. See also *rickettsial diseases*.

**typhus, rat-flea**   See *typhus, murine*.

**typhus, scrub**   A mite-borne infectious disease caused by a microorganism, Rickettsia tsutsugamushi. Characteristic symptoms include fever, headache, a raised (macular) rash, swollen glands (lymphadenopathy), and a dark crusted ulcer, called an eschar or tache noire, at the site of the chigger (mite larva) bite. This disease occurs in the area bounded by Japan, India, and Australia. Also known as Tsutsugamushi disease, mite-borne typhus, and tropical typhus. See also *rickettsial diseases*.

**typhus, tick**   See *Rocky Mountain spotted fever*.

**typhus, tropical**   See *typhus, scrub*.

**typhus, urban, of Malaysia**   See *typhus, murine*.

**typist's cramp**   A dystonia that affects the muscles of the hand and sometimes the forearm, and only occurs during handwriting. See also *dystonia, focal*.

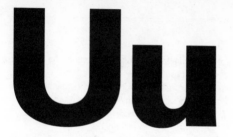

Recent medical advances have increased our understanding of ulcer formation. Improved and expanded treatment options are now available. Treatment involves antibiotics to eradicate H. pyloridus, elimination of risk factors, and prevention of complications.

**ulceration**   The process or fact of being eroded away, as by an ulcer.

**ulcerative colitis**   See *colitis, ulcerative.*

**ulcerative gingivitis**   See *acute membranous gingivitis.*

**ulcerative proctitis**   Ulcerative colitis that is limited to the rectum. See *colitis, ulcerative.*

**ulcerative stomatitis**   See *acute membranous gingivitis.*

**ulocarcinoma**   Cancer of the gums. It is often associated with the use of smokeless (chewing) tobacco. Diagnosis is by observation, and confirmed by biopsy. Treatment may include radiation, chemotherapy, and surgery.

**ultrasonic-assisted liposuction**   See *liposuction, ultrasonic-assisted.*

**ultrasound**   High-frequency sound waves. Ultrasound waves can be bounced off of tissues, using special devices. The echoes are then converted into a picture called a sonogram. Ultrasound imaging allows physicians and patients to get an inside view of soft tissues and body cavities without using invasive techniques. Ultrasound is often used to examine a fetus during pregnancy. There is no convincing evidence for any danger from ultrasound during pregnancy.

**ultraviolet radiation**   Invisible rays that are part of the energy that comes from the sun. Ultraviolet radiation is made up of two types of rays, UVA and UVB, both of which can burn the skin and cause skin cancer. UVB rays are more likely than UVA rays to cause sunburn, but UVA rays pass further into the skin. Scientists have long thought that UVB radiation can cause melanoma and other types of skin cancer. They now think that UVA radiation also may add to skin damage that can lead to cancer. For this reason, skin specialists recommend that people use sunscreens that block both kinds of radiation.

**umbilical cord**   A cord that connects the developing fetus with the placenta while in the womb. The umbilical arteries and vein run within this cord. The umbilical cord is clamped and cut at birth. Its residual tip forms the umbilicus (navel).

**umbilical duct**   See *yolk stalk.*

**umbilicus**   The vestige left behind on a newborn's belly when the umbilical cord is cut; the navel or belly button.

**UAL**   Ultrasonic-assisted liposuction.

**UBT**   Urea breath test.

**UDP-glucuronosyltransferase**   A liver enzyme essential to the disposal of bilirubin, the chemical that results from the normal breakdown of hemoglobin from red blood cells. An abnormality of UDP-glucuronosyltransferase results in a condition called Gilbert syndrome. See also *Gilbert syndrome.*

**ulcer**   A lesion that is eroding away the skin or mucous membrane. Ulcers can have various causes, depending on their location. Ulcers on the skin are usually due to irritation, as in the case of bedsores, and may become inflamed and/or infected as they grow. Ulcers in the GI tract were once attributed to stress, but most are now believed to be due to infection with the bacteria H. pyloridus. They are often made worse by stress, smoking, and other factors, however.

**ulcer, apthous**   See *canker sores.*

**ulcer, duodenal**   A hole in the lining of the first portion of the small intestine: the duodenum. See also *ulcer, peptic.*

**ulcer, esophageal**   A hole in the lining of the esophagus, corroded by the acidic digestive juices secreted by the stomach cells. See also *ulcer, peptic.*

**ulcer, gastric**   A hole in the lining of the stomach, corroded by the acidic digestive juices secreted by the stomach cells. See also *ulcer, peptic.*

**ulcer, peptic**   A hole in the lining of the stomach, duodenum, or esophagus. Peptic ulcer disease is common, affecting millions of Americans yearly. Ulcer formation is related to H. pyloridus bacteria in the stomach, anti-inflammatory medications, and smoking cigarettes. Ulcer pain may not correlate with the presence or severity of ulceration. Complications of ulcers include bleeding, perforation, and blockage of the stomach (gastric obstruction). Diagnosis is made with barium X-ray or endoscopy.

**unconscious** **1** Interruption of awareness of oneself and one's surroundings; lack of the ability to notice or respond to stimuli in the environment. A person may become unconscious due to oxygen deprivation, shock, central nervous system depressants such as alcohol and drugs, or injury. **2** In psychology, that part of thought and emotion that happens outside everyday awareness.

**unconsciousness, temporary** A partial or complete loss of consciousness; interruption of awareness of oneself and one's surroundings. When the loss of consciousness is temporary and recovery is spontaneous, it is referred to as syncope or, more commonly, fainting. Temporary loss of unconsciousness may also occur with some types of seizures, as a result of head injury, or as part of a dissociative state. See *syncope*.

**undulant fever** See *Brucellosis*.

**unicornuate** Having one horn, or being horn-shaped. The uterus is normally unicornuate.

**uniparous** Having one offspring in a birth; as opposed to multiparous, having two or more offspring in a birth. See also *multiparous*.

**unipolar depression** See *depression*.

**unique identifier reporting** In public health, a system that uses a unique code to identify patients who have been tested or treated for an illness. This number is reported instead of the patient's name. Unique identifier reporting is an alternative to named reporting, providing some of the surveillance benefits of reporting by name, such as the elimination of duplicate reports, while reducing privacy concerns. HIV testing facilities in several US states may use unique identifier reporting.

**United Network for Organ Sharing** The US medical agency that coordinates organ donations, including matching potential donors and recipients.

**United States Public Health Service** A part of the Department of Health and Human Services (HHS), the USPHS is responsible for the public health of the American people. It administers a number of important health agencies, including the Food and Drug Administration (FDA), the Centers for Disease Control (CDC), and the National Institutes of Health (NIH).

**universal colitis** See *colitis, ulcerative*.

**UNOS** United Network for Organ Sharing.

**unsteadiness** Loss of one's equilibrium in regard to the environment, often with a feeling of almost falling, or the result of bumping into things. There are many causes for unsteadiness, including problems in the cerebral or cerebellar portions of the brain, the spinal cord, vestibular system, or inner ear. Unsteadiness is medically distinct from dizziness, lightheadedness, and vertigo. See also *dizziness, lightheadedness, vertigo*.

**upper GI series** A series of X-rays of the esophagus, stomach, and small intestine that are taken after the patient drinks a barium solution. See also *barium solution, barium swallow*.

**upper leg** See *leg, upper*.

**urate** A salt derived from uric acid. When the body cannot metabolize uric acid properly, urates can build up in body tissues or crystallize within the joints. See also *gout, uric acid*.

**urban typhus of Malaya** See *typhus, murine*.

**urea** **1** A substance containing nitrogen that is normally cleared from the blood by the kidney, and excreted via the urine. Diseases that compromise the function of the kidney often lead to increased blood levels of urea, which can be measured by the blood urea nitrogen (BUN) test. See also *uremia*. **2** A medical formulation of urea that may be used to remove fluid from body tissues or the skin.

**urea breath test** A procedure for diagnosing the presence of a bacterium, Helicobacter pylori (H. pylori), that causes inflammation, ulcers, and atrophy of the stomach. The test may be used also to demonstrate that H. pylori has been eliminated by treatment with antibiotics. The urea breath test is based on the ability of H. pylori to break down urea, a chemical made of nitrogen and carbon, that normally is produced by the body from excess nitrogen and then eliminated in the urine. For the test, patients swallow a capsule containing urea made from an isotope of carbon. If H. pylori is present in the stomach, the urea is broken up into nitrogen and carbon dioxide. The carbon dioxide is absorbed across the lining of the stomach and into the blood, and then is excreted from the lungs in the breath. Samples of exhaled breath are collected, and the isotopic carbon in the exhaled carbon dioxide is measured. If the isotope is detected in the breath, it means that H. pylori is present in the stomach. If the isotope is not found, H. pylori is not present. When the H. pylori is effectively treated with antibiotics, the test results change from positive to negative. Abbreviated as UBT.

**uremia** The presence of excessive amounts of urea in the blood, which may be a sign of kidney disease or failure. See also *urea*.

**ureters** The tubes that carry urine from each kidney to the bladder.

**urethra** The tube leading from the bladder to transport and discharge urine outside the body. In males, the urethra travels through the penis, and carries semen as well as urine. In females, the urethra is shorter than in the male and emerges above the vaginal opening.

**urethral sphincter** The muscle that controls the release of urine from the bladder.

**urethritis** Inflammation of the urethra. Urethritis can have several causes, including sexually transmitted diseases such as chlamydia, or irritation. Treatment depends on the cause.

**urethroscope** A device for examining the inside of the urethra.

**URI** Upper respiratory infection.

**uric acid** A product produced when proteins are metabolized. In gout, elevated levels of uric acid are often found in the blood (hyperuricemia). However, only a small portion of people with hyperuricemia will develop gout.

**uricaciduria** The presence of excess uric acid in the urine, which may be a sign of gout or kidney stones.

**urinalysis** A test that determines the content of the urine. Because urine removes toxins and excess liquids from the body, it can contain important clues. Urinalysis can be used to detect some types of disease, particularly in the case of metabolic disorders and kidney disease. It can also be used to uncover evidence of drug abuse. Accurate urinalysis usually requires a "clean catch" of urine. If you are giving a urine sample, drink plenty of fluids in advance, and wait until one or two seconds into the flow of urine before urinating into the receptacle. For some tests it is important to get the first urine of the day, which will contain the highest concentration of toxins and other clues.

**urinary** Having to do with the function or anatomy of the kidneys, ureters, bladder, or urethra.

**urinary bladder** See *bladder.*

**urinary calculus** A stone, such as a kidney stone, in the urinary tract.

**urinary incontinence** See *enuresis.* See also *bedwetting.*

**urinary tract** The organs of the body that produce and discharge urine. These include the kidneys, ureters, bladder, and urethra.

**urinary tract infection** Infection of the kidney, ureter, bladder, or urethra. Not everyone with a UTI has symptoms. Common symptoms include a frequent urge to urinate, and pain or burning when urinating. More females than males have UTIs. Underlying conditions that impair the normal urinary flow, such as the formation of cysts within the urinary tract, can lead to complicated UTIs. Treatment is usually with increased fluid intake and antibiotics. In those few cases where physical obstruction is present, special medications or surgery may be necessary.

**urine** Liquid waste. The urine is a clear, transparent fluid. It normally has an amber color, and should be odorless. The average amount of urine excreted in 24 hours is from 40 to 60 oz. Chemically, the urine is mainly a watery solution of salt and substances called urea and uric acid. Normally, it contains about 960 parts of water to 40 parts of solid matter. Abnormally, it may contain sugar (in diabetes), albumin (a protein, as in some forms of kidney disease), bile pigments (as in jaundice), or abnormal quantities of one or another of its normal components.

**urine test** See *urinalysis.*

**urine, blood in the** See *hematuria; hematuria, gross.*

**urogenital** Relating to both the urinary system, and to the interior and exterior genitalia.

**urography** A method for examining the structure and functionality of the urinary system. A special dye is injected, and X-ray machines record its progress through the urinary tract. Urography is particularly useful for discovering cysts or other internal blockages.

**urolithiasis** The process of forming stones in the kidney, bladder, and/or urethra. See also *kidney stone.*

**urologist** A doctor who specializes in diseases of the urinary organs in females, and the urinary and sex organs in males.

**urticaria** See *hives.*

**US National Library of Medicine** See *National Institutes of Health.*

**USFDA** The United States Food and Drug Administration. See *Food and Drug Administration.*

**USPHS**   United States Public Health Service.

**ut dict.**   Abbreviation meaning "as directed." See also *Appendix A, "Prescription Abbreviations."*

**uterine cancer**   See *cancer, uterine.*

**uterine fibroid**   See *fibroid.*

**uterine fornix**   See *fornix uteri.*

**uterine retroversion**   See *uterus, tipped.*

**uterine tube**   See *Fallopian tubes.*

**uterus**   A hollow, pear-shaped organ located in a woman's lower abdomen, between the bladder and the rectum. The narrow, lower portion of the uterus is the cervix; the broader, upper part is known as the corpus. The corpus is made up of three layers of tissue. In women of childbearing age, the inner layer (endometrium) of the uterus goes through a series of monthly changes known as the menstrual cycle. Each month, endometrial tissue grows and thickens in preparation to receive a fertilized egg. Menstruation occurs when this tissue is not used, disintegrates, and passes out through the vagina. The middle layer (myometrium) of the uterus is muscular tissue that expands during pregnancy to hold the growing fetus, and contracts during labor to deliver the child. The outer layer (parametrium) also expands during pregnancy and contracts thereafter.

**uterus, prolapsed**   A uterus that has moved from its normal position in the abdominal cavity, usually into a lower position. Prolapsed uterus may occur because of underlying weak muscles, or simply as a result of repeated term pregnancies. It can sometimes interfere with conception, cause difficulties during pregnancy, or contribute to pelvic pain.

**uterus, tipped**   A slight to dramatic placement of the uterus that orients it toward the back. A tipped uterus is common and usually causes no difficulty. In severe cases, it can affect choice of birth control method and cause pain in the pelvic area, especially during intercourse. Also known as uterine retroversion.

**UTI**   Urinary tract infection.

**utility**   In the analysis of health outcomes, utility is a number between 0 and 1 that is assigned to a state of health or an outcome. Perfect health has a value of 1. Death has a value of 0.

**uvea**   An inner layer of the eye, the uvea includes the iris, the blood vessels that serve the eye (the choroid), and the connective tissue between the two (the ciliary body).

**uveitis**   Inflammation of the uvea.

**uvula**   The anatomic structure that dangles downward at the back of the mouth. It is attached to the rear of the soft palate.

**uvulitis**   Inflammation of the uvula.

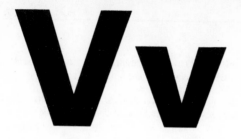

**vaccination** Injection of a weakened or killed microbe intended to stimulate the immune system to produce antibodies to that microbe, thereby preventing disease. The effectiveness of immunizations can often be improved by periodic repeat injections (booster shots). To find out about vaccines for specific illnesses, look under the name of the disease (for example, anthrax immunization, measles immunization, and so on). Also known as immunizations, shots, vaccines. See also *children's immunizations*.

**vaccination, children's** See *children's immunizations*.

**vaccines** Microbial preparations of killed or modified microorganisms that can stimulate an immune response in the body to prevent future infection with similar microorganisms. These preparations are usually delivered by intramuscular injection.

**vagina** The muscular canal extending from the cervix to the outside of the body. It is usually six to seven inches in length, and its walls are lined with mucous membrane. It includes two vaultlike structures: the anterior (front) vaginal fornix and the posterior (rear) vaginal fornix. The cervix protrudes slightly into the vagina, and it is through a tiny hole in the cervix (the os) that sperm make their way toward the internal reproductive organs. The vagina also includes numerous tiny glands that make vaginal secretions.

**vagina, septate** A vagina that is divided, usually longitudinally, to create a double vagina. This situation can be easily missed by the patient and even by the doctor on exam. If the patient becomes sexually active prior to diagnosis, one of the vaginas stretches and becomes dominant. The other vagina slips slightly upward and flush, and is a little difficult to enter.

**vaginal birth after Cesarean section** It was once the rule that after a C-section, the next delivery also had to be by C-section. Now vaginal delivery after Cesarean section is frequently feasible. Abbreviated as VBAC.

**vaginal fornix** The anterior (front) and posterior (back) recesses into which the upper vagina is divided. These vaultlike recesses are formed by protrusion of the cervix into the vagina. Also known as the fornix uteri.

**vaginal hysterectomy** Removal of the uterus through a surgical incision made within the vagina. With a vaginal hysterectomy, the scar is not outwardly visible.

**vaginal introitus** See *vaginal opening*.

**vaginal opening** The exterior opening to the muscular canal that extends from the cervix to the outside of the female body. Also called vaginal introitus, vaginal vestibule.

**vaginal vestibule** See *vaginal opening*.

**vaginitis** Inflammation of the vagina. Vaginitis is a common condition and is often caused by a fungus. Symptoms include itching, burning, and discharge. There are factors that predispose a woman to develop vaginitis. For example, women who have diabetes have vaginitis more often than women who do not. See also *vaginitis, atrophic; yeast; yeast vaginitis*.

**vaginitis, atrophic** Thinning of the lining (the endothelium) of the vagina due to decreased production of estrogen. This may occur with menopause.

**vaginitis, yeast** See *yeast vaginitis*.

**vagus nerve** A remarkable nerve that supplies nerve fibers to the pharynx (throat), larynx (voice box), trachea (windpipe), lungs, heart, esophagus, and the intestinal tract as far as the transverse portion of the colon. The vagus nerve also brings sensory information back to the brain from the ear, tongue, pharynx, and larynx. The vagus nerve is the tenth cranial nerve. It originates in the medulla oblongata, a part of the brain stem, and wanders all the way down from the brain stem to the colon. Complete interruption of the vagus nerve causes a characteristic syndrome in which the soft palate droops on the side where damage occurred, and the gag reflex is also lost on that side. The voice is hoarse and nasal, and the vocal cord on the affected side is immobile. The result is difficulty in swallowing (dysphagia) and speaking (dysphonia). The vagus nerve has several important branches, including the recurrent laryngeal nerve.

**Valium** See *diazepam*.

**Valsalva maneuver** A maneuver in which one tries with force to exhale with the windpipe closed, impeding the return of venous blood to the heart.

**valve, aortic** See *aortic valve*.

**valve, bicuspid** See *mitral valve*.

**valve, mitral** See *mitral valve*.

**valve, pulmonary**   See *pulmonary valve*.

**valve, tricuspid**   See *tricuspid valve*.

**valves, heart**   See *heart valves*. See also *aortic valve, mitral valve, pulmonary valve, tricuspid valve*.

**VAQTA**   A vaccine against hepatitis A. See *hepatitis A, hepatitis A immunization*.

**vara, tibia**   See *tibia vara*.

**variant angina**   See *angina, Printzmetal*.

**variation, observer**   See *observer variation*.

**varicella**   A highly infectious viral disease, known familiarly as chicken pox. It is caused by the herpes zoster virus, which can also cause shingles later in life. See *herpes zoster*.

**varicella vaccination**   See *chicken pox immunization*.

**varicocele**   Elongation and enlargement of veins within the network of veins (pampiniform plexus) leaving the testis to form the testicular vein. A varicocele appears bluish through the scrotum, and feels like a bag of worms. Can cause pain or discomfort.

**varicose veins**   Veins that have enlarged and twisted, often appearing as bulging, blue blood vessels that are clearly visible through the skin. They are most common in older adults, particularly women, and especially on the legs. The veins can cause cramping pain and movement problems, or may simply be a cosmetic concern. Treatment includes elevating the affected limb, wearing support hose to increase pressure on the vein, and in some cases surgery.

**variola**   See *smallpox*.

**varix**   An enlarged and convoluted vein, artery, or lymphatic vessel.

**vasa previa**   A birth in which the umbilical cord vessels are delivered before the fetal head. This can sometimes cause lack of oxygen to the fetus.

**vascular**   Relating to blood vessels of the body.

**vascular bed**   The vascular system, or a part thereof. For example, the pulmonary vascular bed describes the blood vessels of the lungs.

**vascular endothelial growth factor**   A gene responsible for the growth of blood vessels. Abbreviated as VEG-F.

**vascular headache**   See *headache, vascular*. See also *migraine headache*.

**vasculitis**   A general term for a group of uncommon diseases that feature inflammation of the blood vessels. Each of the vasculitis diseases is defined by characteristic distributions of blood vessel involvement, patterns of organ involvement, and laboratory test abnormalities. The actual cause of these vasculitis diseases is usually not known, but immune system abnormality is a common feature. Examples of vasculitis include Kawasaki disease, Behcet disease, polyarteritis nodosa, Wegener granulomatosis, Takayasu arteritis, Churg-Strauss syndrome, giant cell arteritis (temporal arteritis), and Henoch-Schonlein purpura. Vasculitis can also accompany infections, such as hepatitis B; exposure to chemicals, such as amphetamines and cocaine; cancers, such as lymphomas and multiple myeloma; and rheumatic diseases, such as rheumatoid arthritis and systemic lupus erythematosus. Laboratory testing in a patient with active vasculitis generally indicates inflammation in the body. Depending on the degree of organ involvement, a variety of organ function tests can be abnormal. The ultimate diagnosis for vasculitis is typically established after a biopsy of involved tissue demonstrates the pattern of blood vessel inflammation. Treatment depends on the type and severity of the illness, and the organs involved. Treatments are generally directed toward stopping the inflammation and suppressing the immune system. Typically, cortisone-related medications, such as prednisone, are used. Additionally, other immune-suppression drugs, such as cyclophosphamide (brand name: Cytoxan), are considered. These conditions are also known as forms of angiitis or vasculitides.

**vasculitis, allergic**   See *Churg-Strauss syndrome*.

**vasoconstriction**   Narrowing of the blood vessels, resulting from contraction of the muscular wall of the vessels. The opposite of vasodilation.

**vasodepressor syncope**   See *syncope, situational*. See also *vasovagal reaction*.

**vasodilation**   Widening of blood vessels resulting from relaxation of the muscular wall of the vessels. What widens is actually the diameter of the interior (the lumen) of the vessel. The opposite of vasoconstriction.

**vasodilators**   Agents that act as blood vessel dilators, opening blood vessels by relaxing their muscular walls. For example, nitroglycerin is a vasodilator, as are the ACE (angiotensin converting enzyme) inhibitors.

**vasomotor**   Relating to the nerves and muscles that cause the blood vessels to constrict or dilate.

**vasomotor rhinitis**  Inflammation of the nose (rhinitis) due to abnormal neuronal (nerve) control of the blood vessels in the nose. Vasomotor rhinitis is not allergic rhinitis.

**vasopressin**  See *antidiuretic hormone*. See also *ADH secretion, inappropriate*.

**vasovagal attack**  See *vasovagal reaction*.

**vasovagal reaction**  A reflex of the involuntary nervous system that leads the heart to slow down (bradycardia) and, at the same time, affects the nerves to the blood vessels in the legs, permitting those vessels to dilate (widen). As a result, the heart puts out less blood, the blood pressure drops, and what blood is circulating tends to go into the legs rather than to the head. The brain is deprived of oxygen and a fainting episode (syncope) occurs. See also *syncope*.

**vasovagal syncope**  The temporary loss of consciousness in a particular kind of situation (situational syncope, or fainting) due to a vasovagal reaction. See also *syncope*.

**VATER association**  An association of birth defects that include vertebral anomalies, ventricular septal defects, and other heart defects; anal atresia (the lack of an anus at the end of the intestine); tracheoesophageal fistula (communication between the esophagus and trachea) with esophageal atresia (part of the esophagus not being hollow); radial dysplasia (abnormal formation of the thumb or the radius in the forearm); and renal (kidney) abnormalities. This remarkable pattern of malformations has occurred in many babies. The cause of the VATER association is unknown, although it is more common in the children of diabetic mothers. Treatment is by surgery to correct the physical effects, as possible.

**VBAC**  Vaginal birth after Cesarean section.

**VDRL test**  A blood test for syphilis. VDRL stands for Venereal Disease Research Laboratory. A negative (nonreactive) VDRL is compatible with a person not having syphilis. However, a person may have a negative VDRL and still have syphilis since, in the early stages of the disease, the VDRL often gives false negative results. The VDRL test is sometimes positive in the absence of syphilis. For example, a false positive VDRL can be encountered in infectious mononucleosis, lupus, the antiphospholipid antibody syndrome, hepatitis A, leprosy, malaria and, occasionally, pregnancy. See also *syphilis*.

**vector**  In medicine, a carrier of disease or of medication. For example, in malaria a mosquito is the vector that carries and transfers the infectious agent. In molecular biology, a vector may be a virus or a plasmid that carries a piece of foreign DNA to a host cell.

**VEG-F**  Vascular endothelial growth factor.

**vein**  A blood vessel that carries blood low in oxygen content from the body back to the heart. The deoxygenated form of hemoglobin (deoxyhemoglobin) in venous blood makes it appear dark. Veins are part of the afferent wing of the circulatory system, which returns blood to the heart. By contrast, an artery is a vessel that carries blood high in oxygen away from the heart to the body. See also *circulatory system*.

**vein, brachial**  See *brachial vein*.

**vein, external jugular**  See *jugular vein, external*.

**vein, femoral**  See *femoral vein*.

**vein, great saphenous**  See *saphenous vein, great*. See also *saphenous veins*.

**vein, inferior vena cava**  See *vena cava, inferior*.

**vein, internal jugular**  See *jugular vein, internal*.

**vein, jugular**  See *jugular veins*.

**vein, large saphenous**  See *saphenous vein, great*.

**vein, portal**  See *portal vein*.

**vein, pulmonary**  See *pulmonary vein*.

**vein, saphenous**  See *saphenous veins*.

**vein, small saphenous**  See *saphenous vein, small*.

**vein, superior vena cava**  See *vena cava, superior*.

**veins, ophthalmic**  See *ophthalmic veins*.

**veins, spider**  See *spider veins*.

**veins, varicose**  See *varicose veins*.

**Velban**  See *vinblastine sulfate*.

**velo-cardio–facial syndrome**  A congenital syndrome of birth defects that include cleft palate (velum), heart (cardio) defects, an abnormal facial structure, and learning problems. Other less frequent features include short stature, microcephaly, mental retardation, minor ear anomalies, slender hands and digits, and inguinal hernia. Many people with VCF also have mood swings like those seen in bipolar disorders. The cause is usually a microdeletion in chromosome band 22q11.2, as in DiGeorge syndrome, so VCF and DiGeorge syndromes are different clinical expressions of essentially the same chromosome defect. Treatment is by surgery to correct the physical defects, and medication, therapy, and special education to assist with the cognitive and neurological effects, if present. Also known as Shprintzen syndrome. See also *bipolar disorders, DiGeorge syndrome.*

**Velsar** See *vinblastine sulfate.*

**Velpeau hernia** A protrusion of tissue through the muscular wall in the groin, located in front of the femoral blood vessels.

**velvet ant stings** Common in most parts of the world including the Southern and Southwestern United States, velvet ants are actually parasitic wasps. Their sting can trigger allergic reactions that vary greatly in severity. Avoidance and prompt treatment are essential. In selected cases, allergy injection therapy is highly effective.

**vena cava syndrome, superior** See *superior vena cava syndrome.*

**vena cava, inferior** A large vein that receives blood from the lower extremities, pelvis, and abdomen. It then empties this blood into the right atrium of the heart.

**vena cava, superior** The large vein that returns blood to the right atrium of the heart from the head, neck, and both upper limbs. The superior vena cava is located in the middle of the chest, and is surrounded by rigid structures and lymph nodes. Structures bordering the superior vena cava include the trachea, aorta, thymus, right bronchus of the lung and pulmonary artery. Compression of the superior vena cava by disease of any of the structures or lymph nodes surrounding it can cause superior vena cava syndrome. See *superior vena cava syndrome.*

**venereal** Having to do with sexual contact.

**venereal disease** See *sexually transmitted disease.*

**venereal wart** See *genital warts.* See also *human papilloma virus.*

**venlafaxine** A unique antidepressant drug (brand name: Effexor) prescribed to treat depression. It is believed to affect the neurotransmitters serotonin, norepinephrine, and dopamine, but not monoamine oxidase (MAO). It is not usually indicated for use by people with kidney or liver disease, or those with high blood pressure. Common side effects include sleepiness or insomnia, dry mouth, nervousness, nausea, and sexual dysfunction.

**venous aneurysm** A localized widening and bulging of a vein. At the area of an aneurysm, the vein wall is weakened and may rupture.

**venous catheterization** The insertion of a tiny tube (catheter) into a peripheral or central vein to deliver fluids or medication. This is the most frequently used method for administration of intravenous (IV) fluids. The most common complication is infection at the site of the catheter (catheter sepsis).

**ventilator** A machine that mechanically assists patients in the exchange of oxygen and carbon dioxide, a process sometimes referred to as artificial respiration.

**ventral** Pertaining to the front or anterior of a structure. Something that is ventral is oriented toward the belly, toward the front of the body. For example, the belly button (umbilicus) is in the ventral midline. The opposite of ventral is dorsal. See also *Appendix B, "Anatomic Orientation Terms."*

**ventricle** A chamber of an organ. For example, the four connected cavities in the central portion of the brain are called ventricles.

**ventricle, brain** See *ventricle, cerebral.* See also *brain, lateral ventricle, third ventricle, fourth ventricle.*

**ventricle, cerebral** One of a system of four communicating cavities within the brain that are continuous with the central canal of the spinal cord. These are the two lateral ventricles, the third ventricle, and the fourth ventricle. The ventricles are filled with cerebrospinal fluid, which is formed by the choroid plexuses, structures that are located in the walls and roofs of the ventricles. See also *brain ventricle, lateral ventricle, third ventricle, fourth ventricle.*

**ventricle, fourth** See *fourth ventricle.* See also *ventricle, cerebral.*

**ventricle, heart** One of the two lower chambers of the heart. The right ventricle is the chamber that receives blood from the right atrium and pumps it into the lungs via the pulmonary artery. The left ventricle is the chamber that receives blood from the left atrium and pumps it into the system circulation via the aorta.

**ventricle, lateral** See *lateral ventricle.* See also *ventricle, cerebral.*

**ventricle, left** The chamber of the heart that receives blood from the left atrium and pumps it out under high pressure to the body via the aorta. See also *ventricle, heart.*

**ventricle, right** The chamber of the heart that receives blood from the right atrium and pumps it under low pressure into the lungs via the pulmonary artery. See also *ventricle, heart.*

**ventricle, third** See *third ventricle*. See also *ventricle, cerebral*.

**ventricular arrhythmias** Abnormal, rapid heart rhythms (arrhythmias) that originate in the lower chambers of the heart (the ventricles). Ventricular arrhythmias include ventricular tachycardia and ventricular fibrillation. Both are life-threatening arrhythmias most commonly associated with heart attacks or scarring of the heart muscle from previous heart attack.

**ventricular fibrillation** An abnormal, irregular heart rhythm in which very rapid and uncoordinated fluttering contractions of the lower chambers (ventricles) of the heart occur. Ventricular fibrillation disrupts the synchrony between the heartbeat and the pulse beat. Ventricular fibrillation is most commonly associated with heart attacks or scarring of the heart muscle from previous heart attack. It is life-threatening.

**ventricular septal defect** A hole in the wall (septum) between the lower chambers of the heart (the ventricles). Ventricular septal defects (VSDs) are the most common birth defect that involves malformation of the heart. At least 1 baby in every 500 is born with a VSD. A VSD lets blood from the left ventricle, where it is under relatively high pressure, and shunts into the right ventricle, which has to do extra work to handle the additional blood. The right ventricle may have trouble keeping up with the load, enlarge, and fail. The lungs also receive too much blood under too great pressure. The small arteries (arterioles) in the lungs thicken up in response, and permanent vascular damage can be done to the lungs. VSDs that are less than 0.5 square cm in area permit only minimal shunting of blood, so the pressure in the right ventricle remains normal and the heart and lungs function normally. Surgical repair is not recommended for small VSDs. No matter what size a VSD is, it carries an increased risk for infection of the heart walls and valves (endocarditis). To prevent endocarditis, anyone with a VSD should take antibiotics before dental and some other procedures. With a VSD greater than 1.0 square cm in area, there is a significant shunt into the right ventricle, excessive blood flow into the lungs, and elevated pressure in the arteries to the lungs (pulmonary hypertension). The child may have labored breathing, difficulty feeding, and grow poorly. Medically, the heart that has a large VSD should be kept strong. Vascular disease in the lungs must not be allowed to develop. Surgery should be done to close a large VSD. The prognosis for patients with VSD is generally excellent.

**ventricular septum** The wall between the two lower chambers (ventricles) of the heart.

**ventricular tachycardia** An abnormal heart rhythm that is rapid, regular, and originates from an area of the lower chamber (ventricle) of the heart. Ventricular tachycardias are life-threatening arrhythmias most commonly associated with heart attacks or scarring of the heart muscle from previous heart attack.

**venule** A little vein. Venules go from capillaries to veins.

**verbal child abuse** See *child abuse, emotional*.

**vernix** More formally known as vernix caseosa, the vernix is a white, cheesy substance that covers and protects the skin of the fetus. It is still all over the skin of a baby at birth. Vernix is composed of sebum (skin oil) and cells that have sloughed off the fetus' skin.

**vernix caseosa** See *vernix*.

**verruca** See *wart*. See also *human papilloma virus*.

**vertebra** One of 33 bony segments that form the human spinal column. Each vertebra has its own name and/or number. For example, the second cervical vertebra is known as the axis or C2 vertebra. See also *vertebral column*.

**vertebral artery** One of two key arteries located in the back of the neck, a vertebral artery carries blood from the heart to the brain, spine, and neck muscles.

**vertebral column** The 33 vertebrae fit together to form a flexible, yet extraordinarily tough, column that serves to support the back through a full range of motion. It also protects the spinal cord, which runs from the brain through the hollow space in the middle of the vertebral column. There are 7 cervical (C1–C7), 12 thoracic (T1–T12), 5 lumbar (L1–L5), 5 sacral (S1–S5),and 4 coccygeal vertebrae in this column, each separated by intervertebral disks. The first cervical vertebra, known as the atlas, supports the head. It pivots on the odontoid process of the second cervical vertebra, the axis. The cervical vertebrae end at their juncture with the thoracic vertebrae. The seventh cervical vertebra (the prominent vertebra, so named because of its long spiny projection) adjoins the first thoracic vertebrae. The thoracic vertebrae provide an attachment site for the true ribs, and make up part of the back of the chest (thorax). This part of the spine is very flexible, to permit bending and twisting. The thoracic vertebrae join the lumbar vertebrae, which are particularly sturdy and large, as they support the entire structure. The lumbar vertebrae are nonetheless quite flexible. At the top of the pelvis, the lumbar vertebrae join the sacral vertebrae. By adulthood these five bones have usually fused to form a triangular bone called the sacrum. At the tip of the sacrum, the final part of the vertebral column projects slightly outward. This is the coccyx, better known as the tailbone. It is made up of three to five coccygeal vertebrae: small, rudimentary vertebrae that fuse together.

**vertebral compression fracture** A fracture that collapses a spinal vertebra as a result of the compression of bone, leading to collapse of the vertebrae much as a sponge collapses under the pressure of one's hand. Although they may occur without pain, such vertebral fractures often cause a severe, band-like pain that radiates from the spine around both sides of the body. Over many years, spinal fractures lessen the height of the spine and the person becomes shorter. Vertebral compression fractures are often linked to osteoporosis. Treatment is usually with pain medicine, rest, injury avoidance, and bracing, although in some cases surgery can be used. See also *vertebroplasty.*

**vertebral rib** See *false rib.*

**vertebroplasty** A nonsurgical method for the repair of osteoporosis back fractures, such as vertebral compression fractures. Vertebroplasty is performed by a radiologist, without surgery, and involves inserting a glue-like material into the center of the collapsed spinal vertebra to stabilize and strengthen the crushed bone. The glue (methylmethacrylate) is inserted through anesthetized skin with a needle and syringe, entering the midportion of the vertebra under the guidance of specialized X-ray equipment. Once inserted, the glue hardens to form a cast-like structure with the broken bone. Relief of pain comes quickly from this casting effect, and the newly hardened vertebra is then protected from further collapse. The advantages of vertebroplasty, aside from prompt pain relief, include better mobility. Vertebrae that have collapsed to less than 30 percent of their normal height are poor candidates for this procedure.

**vertex** The top of the head. For example, in a vertex presentation at birth, the top of the baby's head emerges first.

**vertical** Upright, as opposed to horizontal. See *Appendix B, "Anatomic Orientation Terms."*

**vertical transmission** Passage of a disease-causing agent (pathogen) from mother to baby during the period immediately before and after birth. Transmission might occur across the placenta, in the breast milk, or through direct contact during or after birth. HIV can be a vertically transmitted pathogen. Also known as perinatal transmission.

**vertigo** A feeling that one is turning around, or that things are turning about you. Vertigo is usually due to a problem with the inner ear. It is medically distinct from dizziness, lightheadedness, and unsteadiness. See also *dizziness, lightheadedness, unsteadiness.*

**vertigo, recurrent aural** See *Ménière disease.*

**VES** Voluntary Euthanasia Society.

**vesical** Refers to the urinary bladder.

**vesicant** A substance that causes tissue blistering. Also referred to as a vesicatory.

**vesicate** To blister.

**vesicatory** See *vesicant.*

**vesicle** 1 In dermatology, a small skin blister. 2 In anatomy, a small pouch.

**vesicular** An adjective indicating the presence of one or more vesicles. A vesicular rash features small blisters on the skin.

**vesicular rickettsiosis** See *rickettsial pox.*

**vesiculitis** Inflammation of a vesicle, and particularly of the seminal vesicles behind the male bladder.

**vesiculography** The use of special X-ray equipment and a dye to examine the seminal vesicles and related structures. Vesiculography is most often used when prostate disease or cancer is suspected.

**vessel** A tube in the body that carries fluids; examples are blood vessels and lymph vessels.

**vessel, afferent** A vessel that carries blood toward the heart; a vein or venule. The opposite of an afferent vessel is an efferent vessel.

**vessel, efferent** A vessel that carries blood away from the heart; an artery or arteriole. The opposite of an efferent vessel is an afferent vessel.

**vestibular** 1 Having to do with a structure that is a vestibule (entrance), such as the vestibule of the ear. 2 Having to do with the body's system for maintaining equilibrium.

**vestibular apparatus** The vestibule and three semicircular canals of the inner ear. Like an internal carpenter's level, these structures work with the brain to sense, maintain, and regain balance and a sense of where the body and its parts are positioned in space. See also *vestibular disorders, vestibular system.*

**vestibular disorders** Many disorders can affect the vestibular system by directly affecting the structure or integrity of the middle ear itself, by interrupting the feedback loop between these structures and the brain, or by affecting those parts of the brain that interpret data from the vestibular apparatus. Conditions known to affect vestibular function include acoustic neuroma, autism, Ménière disease, multiple sclerosis, infection in the middle ear (otitis media), the use of medications that are toxic to the ear (ototoxic), seizure disorders, syphilis, trauma, and vertigo. Diagnosis is by neurological tests, in which the patient's response to movement requests and questions about spacial positioning are observed. It can sometimes be confirmed by imaging or directly viewing inner ear structures or brain function. Treatment depends on the cause of the disorder, but may include medication, surgery, physical therapy, occupational therapy (particularly sensory integration therapy), or lifestyle adjustments.

**vestibular system**   A system comprised of the vestibular apparatus, the vestibulocochlear nerve, and those parts of the brain that interpret and respond to information derived from these structures.

**vestibule**   In medicine and dentistry, a space or cavity at the entrance to a canal, channel, tube, or vessel. For instance, the front of the mouth is a vestibule.

**vestibule of the ear**   A cavity in the middle of the bony labyrinth in the inner ear.

**vestibule, vaginal**   See *vaginal opening*.

**vestibulocochlear nerve**   A nerve that is responsible for the sense of hearing, and which is also pertinent to the senses of balance and body position. Problems with the vestibulocochlear nerve may result in deafness, tinnitus (ringing or noise in the ears), dizziness, vertigo, and vomiting. The vestibulocochlear nerve is the eighth cranial nerve.

**vestigial**   Adjective describing something that is a vestige (remnant) or a primitive structure, and no longer believed to be important. For example, the appendix is considered a vestigial organ, and some infants are born with a vestigial tail.

**VHL**   von Hippel-Lindau. See *von Hippel-Lindau syndrome*.

**viable**   Capable of life: A viable premature baby is one who is able to survive outside the womb.

**Vibrio**   A group of bacteria that includes Vibrio cholerae. Vibrio move about particularly actively.

**Vibrio cholerae**   One of the Vibrio bacteria, V. cholerae is the agent that causes cholera. See also *cholera*.

**vidian neuralgia**   See *cluster headache*. See also *migraine*.

**vinblastine sulfate**   An anticancer drug (brand name: Velban, Velsar) believed to have a unique effect on malignant cells, disrupting one or more metabolic processes within these cells.

**Vincent angina**   See *acute membraneous gingivitis*.

**Vincent gingivitis**   See *acute membraneous gingivitis*.

**Vincent infection**   See *acute membraneous gingivitis*.

**Vincent stomatitis**   See *acute membraneous gingivitis*.

**vincristine**   An anti-cancer drug (brand name: Oncovin) given via IV drip or catheter.

**viral hepatitis**   See *hepatitis, viral*.

**viral infection**   Infection caused by the presence of a virus in the body. Depending on the virus and the person's state of health, various viruses can infect almost any type of body tissue, from the brain to the skin. Viral infections cannot be treated with antibiotics; in fact, in some cases the use of antibiotics makes the infection worse. The vast majority of human viral infections can be effectively fought by the body's own immune system, with a little help in the form of proper diet, hydration, and rest. As for the rest, treatment depends on the type and location of the virus, and may include anti-viral or other drugs.

**virion**   A virus particle.

**virology**   The study of viruses.

**virulence**   The ability of any agent of infection to produce disease. The virulence of a microorganism is a measure of the severity of the disease it causes.

**virulent**   Extremely noxious, damaging, deleterious, disease-causing (pathogenic); marked by a rapid, severe, and malignant course; poisonous.

**virus**   A microorganism smaller than a bacteria, which cannot grow or reproduce apart from a living cell. A virus invades living cells and uses their chemical machinery to keep itself alive and to replicate itself. It may reproduce with fidelity or with errors (mutations)—this ability to mutate is responsible for the ability of some viruses to change slightly in each infected person, making treatment more difficult. Viruses cause many common human infections, and are also responsible for a bevy of rare diseases. Examples of viral illnesses range from the common cold, which is usually caused by one of the rhinoviruses, to acquired immunodeficiency syndrome (AIDS), which is caused by the human immunodeficiency virus (HIV). Viruses may contain either DNA or RNA as their genetic material. Herpes simplex virus and the hepatitis-B virus are DNA viruses. RNA viruses have an enzyme called reverse transcriptase that permits the usual sequence of DNA-to-RNA to be reversed so the virus can make a DNA version of itself. RNA viruses include HIV and the hepatitis C virus. Researchers have grouped viruses together into several major families, based on their shape, behavior, and other characteristics. These include the herpesviruses, adenoviruses, papovaviruses (papilloma viruses), hepadnaviruses, poxviruses, and parvoviruses among the DNA viruses. On the RNA virus side, major families include the picornaviruses (including the rhinoviruses), calciviruses, paramyxoviruses, orthomyxoviruses, rhabdoviruses, filoviruses, bornaviruses, and retroviruses. There are dozens of smaller virus families within these major classifications. Many viruses are host-specific, causing disease in humans or specific animals only.

**virus, attenuated** A virus that has been weakened. A vaccine against a viral disease can be made from an attenuated, less virulent strain of the virus: a virus capable of stimulating an immune response and creating immunity, but not of causing illness.

**virus, Ebola** See *Ebola virus*. See also *filovirus*.

**virus, herpes** See *herpes virus*.

**virus, herpetiform** See *herpetiform virus*. See also *herpesvirus*.

**virus, human immunodeficiency** See *human immunodeficiency virus*.

**virus, human lymphotropic, type III** See *human immunodeficiency virus*.

**virus, lymphadenopathy** See *human immunodeficiency virus*.

**virus, lymphadenopathy-associated** See *human immunodeficiency virus*.

**virus, Marburg** See *Marburg disease*, *Marburg virus*. See also *filovirus*.

**virus, Nipah** See *Nipah virus*.

**virus, respiratory syncytial** See *respiratory syncytial virus*.

**visceral pericardium** The inner layer of the pericardium.

**vision therapy** The use of special eye exercises to address eye defects, such as strabismus. Some vision therapists also claim that eye exercises can help people with neurological or learning disabilities. This approach is not proven for the latter use, although some patients do report improvement.

**vision, central** See *central vision*.

**vision, macular** See *central vision*.

**visual acuity** The clarity or clearness of the vision, a measure of how well a person sees.

**visual acuity test** A test that measures how well you see at various distances: the familiar eye chart test.

**visual field test** A test that measures the extent and distribution of the field of vision. The visual field test may be done by a number of methods, including termed confrontation, tangent screen exam, and automated perimetry. These tests may seem tedious, but are not painful or uncomfortable. Many diseases can adversely affect the visual field, including glaucoma, strokes, high blood pressure (hypertension), diabetes, multiple sclerosis, and overactivity of the thyroid gland (hyperthyroidism). Medications can also affect the visual field, including the antimalarial drugs chloroquine (brand name: Atabrine) and hydroxychloroquine (brand name: Plaquenil).

**visual nerve** See *optic nerve*.

**visual nerve pathways** See *optic nerve pathways*.

**vital** Necessary to maintain life. Breathing is a vital function.

**vitamin B15** An old name for dimethylglycine (DMG, pangamic acid), which is no longer considered to be a vitamin by the strict definition of that word. See *dimethylglycine*.

**vitamin P** An old name for substances now known as bioflavinoids. They are no longer considered to be vitamins by the strict definition of that word. See *bioflavinoids*.

**vitamin therapy** The use of vitamins to prevent or cure disease. Many physicians are now recognizing the beneficial uses of anti-oxidant and other vitamins for a wide variety of conditions, often as a complementary therapy to accompany medication or other treatments. One variant on this theme, megavitamin therapy, is still rather controversial. Always consult your doctor before adding vitamin supplements to your health regimen. See also *Appendix C, "Vitamins."*

**vitamins**   Substances that are essential to life. Vitamins play a part in dozens of crucial activities in the body: some are antioxidants, preventing oxidation of cells and potentially preventing cancer; others permit or deny chemical reactions involved in sight, brain function, metabolism, nucleic acid synthesis, and the like. All vitamins are either available in food, or can be made within the body. However, many people do not eat a diet that contains the minimum daily requirements of certain vitamins. Nutritionists suggest that the best way to ensure appropriate doses of vitamins is to eat a more healthful diet, particularly one that is rich in green, leafy vegetables and carotene compounds. That's because these foods offer many benefits that vitamin supplements cannot, including fiber, and probably including vitamin-like substances that have not yet been isolated. Lack of specific vitamins can lead to deficiency syndromes, such as rickets, beriberi, and anemia. Overconsumption of certain vitamins can also have consequences, ranging from minor to life-threatening. Some vitamins are water-soluble, and any excess is simply excreted in the urine. Others are fat-soluble, and may build up in the body, potentially reaching dangerous concentrations. Vitamins may also interact with prescription and over-the-counter drugs, making them more or less potent. For these reasons, always consult a doctor before adding vitamin supplements to a daily regimen. See also *Appendix C, "Vitamins."*

**vitelline duct**   See *yolk stalk*.

**vitreous humor**   A clear, jelly-like substance that fills the middle of the eye.

**vocal cords**   Two small bands of muscle that form a V-shape within the larynx. When a person breathes, the vocal cords relax and air moves through the space between them without making a sound. When a person talks or sings, the vocal cords tighten up and move closer together. Air from the lungs is forced between them, making them vibrate to produce sound, much like the strings of a guitar. The tongue, lips, and teeth form this sound into words. See also *larynx*.

**voice box**   See *larynx*.

**void**   To urinate. The term is also sometimes used to indicate the elimination of solid waste, or defecation.

**volume, stroke**   See *stroke volume*.

**Voluntary Euthanasia Society**   An organization founded in England in 1935 to advocate for voluntary euthanasia (assisted suicide) and the use of living wills by patients who wish to refuse unwanted life-prolonging medical treatments. See also *active euthanasia, assisted suicide, living will*.

**vomit**   Matter from the stomach that is ejected in tandem with symptoms of nausea. When vomit is reddish or coffee-ground colored, it indicates serious internal bleeding. Also known as vomitus; the process of vomiting is also known as peristalsis.

**vomiting in pregnancy, excess**   See *hyperemesis gravidarum*.

**vomiting of pregnancy, pernicious**   See *hyperemesis gravidarum*.

**von Hippel-Lindau syndrome**   A syndrome characterized by benign blood-vessel tumors that most typically affect the eye and the brain. The eye tumors are termed angiomata, and are in the retina. The brain tumors are termed hemangioblastoma, and are in the cerebellum. There can also be blood-vessel tumors (hemangiomata) in the spinal cord, adrenal glands, liver, and lungs. Pheochromocytoma (a benign tumor of adrenal-like tissue) occurs in some patients. The combination of high blood pressure (hypertension) with angioma may cause bleeding under the skull (subarachnoid hemorrhage). Kidney cancer called renal cell carcinoma (hypernephroma) can metastasize and is a frequent cause of death. An abnormal elevation of red blood cells (polycythemia) can be due to the hemangioblastoma of the cerebellum, or the hypernephroma. Multiple cysts can occur in the pancreas and kidneys. Patients with kidney problems or pancreatic cysts do not have pheochromocytoma, and vice versa. Lab findings in VHL may include high calcium (hypercalcemia) and low potassium (hypokalemia) occurring with the pheochromocytoma. VHL is inherited as an autosomal dominant trait, so one VHL gene is sufficient to cause the syndrome. If a person has VHL, the chance for each of his or her children to receive the VHL gene is 50 percent. The VHL gene has been mapped to chromosome 3 in region 3p26-p25. It has the characteristics of a tumor-suppressor gene, but can be triggered instead to permit tumor growth.

**von Recklinghausen disease**   See *neurofibromatosis*.

**Vrolik disease**   See *osteogenesis imperfecta type II*.

**VSD**   Ventricular septal defect.

**vulva**   The female external genital organs, including the labia, clitoris, and entrance to the vagina.

**vulvar pain, chronic**   See *vulvodynia*.

**vulvitis**   Inflammation of the external genital organs of the female, often caused by the yeast Candida albicans. See also *yeast vulvitis*.

**vulvodynia** Chronic pain in the area of the female vulva. The main symptom is pain, usually a burning irritation or rawness of the genitals. The pain may be constant or intermittent, localized or diffuse. It can last for months or longer, and can vanish as suddenly as it started. The cause of vulvodynia is unknown. Many women with vulvodynia have a history of treatment for recurrent vaginal fungal infections. Treatments being tested include drugs, nerve blocks to numb the vulvar nerves, and biofeedback therapy to relax pelvic muscles. See also *vulvitis, yeast vulvitis.*

# Ww

**Warburg apparatus**   A device used in biochemistry to measure breathing (respiration) by tissues. Tissue slices are enclosed in a chamber in which the temperature and pressure are monitored, and the amount of gas produced or consumed by the tissue is measured.

**Warburg yellow enzyme**   See *enzyme, Warburg yellow*. See also *enzymes, yellow*.

**warfarin**   An anticoagulant medication (brand name: Coumarin, Panwarfin, Sofarin) taken to treat blood clots or overly thickened blood. Some patients also take warfarin to reduce their risk of clots, stroke, or heart attack. It works by suppressing production of some clotting factors. Warfarin interacts with many other drugs, including some vitamins. These interactions can be dangerous, even life-threatening. Talk to your doctor before taking any other prescription or over-the-counter drug. Warfarin can disturb the development of the embryo and fetus and lead to birth defects. Warfarin taken by a woman during pregnancy can cause bleeding into the baby's brain (cerebral hemorrhage), underdevelopment (hypoplasia) of the baby's nose, and stippling of the ends (epiphyses) of the baby's long bones.

**Warren Grant Magnuson Clinical Center**   See *National Institutes of Health.*

**wart**   A local growth of the outer layer of the skin, caused by a papillomavirus. Papillomavirus is transmitted by contact, either with a wart on someone else, or one on oneself (autoinnoculation). Warts that occur on the hands or feet are called common warts. A wart on the sole of the foot is a plantar wart. Genital (venereal) warts are located on the genitals, and are transmitted by sexual contact. Also known as verruca, verruga. See also *genital warts, human papilloma virus.*

**wart, genital**   See *genital warts.*

**wart, venereal**   See *genital warts.*

**warts, plantar**   Warts that grow on the soles of the feet. Plantar warts are different from most other warts. They tend to be flat and cause the buildup of a callus that has to be peeled away before the plantar wart itself can be seen. Plantar warts may attack blood vessels deep in the skin. They can be quite painful. Plantar warts are caused by human papillomavirus (HPV) type 1, and tend to affect teenagers. To avoid plantar warts, a child should be taught never to wear someone else's shoes. If a child gets plantar warts, they should be treated by a doctor. Treatment may include freezing off the wart, excising it, or using an immersible ultrasound device to kill the wart. See also *human papilloma virus.*

**wasp stings**   Stings from wasps can trigger allergic reactions that vary greatly in severity. Avoidance and prompt treatment are essential. In selected cases, allergy injection therapy is highly effective.

**water on the brain**   See *hydrocephalus.*

**water-hammer pulse**   See *Corrigan pulse.*

**wax, ear**   See *ear wax.*

**WBC**   White blood cell.

**WDWN**   Abbreviation for "well developed, well nourished," shorthand used by doctors when jotting down the results of their physical examination. For example, a WDWNWF would be a well developed, well nourished white female.

**Wegener granulomatosis**   See *granulomatosis, Wegener.*

**Wellbutrin**   See *bupropion.*

**Werner-His disease**   See *trench fever.* See also *Bartonella quintana.*

**Western blot**   A technique in molecular biology that is used to separate and identify particular proteins.

**WF**   Doctor's shorthand for white female.

**wheezing**   A whistling noise in the chest during breathing. Wheezing occurs when the airways are narrowed or compressed.

**white blood cells**   Cells that circulate in the blood and lymphatic system, and are harbored in the lymph glands and spleen. They are part of the immune system. White blood cells are responsible for attacking foreign invaders in the body, both directly (in the form of T cells and macrophages) and indirectly (in the form of B cells producing antibodies). Also known as leukocytes. See also *leukocytes.*

**white matter**   The part of the brain that contains myelinated nerve fibers. The white matter is white because it is the color of myelin, the insulation covering the nerve fibers.

**white spots on the nails** See *nails, white spots on the.*

**white subungual onychomycosis, proximal** See *onychomycosis, proximal white subungual.*

**Whitmore disease** See *melioidosis.*

**WHO** World Health Organization.

**whooping cough** See *pertussis.*

**will, living** An advance medical directive that specifies what types of medical treatment are desired. A living will can be very specific or very general. The most common statement in a living will is to the effect that life-sustaining measures that would serve only to prolong one's dying should be withheld or discontinued if a condition is incurable, irreversible, and terminal. More specific living wills may include information regarding an individual's desire for such services as pain relief, antibiotics, hydration, feeding, and the use of ventilators or cardiopulmonary resuscitation.

**Willis, circle of** See *circle of Willis.*

**windpipe** See *larynx.*

**winter depression** See *seasonal affective disorder.* See also *bipolar disorders.*

**wisdom tooth** See *tooth, wisdom.*

**WM** Medical shorthand for white male.

**WNL** Within normal limits. For example, a laboratory test result may be WNL.

**Wolff-Parkinson-White syndrome** A condition caused by an abnormality in the electrical system of the heart, which normally tells the heart muscle when to contract. There is an extra electrical connection inside the heart that acts as a short circuit, causing the heart to beat too rapidly and sometimes in an irregular manner. The syndrome can be life-threatening, although this is unusual. WPW can be treated by destroying the short circuit, using a technique termed radiofrequency catheter ablation, in which wires are put in different places in the heart until the short circuit is found and can be destroyed with radio waves.

**Wolf-Hirschhorn syndrome** A chromosome disorder caused by partial deletion of the short (p) arm of chromosome 4. The syndrome is characterized by midline defects, including a scalp defect; wide-spaced eyes; broad or beaked nose; cleft lip and/or palate; low, simple ears with a dimple in front of the ear; small and/or asymmetrical head; heart defects; and seizures that tend to diminish with age. There is severe to profound developmental and mental retardation. Some patients do learn to walk with or without support, and some achieve sphincter control by day. There is usually very slow progress in development. Nearly 90 percent of cases are due to spontaneous partial deletions. In the remaining 10 percent or so, one of the parents has a balanced chromosome rearrangement involving chromosome 4p, from which the child's deleted 4p (4p–) is derived. Parents of 4p– may wish to seek genetic counseling services. Also known as 4p–syndrome.

**Wolhynia fever** See *trench fever.* See also *Bartonella quintana.*

**womb** See *uterus.*

**word-processor's cramp** A dystonia that affects the muscles of the hand and sometimes the forearm, and only occurs during typing or using the computer. Similar focal dystonias have also been called writer's cramp, pianist's cramp, musician's cramp, and golfer's cramp.

**working memory** See *memory, short-term.*

**World Health Organization** The subagency of the United Nations (UN) concerned with international health. Also known as Organisation Mondiale de la Santé (OMS).

**wormwood** The plant whose essence forms the basis of absinthe, a dangerous, emerald-green liqueur. See also *absinthe.*

**WPW syndrome** Wolff-Parkinson–White syndrome.

**writer's cramp** A dystonia that affects the muscles of the hand and sometimes the forearm, and only occurs during handwriting. Similar focal dystonias have also been called typist's cramp, pianist's cramp, musician's cramp, and golfer's cramp.

**wryneck** See *torticollis.* See also *torticollis, congenital.*

**Wt** Abbreviation for weight. Wt 80 lbs means weight 80 pounds.

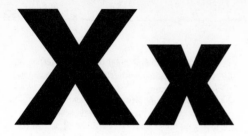

**X** In genetics and medicine, X usually refers to the X chromosome. See *X chromosome, X-linked*.

**X chromosome** The sex chromosome found twice in normal females and singly, along with a Y chromosome, in normal males. The complete chromosome complement consists of 46 chromosomes, including the 2 sex chromosomes, and is thus conventionally written as 46,XX for chromosomally normal females and 46,XY for chromosomally normal males.

**xanthelasma** Tiny, slightly raised, yellowish plaques on the skin surface of the upper or lower eyelids. Xanthelasma is a harmless growth of tissue caused by tiny deposits of fat in the skin, and is often associated with abnormal blood fat levels (hyperlipidemia). It is composed of lipid-laden foam cells called histiocytes.

**xanthinuria** A metabolic disorder caused by lack of an enzyme needed to process xanthine, an alkaloid found in caffeine, theobromine, theophylline, and related substances. Unchecked, xanthinuria can lead to kidney stone formation. Treatment is by avoiding foods and drinks containing xanthine derivatives, such as coffee, tea, and colas.

**xanthoma** One of several conditions characterized by firm yellow, orange, or brown nodules in the skin or mucous membranes. Although xanthomas themselves are harmless, they frequently indicate underlying disease, such as diabetes, lipid disorders (hyperlipidemia), or other conditions. They are composed of lipid-laden foam cells called histiocytes.

**xanthoma tendinosum** Xanthoma that clusters around tendons, and is associated with lipid disorders.

**xanthoma tuberosum** Xanthoma that clusters near joints. It is associated with lipid disorders, cirrhosis of the liver, and thyroid disorders.

**xanthoma, diabetic** Xanthoma associated with poorly controlled diabetes mellitus. Treating the diabetes will cause the xanthomas to disappear.

**xanthoma, disseminatum** A type of xanthoma characterized by orange-to-brown nodules on the skin or mucous membranes.

**xanthoma, eruptive** Xanthoma linked to lipid disorders, and accompanied by a pink-to-red raised rash.

**xanthoma, planar** A type of xanthoma characterized by flat yellow-to-orange patches or pimples that cluster together on the skin.

**xanthomatosis** An accumulation of excess lipids in the body due to disturbance of lipid metabolism, and marked by the formation of xanthomas. See also *xanthoma*.

**xanthopsia** A form of chromatopsia, a visual defect in which objects look as though they have been overpainted with an unnatural color. In xanthopsia, that color is yellow.

**xanthosis** Yellowing of the skin, without yellowing of the eyes as seen in jaundice.

**xenobiotic** Natural substances that are foreign to the body.

**xero-** Prefix indicating dryness. For example, xeroderma is dry skin.

**xeroderma** Abnormally dry skin. Xeroderma can be caused by a deficiency of vitamin A, systemic illness, overexposure to sunlight, or medication. It can usually be addressed by the use of over-the-counter, topical preparations. If these products do not relieve the condition, see an aesthetician or dermatologist for more specific remedies.

**xeroderma pigmentosum** A rare hereditary skin disease characterized by extreme sensitivity to light. If the skin is overexposed to ultraviolet light, growths and benign tumors may form. If tumors form on or near the eyes, they may cause blindness. There is no treatment for xeroderma pigmentosum, but avoiding ultraviolet light and using the highest level possible of sunscreen when exposure cannot be avoided may prevent complications.

**xerophagia** Eating a dry diet.

**xerophthalmia** Dry eyes. Xerophthalmia can be associated with systemic diseases, such as Sjogren syndrome, systemic lupus erythematosus, or rheumatoid arthritis; deficiency of vitamin A; or use of some medications. It results from inadequate function of the lacrimal glands, which produce tears. When xerophthalmia is due to vitamin A deficiency, the condition begins with night blindness and conjunctival xerosis (dryness of the eye membranes), progresses to corneal xerosis (dryness of the cornea), and in its late stages develops into keratomalacia (softening of the cornea). Also known as conjunctivitis arida.

**xerostomia** Dry mouth. Xerostomia can be associated with systemic diseases, such as Sjogren syndrome, systemic lupus erythematosus, and rheumatoid arthritis; or it can be a side effect of medication or poor dental hygiene. Xerostomia results from inadequate function of the salivary glands, such as the parotid glands. Untreated, severe dry mouth can lead to increased levels of tooth decay and thrush.

**xiphoid process** The lower part of the breastbone.

**X-linked** On the X chromosome. An X-linked gene travels with the X chromosome, and therefore is part of the X chromosome. An X-linked disorder is associated with or caused by a gene on the X chromosome.

**X-ray** High-energy radiation; radiation with waves shorter than those of visible light. It is used in low doses for making images that help to diagnose diseases, and in high doses to treat cancer.

**X-ray therapy** The use of X-ray radiation to treat cancer. X-rays may be used inside or outside the body, depending on the type of tumor involved. See also *radiation therapy*.

**X-ray, AP** An X-ray picture in which the beams pass through the patient anteroposteriorly: from front-to-back.

**X-ray, lateral** An X-ray picture taken from the side.

**X-ray, PA** An X-ray picture in which the beams pass through the patient posteroanteriorly: from back-to-front.

**XX** The sex chromosome complement of a normal human female. See also *X chromosome*.

**XXX syndrome** A chromosomal disorder that affects females only, caused by the presence of three X chromosomes rather than the normal two. It may be characterized by mild to moderate mental retardation, tall stature, webbed neck, speech and motor delays, and sterility. Also known as chromosome X syndrome, triple X syndrome.

**XXXX syndrome** A rare chromosomal disorder that affects females only, caused by the presence of four X chromosomes rather than the normal two. It is characterized by mild to severe mental retardation in most cases, sometimes by physical abnormalities, facial features similar to those seen in Down syndrome, and sterility. Also known as poly-X syndrome.

**XXXXX syndrome** A chromosomal disorder that affects females only, caused by the presence of five X chromosomes rather than the normal two. It is characterized by mild to severe mental retardation in most cases, sometimes by physical abnormalities, facial features similar to those seen in Down syndrome, and sterility. Also known as poly-X syndrome.

**XXXXY syndrome** See *Klinefelter syndrome*.

**XXXY syndrome** See *Klinefelter syndrome*.

**XXYY syndrome** See *Klinefelter syndrome*.

**XY** The sex chromosome complement of a normal human male. See also *X chromosome, Y chromosome*.

**xylitol** A sweetener found in plants and used as a substitute for sugar. Xylitol is called a nutritive sweetener because it provides calories, just like sugar. However, it is less likely to contribute to dental caries.

**XYY syndrome** A chromosomal disorder that affects males only, caused by the presence of an extra Y chromosome. Symptoms may include increased height, speech delays, learning disabilities, mild to moderate mental retardation, and behavioral disturbance. Also known as polysomy Y syndrome.

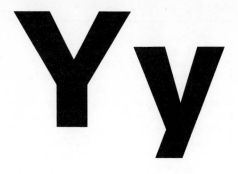

**Y** **1** In chemistry, the symbol for the element yttrium, an ultrarare metal. Yttrium has been used in certain nuclear medicine scans. **2** In genetics, the Y chromosome. See *Y chromosome*.

**Y chromatin** Brilliantly fluorescent body seen in cells stained with the dye quinacrine, which lights up the Y chromosomes most brightly.

**Y chromosome** The male sex chromosome. In normal males, it is found with an X (female) sex chromosome. The Y chromosome contains at least 20 genes, including the unique male-determining gene and male fitness genes that are active only in the testis, which are thought responsible for the formation of sperm. Other genes on the Y have counterparts on the X chromosome, are active in many body tissues, and play crucial "housekeeping" roles with the cell.

**Y fracture** See *fracture, Y*.

**Y map** The array of genes on the Y chromosome.

**YAC** Yeast artificial chromosome.

**Yag laser surgery** **1** The use of a laser to punch a hole in the iris, relieving increased pressure within the eye. Yag laser surgery is an office procedure that may be used for angle closure glaucoma and similar eye conditions. **2** Use of the Yag laser device to remove liver spots, café au lait spots, and some types of tattoos from the skin.

**yard** A measurement of length equal to 3 feet or 36 inches.

**yawn** Involuntary opening of the mouth, accompanied by slowly breathing inward and then outward. Repeated yawning can be a sign of drowsiness, boredom, or depression.

**yaws** A chronic infectious disease that occurs commonly in the warm, humid regions of the tropics. It is characterized by bumps on the skin of the face, hands, feet, and genital area. Almost all cases of yaws are in children under 15 years of age. The organism that causes yaws is a spirochete, Treponema pertenue, which enters the skin at a scraped or cut spot. A painless bump, (the mother yaw) arises and grows at this spot. Nearby lymph glands may become swollen. The mother yaw heals, leaving a light-colored scar. The mother yaw is followed by recurring (secondary) crops of bumps, and more swollen glands. These bumps may be painless, or they may be filled with pus, burst, and ulcerate. In its late (tertiary) stage, yaws can destroy and deform areas of the skin, bones, and joints. The palms and soles tend to become thickened and painful ("dry crab yaws"). Diagnosis is by observation, assuming that the patient lives or has traveled in an area where yaws occurs. Confirmation is by blood tests and by dark-field examination of the spirochete under a microscope. Treatment is by a single shot of penicillin or another antibiotic, usually erythromycin or tetracycline. Also known as granuloma tropicum, polypapilloma tropicum, and thymiosis.

**yd.** Abbreviation for yard.

**yeast** A group of single-celled fungi that reproduce by budding. Most yeast are harmless, and yeast is commonly present without ill effect on normal human skin and mucous membranes, including the digestive (GI) tract. In the GI tract, the amount of yeast is usually controlled by helpful bacteria, although this balance can be upset by illness, immune-system problems, or antibiotic use. Some individuals also report that a diet high in sugars and starches can cause overproliferation, although this has not been medically proven. Extreme overproliferation of yeast can cause discomfort and disease. For example, the common yeast Candida albicans (once called Monilia) causes thrush and rashes, fingernail infections, vaginal infections, and a host of problems in patients with immune deficiency. See also *Candida albicans, candidiasis, thrush, yeast infection, yeast rash*.

**yeast artificial chromosome** A vector created and used in the laboratory to clone pieces of DNA. A YAC is constructed from the telomeric (end), centromeric, and replication origin sequences needed for replication in yeast cells.

**yeast infection** Overgrowth of yeast can affect the skin (yeast rash), mouth (thrush), digestive tract, esophagus, vagina (vaginitis), and other parts of the body. Yeast infections occur most frequently in moist areas of the body. Although Candida albicans and other Candida yeasts are the most frequent offenders, other yeast groups are known to cause illness, primarily in immunocompromised patients. These include Torulopsis, Cryptococcus, Mallasezia, and Trichosporon yeasts. Diagnosis is by observation, and can be confirmed by culturing a stool or mucosa sample, or a scraping from the affected area. Treatment is by topical or oral antifungal medications. Acidopholous, a helpful bacteria that normally helps to keep yeast in check, can also be tried in supplement form or in yogurt with live cultures. See also *Candida albicans, candidiasis, thrush, yeast vaginitis, yeast rash*.

**yeast rash** A slightly raised pink-to-red rash caused by proliferation of yeast, usually in a moist area such as the groin. It is most common in infants, but can also occur on the skin of older children and adults. Treatment is by keeping the affected area clean and dry, and applying topical antifungal medication. Also known as diaper dermatitis, nappy rash.

**yeast vaginitis** Infection of the vagina by Candida albicans, characteristically causing itching, burning, soreness, pain during intercourse and urination, and vaginal discharge. Yeast vaginitis occurs when new yeast are introduced into the vagina, or when the quantity of yeast in the vagina increases relative to the quantity of bacteria. Yeast vaginitis can be exacerbated by injury to the vagina, as from chemotherapy; immune deficiency, as from AIDS or cortisone-type medications; pregnancy or taking birth control pills; antibiotic use; or diabetes. Treatment is by topical or oral antifungal medications. During pregnancy, only the topical creams are used. Patients must take the full course of medication to prevent reinfection. The partners of sexually active women should also be treated. Some patients report that taking acidopholous supplements, eating yogurt with live acidopholous cultures, reducing the amount of sugar and starch in the diet, keeping the affected area clean, and wearing absorbent cotton underwear contribute to prevention of yeast vaginitis. See also *Candida albicans, yeast, yeast infection, yeast vulvitis*.

**yeast vulvitis** A yeast infection of the vulva. Yeast vulvitis commonly goes together with yeast vaginitis. Common symptoms include itching, burning, soreness, pain during intercourse and urination, and vaginal discharge. Treatment is by topical or oral antifungal medications. During pregnancy, only the topical creams are used. Patients must take the full course of medication to prevent reinfection. The partners of sexually active women should also be treated. Some patients report that taking acidopholous supplements, eating yogurt with live acidopholous cultures, reducing the amount of sugar and starch in the diet, keeping the affected area clean, and wearing absorbent cotton underwear contribute to prevention of yeast vulvitis. See also *Candida albicans, yeast, yeast infection, yeast vaginitis*.

**yellow enzyme, Warburg** See *enzyme, Warburg yellow*. See also *enzymes, yellow*.

**yellow enzymes** See *enzymes, yellow*. See also *enzyme, Warburg yellow*.

**yellow fever** An acute, systemic illness caused by the Flavivirus taxon virus. In severe cases, infection causes a high fever, bleeding into the skin, and death of cells (necrosis) in kidney and liver. The liver damage (hepatitis) causes yellowing of the skin from severe jaundice. Yellow fever once ravaged port cities in the US, but is currently most common in tropical areas of Africa and the Americas. The virus is transmitted by a mosquito or, in a very few cases, from monkey bites. Diagnosis is by observation and, if necessary, culturing or examining a blood sample. There is no cure for yellow fever, although antiviral medications may be tried. It usually passes within a few weeks. Nonaspirin pain relievers, rest, and rehydration with fluids will decrease discomfort. The disease can be prevented by vaccination.

**yellow fever vaccination** A live attenuated (weakened) viral vaccine for yellow fever. It is recommended for people traveling to or living in those tropical areas in the Americas and Africa where yellow fever occurs. Because it is a live vaccine, it should not be given to infants or people with immune-system problems.

**yellow jacket stings** Stings from yellow jackets can trigger allergic reactions of varying severity. Avoidance and prompt treatment are essential. In selected cases, allergy injection therapy is highly effective.

**Yersinia** A group of bacteria. The Yersinia family includes Y. pestis, which causes the bubonic, pneumonic, and septicemic plagues; Y. entercolitica, which causes intestinal infections, including mesenteric lymphadenitis, a condition that mimics appendicitis; and Y. pseudotuberculosis, which usually adversely affects only animals but can cause illness in immunocompromised patients. Both Y. entercolitica and Y. pseudotuberculosis have also been implicated in a viral form of arthritis. Infection with Yersinia bacteria can be treated with antibiotics. See also *plague*.

**Y-linked** A gene on the Y chromosome. A Y-linked gene is passed from father to son. See also *Y-linked inheritance*.

**Y-linked inheritance** Inheritance of genes on the Y chromosome. Since only males normally have a Y chromosome, Y-linked genes can only be transmitted from father to son. Also known as holandric inheritance.

**yoga** A relaxing form of exercise developed in India, yoga involves assuming and holding postures that stretch the limbs and muscles, doing breathing exercises, and using meditation techniques to calm the mind. It appears to have benefits for increasing physical flexibility and reducing internal feelings of stress. Yoga may be recommended as an alternative or complementary health-promoting practice.

**yogurt** Milk fermented with a culture of Lactobacillus (the milk bacillus), and often with acidopholous and other helpful bacteria. Some patients with yeast infections, particularly those brought on by taking antibiotics, report that eating yogurt is helpful in alleviating symptoms. See also *probiotics*.

**yolk sac** The membrane outside the human embryo. It is connected by a tube, the yolk stalk, through the umbilical opening to the embryo's midgut. The yolk sac serves as an early site for the formation of blood, and in time is incorporated into the primitive gut of the embryo.

**yolk stalk** A narrow tube present in the early embryo that connects the midgut of the embryo to the yolk sac outside the embryo through the umbilical opening. Later in development, the yolk stalk is usually obliterated, but a remnant of it may persist, most commonly as a finger-like protrusion from the small intestine known as Meckel diverticulum. Found in 2 to 4 percent of people, Meckel diverticulum may become inflamed (much like the appendix) and require surgical removal. Also known as the oomphalomesenteric duct, umbilical duct, or vitelline duct.

**youth** The time between childhood and maturity.

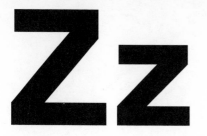

**Z chromosome**   A sex chromosome in certain animals, such as chickens, turkeys, and moths. In humans, males are XY and females XX, but in animals with a Z chromosome, males are ZZ and females are WZ.

**Zantac**   See *ranitidine*.

**Zarontin**   See *ethosuximide*.

**zidovudine**   See *AZT*.

**zinc**   A mineral essential to the body, zinc is a constituent of many enzymes that permit chemical reactions to proceed at normal rates. It is involved in the manufacture of protein (protein synthesis) and in cell division. Zinc is also a constituent of insulin, and is concerned with the sense of smell. Food sources of zinc include meat, particularly liver and seafood; eggs; nuts; and cereal grains. Recently, zinc has been touted as a treatment for the common cold. According to the National Academy of Sciences, the recommended dietary allowance of zinc is 12 mg per day for women and 10 mg per day for men.

**zinc acetate**   A form of zinc that has been used as an emetic.

**zinc deficiency**   Deficiency of zinc is associated with short stature, anemia, increased pigmentation of skin (hyperpigmentation), enlarged liver and spleen (hepatosplenomegaly), impaired gonadal function (hypogonadism), impaired wound healing, and immune deficiency. Among the consequences of zinc deficiency, dermatitis (skin inflammation) and diarrhea are particularly prominent features. A genetic disease called acrodermatitis enteropathica causes impaired zinc uptake from the intestine, leading to deficiency. See also *acrodermatitis enteropathica, zinc*.

**zinc excess**   Too much zinc can cause gastrointestinal irritation (upset stomach), interfere with copper absorption to cause copper deficiency and, like too little zinc, cause immune deficiency. See also *zinc*.

**zinc ointment**   A topical preparation containing zinc that is applied to protect the skin from irritation or sunburn. Zinc ointment is often the basis for commercial preparations for preventing diaper rash. It should not be used on skin that is already broken or irritated, however.

**zinc oxide**   A form of zinc that has antispasmodic qualities.

**zinc sulfate**   A form of zinc that can be administered in eye drops. It is used in some types of eye tests.

**Zinsser disease**   See *Brill-Zinsser disease*. See also *typhus, epidemic*.

**zona pellucida**   The strong membrane that forms around an ovum as it develops in the ovary. The membrane remains in place during the egg's travels through the Fallopian tube. To fertilize the egg, a sperm must penetrate the thinning zona pellucida. If fertilization takes place, the membrane disappears to permit implantation in the uterus.

**zooparasite**   A living parasite, such as a worm or protozoa.

**zoophilia**   A sexual disorder (paraphilia) involving an abnormal desire to have sexual contact with animals. See also *paraphilia*.

**Zyban**   Brand name for bupropion. Zyban is a version developed as a smoking deterrent.

**zygoma**   The bone that forms the prominence of the cheek. Known also as the zygomatic bone, the zygomatic arch, malar bone, yoke bone.

**zygomatic arch**   See *zygoma*.

**zygomatic bone**   See *zygoma*.

**zygomycosis**   A dangerous infection caused by a waterborne fungus. Zygomycosis is seen most often in patients who are already ill with diseases that cause wasting, such as AIDS or poorly controlled diabetes. If unchecked, the fungal infection can spread to the lungs and other organs, the blood, the eyes, and the brain. Treatment is two-fold: controlling the underlying condition, and attacking the infection with antifungal medications.

**zygote**   The cell formed by the union of a male sex cell (sperm) and a female sex cell (an ovum). The zygote develops into the embryo as instructed by the genetic material within the unified cell. The unification of a sperm and an ovum is called fertilization. See *ovum, sperm*.

**zygotic lethal gene**   See *gene, zygotic lethal*.

# APPENDIX A

## Prescription Abbreviations

A number of abbreviations, many derived from Latin terms, are used on prescription forms and medication labels. These include the following:

**ad lib**   Use as much as one desires, or use at your own discretion. From the Latin term *ad libitum*.

**a.c.**   Before meals. From the Latin term *ante cibum*.

**b.i.d.**   Twice a day. From the Latin term *bis in die*.

**cap**   Capsules.

**da**   Dispense as written.

**g, gm, or G**   Gram.

**gtt**   Drops. From the Latin term *guttae*.

**h**   Hour.

**m**   Milligram.

**m**   Milliliter.

**p.c**   Take after meals. From the Latin term *post cibum*.

**p.o**   Take by mouth, orally. From the Latin term *per os*.

**p.r.n**   Take as necessary or when needed. From the Latin term *pro re nata*.

**q.d**   Take once a day. From the Latin term *quaque die*.

**q.i.d**   Take four times a day. From the Latin term *quater in die*.

**q.h**   Take once every hour. From the Latin term *quaque* (every) and the abbreviation for hours.

**q.2h**   Take once every two hours.

**q.3h**   Take once every three hours.

**q.4h**   Take once every four hours.

**t.i.d**   Take three times a day. From the Latin term *ter in die*.

**ut dict**   Take as directed. From the Latin term *ut dictum*.

## Drug Caution Codes

D   Drowsiness

H   Habit Forming

I   Interaction

X   S.O.S. (contains a substance, such as aceta-minophen, that could cause problems—consult your pharmacist)

These code letters are for cautions that apply to all consumers.

You may also see these codes:

A   ASA (contains acetylsalicylic acid: aspirin)

C   Caution

G   Glaucoma

S   Diabetes

These code letters are cautions for patients with specific medical problems. A person with a medical problem, such as high blood pressure, might see the generic "C" code on a prescription bottle if the medication could raise his or her blood pressure.

Patients who see one of these codes on their prescriptions should talk to their pharmacists before using the medication.

In the US, a system of stickers with pictographs may also be used to warn of specific side effects, such as drowsiness.

# *APPENDIX B*

## Anatomic Orientation Terms

In anatomy, certain terms are used to denote orientation. For example, a structure may be horizontal, as opposed to vertical. Commonly used anatomic orientation terms include the following:

**anterior**   The front, as opposed to posterior. The breastbone is part of the anterior surface of the chest.

**anteroposterior**   From front to back, as opposed to posteroanterior. When a chest X-ray is taken with the patient's back against the film plate and the X-ray machine in front of the patient, it is referred to as an anteroposterior (AP) view.

**caudad**   Toward the feet (or tail in embryology), as opposed to cranial.

**cranial**   Toward the head, as opposed to caudad.

**deep**   Away from the exterior surface or further into the body, as opposed to superficial.

**distal**   Farther from the beginning, as opposed to proximal.

**dorsal**   The back, as opposed to ventral.

**horizontal**   Parallel to the floor; a plane passing through the standing body parallel to the floor.

**inferior**   Below, as opposed to superior.

**lateral**   Toward the left or right side of the body, as opposed to medial.

**medial**   In the middle or inside, as opposed to lateral.

**posterior**   The back or behind, as opposed to anterior.

**posteroanterior**   From back to front, as opposed to anteroposterior.

**pronation**   Rotation of the forearm and hand so that the palm is down (and the corresponding movement of the foot and leg with the sole down), as opposed to supination.

**prone**   With the front or ventral surface downward (lying face down), as opposed to supine.

**proximal**   Toward the beginning, as opposed to distal.

**sagittal**   A vertical plane passing through the standing body from front to back. The midsaggital, or median plane, splits the body into left and right halves.

**superficial**   On the surface or shallow, as opposed to deep.

**superior**   Above, as opposed to inferior.

**supination**   Rotation of the forearm and hand so that the palm is upward (and the corresponding movement of the foot and leg), as opposed to pronation.

**supine**   With the back or dorsal surface downward (lying face up), as opposed to prone.

**transverse**   A horizontal plane passing through the standing body parallel to the ground.

**ventral**   Pertaining to the abdomen, as opposed to dorsal.

**vertical**   Upright, as opposed to horizontal.

# APPENDIX C

## Vitamins

The word *vitamin* was coined in 1911 by the Warsaw-born biochemist Casimir Funk (1884–1967). At the Lister Institute in London, Funk isolated a substance that prevented nerve inflammation (neuritis) in chickens raised on a diet deficient in that substance. He named the substance "vitamine" because he believed it was necessary to life and it was a chemical amine. The "e" at the end was later removed when it was recognized that vitamins need not be amines.

The letters (A, B, C, and so on) were assigned to the vitamins in the order of their discovery. The one exception was vitamin K, which was assigned its K (from Koagulation) by the Danish researcher, Henrik Dam. The vitamins include:

**beta carotene** An antioxidant that protects cells against oxidation damage that can lead to cancer. Beta carotene is converted to vitamin A as needed. Food sources of beta carotene include vegetables, such as carrots, sweet potatoes, spinach and other leafy green vegetables; and fruit, such as cantaloupes and apricots. Excessive carotene in the diet can temporarily yellow the skin, a condition called carotenemia, commonly seen in infants fed large amounts of mashed carrots.

**folic acid** An important factor in nucleic acid synthesis, this member of the B vitamin family is essential for cell growth and proliferation, and for proper use of vitamin B12 and vitamin C. Found in leafy green vegetables, organ meats, and whole grains. Deficiency can lead to slow growth, diarrhea, oral inflammation, and megaloblastic anemia; deficiency during pregnancy can cause neural tube defects in the fetus. Also known as folate.

**vitamin A** Retinol. Carotene compounds are gradually converted by the body to vitamin A. A form of vitamin A called retinal is responsible for transmitting light sensations in the retina of the eye. Found in egg yolk, butter, cream, leafy green vegetables, yellow fruits and vegetables, cod-liver oil, and similar fish-liver oils. Deficiency of vitamin A leads to night blindness, and to diseases affecting the eyes and mucous membranes. Overdose of vitamin A can cause insomnia, joint pain, fatigue, irritability, headache, and other symptoms.

**vitamin A2** A slightly different form of vitamin A, found only in the flesh of freshwater fish.

**vitamin B1** Thiamin, which acts as a coenzyme in body metabolism. Found primarily in liver and yeast, but easily destroyed by cooking. Deficiency leads to beriberi, a disease of the heart and nervous system.

**vitamin B2** Riboflavin, essential for the reactions of coenzymes. Found primarily in liver and yeast, but easily destroyed by cooking. Deficiency causes inflammation of the lining of the mouth and skin.

**vitamin B3** Niacin, an essential part of coenzymes of body metabolism. Found primarily in liver and yeast, but easily destroyed by cooking. Deficiency causes inflamma-

tion of the skin, vagina, rectum, and mouth, as well as mental slowing. Also known as nicotinic acid.

**vitamin B5** Pantothenic acid, a B vitamin that is widely distributed in nature. Pantothenic acid is virtually ubiquitous. It is present in foods as diverse as poultry, soybeans, yogurt, and sweet potatoes. No naturally occurring disease due to a deficiency of pantothenic acid has been identified, due to the ease of obtaining this vitamin. An experimental deficiency of pantothenic acid has, however, been created by administering an antagonist to pantothenic acid. This experiment produced disease, thereby demonstrating that pantothenic acid is essential to humans.

**vitamin B6** Pyridoxine, a cofactor for enzymes. Found primarily in liver and yeast, but easily destroyed by cooking. Deficiency leads to inflammation of the skin and mouth, nausea, vomiting, dizziness, weakness, and anemia.

**vitamin B12** An essential factor in nucleic acid synthesis. It may affect vitamin C absorption. Found primarily in liver and yeast, but easily destroyed by cooking. Deficiency leads to megaloblastic anemia, as can be seen in pernicious anemia.

**vitamin B17** Amygdalin, a B vitamin that normally is made in the small intestine. Also found in fresh seeds, some nuts and beans, and bamboo shoots. Overdose can lead to low blood pressure, sweating, nausea, lethargy, respiratory distress, and death. A synthetic (and not identical) version of vitamin B17 is known as laetrile.

**vitamin C** Ascorbic acid, important in the synthesis of collagen, the framework protein for tissues of the body. Vitamin C is found in citrus fruits, tomatoes, berries, potatoes, and most vegetables. It may affect vitamin B12 absorption. Minor deficiency can cause gum bleeding, joint pain, nosebleeds, and easy bruising. Extreme deficiency can lead to scurvy, characterized by fragile capillaries, poor wound healing, and bone deformity in children. Overdose is not possible with this water-soluble vitamin, but overuse can cause diarrhea, painful urination, rash, and nausea.

**vitamin D**  A steroid vitamin that promotes absorption and metabolism of calcium and phosphorus, and that is essential for tooth and bone growth. Under normal conditions of sunlight exposure, no dietary supplementation is necessary because sunlight promotes adequate vitamin D synthesis in the skin. It is added to many common dairy products and breads, and can also be found in saltwater fish and egg yolks. Deficiency can lead to osteomalcia in adults and bone deformity (rickets) in children.

**vitamin D2**  Calciferol, a synthetic form of vitamin D created by treating ergosterol (provitamin D2) with ultraviolet light waves.

**vitamin D3**  Cholecalciferol, a D vitamin needed for proper use of phosphorus, calcium, and vitamin A. It plays a steroid-like role in regulating cellular proliferation and differentiation. Also known as calcitrol.

**vitamin E**  A vitamin that is vital for muscle, skin, blood vessel, and organ development and function. Dietary sources for vitamin E include nuts, nut and corn oils, wheat germ, liver, sweet potatoes, and green leafy vegetables. Deficiency can lead to anemia.

**vitamin H**  Biotin, which is actually considered part of the B vitamin family. It is a coenzyme essential for many enzyme functions. Normally produced by bacteria in the colon, biotin is also found in yeast, organ meats, legumes, egg yolks, whole grains, and nuts.

**vitamin K**  A group of essential factors in the formation of blood clots and in liver function. Vitamin K is normally made within the body by intestinal bacteria, but it is also found in many foods, including leafy green vegetables, yogurt, egg yolk, and fish-liver oils. Deficiency can lead to abnormal bleeding. Overdose can cause anemia in newborns, or kill blood cells in people with glucose-6-phosphate deficiency.

**vitamin P**  Bioflavinoids, a group of substances found with and essential to the use of vitamin C. They are essential for building collagen and capillary walls, among other functions.

# HUNGRY MINDS, INC., END-USER LICENSE AGREEMENT

**READ THIS.** You should carefully read these terms and conditions before opening the software packet(s) included with this book ("Book"). This is a license agreement ("Agreement") between you and Hungry Minds, Inc. ("HMI"). By opening the accompanying software packet(s), you acknowledge that you have read and accept the following terms and conditions. If you do not agree and do not want to be bound by such terms and conditions, promptly return the Book and the unopened software packet(s) to the place you obtained them for a full refund.

1. **License Grant.** HMI grants to you (either an individual or entity) a nonexclusive license to use one copy of the enclosed software program(s) (collectively, the "Software") solely for your own personal or business purposes on a single computer (whether a standard computer or a workstation component of a multiuser network). The Software is in use on a computer when it is loaded into temporary memory (RAM) or installed into permanent memory (hard disk, CD-ROM, or other storage device). HMI reserves all rights not expressly granted herein.

2. **Ownership.** HMI is the owner of all right, title, and interest, including copyright, in and to the compilation of the Software recorded on the disk(s) or CD-ROM ("Software Media"). Copyright to the individual programs recorded on the Software Media is owned by the author or other authorized copyright owner of each program. Ownership of the Software and all proprietary rights relating thereto remain with HMI and its licensers.

3. **Restrictions on Use and Transfer.**

   **(a)** You may only (i) make one copy of the Software for backup or archival purposes, or (ii) transfer the Software to a single hard disk, provided that you keep the original for backup or archival purposes. You may not (i) rent or lease the Software, (ii) copy or reproduce the Software through a LAN or other network system or through any computer subscriber system or bulletin-board system, or (iii) modify, adapt, or create derivative works based on the Software.

   **(b)** You may not reverse engineer, decompile, or disassemble the Software. You may transfer the Software and user documentation on a permanent basis, provided that the transferee agrees to accept the terms and conditions of this Agreement and you retain no copies. If the Software is an update or has been updated, any transfer must include the most recent update and all prior versions.

4. **Restrictions on Use of Individual Programs.** You must follow the individual requirements and restrictions detailed for each individual program in the "About the CD" section of this Book. These limitations are also contained in the individual license agreements recorded on the Software Media. These limitations may include a requirement that after using the program for a specified period of time, the user must pay a registration fee or discontinue use. By opening the Software packet(s), you will be agreeing to abide by the licenses and restrictions for these individual programs that are detailed in the "About the CD" section and on the Software Media. None of the material on this Software Media or listed in this Book may ever be redistributed, in original or modified form, for commercial purposes.

5. Limited Warranty.

   **(a)** HMI warrants that the Software and Software Media are free from defects in materials and workmanship under normal use for a period of sixty (60) days from the date of purchase of this Book. If HMI receives notification within the warranty period of defects in materials or workmanship, HMI will replace the defective Software Media.

   **(b) HMI AND THE AUTHOR OF THE BOOK DISCLAIM ALL OTHER WAR-RANTIES, EXPRESS OR IMPLIED, INCLUDING WITHOUT LIMITATION IMPLIED WARRANTIES OF MERCHANTABILITY AND FITNESS FOR A PARTICULAR PUR-POSE, WITH RESPECT TO THE SOFTWARE, THE PROGRAMS, THE SOURCE CODE CONTAINED THEREIN, AND/OR THE TECHNIQUES DESCRIBED IN THIS BOOK. HMI DOES NOT WARRANT THAT THE FUNCTIONS CONTAINED IN THE SOFTWARE WILL MEET YOUR REQUIREMENTS OR THAT THE OPERATION OF THE SOFTWARE WILL BE ERROR FREE.**

   **(c)** This limited warranty gives you specific legal rights, and you may have other rights that vary from jurisdiction to jurisdiction.

# ABOUT THE CD

The *Webster's New World Medical Dictionary* CD-ROM contains the complete text of the book in searchable electronic format. When you run the installation program, the iMet eBook player and some iMet eLibrary modules will be copied to your hard drive. The Medical Dictionary text remains on the CD, so the *Webster's New World Medical Dictionary* CD-ROM will need to be in your computer's CD-ROM drive before you can access its content through the iMet eBook player.

## Installing the CD

1. Insert the *Webster's New World Medical Dictionary* CD-ROM into your computer's CD-ROM drive.

2. The installation screen should automatically appear. If it doesn't appear after several seconds, please skip to the manual installation instructions.

3. Follow the on-screen instructions to install the software. After the installation, there will be a *Webster's New World Medical Dictionary* shortcut on your desktop.

To manually install the *Webster's New World Medical Dictionary* CD-ROM:

1. Click on the Windows Start Menu.

2. Click on Run.

3. In the Open box, type in *D:\setup.exe,* and click on OK. (*Note:* D is the drive letter for your CD-ROM drive. If your CD-ROM drive is something other than D, such as F, then you would type *F:\setup.exe.*)

4. Follow the on-screen instructions to install the software. After the installation, there will be a *Webster's New World Medical Dictionary* shortcut on your desktop.

## Using the CD

The *Webster's New World Medical Dictionary* CD-ROM is easy to use. Just insert the CD into your CD-ROM drive. After a few seconds, the *Webster's New World Medical Dictionary* window will automatically open. If the CD is already in your CD-ROM drive (or the dictionary window doesn't automatically appear), you can access the CD contents one of the following ways:

Using the Windows Start Menu:

1. Click on the Windows Start Menu.

2. Select Programs.

3. Select iMet eLibrary.

4. Click on *Webster's New World Medical Dictionary.*

Or, you can just doubleclick on the Webster's New World Medical Dictionary desktop shortcut.

## Navigating the CD

There are several ways to navigate the *Webster's New World Medical Dictionary* CD-ROM. Try one of the following:

- Type the term that you want to find in the Search box. The term or its closest match will appear. Click on the term to access the definition.

- Click on the letter of the alphabet under the Medical Dictionary Index. Use the scroll bar to find the term you want. Click on the term to access the definition.

# Useful Tools

The iMet player includes several useful tools. At the top of the window, just under the title, are four buttons[md]*Back, My Bookmark, Find,* and *Exit:*

**Back**—Just like the feature on your web browser, Back returns you to the previous window.

**My Bookmark**—When you find yourself frequently referring to the same entry, you might want to bookmark it for quicker access. When the entry is visible in the window, click on My Bookmark. Follow the instructions for creating and using bookmarks.

**Find**—This feature helps you find all instances of a word in the text. For example, you might want to read every entry that contains the word "Anemia." To do this, click on Find. Type *anemia* in the small box where the cursor is blinking and press enter. The search reports the findings (called hits) organized by the appropriate letter of the alphabet. Double click on one of the hits to find all instances of the word within the text of that letter of the alphabet.

**Exit**—Click on the Exit button to close the *Webster's New World Medical Dictionary* window.